Cancer of the Prostate
and Kidney

NATO Advanced Science Institutes Series

A series of edited volumes comprising multifaceted studies of contemporary scientific issues by some of the best scientific minds in the world, assembled in cooperation with NATO Scientific Affairs Division.

This series is published by an international board of publishers in conjunction with NATO Scientific Affairs Division

A	**Life Sciences**	Plenum Publishing Corporation
B	**Physics**	New York and London
C	**Mathematical and Physical Sciences**	D. Reidel Publishing Company Dordrecht, Boston, and London
D	**Behavioral and Social Sciences**	Martinus Nijhoff Publishers The Hague, Boston, and London
E	**Applied Sciences**	
F	**Computer and Systems Sciences**	Springer Verlag Heidelberg, Berlin, and New York
G	**Ecological Sciences**	

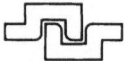

Cancer of the Prostate and Kidney

Edited by

M. Pavone-Macaluso

University of Palermo
Palermo, Italy

and

P. H. Smith

St. James's University Hospital
Leeds, England

Plenum Press
New York and London
Published in cooperation with NATO Scientific Affairs Division

Proceedings of a NATO Advanced Study Institute on
Cancer of Prostate and Kidney, which was also the Fourth Course
of the International School of Urology and Nephrology,
held June 2–12, 1981,
in Erice, Sicily

Library of Congress Cataloging in Publication Data

Main entry under title:

Cancer of the prostate and kidney.

(NATO advanced science institutes series. Series A, Life sciences; v. 53)
    "Proceedings of a NATO Advanced Study Institute on Cancer of the Prostate and
Kidney, which was also the Fourth Course of the International School of Urology and
Nephrology, held June 2–12, 1981, in Erice, Sicily"—Verso t.p.
    "Published in cooperation with.NATO Scientific Affairs Division."
    Includes bibliographical references and index.
    1. Prostate gland—Cancer—Congresses. 2. Kidneys—Cancer—Congresses. I. Pavone-
Macaluso, M. II. Smith, P. H. (Philip Henry). III. NATO Advanced Study Institute on Cancer
of the Prostate and Kidney (1981: Erice, Italy) IV. North Atlantic Treaty Organization.
Scientific Affairs Division. V. Series. [DNLM: 1. Prostatic neoplasms—Congresses. 2. Kid-
ney neoplasms—Congresses. WJ 752 N279c 1981]
RC280.P7C36 1983   616.99′461   82-16505
ISBN 978-1-4684-4351-6   ISBN 978-1-4684-4349-3 (eBook)
DOI 10.1007/978-1-4684-4349-3

© 1983 Plenum Press, New York
Softcover reprint of the hardcover 1st edition 1983
A Division of Plenum Publishing Corporation
233 Spring Street, New York, N.Y. 10013

PREFACE

This book is the record of the proceedings of a NATO Advanced
Study Institute held in Erice, Sicily, from the 2nd - 12th June
1981, during which scientists and clinicians interested in the
problems presented by cancer of the kidney and the prostate were
encouraged to present, to discuss and to challenge the opinions
expressed and the beliefs held by the different contributors.

It is uncommon for scientist, physician, and surgeon to meet
with great regularity or for prolonged periods of time and it must
be exceedingly rare for such people to immerse themselves in each
other's work and company for a period of almost two weeks. For this
to occur in a situation of total isolation such as that provided by
the marvellous Ettore Majorana Centre in Erice, Sicily must be
unique.

The fact that differences of opinion remain will be evident to
all who read the book, as will the wealth of scientific and clinical
work being undertaken within and beyond the NATO countries.

We are very much indebted to the Science Committee of NATO for
their recommendation for support for this meeting and to the Ente
Fiuggi and to several pharmaceutical firms.

We should also like to acknowledge our gratitude to Miss Pinola
Savalli and Dr. Alberto Gabriele, who played such a large part in
making our meeting both pleasant and successful, to the Department
of Medical Illustration at St. James's University Hospital, Leeds,
and to Mrs. S. Conyers, Miss M. Calder, Mrs. S. Purdie, and Miss S.
Stevenson of the Departments of Urology and Oncology of St. James's
University Hospital, Leeds, for the enormous amount of work which
they have undertaken in preparing and typing this volume.

CONTENTS

CONTENTS

CONTENTS

CANCER OF THE KIDNEY

Aetiology, Experimental Tumours, Epidemiology
        Pathology, and Research

CONTENTS

Diagnosis

CONTENTS

RENAL CELL CARCINOMA AND CARCINOMA OF THE PROSTATE;

ACHIEVEMENTS AND CHALLENGES

B. van der Werf-Messing

Rotterdam Radiotherapy Institute
Rotterdam
Holland

RENAL CANCER

In spite of advances in all fields of medical science, the prognosis of renal cell carcinoma has not improved during the last 25 years. The development of more sophisticated diagnostic tools such as arteriography, cavography, ultrasound and C.T. scan facilitate a more accurate assessment of the extent of the primary growth and its spread; however this knowledge has not yet contributed to therapeutic adaptations which result in a better prognosis (Table 1).

Simple nephrectomy and radical nephrectomy yield about the same cure rate. Preoperative irradiation increases local operability and hence local cure rate, but has not contributed to a better prognosis. The same applies to postoperative irradiation (1,2). Apparently prognosis is usually already determined by subclinical metastasis at the time of operation. In a patient with a solitary distant metastasis it remains doubtful whether removal of the primary has any beneficial influence on the course of the disease. Embolisation of the primary, followed by nephrectomy, might improve prognosis in case of limited metastasis (3).

In patients with multiple metastases either at the time of diagnosis or after previous nephrectomy, hormone therapy which seemed to be promising - 17% success up to 1971 - has turned out to be disappointing - 1.6% success after 1971. Chemotherapy, though sometimes producing partial regression or stabilisation has not improved prognosis. Immunotherapy, as the sole type of treatment or in combination with hormone treatment or chemotherapy, seems to be promising but still no proven improvement has yet been demonstrated (4). Radiotherapy delivered to painful or threatening metastases (threatening

1

Table 1. Renal cell carcinoma - survival rates in literature

Author	Type of tumour	No. of patients treated	% 5 year survival
Riches 1964 (5)	Well differentiated	42	70
	Poorly differentiated	42	30
	Renal vein -	60	58
	Renal vein +	26	27
Skinner et al 1972 (6)	T1 T2		
	Renal vein -	102	65
	Renal vein +	59	64
Murphy 1973 (7)	T1 T2	46	57
	T3 T4	40	49
Werf-Messing et al 1978 (2)	Renal vein -	104	65
	Renal vein +	62	28
Syrjänen & Hjelt 1978 (8)	Papillary	53	53
	Glandular/Tubular	31	58
	Undifferentiated	27	37
Sullivan et al 1974 (9)	Simple nephrectomy — T1 T2	24	74
	T3	9	66
	Renal vein + or N1 N2	10	20
	Radical nephrectomy — T1 T2	13	31
	T3	7	86
	Renal vein + or N1 N2	14	29

fracture or paralysis) usually results at least in "partial regression" and - if not given too late - very often in "local control"
(Table 2). Half Body Irradiation (lower half or upper half depending
on the site of the most distressing metastases) can also relieve
pain (10).

As from a prospective study at the Rotterdam Radio-Therapy Institute could be concluded that invasion of the renal vein is the most
important prognostic criterium (2), elective adjuvant therapy seems
justified in these high risk pateints. Adjuvant chemotherapy, immunotherapy or hormone therapy could be considered; however, in view of
their poor results in patients with proven clinical metastases, a
beneficial effect is doubtful but could still be investigated.
Elective irradiation of high risk regions could theoretically improve

prognosis (2). Another approach, elective total body hyperthermia with or without low dose total body irradiation in patients with proven renal vein involvement could be rewarding; this approach is now being investigated at the Rotterdam Radio-Therapy Institute.

PROSTATIC CANCER

Prostatic cancer has been a challenge since the beginning of this century. In 1911 Jean Cauhapé (11) published the results of the first radium implants in prostatic cancer. About three decades later Huggins et al (12) discovered by serendipity the beneficial influence of oestrogens on prostatic cancer. Since that break-through most prostatic cancer patients in the world have been treated endocrinologically and other approaches were only pursued in a few centres. Only after the publication of the Veterans' Administration Study (13,14) which showed that hormone treatment as the initial approach in non-metastatic prostatic cancer was not the ideal type of treatment, was interest again focussed on new possibilities.

Accurate staging, using for instance the TNM classification of the UICC, made it possible to compare treatment results in comparable groups of patients. Improved diagnostic procedures facilitated more accurate staging. However, careful rectal palpation still remains the most accurate diagnostic procedure (15).

In patients with no evidence of distant metastases (MO) radical surgery in the lower T categories yields excellent results. The same can be achieved by interstitial implants of radio-active material. A comparable prognosis is offered by external megavoltage irradiation (Table 3,4). Though results in the same T categories are compared, selection of the cases according to general condition and age does influence the choice of therapy. The main advantage of radiation therapy is the low risk of loss of sexual potency (about 14% after external irradiation and less than 5% after interstitial implant).

There are nearly no complications after interstitial implant in combination with lymphadenectomy; after external irradiation they are acceptable, though multiple transurethral resections or other surgical interventions in the irradiation area do increase the risk of radiation complications (16 - 21).

Survival is largely influenced by the histological grade of the primary. If distant metastases develop hormone therapy can still prolong life considerably in patients with highly and moderately differentiated growths. However, in patients with poorly differentiated lesions the endocrine approach usually fails.

In those with distant metastases and failure of hormone therapy, chemotherapy also appears to be of no substantial value, though some partial responses have been reported (18). Also immunotherapy has been disappointing (22).

Table 2.   Palliative radiotherapy for vertebral metastases of renal cell cancer in the Rotterdam Radio-Therapy Institute

After irradiation

	No pain	Less pain	Same pain	No neurological pathological signs	Same neurological signs
Pain only (28 patients)	19	5	4*	-	-
Pain and neurological signs (32 patients)	19	7	6*+	16	16··
	38 (63%)	12 (20%)	10 (17%)	16 (50%)	16 (50%)

* 1 died during treatment
+ ? pain in 4 patients due to other metastases
·· 9 paralysis > 2 weeks, 1 paralysis within 2 days, 1 progressive

Table 3.   Prostatic cancer - prognosis after interstitial irradiation combined with lymph node dissection or with external irradiation of regional lymph nodes

Type of treatment	Type of growth	No. treated	Prognosis 5 yr. survival	3 yr. survival	Free of disease	Ref. No.
Radical surgery + interstitial therapy 100 mCi 198Au, 2cc diluent	Category T3MO	147	60%			23
Radical perineal surgery	T1,2MO	132	76			24
Radical Perineal surgery	T3,MO	213	64			
Gold grain implant (± 4000 rad) + external megavoltage to a total dose of ± 8000 rad)	Stage C (Category T3MO, T4?MO)					
	Normal serum acid phosph.	13		13	8	25
	Abnormal " "	3		0	0	
	Total stage C (T3MO+T4?MO)	16		13/16	8/16	
	All controlled locally					

(continued)

Table 3 (cont.)

Type of treatment	Type of growth	No. treated	Prognosis	Ref. No.
Retropubic bilateral lymphadenectomy + prostate implant with 125I 16000 rad/1 year = 2023 rets			Crude 5 yr. survival	26
	Category T1M0	65	100%	
	" T2M0	40	100%	
	Limited T3M0	23	77%	
	" T4M0	80	87%	
			Act. 5 yr. survival	
	Lymph nodes negative histologically	102	92%	
	Lymph nodes positive histologically	84	46%	
See above (26)			5 yr. relapse-free survival	27
	Histological grade according to Gleason			
	Well differentiated	19	81%	
	Moderately well diff.	46	69%	
	Poorly differentiated	15	48%	
	Size of the primary			
	<2.5 cm^3	18	89%	
	$2.5 - 7.9$ cm^3	50	65%	
	$8 - 18$ cm^3	32	26%	

Table 4. Prognosis after external supervoltage irradiation in prostatic cancer

Type of treatment and selection	Type of growth	No. treated	Prognosis		Ref. No.
25 MeV Photons (± 40 pts: Co60 or 4 MeV) 4 fields or rotation to prostate + peri-prostatic tissue 60% of patients: 7000-7500 rad/7-7.5 wks	Category T3M0, T4M0 Well differentiated Poorly differentiated	 160 71	5 yr. survival 60% 30%		28
6 MeV Photons 5500 rad/5-7 wks 2 ant. wedge fields, 1 post. field + Hormones Stilboestrol and/or Estradurin (all pts. received antibiotics)	Category T3M0, T4M0 Poorly differentiated	25	3 yr. survival 64% (2 died of other causes)		29
4 MeV Photons 7000-7600 rad/7-7½ wks to prostate and periprostatic tissue (rotation or R + L lat. arc therapy)	Limited to prostate (Category T1M0, T2M0) Extracapsular (Category T3M0, T4M0)	 230 200	5 yr. survival 72% 51%	10 yr. survival 44% 38%	30

(cont.)

Table 4 (con't)

Type of treatment and selection	Type of growth	No. treated	Prognosis 5 yr. survival Free of disease	5 yr. survival With disease	10 yr. survival Free of disease	10 yr. survival With disease	Ref. No.
4 MeV Photons Small field to prostate + periprostatic tissue ± 7000–7500 rad/7–7½ wks	Limited to prostate (Category T1M0, T2M0)	81 28	72%	2%	— 46%	— 4%	19
	Extracapsular extension (Category T3M0, T4M0)	82 23	42%	6%	— 26%	— 5%	
4 MeV Photons Patients ≦ 70 yrs of age lymph node biopsy at lap- arotomy	Stage A, B, C (Category T1M0, T2M0, T3M0, T4M0)		Follow up period 1–50 m. (median: 22 m.)				31
A. Nodes histologically negative ⟶ Random.: a. 7000 rad/7 wks to prostate		17	Free of disease 15				
b. a + pelvic nodes X 4000 rad/7 wks		18	16				
c. a + b + paraortic x		2	1				
		37	32 87%				
B. Pelvic nodes histo- logically pos. ⟶ Random.: b or c		9 5	7 3				
		14	10 72%				

C. Para-aortic nodes
histologically positive
- c.

10   3   30%

Total 61   45   74%

32

22 MeV Photons   Stage C
                      (Category T3MO, T4MO)

                                          5 yr.
                                          survival

I 47 total 7000 rad to prostate   Free of   Alive with
     total 6000 rad to true pelvis   disease   tumour
     total 5000 rad to pelvis inc. L5

97   42%   0

II 50 Idem + hormone therapy   No diff. between I and II
      (orchidectomy + estrogens)

10 MeV Photons   Stage C   33
Whole pelvic fields + (Category T3MO, T4MO)
Booster to prostate

221   5 yr.
                                          survival
                                          58%

                                          Additional hormone therapy
                                          had no bearing on prognosis

22 MeV Photons   Stage B1C1C2   34
Study I. 4 fields (10 x 10   Category T2MO: 4
cm small field to 12 x 15   Category T3MO: 97   Mean follow up: 4 y. 7 m.
cm large field)   Category T4MO: 53   5 yr. survival
Trial 5000 rad/± 5 wks   79   74.7% after X only
Prostate booster 1000-2000   75   61.3% after X + Hormones
rad via ant. + post. field
          Additional hormones   No diff. between 7000 rad and ±
Rand. ⟨ DES 5mg/day   6000-6500 rad.
       No hormones
                                          No diff. between "small" and "large"
Study II. Previous series   X-fields in study I and II
(no trial): 6000-7000 rad/
6-7 wks to true pelvis with
or without hormones.

(continued)

Table 4. (con't)

Type of treatment and selection	Type of growth	No. treated	Prognosis 5 yr. survival	Prognosis Free of disease	Ref. No.
60 Cobalt 6000 rad/6 wks, 5 fields daily Patients ≤ 75 yrs Only patients with negative lymphography are included in study	A (Category T1N0M0)	21	88%	84%	35
	B1 (Category T2N0M0)	43	90%	61%	
	B2 (Category T3N0M0)	30	66%	43%	
	C (Category T4N0M0)	13	39%	37%	
Trial: A. 1 mg Ethinyloestradiol daily	Stage C (Category T3M0, T4M0)	26	65%		36
B. 1 mg Ethinyloestradiol daily + 25 MeV Photons 7000/7 wks by 2 opposing fields covering prostate and surroundings		30	55%		

Type of treatment and selection	Type of growth	No. treated	Act. uncorr. survival 3 yr.	Free of disease	Act. uncorr. survival 5 yr.	Free of disease	Ref. No.
25 MeV Photons 4000 rad + 2 wks split + 3000 rad 4 portals to prostate and surrounding tissue	T3M0 well and mod'ly diff.	40	80%	65%	80%	65%	21
	T3M0 poorly and undiff.	15	55%	35%	fol. up too short		
	T4M0 well and mod'ly diff.	22	65%	65%	65%	63%	
	T4M0 poorly and undiff.	7	50%	25%	fol. up too short		

			No. treated	5 yr. survival	10 yr. survival
6 MeV Photons or Cobalt 60 ± 6000-6800 rad in ±6-7 wks Rotational therapy or 4 field technique or Combination of whole pelvis with additional irradiation With or without hormones.	Stage A (Category T1M0)		13	85%*	-	37
	Stage B (Category T2M0)		21	85%*	-
	Stage C (Category T3M0+T4M0)		112	55%	30%
	T3M0, T4M0 Well + moderately diff.		84	65%*	-
	Undiff.		16	30%*	-
	IVP normal		128	70%*	-
	IVP abnormal		18	25%*	-
	Dose > 6500 rad	All T-categories M0	55	85%*	-
	Dose < 6500 rad	All T-categories M0	91	55%*	-
	Radiotherapy started within 6 m after diagnosis	All T-categories M0	121	70%*	-
	Radiotherapy started after ≥7 m.	All T-categories M0	25	30%*	-
10 MeV Photons or Cobalt 60 Pelvic irradiation 3 or 4 fields 6500-7000 rad/7-8 wks with or without hormones	Stage B (Category T2M0)		36	59%	-	38
	Stage C (Category T3M0+T4M0)		123	58%	30%

No differences between radiation only and X + hormones.

* approximate figures

Radiation therapy of metastases can prevent fractures, eliminate pain and prevent neurological disasters. Pain can also be relieved by pituitary ablation (radiation therapy, implant with radio-active material, injection with alcohol). In case of disseminated painful metastases half body irradiation can yield temporary pain relief (39).

Attempts to improve prognosis can be focussed on improved cure rate of the loco-regional malignancy and on preventing subclinical metastases becoming clinically manifest.

Improvement of loco-regional results by combining hormones and irradiation could not be achieved (Table 4). Increasing the field of irradiation, so as to include all potentially involved regional lymph nodes, has also been unsuccessful (Table 4). The application of multiple daily fractions might offer better results at the cost of more treatment inconvenience to the patient. Theoretically a Pi-meson booster to the prostatic region, after irradiation of the primary and the regional lymph nodes, could improve local cure rate and perhaps prognosis, without increasing the risk of complications. This concept will be implemented at the Pi-meson facility in Villigen. The combination of irradiation with local hyperthermia could theoretically also improve loco-regional results without enhancing the risk of damage.

In prostatic cancer the local cure rate is probably not the main problem though the meaning of persisting positive biopsy or positive cytology after external irradiation is still controversial; as prostatic cancer is a slowly growing malignancy and as after radiation therapy cancer cells only disappear at the time of mitosis, it is possible that non-viable cells will persist for a long time without having any prognostic meaning (17,21,37,40-45). It is most likely that at the time of treatment of the primary sub-clinical metastases already exist. The most reliable indicator for their becoming clinically manifest appears to be an elevated prostatic acid phosphatase in the serum (21). The problem remains whether systemic therapy should be given at the time of the first indicator or at the time of clinical evidence of metastases.

In patients with poorly differentiated lesions about 70% who initially present without clinical evidence of distant metastases will develop metastases within three years (21). As these metastases are usually unresponsive to hormone therapy (or respond only for a short period) and as no really effective chemotherapy or immunotherapy has yet been developed, a pilot study was started in Rotterdam to give elective lower and upper half body irradiation in these high risk cases. The results of the pilot study are presented in Table 5. The procedure is dangerous and requires, in view of the high risk of serious thrombocytopenia (Fig. 1), the facilities of sophisticated hematological support. In a prospective randomised

Table 5. Poorly differentiated prostatic cancer T3,4 MO treated
at the Rotterdam Radio-Therapy Institute electively with 6
Gy lower HBI followed 9 weeks later by 6 Gy upper HBI

Alive 15/20	Dead 5/20	
6 - 12 months : 7	1 month	: sepsis after lower HBI
13 - 18 months : 6 (1 with mets after 18 mths)	6 months	: sepsis in another hospital
	3 months	: Guillain Barré syndrome (PM: no mets)
19 - 24 months : 2	12 months	: lung cancer
	17 months	: mets (evident after 12 mths)

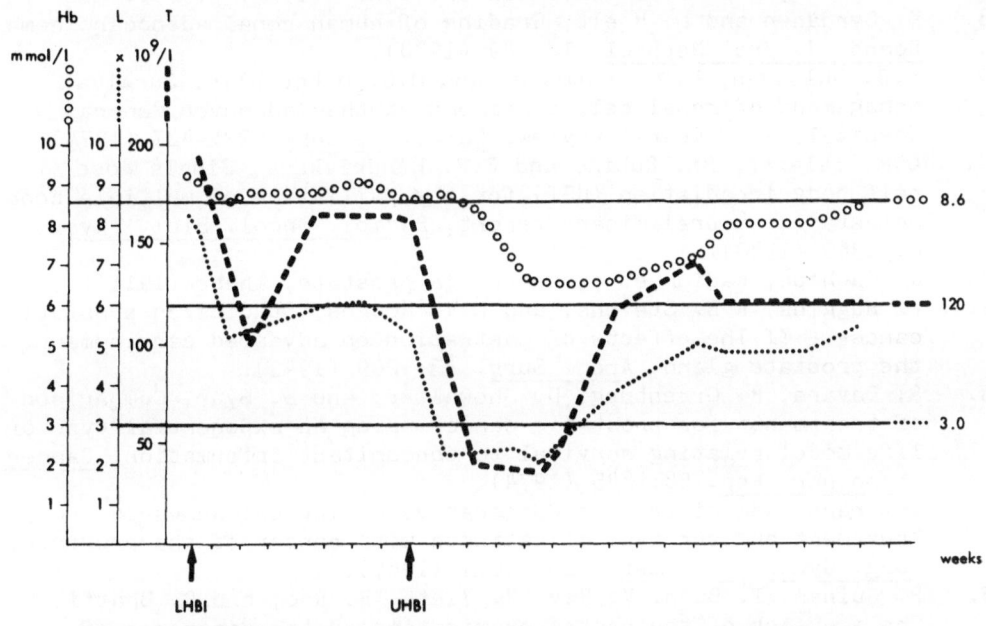

Hb (o o o) – Haemoglobin   L (······) – Leucocytes   T (■ ■ ■) – Thrombocytes

Fig 1. Hematological effects of half body irradiation in
advanced prostatic cancer.

trial the value of this approach is now under investigation at the
Rotterdam Radio-Therapy Institute. It is hoped that in some instances the existing subclinical metastases can be eradicated, and that
in others the treatment may postpone the time at which they become
clinically evident.

REFERENCES

1.   S. Rafla, Renal cell carcinoma. Natural history and results of
     treatment, Cancer 25: 26 (1970).
2.   B. van der Werf-Messing, R.O. van der Heul, and R. Ch. Ledeboer,
     Renal cell carcinoma trial, Cancer Clin. Trials 1: 1 (1978).
3.   S. Wallace, V.P. Chung, D. Swanson, B. Bracken, E.M. Hersh,
     A. Ayala, and D. Johnson, Embolization of renal carcinoma,
     Radiology 138: 563 (1981).
4.   J. Ammon, J.H. Karstens, G. Durben, and K.H. Barth, Carcinoma of
     renal parenchyma, renal pelvis and ureter - radiological diag-
     nosis and treatment planning, Cancer Treat. Rev. 7: 29 (1980).
5.   Sir E. Riches, in: "Tumours of Kidney and Ureter," A. Richards,
     ed., Livingstone, London (1964) p. 295.
6.   D.G. Skinner, C.D. Vermillion, and R.B. Colvin, The surgical
     management of renal cell carcinoma, J. Urol. 107: 705 (1972).
7.   G.P. Murphy, in: "Current results from treatment of renal cell
     carcinoma," 7th Proc. Nat. Cancer. Conf. (1973) p. 751.
8.   K. Syrjänen and L. Hjelt, Grading of human renal adenocarcinoma,
     Scand. J. Urol Nephrol. 12: 49 (1978).
9.   L.D. Sullivan, D.D. Westmore, and M.G. McLoughlin, Surgical
     management of renal cell carcinoma at the Vancouver General
     Hospital, a 20 years' review, Canad. J. Surg. 22: 427 (1974).
10. O.M. Salazar, Ph. Rubin, and F.R. Hendrickson, Single dose
     half body irradiation (HBI) for the palliation of multiple bone
     metastases: a preliminary report, Radiol. Oncol. Biol. Phys.
     6: 1360 (1980).
11. J. Cauhapé, Radium et cancer de la prostate, Thèse (1911).
12. C. Huggins, R.E. Stevens, and C.V. Hodges, Studies on prostatic
     cancer. II The effects of castration on advanced carcinoma of
     the prostate gland, Arch. Surg. 43: 209 (1941).
13. S. Bayard, R. Greenburg, D. Showalter, and D. Byar, Comparison
     of treatments for prostatic cancer using an exponential type of
     life model relating survival to concomitant information, Cancer
     Chemother. Rep. 58: 845 (1974).
14. Veterans' Administration Cooperative Urological Research Group,
     Treatment and survival of patients with cancer of the prostate,
     Surg. Gynecol. Obstet. 124: 1011 (1967).
15. P. Guinan, I. Bush, V. Ray, R. Vieth, R. Rao, and R. Bhatti,
     The accuracy of the rectal examination in the diagnosis of
     prostatic carcinoma, New Eng. J. Med. 303: 499 (1980).
16. C.E. Carlton, Jr., F. Dawoud, P. Hudgins, and R. Scott, Jr.,
     Irradiation treatment of carcinoma of the prostate: a prelim-
     inary report based on 8 years of experience, J. Urol. 108:
     924 (1972).
17. D.R. Hill, Q.E. Cres, Jr., and P.C. Walsh, Prostate carcinoma:
     radiation treatment of primary and regional lymphatics, Cancer
     34: 156 (1974).
18. C.A. Perez, L.V. Ackerman, I. Silber, and R.K. Royce, Radiation
     therapy in the treatment of localized carcinoma of the prostate
     - preliminary report using 22 MeV photons, Cancer 34: 1059 (1974).

19. G.R. Ray and M.A. Bagshaw, The role of radiation therapy in the definitive treatment of adenocarcinoma of the prostate, Annu. Rev. Med. 26: 567 (1975).

20. B. van der Werf-Messing, V. Sourek-Zikova, and D.I. Blonk, Localized advanced carcinoma of the prostate. Radiation therapy versus hormonal therapy, Int. J. Radiol. Oncol. Biol. Phys. 1: 1043 (1976).

21. B. van der Werf-Messing, Prostatic cancer treated at the Rotterdam Radio-Therapy Institute, Strahlentherapie 154: 537 (1978).

22. J.E. Castro, Immunological effects of hormones: a review, J. Roy. Soc. Med. 71: 123 (1978).

23. R.H. Flocks, The treatment of stage C prostatic cancer with special reference to combined surgical and radiation therapy, J. Urol. 109: 461 (1973).

24. F.H. Schröder and E. Belt, Carcinoma of the prostate: a study of 213 patients with Stage C tumors treated by total perineal prostatectomy, J. Urol. 114: 257 (1975).

25. R.C. Chan and A.E. Gutierrez, Carcinoma of the prostate. Its treatment by a combination of radioactive gold-grain implant and external irradiation, Cancer 37: 2749 (1976).

26. B.S. Hilaris, W.F. Whitmore, M. Batata, and W. Barzell, Behavioural patterns of prostate adenocarcinoma following an I ^{125} implant and pelvic node dissection, Int. J. Radiol. Oncol. Biol. Phys. 2: 631 (1977).

27. W. Barzell, M.A. Bean, B.S. Hilaris, and W.F. Whitmore, Jr., Prostatic adenocarcinoma: relationship of grade and local extend to the the pattern of metastases, J. Urol. 118: 278 (1977).

28. S.T. Cantril, J.M. Vaeth, J.P. Green, and A.F. Schroeder, Radiation therapy for localized carcinoma of the prostate; correlation with histopathological grading, Front. Radiat. Ther. Oncol. 9: 274 (1974).

29. F. Edsmyr, P.L. Esposti, B. Littbrand, and L.E. Almgard, Carcinoma of the prostate: the place of radiotherapy, in: "Radiology; Proc. 13th Int. Cong. Radiol., vol. 2, Madrid, 15-20 October 1973," J. Gomez Lopoz and J. Bonmati, eds., Excerpta Medica, Amsterdam (1974) p. 63.

30. M.A. Bagshaw, G.R. Ray, D.A. Pistenma, R.A. Castellino, and E.M. Meares, Jr., External beam radiation therapy of primary carcinoma of the prostate, Cancer 36: 723 (1975).

31. M.A. Bagshaw, D.A. Pistenma, G.R. Ray, F.S. Freiha, and R.L. Kempson, Evaluation of extended field radiotherapy for prostatic neoplasm: 1976 Progress Report, Cancer Treat. Rep. 61: 297 (1977).

32. C.A. Perez, W. Bauer, R. Garza, and R.K. Royce, Radiation therapy in the definitive treatment of localized carcinoma of the prostate, Cancer 40: 1425 (1977).

33. W.J. Taylor, R.G. Richardson, and M.D. Hafermann, Radiation therapy of prostate cancer, Int. J. Radiol. Oncol. Biol. Phys. 2, Suppl. 2 (1977) abstr. 12 and 13.

34.   W.J. Neglia, D.H. Hussey, and D.E. Johnson, Megavoltage radiation therapy for carcinoma of the prostate, Int. J. Radiol. Oncol. Biol. Phys. 2: 873 (1977).

35.   D.G. McGowan, Radiation therapy in the management of localized carcinoma of the prostate. A preliminary report, Cancer 39: 98 (1977).

36.   B. van der Werf-Messing, The experience of the Rotterdam Radio-Therapy Institute (RRTI) in the treatment of urological tumours, in: "The Tumours of Genito-Urinary Apparatus," M. Pavone-Macaluso, ed., Cofese Edizioni, Palermo (1977) p. 93.

37.   L. Harisiadis, R.J. Veenema, J.J. Senyszyn, P.J. Puchner, P. Tretter, N.A. Romas, C.H. Chang, J.K. Lattimer, and M. Tannenbaum, Carcinoma of the prostate: treatment with external radiotherapy, Cancer 41: 2131 (1978).

38.   W.J. Taylor, R.G. Richardson, and M.D. Hafermann, Radiation therapy for localized prostate cancer, Cancer 43: 1123 (1979).

39.   C.G. Rowland, Half body irradiation for treatment of metastatic prostatic carcinoma and plasma cell myeloma, Br. J. Radiol. 54: 372 (1980).

40.   G.H. Jacobi, K.H. Kurth, and R. Hohenfellner, Lokale Hochvolttherapie des Prostatakarzinoms unter kurativer Zielsetzung, Aktuelle Urologie 10: 291 (1979).

41.   A.R. Kagan, J. Gordon, J.F. Cooper, and H. Gilbert, A clinical appraisal of post-irradiation biopsy in prostatic cancer, Cancer 39: 637 (1977).

42.   K.H. Kurth, J.E. Altwein, D. Skoluda, and R. Hohenfellner, Follow-up of irradiated prostatic carcinoma by aspiration biopsy, J. Urol. 117: 615 (1977).

43.   G.R. Ray, J.R. Cassady, and M.A. Bagshaw, Definitive radiation therapy of carcinoma of the prostate. A report on 15 years' experience, Radiology 106: 409 (1973).

44.   R.K. Rhamy, S.K. Wilson, and W.L. Caldwell, Biopsy-proved tumor following definitive irradiation for resectable carcinoma of the prostate, J. Urol. 107: 627 (1972).

45.   H. Sack and E.M. Röttinger, Die Kurative Strahlenbehandlung des Prostata-karzinoms den lokalisierten Stadien, Radiology 17: 263 (1977).

CANCER OF THE PROSTATE

PROSTATIC CANCER: EPIDEMIOLOGY AND ETIOLOGY

C. Bouffioux

Univeristy of Liège
Liège
Belgium

INTRODUCTION

Cancer of the prostate is a very common disease in western
Europe and in the United States: it is one of the leading causes of
death from cancer in man.   However, the incidence of the disease is
sometimes controversial due to a confusion in terminology and methods
of statistical computation.

One must distinguish on the one hand between overt cancers with
urinary or metastatic signs and symptoms and on the other hand latent
cancers which do not manifest any symptomatology and are discovered
by chance or by systematic pathological investigation.

The incidence of microscopic cancer, studied by the "step section
technique" is shown in figure 1: as clearly demonstrated, it increases exponentially and over 50% of men over 80 have some microscopic
areas of cancer in their prostate (1,2).   A routine microscopic
analysis (a few sections at random in the gland) ignores many microscopic cancers, as shown in figure 2.   The striking difference between the curves suggests that the tumor has a long period of biological latency, about 20 years (1).

The clinical incidence of prostatic carcinoma is, happily, far
below the microscopic incidence.   This disproportion is due to many
factors including the fact that prostatic cancer is a disease of the
elderly man and that many such subjects with focal and unsuspected
cancer die of other conditions such as cardio-vascular, respiratory
and other diseases.

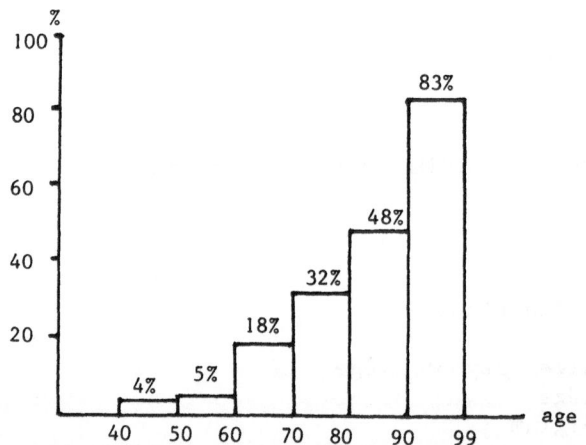

Fig. 1.   Incidence of prostatic cancer, with the step section
          technique.   From Hirst and Bergman (1).

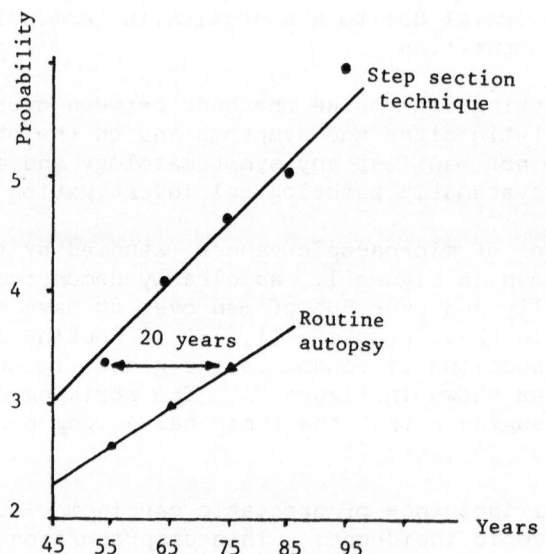

Fig. 2.   Probability of discovering a P.C. with the step section
          technique and with routine autopsy examination.

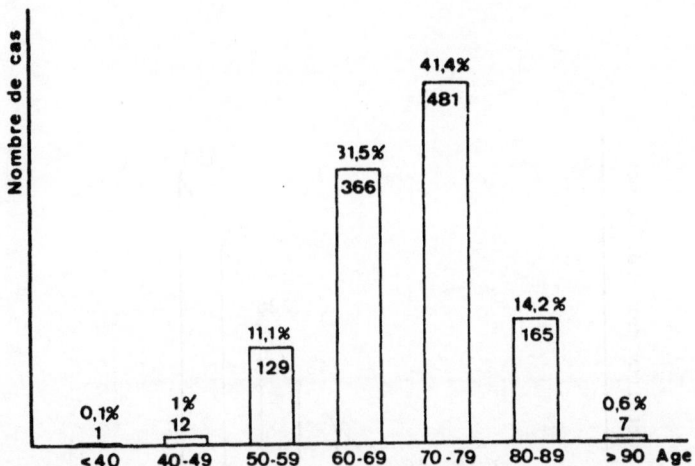

Fig. 3.   Incidence of clinical prostatic cancer with age.

INFLUENCE OF AGE

Figure 3 shows the age distribution of patients in whom prostatic cancer (P.C.) was first discovered in our department (3).   A quick glance leads one to suppose that the incidence of the disease decreases after 80 years.   However, the percentage of distribution by age group is biased by a significant decrease of the population after 80 and probably also by less accurate diagnosis in these older patients.

If one considers the mortality rate by decade, relating the number of deaths in each decade to the living male population in that decade, one observes that the chance of dying of P.C. rises rapidly with age: above 80 years, it is nearly 500 times greater than at 50 years (figure 4).

RACIAL AND GEOGRAPHIC INFLUENCES

Figure 5 shows the mortality rate for P.C. in 16 countries in 1969.   Great differences are observed in the distribution of the malignancy which appears to be very common in Western countries and much more uncommon in Eastern countries, especially Japan.

Such differences are also observed in the United States where the incidence of P.C. increases much faster among blacks than among whites and in the Hawaiian Islands where important discrepancies are noted among racial groups living in the same social conditions.

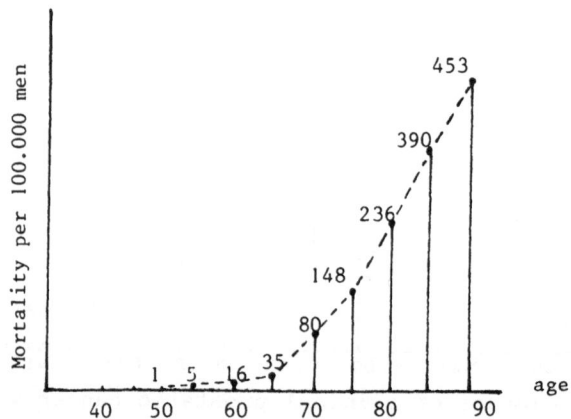

Fig. 4.   Mortality rate for prostatic cancer at differing ages
          (U.S.A. 1958).

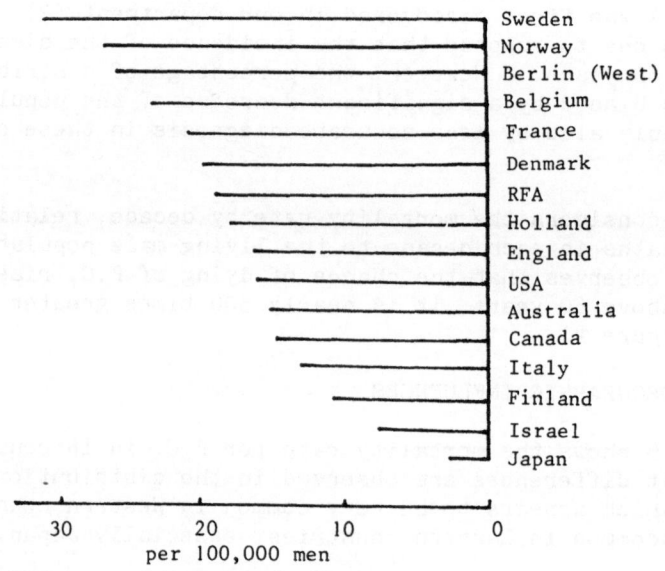

Fig. 5.   Prostatic cancer mortality rate in 16 countries (1969).

Although the results can be biased by several factors, such as quality of medical care, median survival rate, and the organisation of a Cancer Registry, the great discrepancy between caucasians and Japanese is stressed by all epidemiologists (4-7). Therefore, a racial, genetic, perhaps hormonal, factor seems to favour the incidence of the disease.

However, this statement must be tempered by the following considerations:

1. Microscopic prostatic cancer, as demonstrated by autopsy data, is as common in Japanese as in caucasians (8,9). If this is so, the difference in the clinical incidence of the disease would result from a more rapid evolution of in situ cancers among whites, and not from a difference in the oncogenic transformation rate.

2. Racial differences partially disappear when one considers the incidence in immigrants coming from low-risk countries and living in high-risk countries; Haenzel and Kurihara (10) have drawn attention to these differences (Table 1). If substantiated, these data suggest that environmental factors also play a role in the growth of the disease.

TIME TRENDS

An increase in the P.C. mortality rates has been reported during the last decades as shown in figure 6.

It may be questioned whether or not the increase is real. As a matter of fact, we believe, like many others, that the longer life span, better diagnosis and better statistical enquiries can often account for the reported rise. However, in the United States, age-adjusted mortality rates have risen precipitously among blacks, and yet remained unchanged among whites (figure 7).

Table 1. Carcinoma of the Prostate. Percentage
Mortality in Relation to Age (10).

	Mortality % with Age	
	65-74 y.	75 y. and over
Japanese	11.6	28
Issei	40.2	130
American (whites)	92.6	307.5

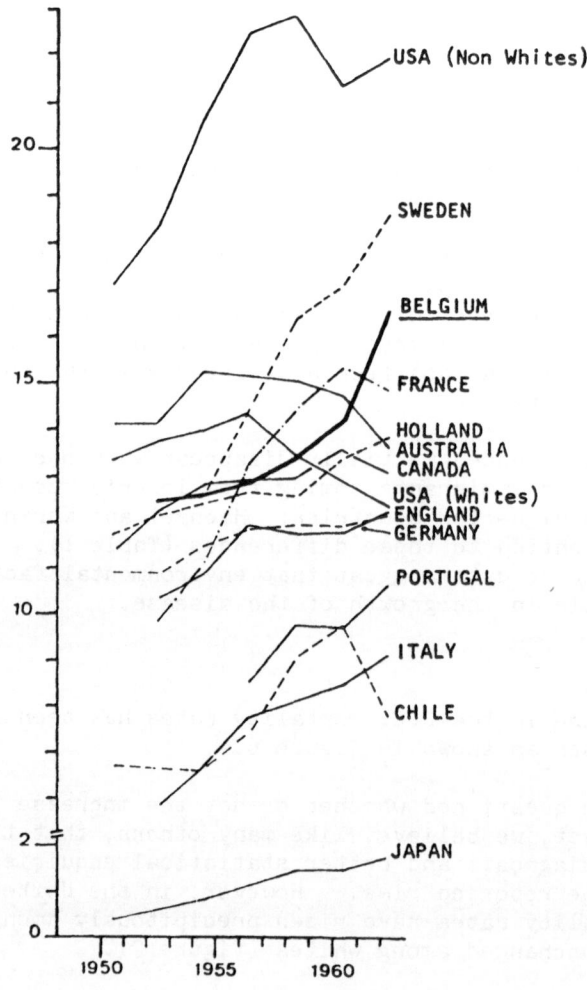

Fig. 6. P.C. mortality rates in 14 countries (1950-1963).

    Ernster, Selvin and Wilkenstein (11) examined the mortality
rates by age and birth cohort and observed that peak rates occured
at every age in the cohort 1896-1900 and declined thereafter (figure 8).   This presages a reversal of time trend, as more recent non-
white cohorts reach the ages of maximum risk.   If this observation
is consistent, it would be of the greatest interest to research the
historical experience of the 1896-1900 cohort in attempting to detect
a common feature which could explain the higher risk in this cohort.

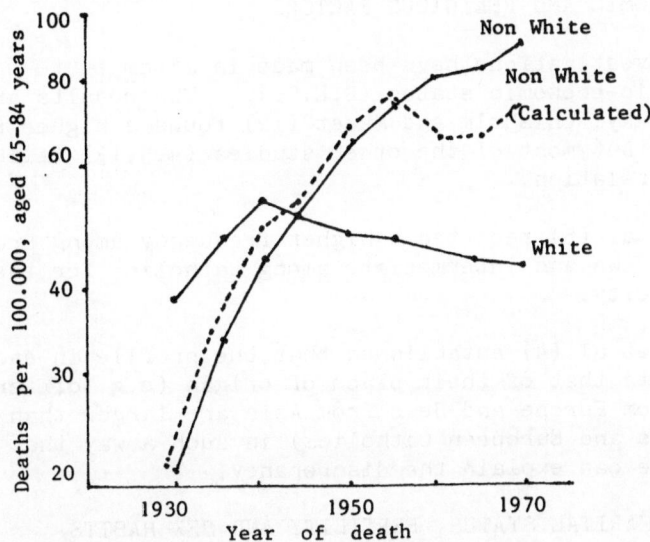

Fig. 7.   Change in mortality of prostate cancer in males in the
United States (11).

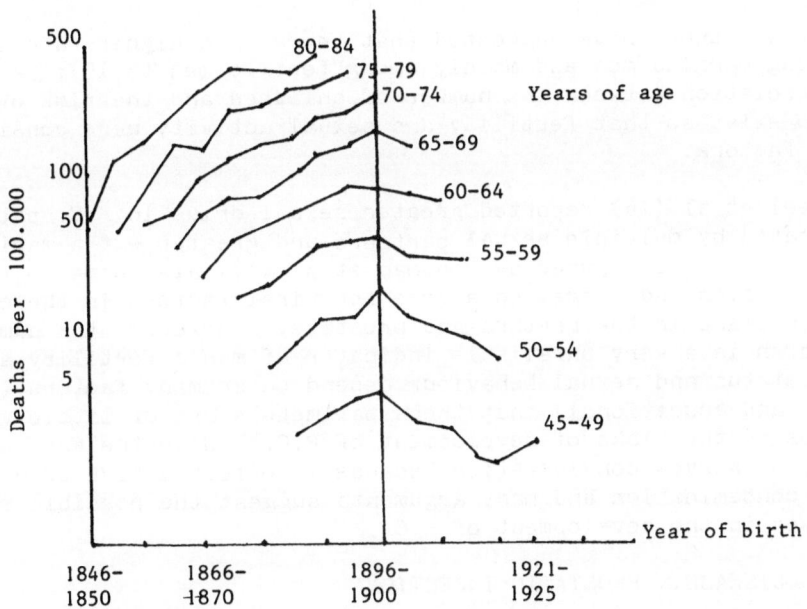

Fig. 8.   Mortality rates for prostatic cancer by age and birth
cohort (11).

SOCIAL, ECONOMIC AND RELIGIOUS FACTORS

Many investigations have been made in attempts to correlate
P.C. and socio-economic status (S.E.S.).   The results are in contradiction: Hakky, Chisholm and Skeet (12) found a higher risk with a
lower S.E.S. but most of the other studies (4,5,13) failed to indicate any correlation.

King et al (5) reported a higher frequency among Protestants,
lower among Jews and intermediate among Catholics for the population
of New York City.

Wynder et al (4) established that the profile in each religion
group reflects that of their place of origin (e.g. differences between Jews from Europe and Jews from Asia are larger than between
European Jews and European Catholics) in such a way that ethnic
factors alone can explain the discrepancy.

MORPHOLOGY, MARITAL STATUS, FERTILITY AND SEX HABITS

The hormonal dependence of P.C. has naturally led investigations
in this direction.

Anthropometric studies including height, weight, somato-type
and hirsutism failed to reveal any statistical difference between
P.C. patients and controls (4,14).

A few authors have suggested that there is a higher rate of
P.C. among married men and mainly among fertile men (5,15): a positive correlation between the number of children and the risk of P.C.
seems to exist so that fertility and sexual activity were considered
as risk factors.

Steel et al (16) reported greater sexual drive in P.C. patients
as indicated by multiple sexual partners and greater extra-marital
activity.   A recent paper by Schuman et al (17) also came to the
same conclusion and suggested a role for viral factors in the causa-
tion of disease in the urethra and prostate.   However, the number
of children is a very unreliable indicator of man's fertility and
marital status and sexual behaviour depend on so many factors (social,
cultural and educational) that these parameters are of little value
in assessing the risks of development of P.C.   Nevertheless, sexual
activity derserves consideration because it offers a risk of urogenital contamination and many arguments suggest the possible role
of viruses in the development of P.C.

VENEREAL DISEASE, PROSTATIC INFECTION

In 1942, on the basis of low incidence of P.C. among Jews,
Ravich (18) presented the concept that it was a venereally trans-

mitted viral disease and that circumcision could protect against it.
In a recent paper (19), the same author incriminates the method of
statistical computation of P.C. in Japan, where early prophylactic
circumcision is not performed and where P.C. is rare, to defend his
opinion.   In fact, circumcision does not seem to protect against
P.C.: Kaplan et al (20) Wynder et al (4) found no statistical difference in the number of circumcisions between non-Jewish cancer patients and controls.

    Chronic prostatic infection as a possible cause of P.C. led some
authors to look for a relationship with a previous history of gonorrhea.   Reports from Wynder (4), Kaplan (20), Steel (16) and Krain
(21) resulted in contradictory conclusions and prompted Heshmat et
al (22) to perform new studies.   These authors presented a very
interesting analysis of association of the incidence of gonorrhea and
prostatic cancer mortality rates in Denmark.   As shown in figure 9,
both curves correlate quite well with a free period of 45 years, as
if gonorrhea could induce local changes transforming prostatic cells
after a long period of latency.

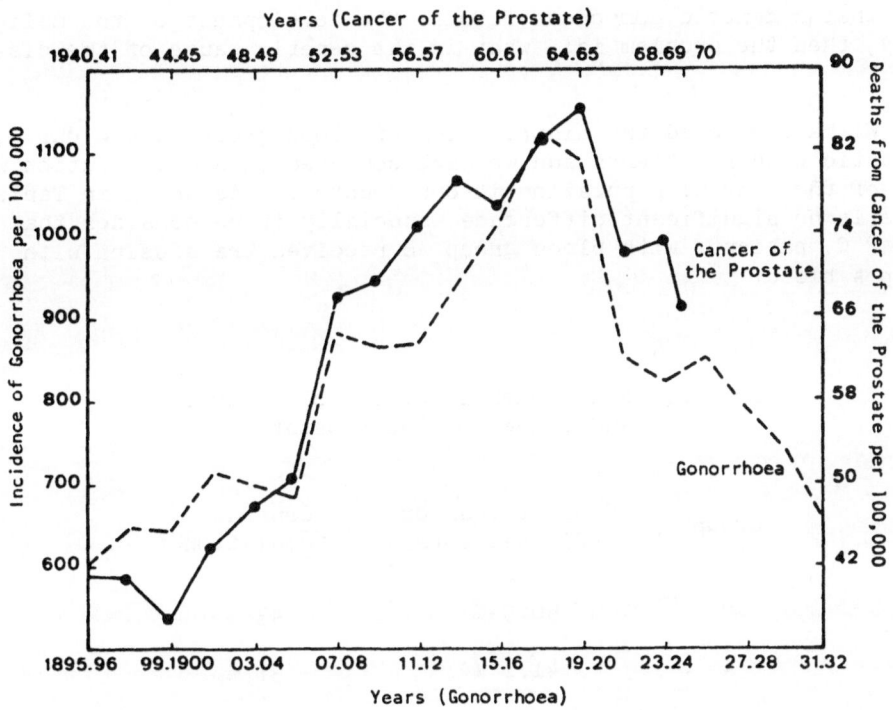

Fig. 9. Relationship between incidence of gonorrhea and mortality
         from prostatic cancer in Denmark (22).

Two hypotheses have been advanced to explain this relationship:

a)   Venereal-viral hypothesis: gonorrhea allows an oncogenic virus to infect prostatic cells and induce potential changes leading to malignant transformation.

b)   Chronic prostatitis hypothesis: bacterial chronic inflammation of the prostate induces atrophic and dystrophic pre-malignant lesions.

If this relationship proves to be true, we would expect a highly significant increase of P.C. around the end of this century, considering the dramatic rise of venereal disease since 1958. However, quick cure of gonorrhea since the advent of antibiotics in 1945 must, in our opinion, considerably limit the influence of this hypothetical factor.

HEREDITY, BLOOD GROUPS

Morganti et al (23) and Woolf (24) clearly demonstrated a higher rate of P.C. among the relatives of P.C. patients. If it is possible that a genetic component favours the development of the malignancy, then the problem is: what is the genetic cause of the disease?

We have studied the distribution of blood groups among our prostatic cancer patients and we have compared this distribution with that of the general population in our country. As shown in Table 2, there is no significant difference especially if we consider that some P.C. patients with blood group AB received transfusion with group A blood.

Table 2.   Relationship Between Blood Group
            and Cancer of the Prostate

Group	Prostate Cancer (250 patients)	General Population
O	50.5 %	43 %
A	41.1 %	37 %
B	7.4 %	7 %
AB	1 %	3 %

ENVIRONMENTAL FACTORS, TOXICITIES, IRRADIATION

Enquiries on tobacco and alcohol consumption among P.C. patients and controls did not show any disproportion (4), and an interesting study performed by Bean et al (25) on routine autopsy material from Hiroshima and Nagasaki showed no relation between the presence of a P.C. and the dose radiation category.

Some workers postulating an association between the degree of urbanization and the incidence of P.C., suggested that the difference between urban and rural areas might be correlated to the level of suspended particulate air pollution (5,26). However, our own analyses on the relative frequency of P.C. by area in Belgium and similar analyses from England and Wales do not provide such evidence. It is possible that the unequal distribution of medical care and an uneven accuracy in the keeping of Cancer Registries in rural and urban areas may account for the differences.

Few data are available concerning the influence of industrial and domestic toxicities but Kippling and Waterhouse (27) drew attention to the high and statistically very significant incidence in P.C. among 248 workers exposed to cadmium dust. Such observations deserve further study.

PROSTATIC ADENOMA AND CARCINOMA

Widely diverging opinions have been put forward regarding the relation between benign prostatic hypertrophy (B.P.H.) and P.C.

Greenwald et al (28) compared the risk of developing a cancer among a group of adenomectomized patients and an age-matched group with prostatic enlargement: they found no differences but Armenian et al (29), in a prospective and retrospective study, found that the relative risk of developing a P.C. was three to five times higher among non-operated B.P.H. patients as compared to controls without prostatic enlargement. Further studies are required to establish a firm correlation but one must admit that the old-fashioned idea that adenoma protect against cancer must be discarded. On the other hand, considering that nearly 50% of the males present some degree of asymptomatic B.P.H. after the age of 60 and that prostatic cancer deaths for these age-groups represent about 1%, one realises that the relationship is far from obvious.

ASSOCIATED DISEASES

To our knowledge, there is no report of extra-genitourinary disease or physical condition significantly associated with P.C., except for the negative relationship with cirrhosis.

Liver cirrhosis provokes hyperestrogenism as a consequence of

decreased liver metabolism of estrogens.   In order to determine the
effect of hyperestrogenism on the incidence of P.C., Glantz (30) compared, by routine autopsies, 550 patients with cirrhosis and 650 patients without liver disease: he observed a 3.3% P.C. rate among the
cirrhotic group and 9.0% in the control group.   The age-group distribution is illustrated in figure 10.

This study confirms the prophylactic effect of estrogens on the
growth of a clinical prostatic cancer but does not demonstrate any
decrease in microscopical cancer as histological examination was not
performed with the step section technique.

VIRUS AND CANCER

Paulson et al (31,32) induced, by viral manipulation (SV-40),
in vitro, the transformation of normal hamster prostatic tissue into
neoplastic tissue, exhibiting the characteristics of an undifferentiated carcinoma.   Transformed cells injected into appropriate hosts
gave rise to cancers showing some analogy with P.C.

Virus-like particles have been identified with electron microscopy in various specimens of P.C. (33).   In addition, many recent
experimental studies provide arguments in favour of the viral-oncogenic hypothesis of Todaro and Huebner (34).   Immunological investigations have detected antibodies against known oncogenic viruses like
SV-40, Herpes 2, Cytomegalovirus (35,36,37) but these antibodies are
often not cancer specific and can be discovered in people without
malignant disease (38).

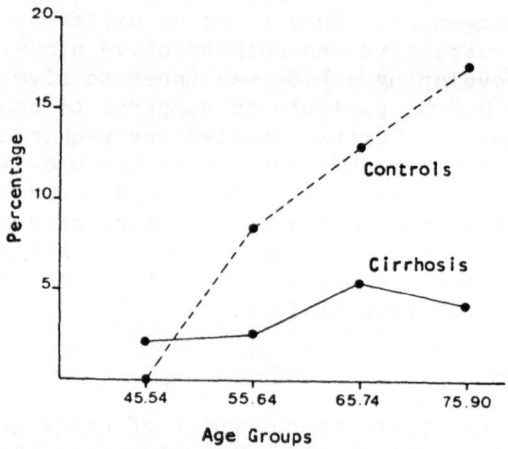

Fig. 10.   Relationship between incidence of prostatic cancer in
          550 patients with cirrhosis and 650 patients without
          liver disease (30).

The role of sexual activity, in particular with partners having genital infections, also provides arguments for the possible influence of viruses.

Although there is no evidence yet of a viral origin of human prostatic cancer we cannot ignore these studies relating prostatic cancer and viruses; the hypothesis of a viral origin of Human Prostate Cancer modulated by genetic, individual and environmental factors cannot be neglected.

ENDOCRINE STATUS

There is no doubt that changes in the hormonal environment influence the evolution of prostatic cancer.   As a reminder, prostatic cancer does not exist among true eunuchoids; hyperestrogenism and post-pubertal castration greatly reduce the incidence of the disease: there is a very close relationship between the geographical distribution of prostate cancer in males and breast cancer in females.

Many workers have attempted to stress changes in the hormonal status of ·prostate cancer patients (39-44).   We have determined the levels of testosterone, LH and FSH in men with P.C., B.P.H. and in men free of prostatic disease.   The relevant data are given in Table 3.   Like many others, we could not find any statistical differences among the three groups.

Similarly, hormonal levels found in low-risk populations like the Japanese and high-risk populations did not reveal any difference.

Table 3. Hormone Levels in Prostatic Cancer, Benign
          Prostatic Hypertrophy and Patients Free of
          Prostatic Disease

Patients	Testosterone (ng/100 ml)	LH (MUI/ml)	FSH (MUI/ml)	No. of Cases	Mean Age
No prostatic disease	414+/-251	16.3+/-9.1	14.4+/-7.2	20	71.1
B.P.H.	439+/-279	11 +/-7.6	13.2+/-5.8	20	70.3
P.C.	444+/-261	12.1+/-4.8	13.8+/-9.7	20	68.8

At the present time, the study of the endocrine status does not provide arguments explaining the relative risk of P.C.   Of course the intra-cellular metabolism of hormones in prostatic cancer cells shows quantitative, if not qualitative, differences with normal prostatic cells but these changes reflect the modifications induced by the neoplastic state rather than the cause of the transformation.

CONCLUSION

Except for age, race and possible but as yet obscure environmental and genetic factors, little is known about the causes favouring the development of carcinoma of the prostate.   It is most probable that the disease, like most other malignancies, does not depend on a single etiology and that we are dealing with complex interactions, some facilitating and other inhibiting any potential oncogenic transformation.

Much work remains to be done to obtain a better understanding of the origin of the disease, so that a more adequate measure can be taken to prevent and detect this common cancer.

REFERENCES

1.   A. Hirst and R. Bergman, Carcinoma of the Prostate in Men 80 or More Years Old, Cancer, 7:136 (1954).
2.   I. Liavag, T. Harbitz and O. Haugen, Latent Carcinoma of the Prostate, in "Recent Results in Cancer Research. Springer Verlag, Berlin, Heidelberg, New York (1972) Vol. 39, p. 131.
3.   C. Bouffioux, Le Cancer de la Prostate, Acta Urol. Belg. 47:189 (1979).
4.   E. Wynder, M. Kiyohiko and W. Whitmore, Epidemiology of Cancer of the Prostate, Cancer, 28:344 (1971).
5.   H. King, E. Diamond and A. Lilienfeld, Some Epidemiological Aspects of Cancer of the Prostate, J. Chron. Dis, 16:117 (1963).
6.   L. Franks, The Incidence of Carcinoma of the Prostate: An Epidemiological Survey, Rec. Res. Cancer Res. 39:144 (1972).
7.   I. Higgins, The Epidemiology of Cancer of the Prostate, J. Chron. Dis. 28:343 (1975).
8.   K. Karube, Study of Latent Carcinoma of the Prostate in Japanese Based on Necropsy Materials, Tohuku J. Exp. Med. 74:265 (1961).
9.   K. Oota, Latent Carcinoma of the Prostate Among Japanese, Acta Un. Int. Cancer, 17:952 (1961).
10. W. Haenszel and M. Kurihara, Studies of Japanese Migrants. 1. Mortality from Cancer and Other Diseases Among Japanese in the United States, J. Natl. Cancer Inst. 40:43 (1968).
11. V. Ernster, S. Selvin and W. Winkelstein, Cohort Mortality for Prostatic Cancer Among United States Nonwhites, Science 200:1165 (1978).
12. S. Hakky, G. Chisholm and R. Skeet, Social Class and Carcinoma of the Prostate, Brit. J. Urol. 51:393 (1979).

13. V. Ernster, S. Selvin, S. Sacks, D. Austin, S. Brown and W. Winkelstein, Prostatic Cancer; Mortality and Incidence Rates by Race and Social Class, Am. J. Epidemiol. 107:311 (1978).

14. P. Greenwald, A. Damon, V. Kirmss and A. Polan, Physical and Demographic Features of Men Before Developing Cancer of the Prostate, J. Nat. Cancer Inst. 53:341 (1974).

15. H. Armenian, A Lilienfeld, E. Diamond and I. Bross, Epidemiologic Characteristics of Patients with Prostatic Neoplasm, Am. J. Epidemiol. 102:47 (1975).

16. R. Steel, R. Lees, A. Kraus and C. Rao, Sexual Factors in the Epidemiology of Cancer of the Prostate, J. Chron. Dis. 24:29 (1971).

17. L. Schuman, J. Mandel, C. Blackard, H. Bauer, J. Scarlett and R. McHugh, Epidemiologic Study of Prostate Cancer: Preliminary Report, Cancer Treat. Rep. 61:181 (1977).

18. A. Ravich, The RElationship of Circumcision to Cancer of the Prostate, J. Urol. 48:298 (1942).

19. A. Ravich, Point of View: Misleading Reports on Japanese Incidence of Prostatic Cancer, Urology, 11:542 (1978).

20. G. Kaplan and V. O'Connor, The Incidence of Carcinoma of the Prostate in Jews and Gentiles, JAMA 196:123 (1966).

21. L. Krain, Epidemiologic Variables in Prostatic Cancer, Geriatrics 28:93 (1973).

22. M. Heshmat, J. Kovi, J. Herson, G. Jones and M. Jackson, Epidemiologic Association Between Gonorrhea and Prostatic Carcinoma, Urology 6:457 (1975).

23. G. Morganti, L. Gianferrarri, A. Cresseri, G. Arrigoni and G. Lovati, Recherches Clinico-statiques et Genetiques sur les Neoplasies de la Prostate, Acta Genet. 6:304 (1956).

24. C. Woolf. An Investigation of the Familial Aspects of Carcinoma of the Prostate, Cancer 13:739 (1960).

25. M. Bean, R. Yatani, P. Liu, K. Fukazawa, F. Ashley and S. Fujita, Prostatic Carcinoma at Autopsy in Hiroshima and Nagasaki Japanese, Cancer 32:498 (1973).

26. W. Winkelstein and S. Kantor, Prostatic Cancer: Relationship to Suspended Particulate Air Pollution, Am. J. Publ. Hlth., 59:1134 (1969).

27. M. Kipling and J. Waterhouse, Cadmium and Prostatic Carcinoma, Lancet 1 :730 (1967).

28. P. Greenwald, V. Kirmss, A. Polan and V. Dick, Cancer of the Prostate Among Men with Benign Prostatic Hyperplasia, J. Nat. Cancer Inst. 53:335 (1974).

29. H. Armenian, A. Lilienfeld and E. Diamond, Relation Between Benign Prostatic Hyperplasia and Cancer of the Prostate. A Prospective and Retrospective Study, Lancet, 2:115 (1974).

30. G. Glantz, Cirrhosis and Carcinoma of the Prostate Gland, J. Urol. 91:291 (1964).

31. D. Paulson, E. Fraley, A. Rabson and A. Ketcham, SV-40 Transformed Hamster Prostatic Tissue: A Model for Human Prostatic Malignancy, Surgery 64:241 (1968).

32. D. Paulson, R. Bonar and Y. Sharief, Properties of Prostatic
    Cultures Transformed by SV 40, Cancer Chemother. Rep. 59:51
    (1975).

33. M. Tannenbaum and J. Lattimer, Similar Virus-Like Particles
    in Cancers of the Prostate and Breast, J. Urol. 103:471 (1970).

34. G. Todaro and R. Huebner, The Viral-Oncogenic Hypothesis: New
    Evidence (N.A.S. Symposium), Proc. Nat. Acad. Sci. USA, 69:1009
    (1972).

35. K. Shah, L. Palma and G. Murphy, The Occurrence of SV40-neutra-
    lizing Antibodies in Sera of Patients with Genitourinary Car-
    cinoma, J. Surg. Oncol. 3:443 (1971).

36. E. Sandford, L. Geder, A. Laychock, T. Rohner and F. Rapp,
    Evidence for the Association of Cyto-Megalovirus with Carcinoma
    of the Prostate, J. Urol. 118:789 (1977).

37. J. Herbert, J. Birkhoff, P. Feorino and G. Caldwell, Herpes
    Simplex Virus Type 2 and Cancer of the Prostate, J. Urol. 116:
    611 (1976).

38. K. Shah, M. Weissmann and G. Murphy, Occurrence of Simian Virus
    40-reacting Antibodies in Sera of Some Patients with Prostatic
    Cancer, J. Surg. Oncol. 4:89 (1972).

39. F. Habib, I. Lee, S. Stitch and P.H. Smith, Androgen Levels in
    Plasma and Prostatic Tissues of Patients with Benign Prostatic
    Hyperplasia and Carcinoma of the Prostate, J. Endocrinol. 71:99
    (1976).

40. J. Frick and G. Bartsch, Hormonal Status in Prostatic Disease,
    in "Prostatic Disease", Alan R. Liss Inc., New York (1976) p.143.

41. O. Djoseland, K. Tveter, A. Attramadal, V. Hanson, H. Haugen and
    W. Mathisen, Metabolism of Testosterone in Human Prostate and
    Seminal Vesicles, Scand J. Urol. Nephrol. 111:1 (1977).

42. F. Di Silverio, V. Gagliardi, G. Sorcini and F. Sciarra, Bio-
    synthesis and Metabolism of Androgenic Hormones in Cancer of
    the Prostate, Invest. Urol. 13:286 (1976).

43. W. Mainwaring, The Relevance of Studies on Androgen Action to
    Prostatic Cancer, in "Steroid Hormone Action and Cancer",
    K.M.J. Menon and J.R. Reel (eds), Plenum Press, New York (1976)
    p. 152.

44. A.L. Houghton, R. Turner and E.H. Cooper, Sex Hormone Binding
    Globulin in Carcinoma of the Prostate, Brit. J. Urol. 49:227
    (1977).

SOME OBSERVATIONS ON INCIDENCE AND NATURAL HISTORY

OF PROSTATIC CARCINOMA

G. Lingårdh, J.E. Johansson, L.B. Schnürer

Regionsjukhuset
Örebro
Sweden

The natural history of prostatic cancer is incompletely known, especially its preclinical and early clinical phases. According to the Swedish Cancer Registry the incidence is increasing but the mortality rate is not rising in a similar manner (1,2). Thus the biological activity of the cancer often seems to be so low that clinical symptoms do not appear.

The frequency of prostatic cancer in the population has previously been evaluated from autopsy studies in which the prostatic glands from all patients, whatever the cause of death, were serially sectioned for histological studies. Liavåg in a Norwegian study in 1968 found 26.5% of histologically detectable cancer in men older than 50 years (3) and in material from Malmö in Sweden from 1970 Lundberg and Berge (4) found a frequency of 39.7%.

During the last decades we have had a fairly constant population in Örebro as a basis for our clinical material of prostatic diseases. For many years all prostatic patients in the district have been sent to us rather than taken care of by other doctors or institutions. It can be calculated that from our population of 170,000 we should have around 26,500 men over the age of 50. Thus from the previous autopsy frequencies of histologically verifiable prostatic carcinoma it can be calculated that we have something between 6,000 and 9,000 cases of prostatic cancer to detect.

In an earlier study from our department (5), it was shown that during the late fifties the annual detection rate was around 40 new cases per 100,000 men. More recent studies show a figure of 70/100,000 men during the late sixties. At present we have almost doubled the detection rate to 130 cases/100,000 men per year within

33

the last decade.   This means that with unchanged diagnostic effort
we are now able to detect approximately 1/3 of all calculated cases
of histologically detectable prostatic carcinoma in our population
while the patients are still alive.

During the three year period March 1977 - April 1980 301 new
cases of prostatic carcinoma were detected and staged according to
the VACURG criteria (6) (Table 1).

Compared to most earlier series, e.g. the VACURG material from
1967 (6) with 13% early stages, the patients with early stage disease
now dominate the picture.   More than half the tumours in our material
are in stage I and II.   Tumours of low grade malignancy dominate
stage I and are fairly common in stage II.   Because of this change
and the fact that the mortality rate for prostatic carcinoma had not
increased to the same amount as the morbidity rate, we decided to
apply a detailed program of observation without treatment to patients
in stage I and those with well differentiated carcinomas in stage II.

Till now, during a mean observation time of three years, 14 of
100 untreated patients have died (none of prostatic cancer).   Most
of them (9 cases) died from cardiovascular diseases.   If some kind
of treatment had been given the deaths would erroneously have been
attributed to the therapy.   However, even selected by the above
criteria, prostatic cancer is by no means a harmless disease as 9
of the patients progressed - one patient in stage I and two patients
in stage II developed osseous metastases after an observation time
of 1 - 3 years, while the others had local progression of tumour
growth.   So far however, all these patients have had a good and prompt
response to therapy instituted at the time when progression was discovered.

Table 1.   Prostatic Cancer, Örebro, March 1977 - April 1980

	Patients	Histological Grade		
		Low	Medium	High
Stage I	53	39	13	1
Stage II	105	49	43	13
Stage III	62	10	38	14
Stage IV	81	13	36	32
Total	301	111	130	60

CONCLUSIONS

An increasing number of prostatic carcinomas, mainly in the
early stages, are diagnosed due to increased watchfulness and easier
and more accessible diagnostic methods, for example fine needle biopsy.
A shift to early detection of the cancer has occurred. Thus, more
than 50% of the patients are now in an early stage of the disease at
diagnosis and this fact may have changed the clinical picture of the
prostatic carcinoma patients taken as a group. Some of the cancers
are detected by chance while the patients are investigated for some
other disease such as cardiovascular or other serious illness. This
will unfavourably influence the patients' life expectancy as compared
to the general population of comparable age. This fact should be
considered in therapeutic trials. Moreover the serious drawbacks of
most kinds of treatment should be carefully weighed against possible
advantages for the patients' quality of life in a group like this, in
which many patients are fragile and others probably will never have
trouble with their cancer during their life time. However, some untreated patients progress rapidly and ordinary histological and cytological methods are not sufficient to discover those in which such
rapid progress will occur. Other methods designed to determine the
biological activity of prostatic carcinoma are urgently needed to
indicate which patients can be safely left without treatment.

REFERENCES

1. National Board of Health and Welfare, Cancer Incidence in Sweden
    1958 - 1976, The Swedish Cancer Registry, Stockholm (1980).
2. National Central Bureau of Statistics, Causes of Death 1958 -
    1976, Official Statistics of Sweden, National Central Bureau of
    Statistics, Stockholm (1978).
3. I. Liavåg, The localization of prostatic carcinoma, Scand. J.
    Urol. Nephrol. 2: 65 (1968).
4. S. Lundberg and T. Berge, Prostatic carcinoma, Scand. J. Urol.
    Nephrol. 4: 93 (1970).
5. T. Dolk and Å. Fritjofsson, Prostate cancer in Örebro County
    from 1958 - 1967, Läkartidningen 71: 3517 (1974).
6. Veterans Administration Cooperative Urological Research Group,
    Treatment and survival of patients with cancer of the prostate,
    Surg. Gynecol. Obstet. 124: 1011 (1967).

ANIMAL MODELS IN PROSTATIC CANCER

J.C. Romijn, G.J. v. Steenbrugge,
M.A. Blankenstein and F.H. Schröder

Erasmus University
Rotterdam
THe Netherlands

INTRODUCTION

Many aspects of human cancer can only be investigated properly by the use of suitable experimental model systems. In the field of prostatic cancer such model systems are relatively scarce. For any model system, it is essential that its properties reflect those of the human situation as closely as possible. Isaacs and Coffey (1) have published a list of requirements that should be fulfilled by an ideal animal model for prostatic cancer. Some of the most important properties of the ideal prostatic cancer model are:

    (i)   histology similar to human prostatic cancer
    (ii) metastatic patterns to lymph nodes and bone
    (iii) slow growth rate
    (iv) initial response to hormonal manipulation
    (v)   ultimate relapse to hormone insensitive state

It is not likely that the ideal model does exist. However, each model should be characterized extensively, especially with respect to the points just mentioned, before treatment studies are performed.

In this paper three types of model systems will be considered:

    (a) models derived from spontaneous animal tumours
    (b) models dervied from induced animal tumors; and
    (c) transplantable human tumors.

37

SPONTANEOUS ANIMAL TUMORS

In contrast to its occurrence in man, the incidence of prostatic cancer in laboratory animals is relatively low (2). Most of the spontaneous animal tumors have been found in aged rats.

Dunning Tumors: In 1961 Dunning (3) discovered a prostatic adeno-carcinoma in an aged Copenhagen rat. This tumor has been passaged by subcutaneous transplantation since its original discovery and gave rise to more than ten distinct sublines (4-6). One of these sublines, R3327-H, appeared to be composed of both androgen-sensitive and androgen-insensitive cells (5,7,8). From this tumor line an androgen-insensitive subline, R3327-HI, has been isolated by long-term passage in castrated male rats (5). Another androgen-independent subline, the rapidly growing anaplastic tumor, R3327-AT, did arise spontaneously from the R3327-H tumor (8). Several studies, especially on the -H, -HI and -AT sublines, have been published in which the histological appearance, the hormonal dependence (5), the tumor kinetics (9), the immunological parameters (9,10) and the biochemical properties (11) were described (for recent reviews, see refs. 1 and 12).

The three related sublines, R3327H, R3327HI and R3327AT are especially suited to search for possible markers for hormonal dependence. As expected, the highest levels of androgen receptor was found in the hormone sensitive subline (1). Also Coffey and co-workers have elaborated a method that employs enzyme activities, rather than receptor concentrations. A so-called relative enzyme index, R.E.I., has been defined as follows:

$$R.E.I. = \frac{(3\,\alpha\,HSD) \times (LAP) \times (LDH)}{(5\,\alpha\,reductase)(7\,\alpha\,6\,\alpha\,hydroxylase)\,(Alk\,P)} \quad (11)$$

(HSD = hydroxysteroid dehydrogenase; LAP = leucin amino peptidase; LDH = lactate dehydrogenase; Alk P = alkaline phosphatase).

The enzyme activities were normalized to those measured in the normal dorsolateral prostate of the rat. As shown in Table 1, the values of the R.E.I. are widely different for the three different sublines. It is worthwhile to check whether a similar method might be applied to human tumors as well.

The heterogeneity of the Dunning tumor sublines may well reflect the variability observed with human prostatic cancer, e.g., with respect to its biological behavior or to its response to therapy. The natural history of the H and the HI sublines demonstrates that the well known phenomenon of change to the hormone insensitive state could be the result of a selection process.

Table 1:   Relative enzyme index in Dunning tumor sublines
(after ref. 11)

	range	average R.E.I.
R3327H	0.7-4	0.89
R3327HI	26-110	41.4
R3327AT	2337-9260	2533

Pollard Tumors: Other interesting prostatic tumor lines have been
developed from three spontaneous tumors detected by Pollard in aged
germ-free Lobund-Wistar rats (13). The tumor lines, that were
designated as PA-I, PA-II and PA-III, differ on the basis of morphology, histology and the pattern of metastasis (14). Male rats
appear to be somewhat more susceptible to tumor transplants than
females, but a detailed endocrinological characterization has not
yet been accomplished. In all lines there is a partial response to
DES. An important feature of the Pollard lines is their ability
to metastasize to the lymph nodes and the lungs (15,16). Some
studies on the modulation of metastasis have been carried out (16).

INDUCED ANIMAL TUMORS

In addition to the spontaneous tumors, a few models based on
induced prostatic tumors have been described. Most important of
these are the tumors, described by Noble, initiated by prolonged
exposure of Nb rats to steroid hormone implants. Such treatment
has resulted in a number of transplantable tumor lines originating
from the dorsolateral prostate (17,18,19). The tumors were either
androgen-dependent, estrogen-dependent, or autonomously growing (20).
The growth rate is not much different for the three types of tumor
(doubling time around five days). The autonomous lines tend to
metastasize more readily than the hormone-dependent lines. The
tumors have also been grown in nude mice (21) where the hormone
dependency is similar to that in the rat.

A very interesting observation with the hormone-dependent Nb
tumors is the prevention of autonomous growth by a low dose of
hormone. Complete withdrawal of hormones (by removal of the
steroid implant) did ultimately result in the recurrence of a
hormone unresponsive tumor. However, if the original steroid implant was replaced by an implant containing a lower dose of the
same steroid (20%), the tumor that recurred appeared to have retained its hormone responsiveness (22). Thus, the change to
autonomy could be prevented by means of a low maintenance dose of
steroid. This finding could imply that hormone dependence is a
property that might be influenced by the endocrine environment.
This is in contrast with the view, supported by the establishment

of the Dunning R3327H sublines, that the change to autonomy is due
to a selection process. It is obviously of greatest interest to
find out whether either of these mechanisms, or perhaps both, is
operative in human prostatic tumors.

TRANSPLANTABLE HUMAN TUMORS

     Although valuable information about the biological and bio-
chemical properties of prostatic cancer will be obtained from the
studies using the models mentioned above, these models all share
a common disadvantage, their non-human origin. For that reason
several attempts have been made to propagate human tumors in
immunodeficient animals, such as the athymic nude mouse. So far,
however, very few successes have been reported in this line of
research.

     In vitro cell lines that originate from the human prostate, such
as EB33 (23), DU145 (24), PC-3 (25) and LNCaP (26), will in most
cases induce tumors in nude mice. With the possible exception of
the recently established LNCaP cell line, there are serious doubts
whether these cell lines can be considered as meaningful representatives of prostatic carcinoma.

     Only a few reports exist on the successful heterotransplant-
ation of prostatic tissue in nude mice. Shimosako et al (27) and,
very recently, Jones et al (28) have reported the establishment of
rather undifferentiated, hormone-independent tumor lines. Reid et
al (29) have described a transplantable line derived from a moderately differentiated adenocarcinoma of the prostate. This tumor
has a slow growth rate and is at least partly dependent on androgens
(29). In our laboratory the transplantable line PC82 was developed
in 1977 from a moderately differentiated carcinoma (30). Some of
the characteristics of this tumor line are summarized in Table 2.

Table 2: Characteristics of the PC82 Prostatic Cancer (30)

Histology:	adenocarcinoma; cribriform
Function:	secretion present human prostatic acid phosphatase human LDH-isoenzymes
Growth:	doubling time 15.8 ± 2.5 days
Endocrinology:	no growth in females no growth in castrated males regression after castration androgen receptor present

Table 3: Some Important Properties of Tumor Model Systems

	Dunning R3327 H	HI	AT	Pollard PA I-III	Nb tumors 2Pr	13Pr	Nude mouse PC82
ORIGIN	rat probably dorsal lobe			rat ?	rat dorsal lobe		human primary prostatic tumor
ADENOCARCINOMA	yes			yes	yes		yes
RATE OF METASTASIS (lymph nodes, lungs)	low			high	moderate	high	absent
GROWTH RATE (doubling time in days)	15-20	15-20	2	1	5.3	4.3	16
HORMONE SENSITIVITY Androgen required	yes	no	no	?	yes	no	yes
Response to castration	partial	-	-	?	partial	-	yes
Recurrence after regression	yes				yes		?

The histology of the tumor shows that it is an adenocarcinoma with a cribriform pattern that resembles the structure of the original tumor quite well. The tumor contains a large amount of human prostatic acid phosphatase as demonstrated by immunohistochemistry (30). Serum levels of acid phosphatase are significantly increased in mice bearing the PC82 tumor. Also the presence of human LDH-isoenzymes could be demonstrated in the tumor as well as in the mouse serum.

The growth rate is relatively slow and has, until now, not changed in subsequent passages. The PC82 tumor is, so far, completely dependent upon the presence of androgens since it did in no case grow on female nude mice, nor on castrated male mice. Castration of a male nude mouse bearing a PC82 tumor did result in regression of the tumor. So far, recurrence after regression has not been observed.

CONCLUSIONS

Some of the most important properties of the tumor models discussed above, are compared in Table 3. This table shows that there is a variety of models that differ with respect to rate of metastasis, growth rate and hormonal dependence. This situation does well reflect the differences in human prostatic tumors clinically presented. It is therefore advisable to use different appropriate models to study different aspects of human prostatic cancer. The question of which of the presented models should be considered as a realistic model for human cancer is very difficult to answer at the present time. In this regard it should be noticed that the big advantage of the PC82 model over all other models is its human origin. Therefore the PC82 model might be considered as a suitable model for human prostatic cancer, especially for studies on the effect of hormonal manipulations.

REFERENCES

1. J.T. Isaacs and D.S. Coffey, Spontaneous animal models for prostate cancer, in: "Prostate Cancer," UICC Technical Report Series, Vol. 48, D.S. Coffey and J.T. Isaacs, eds, Geneva, 195-219 (1979).
2. A. Rivenson and J. Silverman, The prostatic carcinoma in laboratory animals. A bibliographic survey from 1900 to 1977, Invest. Urol. 16:468-472 (1979).
3. W.F. Dunning, Prostate cancer in the rat, National Cancer Institute Monograph 12:351-369 (1963).
4. A.J. Claflin, E.C. McKinney and M.A. Fletcher, The Dunning R3327 prostate adenocarcinoma in the Fischer-Copenhagen F1 rat: a useful model for immunological studies, Oncology 34:105-109 (1977).

5. J.T. Isaacs, W.D.W. Heston, R.M. Weissman and D.S. Coffey, Animal models of the hormone-sensitive and insensitive prostatic adenocarcinomas, Dunning R3327-H, R3327-HI and R3327-AT, Cancer Res. 38:4353-4359 (1978).

6. G. Seman, G. Meyers, J.M. Bowen and L. Dmochowski, Histology and ultrastructure of the R3327 C-F transplantable prostate tumor of Copenhagen-Fischer rats, Invest. Urol. 16:231-236 (1978).

7. J.K. Smolev, D.S. Coffey and W.W. Scott, Experimental models for the study of prostatic adenocarcinoma, J. Urol. 118:216-220 (1977).

8. J.K. Smolev, W.D.W. Heston, W.W. Scott and D.S. Coffey, Characterization of the Dunning R3327H prostatic adenocarcinoma: an appropriate animal model for prostatic cancer, Cancer Treatment Rep. 61:273-287 (1977).

9. R.M. Weismann, D.S. Coffey and W.W. Scott, Cell kinetic studies of prostatic cancer: adjuvant therapy in animal models, Oncology 34:133-137 (1977).

10. B.R. Rao, A. Nakeff, C. Eaton and W.D.W. Heston, Establishment and characterization of an in vitro clonogenic cell assay for the R3327-AT Copenhagen rat prostatic tumor, Cancer Res. 38:4431-4439 (1978).

11. J.T. Isaacs, W.B. Isaacs and D.S. Coffey, Models for development of non-receptor methods for distinguishing androgen-sensitive and -insensitive prostatic tumors, Cancer Res. 39:2652-2659 (1979).

12. D.M. Lubaroff, L. Cranfield and C.W. Reynolds, The Dunning tumors, in: "Models for Prostate Cancer," G.P. Murphy, ed., Alan R. Liss, Inc. New York, 243-263 (1980).

13. M. Pollard, Spontaneous prostate adenocarcinomas in aged germ-free Wistar rats, J. Natl. Cancer Inst. 51:1235-1241 (1973).

14. M. Pollard and P.H. Luckert, Transplantable metastasizing prostate adenocarcinomas in rats, J. Natl. Cancer Inst. 54:643-649 (1975).

15. M. Pollard, The Pollard tumors, in: "Models for Prostate Cancer," G.P. Murphy, ed., Alan R. Liss, Inc. New York, 293-302 (1980).

16. M. Pollard, C.F. Chang and P.H. Luckert, Investigations on prostatic adenocarcinomas in rats, Oncology 34:129-132 (1977).

17. R.L. Noble, The development of prostatic adenocarcinoma in the Nb rat following prolonged sex hormone administration, Cancer Res. 37:1929-1933 (1977).

18. R.L. Noble, Development of androgen-stimulated transplants of Nb rat carcinoma of the dorsal prostate and their response to sex hormones and tamoxifen, Cancer Res. 40:3551-3554 (1980).

19. R.L. Noble, Sex steroids as a cause of adenocarcinoma of the dorsal prostate in Nb rats, and their influence on the growth of transplants, Oncology 34:138-141 (1977).

20. R.L. Noble, Hormonal control of growth and progression in tumors of Nb rats and a theory of action, Cancer Res. 37:82-94 (1977).

21. J.R. Drago, M.E. Gershwin, R.E. Maurer, R.K. Ikeda and
     D.E. Eckels, Immunobiology and therapeutic manipulation of
     heterotransplanted Nb rat prostate adenocarcinoma into con-
     genitally athymic (nude) mice, J. Natl. Cancer Inst. 62:
     1057-1066 (1979).

22. R.L. Noble, Production of Nb rat carcinoma of the dorsal
     prostate and response of estrogen-dependent transplants to
     sex hormones and tamoxifen, Cancer Res. 40:3547-3550 (1980).

23. K. Okada, F.H. Schröder, W. Jellinghaus, K.H. Wullstein and
     H.M. Heinemeyer, Human prostatic adenoma and carcinoma:
     transplantation of cultured cells and primary tissue fragments
     in nude mice, Invest. Urol. 13:395-403 (1976).

24. D.D. Mickey, K.R. Stone, H. Wunderli, G.H. Mickey, R.T. Vollmer
     and D.F. Paulson, Heterotransplantation of a human prostatic
     adenocarcinoma cell line in nude mice, Cancer Res. 37:4049-
     4058 (1977).

25. M.E. Kaighn, K.S. Narayan, Y. Ohnuki, J.F. Lechner and
     L.W. Jones, Establishment and characterization of a human
     prostatic carcinoma cell line (PC-3), Invest. Urol. 17:16-23
     (1979).

26. J.S. Horoszewicz, S.S. Leong, M.T. Chu, M. Friedman, U. Kim,
     L.S. Chai, S. Kakita, S.A. Arya and A A. Sandberg, A new model
     for studies on human prostatic carcinoma, Proc. AACR 20:212
     (1979).

27. Y. Shimosato, T. Kameya, K. Nagai, S. Hirohashi, T. Koide,
     H. Hayashi and T. Nomura, Transplantation of human tumors in
     nude mice, J. Natl. Cancer Inst. 56:1251-1260 (1976).

28. M.A. Jones, G. Williams and A.J.S. Davies, Value of xenografts
     in the investigation of prostatic function: preliminary
     communication, J. Roy. Soc. Med. 73:708-712 (1980).

29. L.C.M. Reid and S. Shin, Transplantation of heterologous
     endocrine tumor cells in nude mice, in: "The Nude Mouse in
     Experimental and Clinical Research," J. Fogh and B.C. Giovanella,
     eds., Academic Press, New York, 313-351 (1978).

30. W. Hoehn, F.H. Schroeder, J.F. Riemann, A.C. Jobsis and
     P. Hermanek, Human prostatic adenocarcinoma: some character-
     istics of a serially transplantable line in nude mice (PC82).
     The Prostate 1:95-104 (1980).

TISSUE CULTURE IN PROSTATIC CANCER

C. R. Bouffioux

University of Liège
Liège
Belgium

INTRODUCTION

The aim of this presentation is to give an overview of the studies performed in vitro with prostatic tissue and also to give a summary of our own work in this field.

"In vitro" culture of prostatic tissue is not a new technique since Burrows et al (1) reported in 1917 the growth of cells from an explant of human prostatic adenocarcinoma. After sinking into oblivion for some decades, the method has been steadily developed with the progress of technology. The increasing interest of tissue culture techniques as a model for studying human prostatic adeno-carcinomas is partially due to the lack of suitable animal models.

The theoretical advantages of "in vitro" techniques are numerous:
- many experiments can be made with a minimum of tissue material;
- the medium surrounding the cells can be more or less precisely defined and cells are not submitted to systemic influences;
- numerous drugs can be tested alone or in association;
- the tissue can be endocrinologically manipulated and direct cellular influences can be studied;
- relations between epithelial cells and stroma can be studied according to the type of the culture (cell or organotypic culture);
- the growth can be monitored by rather simple cell counts;
- culture is the only way to study simunltaneously or repeatedly the influences of drugs or hormones on human prostatic tissue.

On the other hand, culture of prostatic tissue suffers many

shortcomings and limitations resulting from its highly artificial
nature and despite the abundance of in vitro studies, little knowledge of practical value has so far been obtained.

CULTURE OF ANIMAL PROSTATIC TISSUE

Culture of Normal Rodent Prostatic Tissue

In the 1950's, Lasnitzki, Franks, and Bengmark et al (2-4)
were among the first who succeeded in culturing prostatic tissue
from rats and mice. Following this pioneer work, many studies have
defined the influence of the medium, hormones, and vitamins on
growth, maintenance of the morphology and metabolism of prostatic
tissue (3,5-17). Although some discrepancy in the response was
noticed in relation to the origin (ventral or dorsal prostate) or
the age of the donor, general conclusions can be drawn from those
studies: in vitro, animal prostate usually exhibits an androgen
dependence; different metabolites of testosterone may produce
different effect; the serum diminishes the effect of the androgens,
probably due to binding of the hormones by the globulins; prolactin
increases the effect of testosterone; vitamin A is necessary to the
maintenance of the secretory activity of the epithelium; estrogens
have variable effects, sometimes inhibiting the growth of the cells
but sometimes enhancing it; insulin and hydrocortisone have a stimulating effect. Potentially therapeutic agents have also been tested
on organ cultures of rodent prostates with various results (18-20).

Influence of Carcinogens

As early as 1950, Lasnitzki studied the influence of methyl-
cholanthrene on explants of young rat prostates. She noticed that
the carcinogen induced epithelial hyperplasia with squamous metaplasia and increased mitotic activity. Estrogens increased the
effect of the carcinogen but cortisone, testosterone and vitamin A
had a protecting influence (21-26). Thereafter, some authors produced
malignant transformation "in vitro" by culturing normal prostatic
tissue of rats with carcinogenic hydrocarbons (27-31); but the
tumors induced were fibrosarcomas or epidermoid epitheliomas without
any hormonal dependence.

Effect of Oncogenic Viruses

Paulson, Fraley and Ecker (32) produced "in vitro" malignant
transformation of normal hamster prostate by introduction of a DNA
oncogenic virus (SV-40) within the culture. Transformed cells
injected into homologous hamsters produced epithelial tumors

secreting acid phosphatases and metastasizing.

This experience opened new fields in the study of the role of viruses in the occurrence of prostatic cancers but produced an imperfect model for human prostatic cancer as the hormonal dependence was variable and different from that of the human cancer (33).

Spontaneous Transformation "In Vitro"

After many subcultures of epithelial cells from adult C3H rat prostates, Chen and Heidelberg (34) observed a spontaneous malignant transformation (cells growing quickly, in multiple layers). Injected into autologous hosts, these cells, although having an epithelial appearance, produced fibrosarcomas.

Once more, these experiences, though interesting for the study of some oncogenic mechanisms, gave models of very limited interest for the study of human prostatic adenocarcinoma.

Cultures of Natural Animal Adenocarcinomas

In some instances, spontaneous rodent prostatic tumors have been discovered and transplanted to successive generations of syngenetic hosts: Dunning's tumors, Noble's tumors and Pollard's tumors. Many studies have been performed on these animal models (35-37).

In some cases, in vitro sutdies were made with these tumours in order to identify morphological or biochemical markers of cancerous transformation (38,39). They were not very conclusive.

Cultures of Prostatic Tissue from Dogs and Primates

More recently, studies "in vitro" used prostatic tissue from the dog and the Rhesus monkey (40,41). This material was chosen because of its closer relation to human prostate. Indeed rodent prostates have anatomical, histological and biochemical differences from the human prostate and their behaviour "in vitro" shows some striking differences in such a way that an extrapolation of the experimental results to the human situation can be misleading. So far these recent studies have not led to any development of great significance or practical relevance.

CULTURE OF HUMAN PROSTATIC TISSUE

After the pioneer work of Burrows et al in 1917 (1) Röhl published his experience of the culture of adenomatous and cancerous human prostatic tissue (42). Since then, culture of human prostatic tissue (normal, adenomatous or carcinomatous) has elicited a sustained interest in many centers, mainly in the United States, in Scandinavia, in Great Britain and in Germany. A great deal of information has been collected, often scattered, sometimes contradictory, always optimistic; but the objective analysis of the data is rather disappointing and inspires a pessimistic view as to their practical application.

A review of the literature on human prostatic models in vitro reveals a broad variety of techniques, each center trying to resolve a specific question and conceiving an artificial system fitted to its preoccupations.

a) At the beginning of the 1970's, efforts were made to define the optimal conditions for reproducing short-term cultures of human adenoma and carcinoma (43-51). The nutritional needs, the influence of the serum and the role of hormones have been widely investigated (52-61). The results were often contradictory: the stimulating effects of androgens and the inhibiting effects of estrogens on the growth were not the rule and the response of the explants varied considerably in relation to the age of the donor, the origin of the tissue (normal, adenomatous or cancerous) and the type of experimentation.

b) Studies in electron microscopy tried to define some morphological differences between normal, adenomatous and cancerous cells "in vitro"; these works were not convincing (62), but it was clearly demonstrated that submicroscopic alteration occurred with the ageing of the cultures (lysosmal, mitochondrial alterations, and increase of cytoplasmic microfilaments ...) (63-65).

c) The metabolism of androgens has been widely studied "in vitro" (66,67). The major role of DHT has been established; but the results of hormonal influences on the human prostate "in vitro" were inconsistent and sometimes contradictory.

d) The prostate is constituted of smooth muscle, a vascular stroma and epithelial acini. The latter are responsible for the malignant transformation, adenocarcinoma representing more than 95% of all prostate cancers. Prostatic adenocarcinoma is very heterogeneous: stromal areas, normal epithelium, adenomatous foci and adenocarcinoma are often intimately mixed.

Although preliminary work from Franks et al (45) indicated that epithelial cells separated from their stroma cannot grow "in vitro", many authors, considering that epithelial cells alone were necessary for the study of the cancer, used technical artifices (mechanical separation, trypsin, collagenase or viokase enzymatic digestion or gradient sedimentation) to isolate epithelial cells and to obtain pure epithelial cell cultures (68,77). As stressed by Schroeder (74), most of these techniques proved to be ineffective.

e) Because of the heterogeneity of the material, one of the major problems with culture of human prostatic adenocarcinoma is the identification of the growing cells: are they stromal cells or epithelial cells and if the latter, are they normal or cancerous cells? Indeed, if one aims to draw practical conclusions from the behaviour of human prostate cancer "in vitro", it is fundamental to make sure that the material studied is actually cancerous. In this respect, electron microscopy (62), histochemical and immunochemical studies can distinguish epithelial cells and fibroblasts (78,79), but up to now, there is no specific marker to distinguish normal epithelial cells from cancer cells.

Furthermore, some works seem to prove that, paradoxically, when explants of cancerous prostates are grown "in vitro", the growth around the explant is due to the proliferation of basal cells from normal glands while cancer cells degenerate (64,80,81). Chromosome counts (82) on cells surrounding the explant give uniform diploid values. Two explantations can be advanced: either these cells correspond to a well-differentiated carcinoma in which diploidy is usual; or we have another argument in favor of the benign origin of cells growing in monolayer around the original explant of prostatic cancer tissue.

f) An "in vitro" model can give practical information if it reflects the characteristics of the cancer in vivo. As proved by the above considerations, the culture of human prostate cancer meets major problems in this regard and the uncertainty of the cancerous nature of the growing cells is surely not one of the least!

g) Recent work from Romijn and Schroeder (83) and Cowan et al (84) using separated pure epithelial and pure stromal cells originating from prostatic tissue, showed that 5-α-reductase (transforming testosterone into DHT) is essentially localized within the stroma where the transformation of active hormones, necessary to the epithelial cells, occurs. These investigations illustrate the highly artificial condition of cell cultures which nevertheless have been widely used to try to determine the hormonal response of prostatic cancer to various hormonal compounds.

h) As in animals, human prostatic tissue has been submitted "in vitro" to oncogenic compounds and oncogenic viruses (85-87). Cellular alterations and transformations suggesting cancerous potentialities were observed but these cancers were, once more, very different from human prostatic adenocarcinoma and could not be used for clinical applications.

i) Permanent cell lines have also been widely studied. Many

permanent cell lines derived from primary cultures of normal or
cancerous human prostates are available and are often considered
useful models for the investigation of potential therapeutic
agents. The better known are:
  Line MA-160 (Fraley and Ecker) (88-90)
  Line EB-33 (Schroeder et al)   (91-93)
  Line HPC-36 (Lubaroff) (94)
  Line NP-2 (Webber) (95)
  Line DU-145 (Stone et al) (96)
  Line PC-3 (Kaighn et al) (97)
  Line LNCaP (Horoszewick et al) (98)

     Colleagues interested in the origin and the properties of these
lines will find all the details in the original papers of the
authors. Although many authors claim the usefulness of those lines,
we believe that the greatest care is necessary when they are manipulated. Some of these lines are of uncertain origin (line MA-160 and

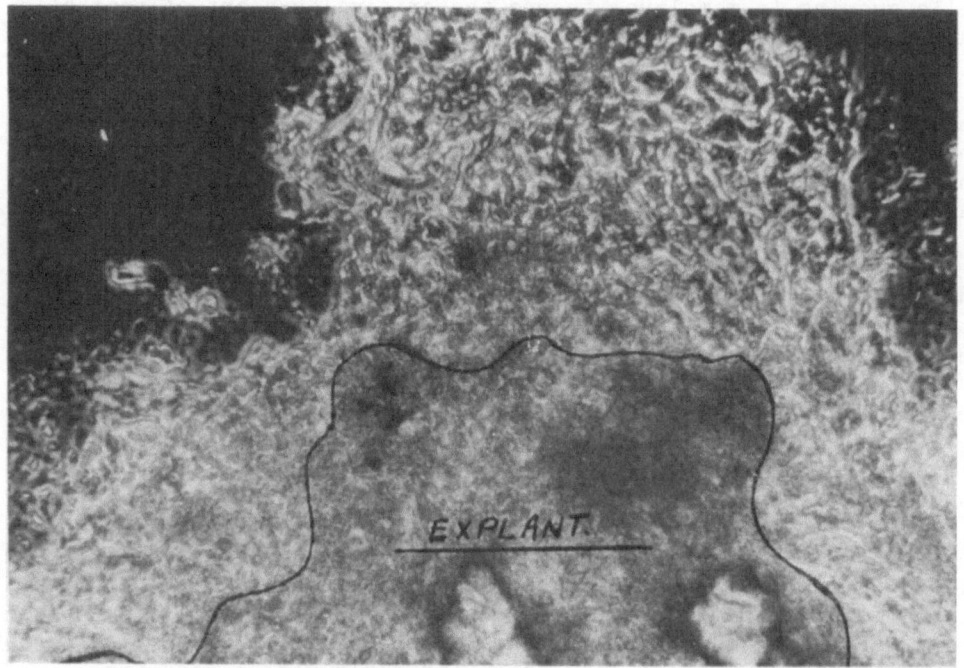

Fig. 1. Human prostatic adenoma.
         7th day of culture. Area of growth surrounding an explant.
         (phase contrast).

perhaps line EB-33 should not be prostatic cell lines but the result
of a contamination by HeLa cells!); there is no doubt that these
lines have modified their nutritional needs and their enzymatic
system with prolonged culture and that most of them do not have a
clear hormonal dependency. It would be dangerous, in our view, to
extrapolate the therapeutic results obtained with these highly
selected lines to human prostatic cancers, even to those which are
hormone resistant, in vivo.

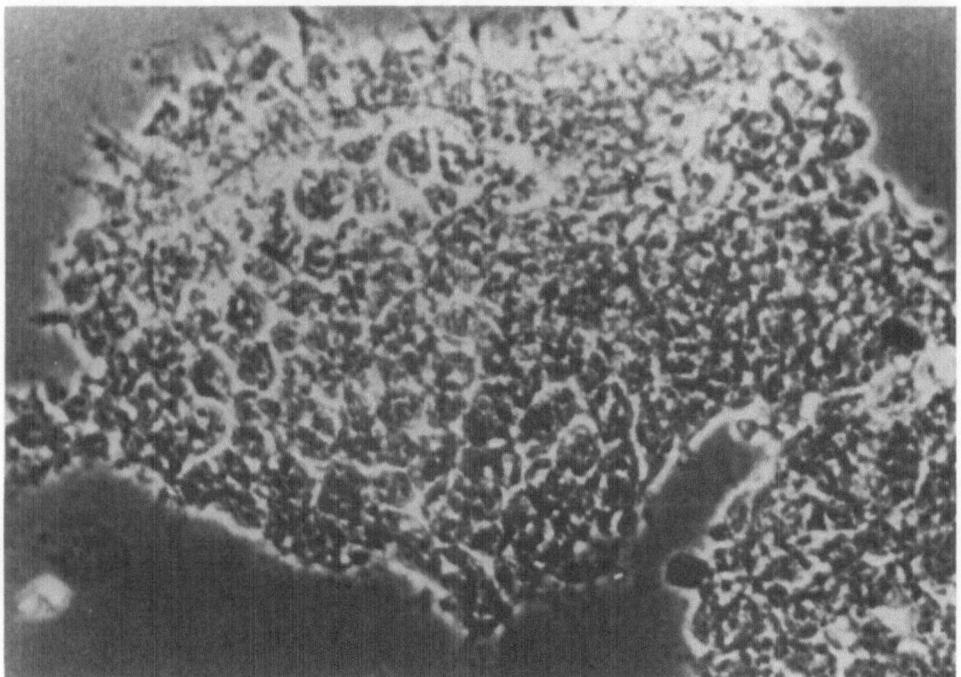

Fig. 2.   Culture of human prostatic adenoma.
          23rd day of culture. One notices a diffuse cellular
          necrosis in this islet at the periphery of one explant
          (phase contrast x 400).

Our Experience of the Culture of the Human Prostate

     Preliminary studies were performed with human prostatic adenoma
obtained either by suprapubic surgery, or by trans-urethral resection
(TUR). Cultures were performed at $37^{\circ}C$, in a closed atmosphere
(without adding carbon dioxide) and a synthetic buffer (HEPES) was
added to the medium to prevent changes of the pH.

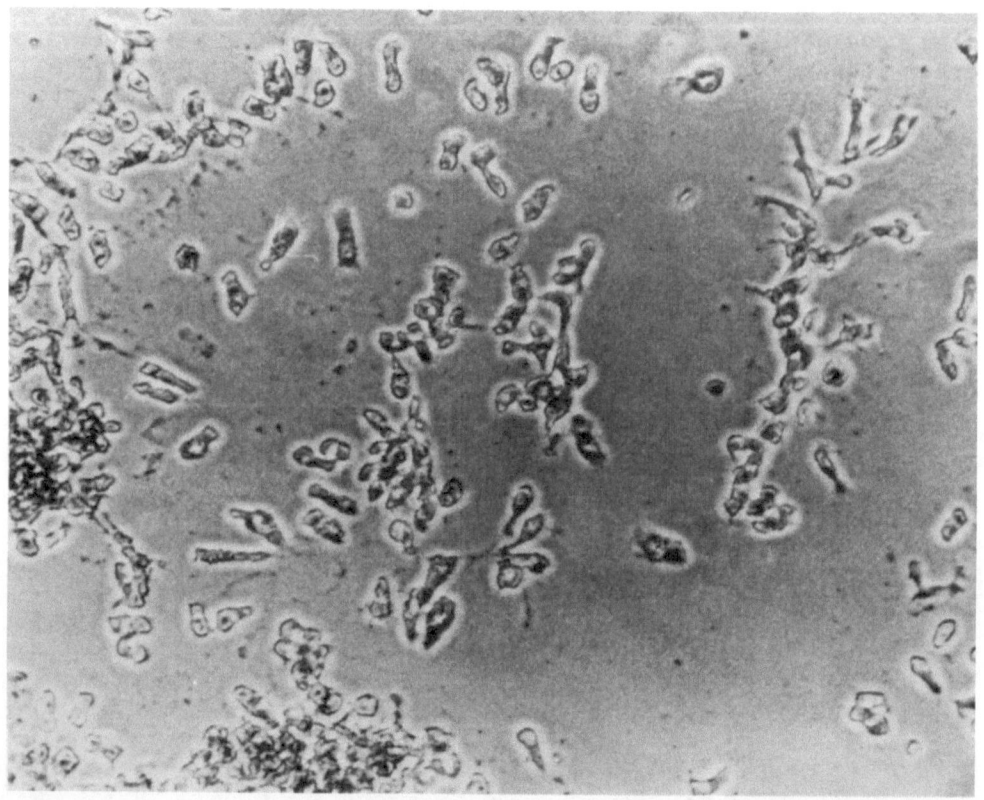

Fig. 3. Epithelial prostatic cells isolated according to our
          mechanical method (phase contrast: G x 200)

    In these preliminary studies, we have tried to define the
optimal nutritional needs, the patterns of growth of organ cultures
and the behaviour of isolated epithelial cells.

    a) Organ Cultures. The medium was composed of BME (Basal
Eagle's medium) or MEM (Minimum Essential Medium) or Medium 199 (Flow
Laboratories) to which was added glutamine, serum (HS or FCS, at
concentrations of 5 to 20%), and antibiotics (Gentamycin, 50 μg/ml).
We observed a peripheral growth in nearly 40% of the explants, as is
shown in Figure 1.

    The growth was usually epithelial and not fibroblastic but the
cell population surrounding the explants was not pure. Growth

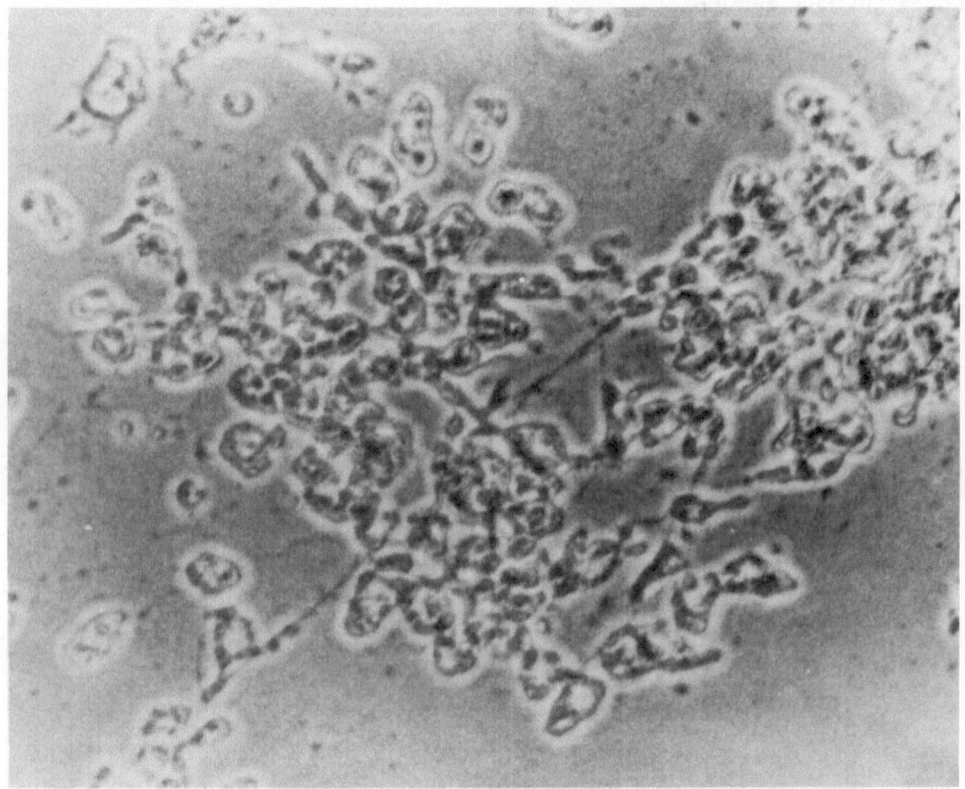

Fig. 4.   Cell culture: 5th day.   Most cells appear viable
          (contrast x 400)

usually started after 48 to 72 hours. It was always slow and we
never observed a confluence of the cell sheets in the Petri dishes.
In most cases, after two to three weeks, toxic signs appeared with
pyknosis of the nuclei, accumulation of cytoplasmic granulations and
death of the cells. We never succeeded in obtaining subcultures
(Fig. 2).

        Significant bacterial contamination occurred in many explants
obtained by TUR in spite of aseptic and antiseptic measures.

        The type of serum (HS or FCS) and its concentration (5 to 20%)
or the type of medium (BME, MEM or 199) had no very significant
influence on the growth. However insulin (at a concentration of

0.08 U/ml) and vitamin C (150 g/ml) seemed to have a stimulating
effect on the growth.

b) Cell Cultures. Epithelial cells were obtained by applying
pressure and irrigation between two slides of prostatic tissue
samples. The cell suspension was then centrifuged for ten minutes
at 800 r/min. and the pellet was put in culture (Fig. 3). During

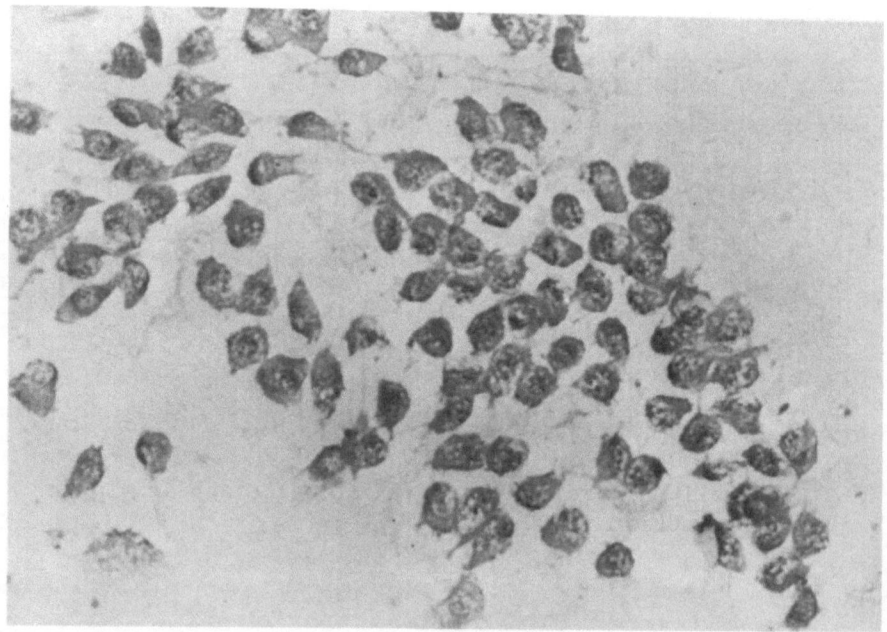

Fig. 5. Prostatic adenoma cell culture fixed and stained after
         23 days of culture. Many cells exhibit necrosis with
         vacuolization and rupture of the cytoplasm (G x 375)

the first days, the cells seemed viable (Fig. 4), but after eight to
ten days, they showed degenerative alterations and a large percentage
of cells exhibited necrosis after 20 days of culture (Fig. 5).

We never observed significant cell multiplication and the
addition of colcemid (between the 6th and 12th day) to the culture
very rarely showed evidence of blocked metaphase. Therefore, our

work seems to indicate that it is difficult if not impossible to grow epithelial cells "in vitro" after mechanical separation from their stroma.

These conclusions are in accord with those of Franks et al (45) but in contradiction with other experiments (69-71, 76) in which epithelial cell cultures were successful. It is probable that our mechanical method used to separate the epithelial cells, only releases superficial secreting cells with high exfoliative capacity from the acini - and these cells have lost the property to divide - while other methods (such as the enzymatic) may release basal cells of the acini which can divide actively and are probably responsible of the growth.

In a second phase, we repeated organ cultures of adenoma and carcinoma of the prostate, in more classical conditions, using a gas incubator. In these conditions, nearly 50% of the explants showed a peripheral growth but, as previously, growth was always slow and limited and after two or three weeks, most cultures died; our attempts to produce subcultures were unsuccessful.

Studying the influence of the medium on the growth, we did not notice significant differences between BME, MEM and medium 199 as shown in Fig. 6. The influence of antibiotics added to the medium was also investigated. As shown in Table 1, the best results were achieved with Gentamycin at the concentration of 50 μg/ml. At this concentration, no cytotoxicity was noticed although Gentamycin at 200 μg/ml slightly reduced the growth.

It was also clear, in these experiments, that the method of collecting the tissue played an important role in the capacity for growth; only 30% of tissue samples provided by TUR against 55% of the samples obtained by retropubic surgery grew "in vitro".

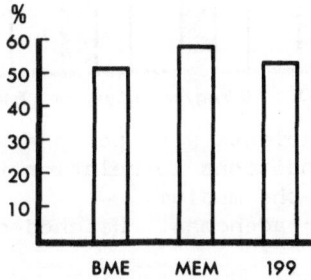

Fig. 6.   Percentage of growing explants from prostate adenomas in relation to type of medium used.

Table 1. Influence of Antibiotics Added to the Medium on the Growth
(P. = Penicillin, S. = Streptomycin, G = Gentamycin)

Antibiotic	Number of Cultures	Number of Infections	Percentage of growing Explants	Percentage of Growing Explants in Non Infected Medium
None	24	12	19%	38%
P. 10 U/ml S. 10 μg/ml	24	10	23%	40%
P. 100 U/ml S. 100 μg/ml	24	6	29%	39%
G. 50 μg/ml	24	5	33%	42%
G. 200 μg/ml	24	5	24%	30%

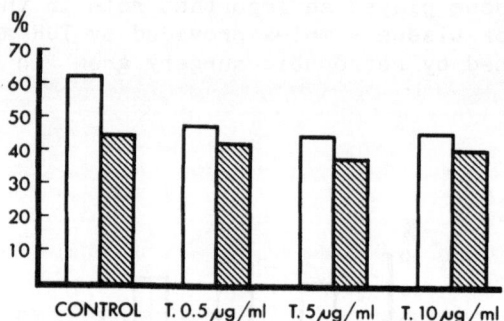

Fig. 7.   Percentage of explants with peripheral growth in our
experimental conditions in relation to concentration of
testosterone in the medium.
(Blank columns = adenomas.   Hatched columns = carcinomas)

The influence of testosterone added to the medium was
investigated. At concentrations of 0.5, 5 and 10µg/ml, testosterone
had an inhibiting effect on the growth of the adenomas while it did
not influence the carcinoma (Fig. 7). However the relevance of the
hormonal influence assessed by counting the number of growing
explants as we did, is subject to criticism on two points: firstly
the hormonal concentrations were 50 to 1000 times higher than
physiological levels; secondly we did not take into account the
percentage of initially nongrowing explants, due to the quality of
the tissue.

In a second experiment, we used testosterone at lower concentrations (0.01, 0.1 and 0.5 µg/ml) and we measured the area of
growth surrounding explants of adenoma and carcinoma, at the
seventh day of culture, on fixed material. We observed no effect,
either stimulating, or inhibiting as compared with controls.

Two explanations can be suggested:
1. In vitro, human prostatic tissue loses its hormonal dependency,
   which seems unlikely in short term organ culture.
2. The determination of the androgen dependency was not correctly
   appreciated, i.e. the medium without addition of hormones can
   indeed possess enough testosterone to allow a normal metabolic
   activity of the cells.

To verify this latter hypothesis, we measured the level of
testosterone, dihydrotestosterone (DHT) and androstenedione ($\Delta 4$)
in the culture medium before and after two, six and nine days of
culture in two different conditions: in a control medium (no
testosterone) and in a medium with added testosterone (0.1 ug/ml).
The results are given in Table 2.

Therefore it appears that the explants contain hormonal reserves
and that a medium not supplemented with hormones is rich enough,
during the first few days, to allow a normal metabolism of the
prostatic tissue, and that addition of testosterone to the medium is
not a valuable method for the study of hormonal influence on the
growth in short term organ culture.

DETERMINATION OF THE INDIVIDUAL RESPONSE OF PROSTATIC CARCINOMA TO
THERAPEUTIC AGENTS BY IN VITRO ASSAYS

Whilst randomized clinical trials are fundamental to determine
the overall value of different compounds, one knows that individual
response is sometimes very different from one patient to another.
The purpose of our "in vitro" experiments with human prostatic
carcinoma was to investigate some of these variations.

Table 2. Levels of Testosterone, DHT, and 4 in Horse Serum and
          Control Medium With and Without Added Testosterone
          (Results in Picogram/ml).

Medium	Testosterone	ΔDHT	Δ4
Horse serum	100	< 40	60
Control medium before culture	< 40	< 30	< 30
after 2 days culture	4.100	360	< 50
6 days culture	5.200	720	65
9 days culture	2.200	320	< 50
Control + Testosterone, 0.1 μg/ml			
after 2 days culture	57.000	4.250	620
6 days culture	86.000	4.415	560
9 days culture	77.000	5.390	720

This shows clearly that:
 - Horse serum and control were very poor in T. and DHT.
 - After incubation of the explants, the control medium
   becomes very rich in T. and DHT.

Table 3. Response of Tissue Cultures From Patients with Prostatic
          Cancer Refractory to Stilboestrol to the Addition of
          Hormonal Agents.

Drug Added to the Medium	Number of Explants Evaluated	Number of Growing Explants	Percentage Growing
Control	48	21	43%
Estracyt (100 μg/ml)	52	24	46%
DES (1 μg/ml)	61	14	23%
MPA (10 μg/ml)	55	20	36%
RO-6-1963 (10 μg/ml)	43	17	39%

Whilst undertaking these "in vitro" studies, we became aware of the severe practical limitations of the technique:

1. The collection of prostate cancer tissue suitable for culture raises problems: in cases suitable for hormonal treatment or chemotherapy, the only way to obtain tissue samples for culture is by needle biopsy or TUR which provide great risks of infected or non viable tissue.

2. Independently of any therapeutic effect, nearly 60% of the explants do not grow in vitro and it is difficult to draw the distinction between the inhibiting effect of the drug and the initial alteration of the tissue.

3. In vitro, systemic influences are suppressed: the hypothalamic control, so important in the hormonal effect is no longer present, and the influence of serum binding globulins and the possible potentiation of the effect by substances like insulin, corticosteroids, growth hormone, and prolactin are also absent.

4. Last but not least, prostate cancer is very heterogeneous and one does not know whether the cells growing are true cancer cells or normal basal cells present in the explant. The lack of specific markers for prostatic cancer cells is another important shortcoming.

In spite of these limitations, but aware of them, we tried to evaluate "in vitro" the therapeutic value of different compounds on explants of individual prostatic carcinomas. The following drugs were tested: Estracyt, Stilbestrol (DES), Medroxyprogesterone acetate (MPA), and RO-6-1963 (an inhibitor of 5-α-reductase).

Unfortunately, the detailed results of the experiments performed on nearly 600 explants from 10 prostatic carcinomas did not allow us to draw any practical conclusions. Perhaps it is reasonable to give one example:-

M.L., 71 years old was treated for prostatic cancer with DES (5 mg/day) for two years. The patient deteriorated despite treatment and bone metastases appeared together with a right hydronephrosis.

A TUR was performed and tissue was put in culture to evaluate the response to the previously mentioned drugs. The results appear in Table 3.

The inhibition of growth was the greatest with DES "in vitro", but in vivo the disease still progressed aggressively. In vitro, the least response was observed with Estracyt, but with Estracyt, the patient showed an excellent objective response for 18 months.

CONCLUSION

       We do not believe that "in vitro" models can, at the present
time, provide us with information of practical value in the clinical
management of prostatic cancer. We do not claim that culture of
normal or cancerous tissue is useless; indeed, it has contributed to
the elucidation of some important problems in normal and cancer cell
biology. However we caution against the premature extrapolations of
experimentors who, using specific systems in specific situations,
believe that they can draw direct clinical conclusions, ignoring
the fundamental practical problems.

       Thus, our conclusions are the same as those of Schroeder and
Oishi who stated, in a recent review of the problem (74), that "On
the whole, attempts to use tissue culture techniques in research
related to prostatic cancer have been disappointing. They have
contributed minimally to the understanding of this tumor and to its
better management".

REFERENCES

1. M. Burrows, J. Burns, and Y. Suzuki, Studies on the growth of
    cells: cultivation of bladder and prostatic tumors outside the
    body, J. Urol. 1:3 (1917).
2. I. Lasnitzki, The effect of testosterone proprionate on organ
    cultures of mouse prostates, J. Endocrin. 12:236 (1955).
3. L. Franks, The effect of age on the structure and response to
    estrogens and testosterone of the mouse prostate in organ
    cultures, Brit. J. Cancer 13:59 (1959).
4. S. Bengmark, B. Ingemanson, and B. Kallen, Endocrine dependence
    of rat prostatic tissue in vitro, Acta Endocrin 30:459 (1959).
5. L. Franks, A factor in human serum that inhibits epithelial
    growth in organ culture, Exp. Cell Res. 17:579 (1959)
6. L. Franks and A. Barton, The effects of testosterone on the
    ultrastructure of the mouse prostate in vivo and in organ
    culture, Exp. Cell Res. 19:35 (1960).
7. L. Franks, The growth of mouse prostate during culture in vitro
    in chemically defined and natural media, and after transplant-
    ation in vivo, Exp. Cell Res. 22:56 (1961).
8. I. Lasnitzki, The effect of hydrocortisone on the ventral and
    anterior prostate gland of the rat grown in culture,
    J. Endocrin. 30:225 (1964).
9. P. Gyorkey and D. Brandes, Reactions of mouse prostate, Lab.
    Invest. 11:260 (1962).
10. R. Santti and R. Johansson, Some biochemical effects of insulin
    and steroid hormones on the rat prostate in organ culture, Exp.
    Cell Res. 77:111 (1973).

11. S. Calame and A. Lostroh, Effect of insulin and lack of
     effect of testosterone on the proteins of ventral prostate from
     castrated mice maintained as organ cultures, Proc. Nat. Acad.
     Sci. (Wash.) 75:451 (1964).
12. A. Lostroh, Effect of testosterone and insulin in vitro on
     maintenance and repair of the secretory epithelium of the
     mouse prostate, Proc. Nat. Acad. Sci. (Wash.) 88:500 (1971).
13. J. Simnett and A. Morley, A comparison of mitotic activity in
     mice of different ages in vivo and in organ cultures, Exp. Cell
     Res. 46:29 (1967).
14. J. Gittinger and I. Lasnitzki, The effect of testosterone and
     testosterone metabolites on the fine structure of the rat
     ventral prostate gland in organ culture, J. Endocrin. 52:459
     (1972).
15. I. Lasnitzki, J. Dingle, and S. Adams, The effect of steroid
     hormones on lysosomal activity of rat ventral prostate gland
     in culture, Exp. Cell Res. 43:120 (1965).
16. R. Johansson and M. Niemi, DNA and protein synthesis of
     prostatic cultures in relation to histological response under
     the influence of testosterone and its metabolites, Acta
     Endocrin. 78:766 (1975).
17. W. Edwards, R. Bates, and S. Yuspa, Organ culture of rodent
     prostate. Effects of polyamine and testosterone, Invest. Urol.
     14:1 (1976).
18. A. Hoisaeter, Incorporation of 3-H-thymidine into rat ventral
     prostate in organ culture. Influence of hormone-cytostatic
     complexes, Personal Communication (1979).
19. M. Blend, In vitro uptake of labelled androgens by prostate
     tissue in presence of dieldrin, Bull. Encironm. Contam. Toxic.
     13:80 (1975).
20. R. Johannsson, Effects of some synandrogens and antiandrogens
     on the conversion of testosterone to DHT in cultured rat
     ventral prostate, Acta Endocrin. 81:393 (1976).
21. I. Lasnitzki, Precancerous changes induced by 20-Methyl-
     cholanthrene in mouse prostate grown in vitro, Brit. J. Cancer
     5:345 (1952).
22. I. Lasnitzki, The influence of hypervitaminosis on the effect
     of 20-MC on mouse prostate glands grown in vitro, Brit. J.
     Cancer 9:434 (1955).
23. I. Lasnitzki, The effect of estrone alone or combined with
     20-MC on mouse prostate glands grown in vitro, Cancer Res.
     632 (1955).
24. I. Lasnitzki and S. Pelc, Effects of 20-MC on DNA synthesis
     in mouse prostates grown in vitro, Exp. Cell Res. 13:140 (1957).
25. I. Lasnitzki, Growth pattern of the mouse prostate gland in
     organ culture and its response to sex hormones, vitamin A and
     3-MC, Nat. Canc. Inst. Monogr. 12:381 (1963).

26. I. Lasnitzki and S. Goodman, Inhibition of the effects of MC
     on mouse prostate in organ culture by vitamin A and its analogs,
     Canc. Res. 34:1564 (1974).
27. Y. Berwald and L. Sachs, In vitro transformation of normal cells
     to tumor cells by carcinogenic hydrocarbons, J. Nat. Cancer
     Inst. 25:641 (1965).
28. M. Roller and G. Heidelberg, Attempts to produce carcinogenesis
     in organ cultures of mouse prostates with polycyclic hydro-
     carbons, Int. J. Canc. 2:509 (1967).
29. C. Heidelberger and P. Iype, Malignant transformation in vitro
     by carcinogenic hydrocarbons, Science 155:214 (1967).
30. T. Chen and C. Heidelberger, In vitro malignant transformation
     of cells derived from mouse prostate in presence of 3-MC,
     J. Nat. Canc. Inst. 42:915 (1969).
31. T. Chen and C. Heidelberger, Quantitative studies on the malig-
     nant transformation of mouse prostate cells by carcinogenic
     hydrocarbons in vitro, Int. J. Canc. 4:166 (1969).
32. D. Paulson, E. Fraley, A. Rabson and A. Ketcahm, SV-40 trans-
     formed hamster prostatic tissue: a model of human prostatic
     malignancy, Surgery 64:241 (1968).
33. A. Abdalla and J. Oliver, SV-40 transformed prostatic carcinoma
     in the hamster: effect of hormonal manipulation on the growth
     rate, Cancer 27:468 (1971).
34. T. Chen and C. Heidelberger, Cultivation in vitro of cells
     derived from adult C3H mouse ventral prostate, J. Nat. Canc.
     Inst. 42:903 (1969).
35. D. Lubaroff, L. Canfield and W. Reynolds, The Dunning tumors,
     in "Progress in Clinical and Biological Research, vol. 37,
     Models for Prostate Cancer", Alan R. Liss, New York (1980).
36. J. Drago, L. Goldman and R. Maurer, The Nb rat prostatic adeno-
     carcinoma, in "Progress in Clinical and Biological Research,
     vol. 37, Models for Prostate Cancer", Alan R. Liss, New York
     (1980).
37. M. Pollard, The Pollard tumors, in "Progress in Clinical and
     Biological Research, vol. 37, Models for Prostate Cancer", Alan
     R. Liss, New York (1980) p.293.
38. F. Feuchter, D. Rowley and P. Heidger Jr., Isolation, in vitro
     cultivation and electron microscopy of normal and malignant
     epithelial cells from the Copenhagen rat, Urol. Res. 8:139
     (1977).
39. C. Chang and M. Pollard, In vitro propagation of prostate adeno-
     carcinoma cells from rats, Invest. Urol. 14:331 (1977).
40. K. Herwig, T. Fischer, W. Burkel and R. Kahn, Organ culture of
     canine prostate, Invest. Urol. 15:291 (1978).
41. R. Lewis and B. Kaack, Non human primate prostate culture, in
     "Progress in Clincal and Biological Research, vol. 37, Models
     for Prostate Cancer, Alan R. Liss, New York (1980) p.39.
42. L. Roehl, Prostatic hyperplasia and carcinoma studied with
     tissue culture technique, Acta Chir. Scand. Suppl. 240:1 (1959).

43. B. Kallen and L. Roehl, Tissue culture studies of endocrine
     dependency of human prostatic hyperplasia, Urol. Int. 10:329
     (1960).

44. T. Harbitz, Organ culture of benign nodular hyperplasia of human
     prostate in chemical defined medium, Scand. J. Urol. Nephrol.
     7:6 (1973).

45. L. Franks, P. Riddle, A. Carbonnel and G. Gey, A comparative
     study of the ultra-structure and lack of growth capacity of
     adult human prostate epithelium mechanically separated from its
     stroma, J. Path. 100:113 (1970).

46. O. Stonnington and M. Hemmingsem, Culture of cells as a mono-
     layer derived from epithelium of the human prostate: a new cell
     growth technique, J. Urol. 106:393 (1971).

47. V. Lerch, J. Todd, J. Lattimer and M. Tannenbaum, A technique
     for the study of human prostatic epithelial cells in vitro by
     time-lapse cinematography, J. Urol. 104:564 (1970).

48. M. Webber, Effect of serum on the growth of prostatic cells in
     vitro, J. Urol. 112:798 (1974).

49. F. Schroeder, G. Sato and R. Gittes, Human prostatic adeno-
     carcinoma: growth in monolayer tissue culture, J. Urol. 106:734
     (1971).

50. R. Schrodt and C. Foreman, In vitro maintenance of human hyper-
     plastic prostate tissue, Invest. Urol. 9:85 (1971).

51. B. Brehmer and O. Madsen, Kulturen menschlicher zellen aus
     prostataadenom-und-karzinomgewebe und ihre unterscheidungsmerk-
     male in vitro, Urol. Intern. 28:338 (1973).

52. A. Wojewski and D. Przeworska-Kaniewicz, The influence of stil-
     boestrol and testosterone on the growth of prostatic adenoma
     and carcinoma in tissue culture, J. Urol. 106:734 (1965).

53. M. McMahon and G. Thomas, Morphological changes of benign
     prostatic hyperplasia in culture, Brit. J. Cancer 27:323 (1973).

54. R. Ghanadian, G. Chisholm and I. Ansell, 5-DHT stimulation of
     human prostate in organ culture, J. Endocrin. 65:253 (1975).

55. C. McRae, R. Ghanadian, K. Fotherby and G. Chisholm, The effect
     of testosterone on the human prostate in organ culture, Brit.
     J. Urol. 45:156 (1973).

56. D. Fuller, S. Colleshill, K. Chan and G. Thomas, Insulin and
     testosterone responses in cultured prostates, Proc. Soc. End.
     59 (1974).

57. I. Lasnitzki, R. Whitaker and J. Withycombe, The effect of
     steroid hormones on the growth pattern and RNA synthesis in
     human benign prostatic hyperplasia, Abstract. Brit. J. Cancer
     32:168 (1975).

58. M. McMahon and G. Thomas, An organ culture technique for the
     investigation of hormonal dependence in human prostatic neo-
     plasia, Abstract. Brit. J. Surg. 57:860 (1970).

59. M. McMahon, A. Butler and G. Thomas, Morphological responses
     of prostatic carcinoma to testosterone in organ culture, Brit.
     J. Cancer 26:388 (1972).

60. M. Madsen, B. Brehmer, M. Westenfelder and A. Mosegaard, In
    vitro studies on human prostatic cells in monolayer tissue
    culture, Urol. Nephrol. 12:138 (1973).
61. A. Sinha, C. Blackard, R. Doe and U. Seal, The in vitro local-
    ization of H3 estradiol in human prostatic carcinoma, Cancer
    31:682 (1973).
62. B. Brehmer, J. Riemann, J. Bloodworth and P. Madsen, Electron
    microscopic appearance of cells from carcinoma of the prostate
    in monolayer tissue culture, Urol. Res. 1:27 (1973).
63. M. Webber and O. Stonnington, Ultrastructural changes in human
    prepubertal prostatic epithelium growth in vitro, Invest. Urol.
    12:389 (1975).
64. M. Webber, O. Stonnington and P. Poche, Epithelial outgrowth
    from suspension cultures of human prostatic tissue, In Vitro
    10:196 (1974).
65. M. Webber, Ultrastructural changes in human prostatic epithelium
    grown in vitro, J. Ultrastruct. Res. 50:89 (1975).
66. I. Lasnitzki, Metabolism and action of steroid hormones on human
    benign prostatic hyperplasia and prostatic carcinoma grown in
    organ culture, Steroid Biochem. 11:625 (1979).
67. M. Boileau, E. Keenan, E. Kemp, R. Lawson and C. Hodges, The
    effect of human serum on 3H thymidine incorporation in human
    prostate tumors in tissue culture, J. Urol. 119:777 (1978).
68. M. Kaingh and M. Babcock, Monolayer cultures of human prostatic
    cells, Canc. Chemo. Rep. 59:59 (1975).
69. K. Stone, M. Stone and D. Paulson, In vitro cultivation of
    prostatic epithelium, Invest. Urol. 14:79 (1976).
70. N. Rose, B. Choe and J. Pontes, Cultivation of epithelial cells
    from the prostate, Canc. Chemo. Rep. 59:147 (1975).
71. E. Sandford, L. Geder, R. Jones, T. Rohner and F. Rapp, In vitro
    culture of human prostatic tissue, Urol. Res. 5:207 (1977).
72. T. Malinin, A. Claffin, N. Block and A. Brown, Establishment
    of primary cell cultures from normal and neoplastic human pros-
    tate gland tissue, in "Progress in Clinical and Biological
    Research, vol. 37, Models for Prostate Cancer, Alan R. Liss,
    New York (1980) p.161.
73. M. Webber, Growth and maintenance of normal prostatic epithelium
    in vitro; a human cell model, in "progress in Clinical and
    Biological Research, vol. 37, Models for Prostate Cancer,
    Alan R. Liss, New York (1980) p.181.
74. F. Schroeder and K. Oishi, The application of cell culture
    technique to human prostatic carcinoma, in "Prostate Cancer,
    UICC, Technical Report Series" vol. 48, UICC, Geneve (1979)
    p. 145.
75. O. Stonnington, N. Szwec and M. Webber, Isolation and identifi-
    cation of the human malignant prostatic epithelial cell in pure
    monolayer culture, J. Urol. 114:903 (1975).

76. T. Pretlow 11, Disaggregation of prostates and purification of epithelial cells from normal and cancerous prostates, Canc. Chemo. Rep. 59:143 (1975).

77. M. Webber and O. Stonington, Stromal hypocellularity and encapsulation in organ cultures of human prostate: application in epithelial cell isolation, J. Urol. 114:246 (1975).

78. J. Pontes, B. Choe, N. Rose, and J. Pierce, Immunochemical identification of prostatic epithelial cells in culture, J. Urol. 119:801 (1978).

79. R. Williams, D. Bronson, E. Elliott, C. Gehrke, K. Kuo, and E. Fraley, Biochemical markers of cultured human prostatic epithelium, J. Urol. 119:768 (1978).

80. F. Schroeder and W. Jellinghaus, Prostatic adenoma and carcinoma in cell culture and heterotransplantation, in:"Prostatic Disease," Alan R. Liss, New York (1976) p.301.

81. D. Merchant, A. Johnson, and S. Clarke, Characterization of prostate cells, in:"Progress in Clinical and Biological Research, vol. 37, Models for Prostate Cancer", Alan R. Liss, New York (1980) p.233.

82. W. Jellinghaus, K. Okada, C. Ragg, H. Gernardt, and F. Schroeder, Chromosal studies of human prostatic tumors in vitro, Invest. Urol. 14:16 (1976).

83. J. Romijn, Personal Communication (1980).

84. R. Cowan, S. Cowan, J. Grant, and H. Elder, Biochemical investigations of separated epithelium and stroma from benign hyperplastic prostatic tissue, J. Endocrinol. 74:111 (1977).

85. W. Noyes, Effect of 3-methylcholanthrene on human prostate in organ culture, Cancer Chemo. Rep. 59:67 (1975).

86. E. Sandford, L. Geder, A. Laychock, T. Rohner, and F. Rapp, Evidence for the association of cytomegalovirus with carcinoma of the prostate, J. Urol. 118:789 (1977).

87. R. Jones, E. Sandford, T. Rohner, and F. Rapp, In vitro viral transformation of human prostatic carcinoma, J. Urol. 115:82 (1976).

88. E. Fraley and S. Ecker, Spontaneous in vitro neoplastic transformation of adult human prostatic epithelium, Science, 170:540 (1970).

89. R. Ban, J. Cooper, H. Imfeld, and A. Foti, Hormonal effect on prostatic acid phosphatase synthesis in tissue culture, Invest. Urol. 11:308 (1974).

90. M. Webber, P. Horan, and T. Bouldin, Present status of MA-160 cell line, Invest. Urol. 14:335 (1977).

91. K. Okada, I. Laudenbach, and F. Schroeder, Human prostatic carcinoma in cell culture: preliminary report on the development and characterization of an epithelial cell line (EB33), Urol. Res. 2:111 (1974).

92. K. Okada, I. Laundenback, and F. Schroeder, Human prostatic epithelial cells in culture: clonal selection and androgen dependence of cell line EB33, J. Urol. 115:164 (1976).

93. F. Schroeder, A last word about EB - EE, Abastract No 405, Congress AUA, (1979).

94.   D. Lubaroff, Development of an epithelial tissue culture line
      from human prostatic adenocarcinoma, J. Urol. 118:612 (1977).
95.   M. Webber, In vitro models for prostatic cancer, in:"Progress
      in Clinical and Biological Research, vol 37, Models for
      Prostate Cancer", Alan R. Liss, New York, (1980) p.133.
96.   D. Mickey, K. Stone, H. Wunderli, G. Mickey, and D. Paulson,
      Characterization of a human prostate adenocarcinoma cell line
      (DU 145) as a monolayer culture and as a solid tumor in athymic
      mice, in:"Progress in Clinical and Biological Research, vol 37,
      Models for Prostate Cancer", Alan R Liss, New York, (1980) p.62.
97.   M. Kaighn, J. Lechner, M. Babcock, M. Marnell, Y. Ohnuki, and
      K. Narayan, The Passadena Cell Lines, in:"Progress in Clinical
      and Biological Research, vol. 37, Models for Prostate Cancer",
      Alan R Liss, New York, (1980) p.85.
98.   J. Horoszewicz, S. Leong, T. Ming Chu, Z. Wajsman, P. Friedman,
      L. Papsidero, U. Kim, L. Chai, S. Kakati, S. Arya, and
      A. Sandberg, The LNCaP cell line: a new model for studies on
      human prostatic carcinoma, in:"Progress in Clinical and
      Biological Research, vol. 37, Models for Prostate Cancer",
      Alan R. Liss, New York (1980) p.115.

HISTOPATHOLOGY OF THE HUMAN PROSTATE GLAND

M. Tannenbaum and S. Tannenbaum

Columbia-Presbyterian Medical Center
New York
U.S.A.

INTRODUCTION

In the past, the modality of treatment, whether it be surgical, hormonal or chemotherapeutic, depended on the histological type and organ system from which the tumor cells were derived. Unfortunately, at the present time, we have no clear-cut definitive explanations as to why some prostatic carcinomas, in many institutions, are not usually defined as to histological type, extent or grade. Also, why some tumors act in a more benign clinical fashion in one patient and in a more malignant manner in another. Many of these prostatic carcinomatous patterns should be diagnosed as to their type and also their extent both in terms of volume and percentage of the involved prostate gland. Perhaps, some time in the near future, the various histological types and grades as well as their extent will also be correlated with the regions of the world in which the patient dwells and with other epidemiological factors. Without these multispectral analyses, the pathobiology of prostate carcinoma will remain an enigma as it has for the last 40 years.

HISTOPATHOLOGICAL PROCESSING OF TISSUE WITH INCIDENCE OF CARCINOMA OF THE PROSTATE IN SURGICAL SPECIMENS

The histopathology of prostate carcinoma is extremely frustrating as compared to that of many other organ systems, such as the cervix, endometrium, and breast. Equally frustrating in many institutions is the manner in which the prostatic tissue has been processed whether from a whole surgical specimen obtained by suprapubic prostatectomy or by means of a transurethral resection (TUR).

There is a high incidence of cancer, from 16 to 30% depending

on the age group.   It is the dictum of our institution [Columbia-
Presbyterian Medical Center (CPMC)] that one section be taken for
every 5 gms. of prostatic tissue obtained from either a suprapubic
or retropubic prostatectomy specimen.   In the case of a TUR of the
prostate, every gram of prostatic tissue must be put through for
processing.   When this is done, the incidence of carcinoma of the
prostate at CPMC varies between 23 and 28% depending on the surgical
procedure.   The question then arises: what does the urologist do
next?   It is easily demonstrated that there is tremendous variation
in histological pattern and involvement of the different forms of
prostatic carcinoma.   In many institutions at the present time the
exact histological type of prostate carcinoma and/or the extent to
which it is present within the prostatic tissue unfortunately is not
determined.   The urologist needs to know the extent of the carcinoma as well as the morphological type.   These factors can be expressed in different grading systems (1-3).   Many pathologists have
demonstrated that the degree of cellular grading may also indicate
to the urologist that he or she is dealing with a more biologically
active form of prostate carcinoma.

DIAGNOSTIC CRITERIA FOR HISTOPATHOLOGICAL EVALUATION
OF PROSTATIC TISSUE FOR CANCER

     Most pathologists and urologists who examine histological
sections see many different patterns of carcinoma of the prostate.
These patterns, if unfamiliar, are often dismissed as being non-
carcinomatous.   This is not only disastrous to the patient, but
also allows many false therapeutic interpretations to be perpetuated.
Many pathologists and urologists are now aware of the time-proven
pattern recognitions of prostate carcinoma (1,4).   At the time of
surgery or autopsy, these patterns are seen in the histological
sections of the prostate gland.   In many instances it may be
extremely difficult to define the grade or neoplastic potential of
the prostate tissue because of the large numbers of patterns displayed even within one microscopic field in a TUR specimen.   Also,
the diagnosis is further complicated if the TUR material is severely
traumatized, i.e., either crushed or cauterized.   The patterns seen
may include carcinoma-in-situ of the small or large glandular type,
Indian file and a cribriform pattern.   Recently three other forms
of prostatic carcinoma have been clinically recognized, the periurethral ductal transitional cell tumors, endometrioid tumors and
carcinoid tumors of the prostate gland (5-7).   They are now being
defined by their biological activity and by immunological determinations for acid phosphatase.

     Numerous atlases and texts present in detail the various pat-
terns and histological types seen within most carcinomas of the
prostate (1,4).   For the urologist or prostatic specialist evaluating a biopsy or tissue section taken from a surgically removed
prostate, the following histological structural changes are indica-

tive of prostatic malignancy: (a) prostatic acini are back-to-back, (b) the cells lining the acini are often in a single layer. The basal layer is usually not present, and if present, there is a great tendency on the part of many pathologists to consider these glands as non-neoplastic, (c) large prominent eosinophilic nucleoli are usually present in carcinomatous cells. To observe these nucleoli the tissue sections must be quickly and properly fixed either in formalin or in Bouin's solution, (d) prostatic acini are seen in a linear infiltrate entering the surrounding fibromuscular tissue. This streaming pattern resembles rowboats racing up and down a river, (e) nuclear hyperchromatism may or may not be seen depending on the quality of tissue fixation. For this reason, we do not believe that nuclear hyperchromatism can be evaluated from laboratory to laboratory unless there is uniform fixation. Cautery artifact is often seen in the TUR specimen and quite often may lead to misdiagnosis when hyper- chromatism is entertained as a diagnostic feature, (f) perineural invasion may or may not be discernible. When detected, especially in a frozen section, it is usually indicative of the malignant potential of a well-differentiated prostatic glandular pattern. All of these patterns may vary from one microscopic field to another. The tumor may also be seen as a solid mass resembling a granuloma. Fortunately, the Indian file and the signet ring patterns are usually not the predominant cell pattern (4). These two patterns of pros- tatic carcinoma are easily obscured by too much electrical cutting current within the resectoscope and are obliterated by cautery arti- fact. Extreme caution must also be used because some of the fea- tures mentioned above may be present and still the diagnosis may be that of benign disease (4). On the other hand, in many instances, not all the criteria need to be present for the diagnosis of malignancy.

Microacini are often present in the posterior lobe of the prostate and yet the gland is benign. These microacini are also frequently associated with prostatitis. When carefully examined, many of these microacini are not back-to-back and under the high-power objective in the microscope, they are usually seen to be lined by a double layer of cells (4).

In many instances, where there is adequate tissue sampling as described previously, the periacinar ducts of the prostate as well as the periurethral ducts may be filled with bizarre cells that are very active mitotically and yet, in many institutions, when they are seen in a TUR specimen, they are signed out as carcinomas of the prostate. This lesion which is of a transitional cell nature in many cases is often misdiagnosed and treated as a regular carcinoma of the prostate. The periurethral ducts as well as the glands around an area of infarction may show extensive squamous cell metaplasia and nuclei with prominent nucleoli. When care is not taken, this is often misdiagnosed as a malignancy (4). Many times diethylstilbestrol may induce squamous metaplasia as well as obscure

the carcinomatous cells in the fibromuscular tissue sections (4).
Thus great care must be taken as a consortium of many factors influence the diagnosis of carcinoma of the prostate.

A group of bizarre cells with pleomorphic nuclei will most
likely be seminal vesicular epithelium.   The pathologist should
look for the brownish refractile cytoplasmic pigment that is
characteristic of seminal vesicular epithelial cells (4).

The mechanical distortion or compression of nuclei that makes
them appear hyperchromatic, is the one consistent problem that most
pathologists see in evaluating prostatic cancer in needle biopsies,
especially in those patients who have elevations of acid phosphatase
(4).   This effect will usually confuse the diagnosis in either
direction, i.e., malignancy or benignity.   If there is a question
as to diagnosis, the surgical pathologist should request additional
tissue levels from the biopsy or ask for another biopsy.

PROSTATIC CARCINOMA-IN-SITU

The term "carcinoma-in-situ" denotes an incidental carcinoma with
an intraacinar neoplasm.   We tend to favor this term of carcinoma-
in-situ although others do not (1).   Usually there is no apparent
light microscopic invasion of the surrounding fibromuscular tissue.
However, when these microscopic foci of carcinoma-in-situ are seen,
the surgical pathologist should do extensive sectioning of the
remaining tissue that might be left over from the suprapubic or
retropubic prostatectomy.   When serial sections are taken, the
incidence of prostate carcinoma increases from 14 to 34%.   Therefore,
it is important that all of the prostatic tissue be embedded, cut
properly and each section examined.   If this examination is carefully executed then at least 24% of the tissue so examined will reveal different patterns of carcinoma.   In many instances, there is
only carcinoma-in-situ and no other form of prostate cancer.   In
these cases, the surgical pathologist should indicate in the diagnosis that there is a carcinoma-in-situ present only in one chip
out of whatever number of chips were placed on the microscope slide.

TRANSITIONAL CELL CARCINOMA OF THE PROSTATE GLAND

Until very recently, periurethral ductal or transitional cell
carcinomas of the prostate were seldom recognized or categorized as
a special classification in the pathology section of the Urology
boards.   However, this classification is justified since these
types of prostatic carcinomas are much more biologically active
than the regular acinar forms.   The initial reports in the literature stated that out of 200 consecutive carcinomas of the prostate,
seven arose in the periurethral prostatic duct (6).   The percentage
at our institution is almost double because of our awareness of the
lesion and the numerous histological levels that are taken.   In

the original report, these lesions were not associated with chemical elevations of serum acid phosphatase (4). Although the data were scant at that time, these lesions did not appear to have an innocuous course. Ende et al (6) noted that the lesions paradoxically extended into the retroperitoneal lymph nodes with subsequent obstructive uropathy and ensuing uremia. In numerous cases, they did not find any associated urothelial neoplasm elsewhere in the urinary tract.

ENDOMETRIAL TUMORS OF THE PROSTATE GLAND

Endometrial neoplasms of the prostate arise not only in the verumontanum of the prostate but also in the periurethral prostatic ducts. Periurethral lesions may also be of an adenocarcinomatous variety and as such may be papillary in form and spread intraductally as some carcinomas of the breast do. This is another variety which is the subject of much controversy (1, 4, 7). In many instances, it can arise from the prostatic utricle which is the colliculus seminalis and is derived from the müllerian duct. These tumors and those that originate in the periurethral prostatic ducts may demonstrate a pattern that is very similar histologically to the endometrium of the uterus. When they arise from the müllerian duct, the histology is like that of the endometrium and is indicative of a non-metastasing neoplasm. In the majority of these types of tumors, there is an associated carcinoma of the prostate which is contiguous but not continuous with the endometrial tumors. There was no metastasizing potential with the exception of two out of 100 cases of endometrial tumors seen at this institution. When they do arise in the peri-urethral prostatic ducts and not in the prostatic utricle, they may have an endometrioid pattern in conjunction with a regular trans-itional carcinomatous pattern. In these malignant lesions, there is usually a wide variation in patterns in the papillary portions of the periurethral prostatic ducts which may be clinically exophytic into the prostatic urethra. In such cases, these lesions may also demonstrate, in some focal areas, a regular adenocarcinomatous pattern of the cribriform or transitional cell type as well as an endometrioid pattern. In these lesions, it is not uncommon to find an associated elevation of serum acid phosphatase as determined by immunological methods.

MIXED ADENOCARCINOMA-CARCINOID TUMORS (THE ENDOCRINE COMPONENT OF PROSTATIC CARCINOMAS)

In normal and hyperplastic prostatic epithelium, the occurrences of argyrophil and argentaffin cells have been long recognized. Recently Capella et al. have published an extensive report dealing both with the ultrastructure and histochemical identification of these endocrine cells in prostatic carcinomas (5). They have identified two different types of endocrine paracrine cells in normal and hyperplastic prostate cells. The type 1 cells resemble

enterochromaffin cells (EC) and the type 2 cells are similar to
urethral endocrine-paracrine cells previously reported by Casanova et
al (8).   Capella et al (5) noted that about one third of the 40
prostatic carcinomas contained EP cells and four tumors showed a very
extensive number of these cells.   Two of the tumors were composite
tumors exhibiting both adenocarcinomatous and carcinoid patterns.
The tumors were studied ultrastructurally and histochemically and the
presence of ACTH and beta-endorphin immunoreactive cells ultrastructurally resembling pituitary corticotrophic cells were noted.

SUMMARY

With the advent of immunohistochemical light histology and ultrastructural techniques applied to the prostate, the future may reveal
that there are certain tumors that are immunoreactive for certain
chemical constituents like acid phosphatase and other substances such
as beta-ACTH.   At the present time, there have been no histological
pattern and grade correlations with these immunological histochemical
and ultrastructural findings.   If these correlations are forthcoming
along with a better understanding of tumor biology, then the future
seems very promising.

REFERENCES

1.   F.K. Mostofi and E.B. Price, Atlas of Tumor Pathology: Tumors
      of the Male Genital System, Armed Forces Institute of Pathology,
      Washington, D.C. (1973).
2.   D.F. Gleason and The Veterans Administration Cooperative Urolo-
      gical Research Group, Urologic Pathology: The Prostate, Lea &
      Febiger, Philadelphia (1977).
3.   J.F. Gaeta, Glandular Profiles and Cellular Patterns in Prostatic
      Cancer Grading.   National Prostatic Cancer Project System,
      Urology, 17:33 (1981).
4.   M. Tannenbaum, Urologic Pathology: The Prostate, Lea & Febiger,
      Philadelphia (1977).
5.   C. Capella, L. Usellini, R. Buffa, B. Frigerio and E. Solcia,
      The Endocrine Component of Prostatic Carcinomas, Mixed Adeno-
      carcinoma-Carcinoid Tumors, and Non-tumor prostate.   Histo-
      chemical and Ultrastructural Identification of the Endocrine
      Cells, Histopathology, 9:175 (1981).
6.   N. Ende, L.P. Woods and H.S. Shelley, Carcinoma Originating in
      Ducts Surrounding the Prostatic Urethra, Am. J. Clin. Pathol.
      40:183 (1963).
7.   M.M. Melicow and M. Tannenbaum, Endometrial Carcinoma of Uterus
      Masculinus (prostatic Utricle).   Report of Six Cases, J. Urol.
      106:892 (1971).
8.   S. Casanova, F. Corrado and G. Vignoli, Endocrine-Like Cells in
      the Epithelium of the Human Male Urethra, J. Submicroscopic
      Cytology, 6:435 (1974).

CYTOLOGY OF THE PROSTATE

H.J. de Voogt

Free University Hospital
Amsterdam
The Netherlands

As early as 1930 Ferguson described a method of needle puncture and aspiration of the prostate for diagnostic purposes (1). From his work mainly originated the so-called thick needle biopsy for which several instruments were designed. The best known are the Vim-Silverman needle, the Veenema needle and that most commonly used now, the Tru-cut needle. All give punch-biopsies which can be used for histological examination as well as for histochemical reactions (acid phosphatase, peroxidase, etc.). For several decades this was the recognized method for pathological diagnosis of prostatic carcinoma, the diagnosis being based mainly on the structure and architecture of the malignant epithelial cells in relation to the stroma and on some cytologic criteria.

However there were a number of disadvantages. The puncture, whether transperineal or transrectal, is usually painful and cannot be done without some kind of anaesthesia. Local anaesthesia is sufficient in most cases but there are urologists who demand general anaesthesia, which in turn carries a certain risk factor. Also one needle puncture could accidentally miss the cancer nodule and as pathologists sometimes have great difficulty in making a diagnosis on a small piece of tissue, they often require more than one puncture biopsy, preferably from different sites which of course makes it more disagreeable for the patient. Finally the procedure is not convenient for follow up histological observations of a certain treatment.

It is not surprising therefore, that aspiration biopsy cytology as it was first presented by Franzén et al in 1960 (2) has attracted more and more attention in the last 10 years. The method is simple and can be done on a routine out-patient basis. The instrument was

designed by Franzén. It consists of a syringe with a special holder
to apply a vacuum with one hand whilst a thin needle, in which the
cells are aspirated is guided by a needle guide that fits the index
finger of the other hand, transrectally, to the cancer nodule in the
prostate. The needle can be directed very accurately to the right
place, i.e. to the nodule and to any other part of the prostate from
which it is felt necessary to get material from different sites of a
nodule or of the prostate. The patient feels no more than a little
unpleasantness and anesthesia is not required.

By applying a vacuum and making back and forth movements, the
epithelial cells and some prostatic fluid with erthrocytes are drawn
into the needle. Stromal cells are never aspirated. Care must be
taken to equalize the pressure before withdrawing the needle to
prevent the aspiration of rectal contents and epithelium. It is wise
to use a sterilized instrument to prevent the introduction of hospital bacteria into the patient. By a careful technique and by
avoiding the use of the Franzén needle for diagnosing prostatitis
the risk of infection for the patient is extremely small as is the
risk of transplanting cancer cells. Infections and transplant
metastases have been reported in thick needle biopsies, but in large
series of aspiration cytology they are virtually absent (3).

The cellular material is expressed from the needle onto glass
slides and smears are made of it. They can be fixed by air-drying
and then stained using the M.G. Giemsa technique which is used universally and gives satisfactory results. However some cytologists
prefer the Papanicolaou-stain.

The cytologic patterns of normal, hyperplastic and carcinomatous
epithelium are described in detail by Esposti (4) and Staehler (5).
They stated that grading according to cytological criteria is more
accurate than can be done on tissue-sections. The main criteria for
malignancy are:

1.   decreasing cellular adhesiveness.
2.   decreasing cytoplasmic/nuclear ratio.
3.   nuclear atypia and prominent nucleoli.

As we will hear more about grading in other lectures of this
course the subject will not be pursued here. However the question
remains whether cytology and histology are adequate for diagnosis.
To that end in Leiden in 1979 the results of histology and cytology
of 294 patients were reviewed and compared. They are given in
Table 1. Our conclusion from this study was that on a routine basis
histology and cytology are nearly aequal, but from the academic
standpoint the two are complementary.

At the time of initial diagnosis both methods are desirable to
get a complete picture and give a reliable grading and staging

Table 1. Comparison of Diagnoses by Histology (Needle Biopsy)
          and by Cytology (Thin Needle Aspirates) of 294 Patients,
          Suspected of Prostate Cancer

Histology

Cytology	negative	positive	dysplasia	not enough material	number of patients
Negative	125	3	-	-	128
Positive	6	140	8	-	154
Not enough material	-	-	-	12	12
Total	131	143	8	12	294

In 10% of cases disagreement

4% by not enough or no proper material

3% by dysplasia

3% by false-negative, c.q. false positive

(6,7,8). However for follow-up purposes we should resort to and
confine ourselves to cytology, as it has the advantage of being
tolerated well by the patient and of indicating whether a tumour is
responding to a given treatment or not.

Finally the cellular material, obtained by aspiration, can be
used for different kinds of sophisticated research, such as cytomorphometry and karyometry, flow-cytometry and cell-sorting. In
these methods cells are stained with one or more fluorescent stains,
which can then be measured by fluorescence microscopy. Also other
methods of cytochemistry can be applied of which the method of using
fluorescent steroids (fluoresceine-steroid conjugates) to locate
steroid receptors is very interesting. Last but not least cell-
kinetic techniques can be employed. Some of these methods will be
considered further in this course.

In conclusion, it is my opinion that cytology of the prostate
will become more and more important, because of the:

1. Simplicity of the procedure, which is well tolerated by the
    patient.

2. Diagnostic reliability and possibility of accurate grading of prostatic cancer.
3. Usefulness for follow-up evaluation of different forms of therapy, and
4. Possibilities for more sophisticated research.

REFERENCES

1. R.S. Ferguson, Prostatic neoplams. Their diagnosis by needle puncture and aspiration, Amer. J. Surg. 9:507 (1930).
2. S. Franzén, G. Giertz, J. Zajicek, Cytological diagnosis of prostatic tumours by transrectal aspiration biopsy, Brit. J. Urol. 32:193 (1960).
3. J. Zajicek, Aspiration biopsy cytology, Mon. Clin. Cytol. 4:20 (1974).
4. P.L. Esposti, Cytologic malignancy grading of prostatic carcinoma by transrectal aspiration biopsy, Scand. J. Urol. Nephrol. 5:199 (1971).
5. W. Staehler, H. Ziegler, D. Völter, Zytodiagnostik der Prostata, Schattauer Verlag, Stuttgart (1975).
6. E. Altenähr, Zytodiagnostik der Prostata, Ärzt Lab. 21:399 (1975).
7. Ch. Voeth, M. Droese, and G. Steuer, Erfahrungen mit dem Zytologischen Grading beim Prostata Karzinom, Urologe A 17: 367 (1978)
8. P.J. Spaander, D.J. Ruiter, J. Herman, H.J. de Voogt, J. Brussee, and M.E. en Boon, The implications of subjective recognition of malignant cells in aspirations for the grading of prostatic cancer using cell image analysis, 5e Symposium für Exp. Urologie, (1980).

THE ESTIMATION OF DNA BY ABSORPTION CYTOPHOTOMETRY ON SMEARS OF TRANS-RECTAL FINE NEEDLE ASPIRATION OF THE PROSTATE

C.R. Bouffioux

Department of Urology
University of Liège
Belgium

INTRODUCTION

Mitosis, the predominant step of cell multiplication, occurs when a cell has doubled its metabolic and genetic contents.

Among the synthesis mechanisms preceding mitosis, the synthesis of DNA, a major component of the chromosomes, plays an important role.

Normal human tissue, not actively dividing, consists predominantly of cells in the pre-synthesis phase or "resting"-phase (G1) with diploid chromosomes (2 c = 46) and a corresponding content of DNA (about seven picograms in human cells). During the phase of synthesis (S), the DNA content increases up to a tetraploid value corresponding to a double set of chromosomes (4c). When the cell has reached this tetraploid value, it does not divide immediately: there is a post-synthesis phase (G2) during which other protein formation occurs.

During mitosis (M), the DNA content is equally distributed between both daughter cells and returns to diploid values, and the cell-cycle continues (1,2).

Fig. 1. shows that, in normal tissues, most of the cells are in G1 and have a diploid content of DNA. Few cells are in S-phase or G2 with an intermediate or a tetraploid value of DNA.

In actively growing cancer tissues the percentage of cells in the S- and G2-phase is increased and, due to pathologic division of the nuclei, heteroploid or aneuploid cells can be encountered.

77

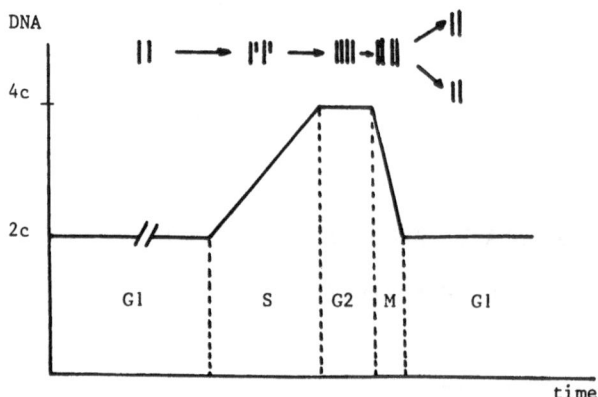

Fig. 1.   Schematic representation of the modifications in DNA
          content during the cell cycle.

Therefore, the number of cells with intermediate DNA content (between
2 c and 4 c) increases (aneuploid cells or cells in S-phase) and
the number of cells with tetraploid DNA content also increases (basal
tetraploid cells or diploid cells in phase G2) and hexa- or octoploid
cells (e.g. tetraploid cells in phase G2) or even hexadecaploid
cells can be encountered (3-7).

     Generally speaking, the lesser differentiated the cancer the
more aggressive it is; the percentage of non diploid cells is increased accordingly. Therefore, the measurement of DNA is of value
in the evaluation of the initial aggressiveness of a tumor and in
the study of its response to treatment.

MATERIAL AND METHODS

     Material provided by trans-rectal fine-needle aspiration of the
prostate was divided into two slides to allow a comparison. One of
the slides was air-dried and stained with May-Gruenwald-Giemsa,
while the other was fixed in an equal volume of acetone and absolute
ethanol at 4°C for 24 hours. Thereafter, the slide was plunged into
absolute alcohol at 4°C for 24 hours minimum; after drying, it was
stored in darkness until staining with Feulgen reaction (8,9). The
measurement of DNA in the individual cells of the smear was performed on a Vickers M86 Scanning Microdensitometer. Completely
automated, this apparatus determines the DNA content of the examined
nucleus in five seconds.

The value is expressed in abitrary units, but the presence of segmented white blood cells, which are always diploid, in the smear allows an easy conversion of these arbitrary units. At the same time, the densitometer provides a measure of the area of the nucleus. DNA histograms were performed in each case, on a minimum of 100 nuclei.

RESULTS

We have analyzed:

1. The DNA histograms in adenomas, prostatitis and adenocarcinomas of the prostate.
2. The relation, in prostate adenocarcinomas, between the cytological grade and the corresponding histogram.
3. The changes occurring in the histograms following the treatment.
4. The practical significance of DNA cytophotometry for the diagnosis, grading, and prognosis of prostatic cancer.

DNA Histograms in Adenomas, Prostatitis and Untreated Carcinomas

Adenomas. Sixteen cases of benign prostatic hypertrophy were examined. The histograms always show an obvious peak corresponding to the diploid value of DNA. Less than 5% of the nuclei have aneuploid values deviating more than 20% from the diploid value (Figs. 2 and 3).

This finding means that in prostatic adenoma, very few cells are dividing and that the disease is more likely a dysplasic phenomenon than a true benign tumor in which an increase of the tumor mass should be correlated with an increased mitotic activity.

Prostatitis. Chronic prostatitis was investigated in 10 patients. In some cases, the histograms are the same as in the adenomas, exhibiting a great majority of cells with diploid values of DNA (Fig.4). In others however, the DNA content spreads beyond the diploid value with a few nuclei exhibiting tetraploid values (Fig. 5). This appearance is identical to that observed in well-differentiated carcinoma and results from an increased mitotic activity in an attempt to restore the epithelium destroyed by the microbial infection. In this situation, the DNA histogram cannot provide a differential diagnosis between well differentiated carcinoma and prostatitis but it can help when the histogram returns to normal after a few weeks of treatment with antibiotics (Fig. 6).

The following case illustrates the situation:

M.B. is 76 years old. Rectal examination reveals a limited induration of the prostate. Cytology is performed and cannot exclude a well differentiated cancer although the presence of

numerous segmented neutrophils and lymphocytes suggests a
prostatitis.

The DNA histogram shows many aneuploid nuclei close to the
tetraploid value (Fig. 5) but after six weeks of treatment with
tetracyclines, a further DNA histogram shows uniformly diploid values
(Fig. 6) and virtually excludes a diagnosis of carcinoma.

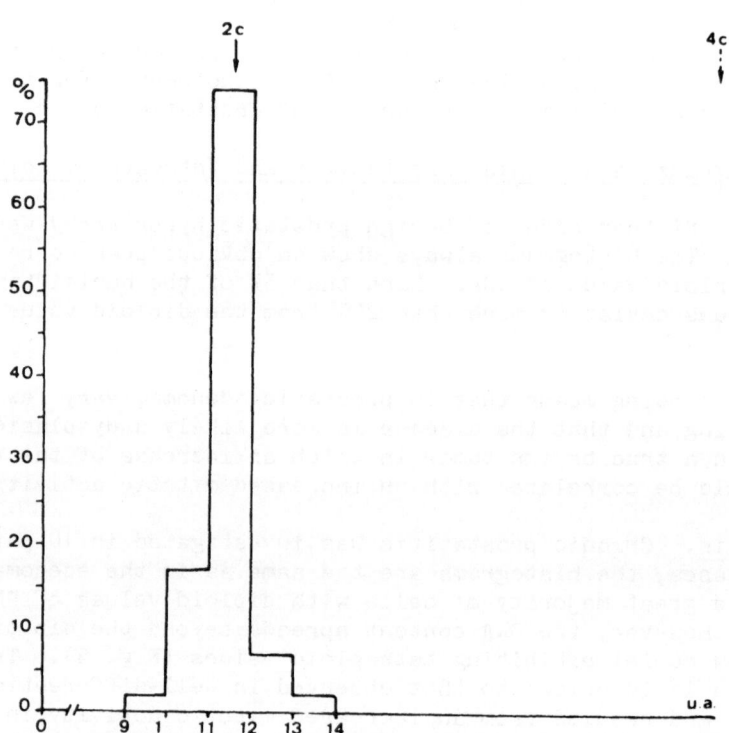

Fig. 2.   DNA content in a smear of epithelial cells from prostatic
           adenoma, obtained by transrectal aspiration, 102 nuclei
           were successively studied by absorption cytophotometry
           after Feulgen reaction.
           Abscissa, the value in DNA expressed in arbitrary units (u.a.).
           Ordinate, the percentage of nuclei.
           The full line above the histogram indicates the mean diploid
           value calculated (2 c = 2 DNA). The broken line indicates
           the mean tetraploid value (4 c) obtained by multiplication
           of the diploid value by two.

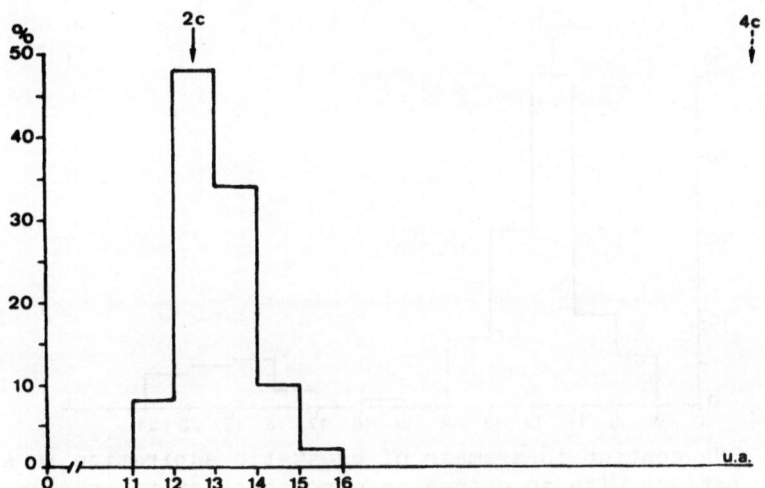

Fig. 3.   DNA content in a smear of epithelial cells from a prostatic
          adenoma (n = 100) For details, cf legend Fig. 2)

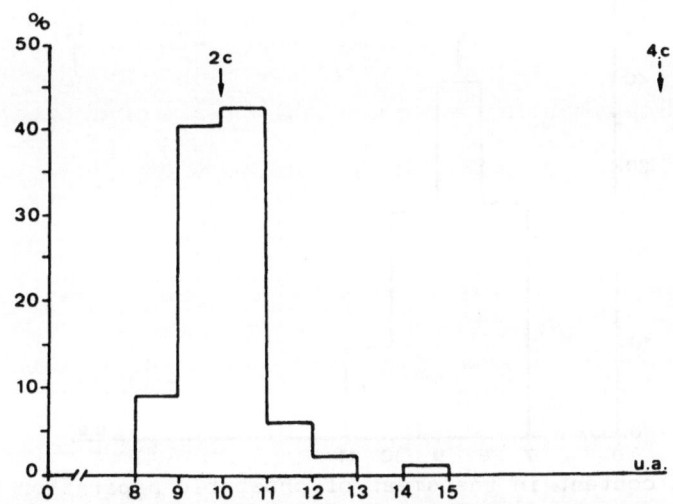

Fig. 4.   DNA content in a smear of epithelial cells in a case of
          chronic prostatitis (n = 102) For details, cf legend Fig.2).

C. R. BOUFFIOUX

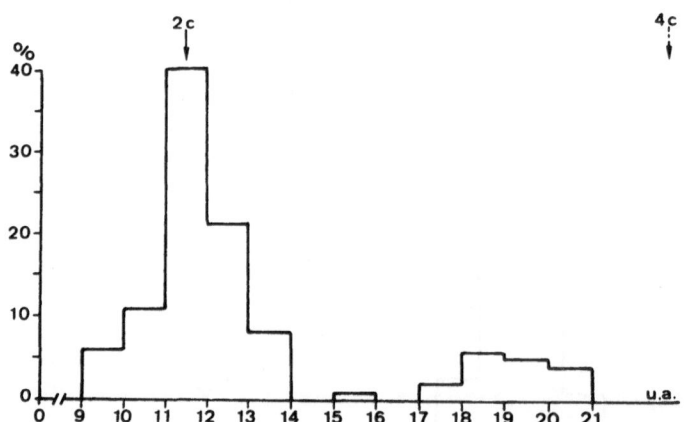

Fig. 5. DNA content in a smear of prostatic aspiration in a
         patient with an untreated chronic prostatitis (n = 104)
         For details, cf legend Fig. 2).

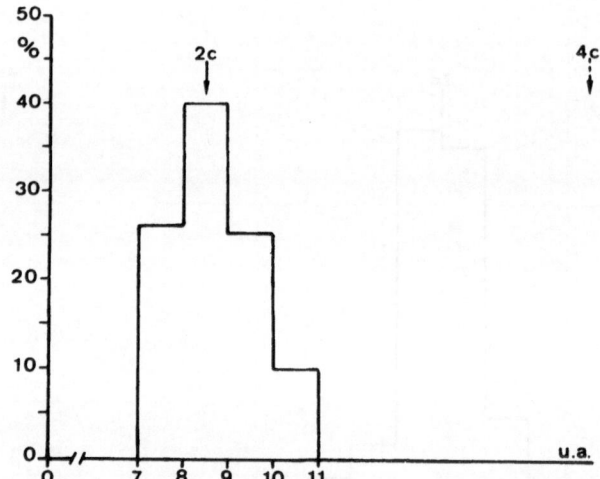

Fig. 6. DNA content in the smear of prostatic aspiration in the
         same patient (cf Fig. 5) after antibiotic therapy (n = 102)
         For details, cf legend Fig. 2.

<u>Carcinomas</u>. Untreated carcinomas were investigated in 32 patients.
The DNA histogram allows a classification into three categories:

Category 1 - cancers in which at least 80% of the cells display
diploid values of DNA (Fig. 7).

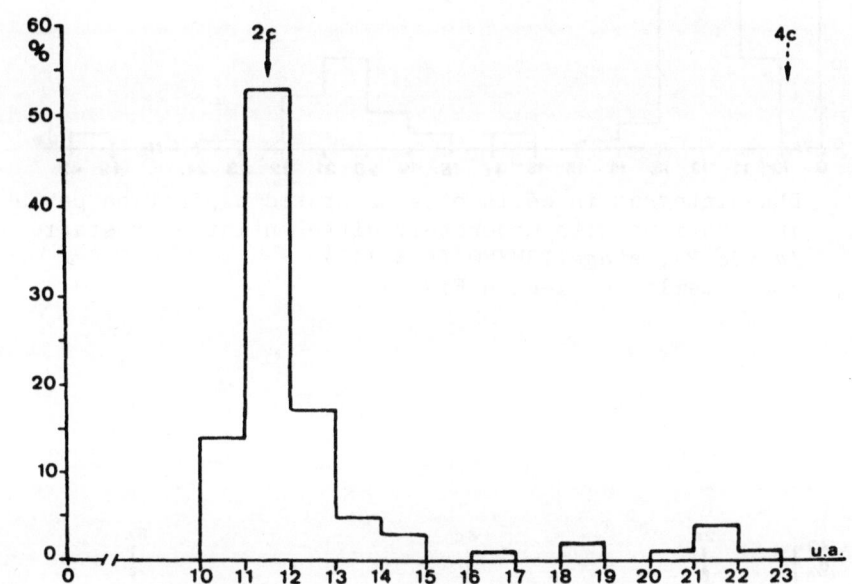

Fig. 7.   DNA-histogram in a smear of prostatic aspiration
          performed in a patient with a well differentiated
          prostatic cancer (grade 1), stage T2 NX MO (n = 11).
          For details, cf legend Fig. 2.

Category 2 - cancers in which less than 80% but more than 50% of the
nuclei display diploid values of DNA (Fig. 8).

Category 3 - cancers in which less than 50% of the nuclei show
diploid values of DNA. Many cells are aneuploid or tetraploid(Fig. 9).

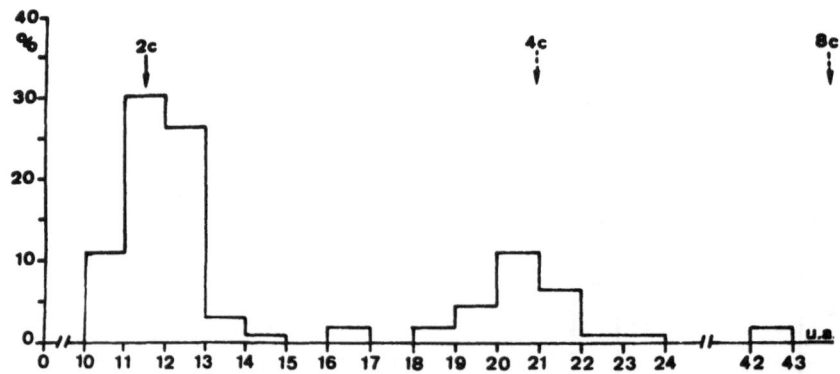

Fig. 8. DNA-histogram in cells of a prostatic aspiration performed
         in a patient with moderately differentiated prostatic cancer
         (grade 2), stage T3NXMO (n = 110).
         For details, cf legend Fig. 2.

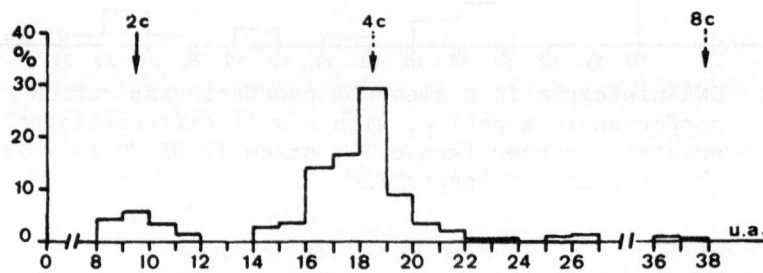

Fig. 9. DNA-histogram in a smear of prostatic aspiration performed
         in a patient with a poorly differentiated prostatic cancer
         (grade 3) T3NXM1 (n = 184).
         For details, cf legend Fig. 2.

Relation Between the Cytological Grade and the DNA Histogram

In the 32 cases of untreated carcinomas we have compared the cytological grade and the histogram category, the aspirate having been distributed on two slides, one for cytological examination and one for DNA cytophotometry. The results are expressed in Table 1.

In 21 of the 32 cases (66%), the cytological grade and the histogram category are in agreement. Also none of the grade 1 cancer enters the category 3 of ploidy and none of the poorly different-iated cancers enters the category 1 of ploidy. It appears there-fore that cytology is a good parameter for the study of tumor aggression.

One must particularly notice that among cytological grade 2 cancers, the DNA histograms allow stratification which distinguishes actively, moderately and poorly dividing cancers. Zetterberg and Esposti (10) have already shown an excellent correlation between ploidy, therapeutic response and survival.

When studying the prognosis of prostatic cancer in correlation with the histological or the cytological grade (11), correlation is excellent for poorly or well differentiated carcinomas but is less evident for the moderately differentiated tumors. The use of cytophotometric dosage of DNA, which distinguishes, in this group, cancers with different evolutive patterns, adds an important prognostic refinement.

Table 1: Relationship between cytological grade and DNA-histogram on 32 patients with untreated prostatic cancer

Cytological grade	Well diffd.	Moderately diffd.	Poorly diffd.	Total
	G1	G2	G3	
DNA histogram				
Category 1	5	7	-	12
Category 2	1	13	1	15
Category 3	-	2	3	5
Total	6	22	4	32

Changes Occurring in DNA Histograms during Treatment

In 24 patients with a prostatic carcinoma we have carried out cytophotometric studies during treatment. In 12 other patients we have obtained DNA histograms before and during treatment.

In 19 of the 24 patients examined during treatment, DNA histograms displayed normal patterns, all the nuclei showing DNA values ranging around the diploid value. In all these patients, the clinical response to treatment was very good.

In five of the 24 patients, histograms showed marked aneuploidy and polyploidy. In three of them, clinical signs of progression were obvious. In two, the clinical response seemed to be good at the time of examination but one progressed three months later.

In the 12 patients in whom we performed DNA-histograms at the time of diagnosis and during the treatment, an objective clinical response was observed in eight. Comparison of DNA-histograms before and during treatment shows a striking reduction of poly- and aneuploidy during therapy (Figs. 10 and 11).

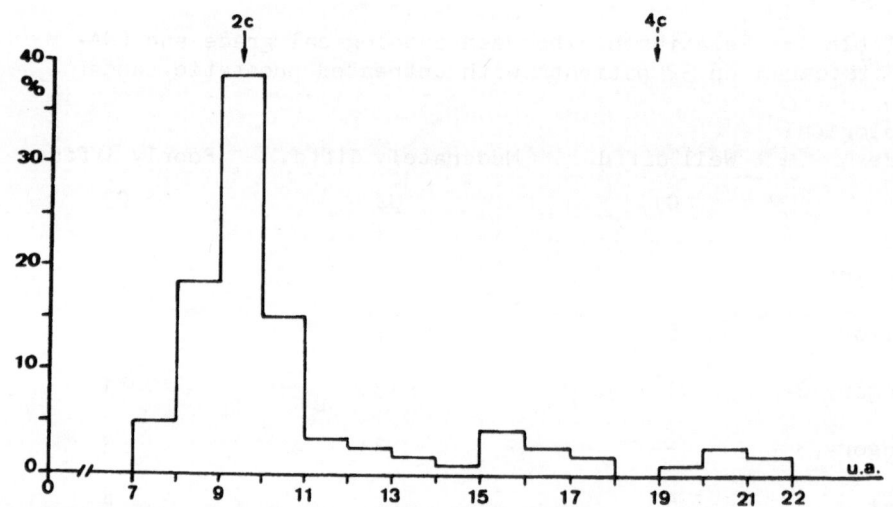

Fig. 10. DNA-histogram is a smear of prostatic aspiration performed in a patient with a moderately differentiated prostatic cancer (G2), stage T2N+M0, before treatment (n = 118). For details, cf legend of Fig. 2.

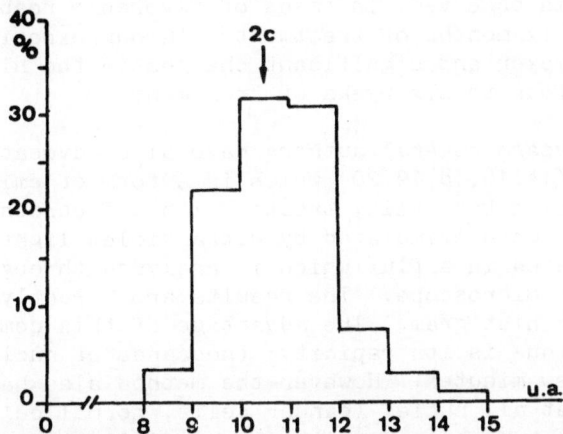

Fig. 11. DNA-histogram in the same patient (n = 108), six months
          after orchiectomy. One notices a normalisation of the
          histogram; the clinical response is excellent.

In three patients, the DNA-histogram showed a partial reduction
of aneuploidy and polyploidy . Although the immediate clinical
evolution was good in two patients, progression occurred within
six months. In the third patient in this group, who did not exhibit
response to the estrogenic treatment, the DNA histogram remained
unchanged, revealing an important percentage of non diploid cells.

DISCUSSION

There have been a few reports of measurement of DNA in prostatic
cancer (10,12,13,14,15). Our results are in agreement with them and
indicate that the use of absorption cytophotometry for the measurement of DNA in prostatic cancer cells yields information which is of
value in the classification and the prognosis of the disease.

Modifications of the DNA-histograms during treatment constitute,
in our experience, one of the earliest and the most reliable signs
of objective response to the treatment: a normalization of the
histogram is always a sign of a good therapeutic response while the
persistence or the reappearance of abnormalities in the DNA histogram is proof of an incomplete response or a premonitory sign of
impending progression which invites a change of the treatment.
Kjaer et al (16) and Leistenschneider and Nagel (17) draw the same
conclusions but consider that the return of the histogram to the

normal pattern is observed, in cases of favorable response, only
after three to six months of treatment. In our experience, this
evolution is quicker and significant changes in the histograms are
observed after four to six weeks of treatment.

In recent years several authors have also advocated pulse
cytophotometry (14,16,18,19,20) which is a form of emission cytophotometry in which the cells, treated with a fluorochromic compound, fluoresce when stimulated by ultra violet light. These
cells are aspirated in a flux which is analyzed through the lens
of a photometric microscope. The results are directly expressed
by computer on a histogram. The advantage of this completely
automated technique is its rapidity; thousands of nuclei can be
analyzed in a few minutes. However the method also has the disadvantage in that all nuclei (cancer cells, normal cells, white
blood cells ...) are analyzed without any distinction, aggregates
or fragments of cells can alter the results, and lastly, this
technique gives no information on the morphological aspect of the
cells. On the other hand, our technique of absorption-cytophotometry
on single cells after Feulgen staining gives important morphological
information.

CONCLUSION

The measurement of DNA by microdensitometry is a technique
providing important information for the diagnosis, classification
and prognosis of prostatic cancer. It is a relatively simple and
quick technique, which is easily performed in centers equipped
with scanning microdensitometers. It has the advantage over
pulse cytophotometry of providing morphological information.

REFERENCES

1. R. Bassleer, Recherches sur les protéines nucléaires totales et
   les acides désoxyribonucléiques dans les fibroblastes cultivés
   in vitro et dans les cellules tumorales d'Ehrlich. Une étude
   cytochimique quantitative réalisée par micro-interférométrie et
   cytophotométrie. (Thèse d'agrégation de l'Enseignement
   Supérieur). Arch. Biol. 79:2 181-325 (1968).
2. I. Cameron, Is the duration of DNA synthesis in somatic cells
   of mammals and birds a constant? J. Cell. Biol. 20:185-187
   (1964).
3. L. Adams, S. Dahlgren, Cytophotometric measurements of the DNA
   content of lung tumours, Acta Path. Microbiol. Scand.,
   72:561-574 (1968).
4. N. Atkin, Nuclear size in carcinoma of the cervix; its relation
   to DNA content and prognosis, Cancer 17:1391-1394 (1964).
5. N. Inui, and K. Oota, DNA content of human tumor cell nucleus.
   A study on gastric carcinoma, with special reference to its
   histological features, Gann 56:567-574 (1965).

6. C. Leuchtenberg, R. Leuchtenberg and A. Davis, A microspectro-
    photometric study of the desoxyribose nucleic acid (DNA)
    content in cells of normal and malignant human tissues,
    Am. J. Path. 30:65-85 (1954).

7. W. Sandritter, M. Carl and W. Ritter, Cytophotometric measure-
    ments of the DNA content of human malignant tumors by means of
    Feulgen reaction, Acta Cytol. 10:26-30 (1966).

8. R. Feulgen and H. Rossenbeck, Mikroskopisch-chemischer Nachweis
    einer Nukleinsäure vom Typus der Thymokleinsäure und die darauf
    berukende elektive färbung von Zelkernen in microskopischen
    Präparten. Hoope Seylers. Z. Phys. Chem. 135:203-248 (1924).

9. F. Kasten, The Feulgen reaction. An enigma in cytochemistry,
    Acta Histochem. 17:88-99 (1964).

10. A. Zetterberg and P. Esposti, Cytophotometric DNA analysis of
    aspirated cells from prostatic carcinoma, Cytol.(Baltimore)
    20:46 (1976).

11. C. Bouffioux, Le cancer de la prostate, Acta Urol. Belg.
    47, V. 344-348 (1979).

12. L. Persky and C. Leuchtenberger, Cytochemical studies of
    prostatic epithelium: I. The desoxyribose nucleic (DNA)
    content in individual cells, J. Urol.78:788-795 (1957).

13. E. Sprenger, L. Volk and W. Michaelis, Die Aussagekraft der
    Zelkern-DNS-Bestimmung bei der Diagnostik des Prostata-
    karzinoms, Beitr. Path.Bd. 153:370-378 (1974).

14. P. Bichel, P. Frederiksen, T. Kjaer, P. Thommesen and
    L. Vindeløv, Flow micro-fluorometry and transrectal fine
    needle biopsy in the classfication of human prostatic carcinoma,
    Cancer 40:1206-1211 (1977).

15. A. Tavares, J. Costa, A. de Carvalho and M. Reis, Tumour
    polyploidy and prognosis in carcinomas of the bladder and
    prostate, Brit. J. Cancer 20:438-441 (1966).

16. T. Kjaer, P. Thommesen, P. Frederiksen and P. Bichel, DNA
    content in cells aspirated from carcinoma of the prostate
    treated with oestrogenic compounds, Urol. Res. 7:249-251 (1979).

17. W. Leistenschneider and R. Nagel, Estracyt therapy of advanced
    prostatic cancer with special reference to control of therapy
    with cytology and DNA cytophotometry, Eur. Urol. 6:11-115
    (1980).

18. L. Vindeløv, Flow microfluorometric analysis of nuclear DNA
    in cells from solid tumors and cell suspensions. A new method
    for rapid isolation and staining of nuclei. Virchows Arch.
    B. Cell Path. 24:227-242 (1977).

19. A. Zimmerman and F. Truss, Flow-through-Cytophotometry,
    Urol. Res. 7:1-3 (1979).

20. B. Tribukait, P.L. Esposti and L. Rönström, Tumour ploidy for
    characterization of prostatic carcinoma: Flow cyto-fluoro-
    metric DNA studies using aspiration biopsy material,
    Scand. J. Urol. Nephrol., Suppl. 55:59-64 (1980)

ASPIRATION BIOPSY CYTOLOGY IN THE MANAGEMENT OF PROSTATIC CARCINOMA AND IN MONITORING RESPONSE TO TREATMENT

P.L. Esposti, S. Franzén, L. Andersson

Karolinska sjukhuset
Stockholm,
Sweden

INTRODUCTION

Transrectal fine needle aspiration biopsy of the prostate (1) is a fast, safe and accurate method of identifying malignant disease and also of assessing the grade of malignancy (2). At the Karolinska sjukhuset an annual average of 800 aspiration biopsies of the prostate have been performed for the last twenty years. The fine needle of the Franzén instrument gives minimal trauma and the procedure can be performed repeatedly without causing undue discomfort to the patient. This allows the response to therapy to be monitored by repeated biopsies.

In patients not given active treatment for various reasons, but checked regularly, biopsies have given identical findings over a long period of time in the majority of the cases, indicating that the method is reproducible. In some cases, however, there was an increase of malignancy grade with time; a well-differentiated carcinoma becoming more polymorphous and less well differentiated (Fig. 1). In others, in patients with reduction of the local tumour following therapy, a gradual disappearance of the malignant cell population occurred.

MONITORING OF RESPONSE TO THERAPY

After Radical Surgery

In patients subjected to radical prostatectomy where pelvic nodules were palpable per rectum, aspiration biopsy verified local recurrence of the tumour.

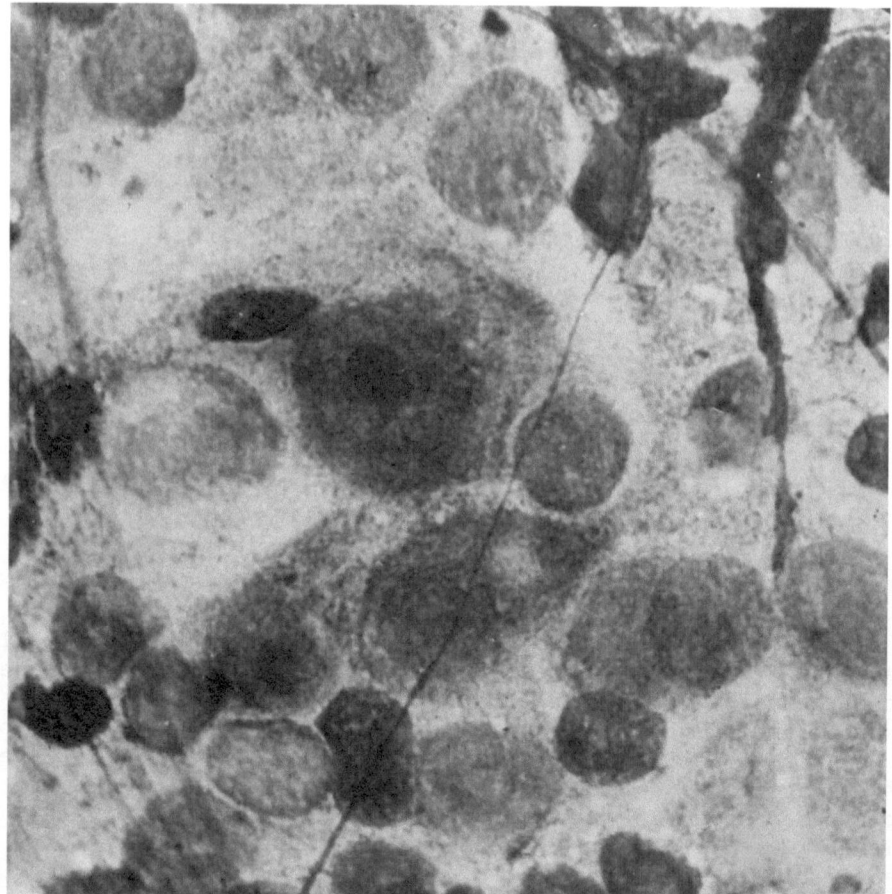

Fig. 1. Poorly differentiated prostatic carcinoma, with polymorphous
         nuclei and evident nucleoli. Recurrence after estrogen
         therapy. MGG-stained smear from prostatic aspirate.

Hormone Therapy

     The cellular changes in histologic sections of prostate carci-
noma following estrogen therapy were first demonstrated by Kahle,
Schenken and Burns in 1943 (3). These changes can easily be studied
by transrectal aspiration biopsy of the malignant gland. The nuclei
become uniformly dark and lose their chromatin details. Large
squamous cells with pyknotic nuclei appear together with the so-
called glycogenic cells (Fig. 2). The latter are probably the most
characteristic cells of a prostatic smear after estrogen therapy.
They are round or oval, appear single or in small groups and in
special staining prove to contain glycogen. They are never seen in
the prostatic aspirate before therapy and they disappear if the
patient stops his medication.

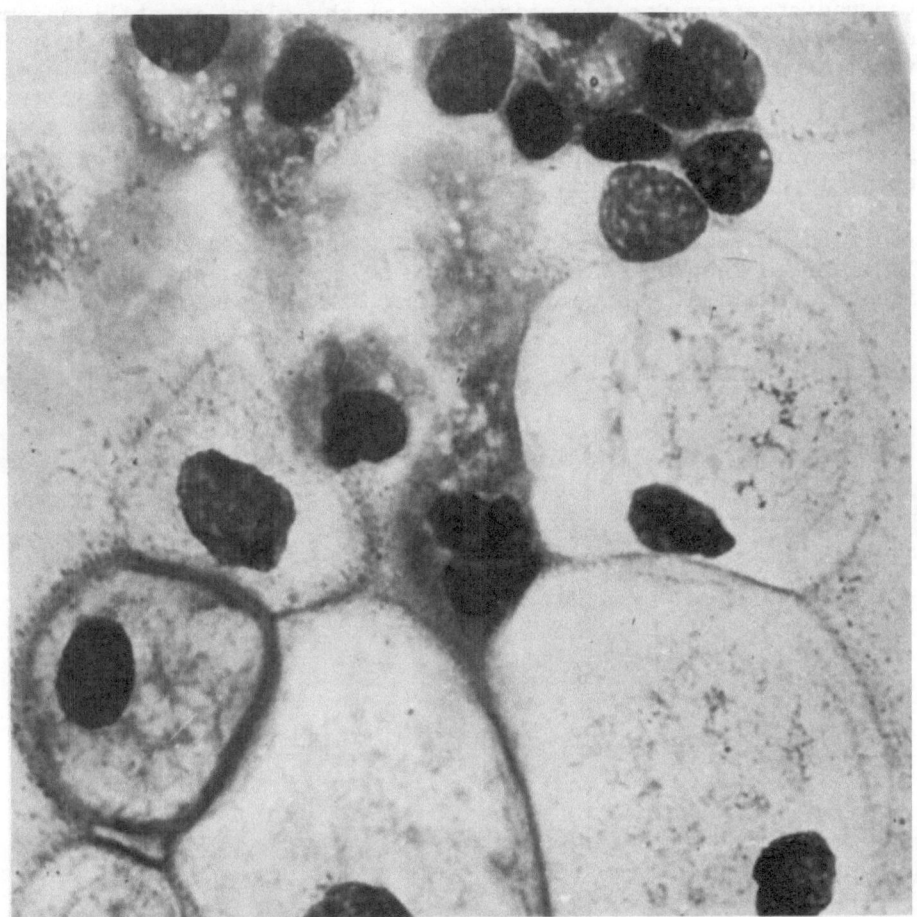

Fig. 2. Cytologic changes in prostatic carcinoma after estrogen
therapy: altered carcinoma cells with pyknotic nuclei and
glycogenic cells. MGG-stained smear from prostatic
aspirate.

In patients in whom long term hormonal therapy is successful it
is increasingly more difficult to identify obvious carcinoma cells,
while squamous metaplastic and glycogenic cells will dominate in
the smear. On the other hand, the response to therapy is classified
as poor when the smears on check-up are dominated by unmodified
cancer cells.

Radiation Therapy

Morphological changes in the malignant cell population occur
slowly after radiotherapy and in our experience a control biopsy of
the prostate should not be carried out earlier than four months

after radiotherapy for two reasons - (a) the gland is still oedema-
tous, bleeds easily and there is a danger of complications, and (b)
several atypical cells are still present, morphologically resembling carcinoma cells but not viable. In fact they disappear later on.
When performing a control biopsy too soon there is a risk of a false
positive diagnosis. The ideal time for a check biopsy after radiotherapy is probably between four and six months.

If the therapy has been successful, unmodified carcinoma cells
will later on become less numerous while radiation changes become
evident: cytoplasmic vacuolization, and markedly enlarged nuclei of

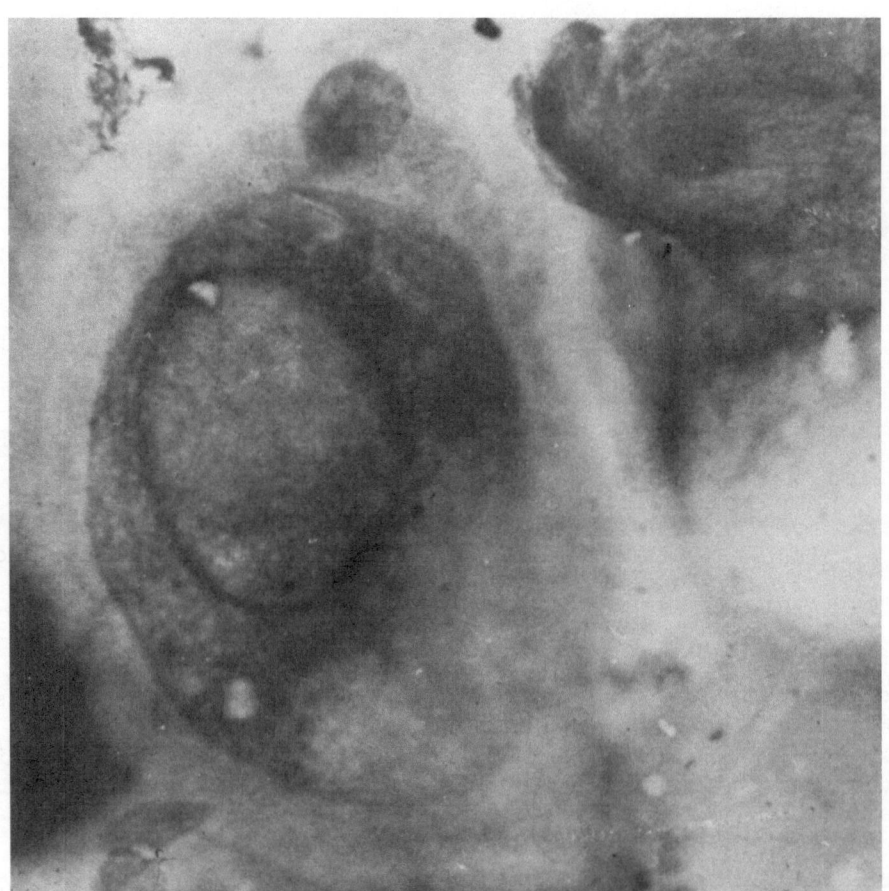

Fig. 3. Radiation changes in prostatic carcinoma cells: enlarged
         nuclei with vacuolisation. MGG-stained smear from prostatic
         aspirate.

bizarre shape, exhibiting signs of nuclear damage such as large
vacuoles (Fig. 3). The cellularity of the irradiated gland decreases
gradually and, with full effect, a control biopsy will yield scant
material and no carcinoma cells.

REFERENCES

1. S. Franzén, G. Giertz, and J. Zajicek, Cytological diagnosis of
    prostatic tumours by transrectal aspiration biopsy: A preliminary
    report, Br. J. Urol. 32: 193 (1960).
2. P.L. Esposti, Cytologic malignancy grading of prostatic carcinoma
    by transrectal aspiration biopsy, Scand. J. Urol. Nephrol. 5:
    199 (1971).
3. P.J. Kahle, J.R. Schenken, and E.L. Burns, Clinical and patholog-
    ical effects of diethylstilbestrol and diethylstilbestrol di-
    propionate on carcinoma of the prostate gland, J. Urol. 50: 711
    (1943).

THE ROLE OF ASPIRATION BIOPSY IN FOLLOWING PATIENTS TREATED WITH CHEMOTHERAPY AND RADIATION

S. Brosman

Bay Urologic Medical Group
Santa Monica,
California, USA

INTRODUCTION

The value of fine needle aspiration biopsy (FNA) in the diagnosis of prostate cancer has been confirmed repeatedly from numerous studies (1,2). The technique has a high degree of efficiency in that the sensitivity (true positive) and specificity (true negative) correlate well with the standard needle biopsy. The FNA is not recommended as a general screening test for prostate cancer but to help establish the diagnosis in patients whose prostates are suspicious for carcinoma. An additional use of the test may be to help determine response to therapy.

The method has several advantages as a diagnostic study. Anaesthesia is not required, the complication rate is low, the study can be repeated at frequent intervals, and very small areas of the prostate can be examined. As experience with the technique has increased, cytologic grading has improved and can be correlated with over 90% of the histologic specimens (1,3).

Based on cytomorphologic criteria, Esposti and others have described the characteristics associated with tumor grade (3,4). Cytologic aspiration of well differentiated tumors (Grade 1) tends to demonstrate clusters of cells, nuclear polymorphism of a moderate degree and nucleoli which are distinct and not enlarged. The cells are often grouped into an adenomatous complex with the nuclei on the periphery.

Moderately differentiated (Grade 2) lesions show an increase in nuclear polymorphism and less cellular adherence. Poorly differentiated lesions (Grade 3) are characterized by extreme nuclear polymorphism, enlarged nucleoli and cellular dissociation.

RESULTS

We have evaluated serial FNA biopsies in patients who have been
treated with external beam irradiation, implantation of 1^{125} seeds,
hormonal therapy and combination chemotherapy.

Changes following hormonal therapy (5,6) have been adequately
reported and this discussion will be confined to a small series of
patients who were treated with irradiation or chemotherapy.

The patients were biopsied prior to the initiation of treatment
and at regular intervals (3 - 6 months) depending on the type of
treatment. Four to six slides were obtained from each patient. The
slides were labelled according to the site of the aspiration and compared to previous biopsies.

RADIATION THERAPY

There have been 39 patients with localised prostate cancer
treated with some form of irradiation. Twelve received external beam
irradiation 6500r and 27 patients were treated with interstitial irradiation using 1^{125}. The dose varied between 28,000 and 42,000r.
These patients were biopsied every six months following completion
of their therapy. Grade 1 tumor, as determined by a combination of
FNA and histologic biopsy, was the predominant grade in 18 patients,
Grade II in 14 patients and Grade III in 7 patients.

The cytologic effect of irradiation was the same in patients
receiving external beam or interstitial irradiation. The predominant
effects characteristic of radiation change are the 'smudging' or
indistinctiveness of cellular fractures and boundaries, pyknotic
nuclei and small or absent nucleoli (7).

All twelve patients treated with external beam irradiation
demonstrated malignant appearing cells six months following therapy
(Table 1). Ten patients (87%) had a definite radiation response
with altered cytology. The remaining two patients showed no apparent
change from their original biopsy. At 12 months all of the patients
had biopsies disclosing abnormal, irradiated cells. Eighteen months
following therapy, no malignant or radiation altered cells could be
found in five (40%) patients. The remaining patients demonstrated
radiation altered cells. There were changes in the predominant cell
pattern which were attributed to a beneficial therapeutic response.
There were six patients originally considered to have Grade 2 tumors.
Following irradiation, three of these patients had a predominant
Grade 1 tumor. One of the three patients with a Grade 3 tumor had
a change in the predominant cell pattern in Grade 1. After twenty-
four months, seven patients (58%) had no evidence of radiation

altered cells or neoplastic cells. Two of the remaining five patients demonstrated neoplastic cells which did not seem to be altered by radiation, while the last three had bizarre cells due to radiation effect. None of the 12 patients in this group has yet shown evidence of metastatic disease.

The group of 27 patients treated with interstitial irradiation were biopsied six months following surgery. The biopsies revealed radiation effect in all the patients (Table 2). At 12 months, 9 patients (35%) had no evidence of carcinoma, 8 patients had only scattered cells showing severe radiation effect, and 10 patients demonstrated numbers of irradiated cells, of whom three also had neoplastic appearing cells which did not have a radiation effect.

At eighteen months, 14 patients showed no evidence of carcinoma in their biopsies, eight patients had neoplastic cells showing radiation effect and five patients demonstrated 'healthy' neoplastic cells in addition to cells with radiation effect.

Twenty-four months following surgery, no tumor could be identified in 18 (66%) patients and nine continued to show neoplastic cells with radiation effect. Five of these patients also demonstrated unaffected cancer cells.

The presence of apparently unaltered cancer cells in addition to the continued presence of irradiated cells has led us to believe that these patients may not have had a good distribution of the 1^{125} seeds. None of the patients has received additional therapy and there has been no evidence of recurrence.

Table 1.   Results of fine needle aspiration biopsy (FNA)
           in 12 patients receiving radiotherapy (6500r)

Result of FNA	Months after radiotherapy			
	6	12	18	24
Positive with XR response	10	12	7	3
Positive without XR response	2	-	-	2
No tumor	-	-	5	7
Decrease in grade (8)	-	-	4	2

Table 2. Results of FNA in 27 patients treated with I^{125}

Result of FNA	Months after I^{125} therapy			
	6	12	18	24
Positive with XR response	27	18	8	9
Positive without XR response	0	3	5	5
No tumor	0	9(33%)	14(52%)	18(66%)
Decrease in grade (13)	0	5	2	2

Tumor grade could be evaluated in 13 patients. Twelve months following therapy, an alteration in the predominant cell grade could be seen in five patients and an additional two patients had an alteration in their cell grade at 18 months. These instances of downgrading are not likely to reflect an actual decrease in the grade of the malignancy, but a change in the predominant cell pattern. This change may be due to an absence of higher grade tumor cells or a reflection of sampling.

CHEMOTHERAPY

Fifty-six patients were treated with a combination of cis-platinum (100 mg/m^2), cytoxan (0.8 gm/m^2) and stilphostrol (0.8 gm/m^2) (Table 3). Full dose therapy was given monthly for 2 - 4 months, followed by lesser doses of maintenance therapy at monthly intervals. Forty-two patients had received prior irradiation or hormonal therapy. Fourteen patients had newly diagnosed disease and had received no prior therapy. Grade 1 tumor was present in 21, Grade 2 in 23, and Grade 3 in 12 patients. Serial FNA was performed every three months to evaluate the effect of therapy.

The cytologic changes related to chemotherapy have been difficult to interpret because of the combination of therapies. The major cytologic changes were a change in the predominant tumor grade and an absence of cancer cells on biopsy. Hormonal changes were noted in some cells. Although the cytologic morphology appears to be altered by chemotherapy in the majority of patients, we have not been able to identify uniform or specific changes. Many patients showed no change in their cellular morphology.

The alterations in the tumor located within the prostate did not always correlate with those in tumor located elsewhere. In some instances there was a good response within the prostate as indicated

Table 3. Chemotherapy (56 patients)
DDP - CTX - Stilphostrol

Months	Patients	Morphological Change	Grade	No Tumor
3	56	31(55%)	9(16%)	0
6	48	35	18	4
12	37	22(59%)	18(48%)	8(21%)
18	25	16	15	7
24	16	11(68%)	11(68%)	5(31%)

by a reduction in prostate size, a softening of the gland, and a
decrease in tumor grade or an absence of tumor whilst tumor in the
bone or other locations was progressing. If we assume that prostate
cancer is a polyclonal tumor, the therapy may be effective in eradic-
ating some clones but ineffective in others.

A morphologic change attributed to the effects of chemotherapy
was seen in 55% of patients at three months, 59% at 12 months and
68% at 24 months.

The predominant cell pattern had a decreased tumor grade in
16% of patients at three months, 48% at 12 months and 68% at 24
months. No tumor was seen on biopsy in 21% of patients at 21 months
and 31% at 24 months. This table does not reflect patient survival
but only changes in the results of FNA. The patients are heterogeneous - some had prior therapy and others had not been treated
previously.

DISCUSSION

The value of FNA in monitoring the results of therapy is dependent upon the use of the data and the implication of residual cellular material in the prostate. If the presence of altered cells in
an irradiated prostate has no clinical meaning, there is no need to
perform biopsies. The presence of such cells does not necessarily
imply that they are active or will contribute to metastatic disease.
However, if unaltered cancer cells are identified two years following
radiation, consideration could be given to the institution of additional therapy. A decrease in the predominant cell grade may suggest
only a partial benefit from therapy.

FNA in patients receiving chemotherapy may be considered in the
same manner. A variety of techniques are available to assess thera-

peutic response. An absence of tumor cells or a decrease in the
predominant cell grade may reflect a benefit of treatment particularly
if this corresponds to changes in other parameters.

There is not enough data to determine the specificity, sensitivity and efficiency of FNA as a sole diagnostic aid. Therefore
caution must be exercised before one uses the results of FNA in
making therapeutic decisions. At the present time the use of FNA
should be as an adjunct in determining response to therapy.

REFERENCES

1.   P.L. Esposti, Transrectal aspiration biopsy of the prostate
     with Franzen's instrument, in: "Bladder tumors and other topics
     in Urological Oncology," M. Pavone-Macaluso, P.H. Smith, and
     F. Edsmyr, eds., Plenum Press, London and New York (1980), p. 459.
2.   B.P. Lin, W.E. Davies, and P.A. Harmata, Prostatic aspiration
     cytology, Pathology 11: 607 (1979).
3.   P.L. Esposti, Cytologic malignancy grading of prostatic carc-
     inoma by transrectal aspiration biopsy, Scan. J. Urol. Nephrol.
     5: 199 (1971).
4.   C. Voeth, M. Drosse, and G. Steur, Cytologic grading of
     prostatic carcinoma, Urologe 17: 367 (1978).
5.   F. Paul, E. Schmidt, and R. Kerr, The prognostic significance
     of cytologic differentiation grades of estrogen-treated pros-
     tatic carcinoma. Follow-up of 496 patients treated with
     estrogen for 5 years, Urologe 17: 377 (1978).
6.   W. Leistenschneider and R. Nagel, Cytologic grading of regres-
     sion in conservatively treated prostate carcinoma and its
     prognostic significance, Aktuel Urol. 11: 263 (1980).
7.   K.H. Kurth, J.E. Altwein, D. Skoluda, and R. Hohenfellner,
     Follow-up of irradiated prostatic carcinoma by aspiration
     biopsy, J. Urol. 117: 615 (1977).

Editorial Note (M.P.M.)

Stilphostrol is a trade name for phospho-oestrol or stilboestrol
diphosphate (honvan in most european countries), whereas cytoxan
(endoxan in Europe) corresponds to cyclophosphamide. It is a pity
that this study does not correlate the cytological response with the
clinical response or the survival rate.

EPITHELIUM AND STROMA IN PROSTATIC

CANCER AND HYPERPLASIA

M.A. Blankenstein, J.C. Romijn, G.J. van Steenbrugge,
and F.H. Schröder

Erasmus University
Rotterdam
The Netherlands

The normal morphogenesis and cytodifferentiation of rodent prostatic epithelium is strongly dependent on the continuous association with mesenchymal cells of proper (i.e. urogenital) origin (1,2). The inductive capacity of urogenital stroma has been tested on different epithelia, and it was found that, in the presence of androgens, integumental epithelium was transformed by urogenital stroma into a glandular epithelium characteristic of the source of the stroma (1,3). Moreover, adult bladder epithelium could be induced to form prostate-like acini by embryonic stroma of urogenital origin (3). From these observations McNeal (4) hypothesized that the formation of prostatic acini during the development of benign prostatic hyperplasia may be the result of a re-expression of embryonic inductive capacity. Cunha et al. (5) summarized the pre-requisites for prostatic development to be i) the presence of androgens; ii) the presence of "inductive" stroma and iii) the ability of the epithelium to respond to the inductive influences.

According to the generally accepted mechanism of steroid hormone action, androgens exert their effect(s) on target tissues through specific receptors present in the cytoplasm, which translocate to the nucleus after binding the androgen. In the nucleus, mRNA and protein synthesis are stimulated, leading ultimately to the observed hormonal effects (6). Prior to receptor binding, testosterone is reduced to 5α-dihydrotestosterone (7), which has a higher affinity for the androgen receptor. Androgen receptors (8-11) and 5α-reductase (11-14) are indeed present in human prostatic tissue.

CELL SEPARATION

For the study of possible biochemical interactions between
stroma and epithelium from human prostatic tissue, the availability
of a method to separate the two tissue compartments is essential.
Mechanical (15,16) and enzymatic (17,18) methods have been used for
the separation of human prostatic epithelium and stroma. Generally,
however, the yield was low and the cells obtained lacked viability.
In our laboratory a method was developed for the isolation of human
prostatic epithelial cells, which is based on squeezing of finely
minced tissue and purification of the epithelium by a series of
sedimentation steps at unit gravity (19). Although 95% of the cells
excluded trypan blue and about 45% of the cells incorporated uridine,
it has not yet been possible to maintain the cells in culture. As an
alternative to separation of cells, selective cultivation of fibroblasts, which are assumed to represent the stroma, and epithelium
(20,21) have been used to obtain separated cell types. A possible
disadvantage of these methods is that the cells obtained may not
properly reflect the cells present in the original prostatic tissue
sample.

MARKERS

The prostate is known to be rich in acid phosphatase and
ornithine decarboxylase (22). Acid phosphatase is generally accepted
to be a marker for prostatic epithelial cells (23-25) and its
activity was found to be 25 times higher in epithelial cells than in
the remaining stroma (19). Although the activity of prostatic acid
phosphatase in the serum of patients with advanced prostatic carcinoma
decreases after castration, the dependency of the enzyme activity on
hormones has not yet been established unequivocally. Using the
prostatic cell line MA 160, Ban et al, (26) showed that both androgens and oestrogens decreased acid phosphatase activity. There are,
however,serious doubts whether this cell line is still to be considered as being prostatic (for review, see 27).

In 25% of patients with prostatic cancer and 8% of patients with
benign prostatic hyperplasia elevated serum levels of spermidine have
been detected (28). Because of the abundancy of ornithine decarboxylase in the prostate, this enzyme, which catalyses the first step in
polyamine biosynthesis, may be useful for the study of androgen
dependency of prostatic tumours. Carcinoembryonic antigen secretion
has also been used as a marker for prostatic epithelial cells in
culture (29). In the same study, the polyamine concentration of the
culture medium was found to be of no value as a marker for prostatic
epithelial cells.

BIOCHEMICAL PROPERTIES

Andogen receptors appear to be distributed evenly over epithelium and stroma, as does dihydrotestosterone (11). Sex hormone binding globulin (SHBG) was found to be associated exclusively with the stroma (16). These results could be explained by assuming that the SHBG provides a high testosterone concentration to the stromal 5α-reductase and that the DHT formed in the stroma moves to the epithelium where it interacts with the androgen receptor. Recent findings (14,30,31) that 5α-reductase is almost exclusively confined to the stroma are in agreement with such a model. The observation reported by Habib et al. (32) that stromal and epithelial 5α-reductase activites were of a similar order of magnitude, is in sharp contrast to these findings. Differences in the methods used for the separation of the cells and estimation of the enzyme activity may well be responsible for the differences in the reported results. In prostatic carcinoma tissue the 5α-reductase activity is lower than in BPH-tissue (33,34). This difference appears to be due to changes in the enzyme activity in the stroma, since the activity was much higher in fibroblasts and stroma from hyperplastic tissue than in fibroblasts and stroma from carcinoma tissue (35,36). The distribution of steroid receptors over the tissue compartments has also been studied by Pertschuk et al. (37,38). Using incubation of tissue slices with a fluorescent testosterone derivative, they found most fluorescence to be localized in the epithelium. There is, however, still serious doubt about the nature of the protein(s) which bind fluorescent steroid derivatives (39) and a proper biochemical study still needs to be carried out. Oestrogen (40), progesterone (41) and prolactin (42) receptors have been identified in human prostatic tissue. The concentration of oestrogen receptors appears to be higher in carcinoma tissue than in hyperplastic tissue (40). Krieg et al. (31) reported that oestrogen receptors could be identified more often in isolated stroma than in epithelium or in whole tissue preparations.

The distribution of all receptors over the prostatic tissue compartments as well as their possible role in stromal-epthelial interactions needs to be studied further.

CONCLUSION

In order to determine if stromal-epithelial interactions play a major role in the development of benign prostatic hyperplasia and/or prostatic cancer, future research must be directed towards:

1. improvement of techniques for the separation of prostatic epithelium and stroma, with special emphasis on the viability of the cells obtained;
2. the identification of proper markers for the stroma;

3.   the study of possible effects of isolated stroma on the
      biochemical properties of the isolated epithelium, and, if
      such effects should indeed be observed;
4.   identification of the factor(s) which may be responsible for
      these effects.

REFERENCES

1.   G.R. Cunha, Tissue interactions between epithelium and mesenchyme
      of urogenital and integumental origin, Anat.Rec. 172:529 (1972).
2.   I. Lasnitzki and T. Mizuno, Induction of the rat prostate gland
      by androgens in organ culture, J.Endocr. 74:47 (1977).
3.   G.R. Cunha and B. Lung, The importance of stroma in morphogenesis
      and functional activity of urogenital epithelium, In vitro
      15:50 (1978).
4.   J.E. McNeal, Origin and evolution of benign prostatic enlarge-
      ment, Invest.Urol. 15:340 (1978).
5.   G.R. Cunha, B. Lung and B. Reese, Glandular epithelial induction
      by embryonic mesenchyme in adult bladder epithelium of Balb/c
      mice, Invest.Urol. 17:302 (1980).
6.   W.I.P. Mainwaring, "The Mechanism of Action of Androgens,"
      Springer-Verlag, New York (1977).
7.   N. Bruchovsky and J.D. Wilson, The conversion of testosterone
      to 5 -androstan-17β-ol-3-one by rat prostate in vivo and in
      vitro, J.Biol.Chem. 243:2012 (1968).
8.   M.Menon, C.E. Tananis, M.G. McLoughlin, and P.C. Walsh, Androgen
      receptors in human prostatic tissue-review, Cancer Treatment
      Rep. 61:265 (1977).
9.   L.L. Hicks and P.C. Walsh, A microassay for the measurement of
      androgen receptors in human prostatic tissue, Steroids 33:389
      (1979).
10.   M. Snochowski, A. Pousette, P. Ekman, D. Bression, L. Andersson,
      B. Hogberg, and J.A. Gustafsson, Characterisation and measurement
      of androgen receptor in human benign prostatic hyperplasia and
      prostatic carcinoma, J.Clin.Endocr.Metab. 45:920 (1977).
11.   D.A.N. Sirett, S.K. Cowan, A.E. Janeczo, J.K. Grant, and
      E.S. Glen, Prostatic tissue distribution of 17β-hydroxy-5α-
      androstan-3-one and of androgen receptors in benign hyperplasia,
      J.Steroid Biochem. 13:723 (1980).
12.   P.K. Siiteri and J.D. Wilson, Dihydrotestosterone in prostatic
      hypertrophy, J.clin.Invest. 49:1737 (1970).
13.   R.F. Morfin, S. DiStefano, J.P. Bercovici, and H.H. Floch,
      Comparison of testosterone, 5α-dihydrotestosterone and 5 -
      androstane-3β, 17β-diol metabolisms in human normal and
      hyperplastic prostates, J.Steroid Biochem. 9:245 (1978).
14.   J.C. Romijn, K. Oishi, J. Bolt-de Vries, H.U. Schweikert,
      E. Mulder, and F.H. Schröder, Androgen metabolism and androgen
      receptors in separated epithelium and stroma of the human pros-

tate, in:"Steroid Receptors, Metabolism and Prostatic Cancer,"
F.H. Schröder and H.J. de Voogt, eds., Exerpta Medica, Amsterdam,
(1980) p. 134.

15. L.M. Franks, P.N. Riddle, A.W. Carbonell, and G.O. Gey, A
comparative study of the ultrastructure and lack of growth
capacity of adult human prostate epithelium mechanically
separated from its stroma, J.Pathol. 100:113 (1970).

16. R.A. Cowan, S.K. Cowan, C.A. Giles, and J.K. Grant, Prostatic
distribution of sex hormone-binding globulin and cortisol-
binding globulin in benign hyperplasia, J.Endocr. 71:121 (1976).

17. S.R. Helms, R.I. Brazeal, A.J. Bueschen, and T.G. Pretlow,
Separation of cells with histochemically demonstrable acid
phosphatase activity from suspensions of human prostatic cells,
Am.J.Pathol. 80:79 (1975).

18. T.G. Pretlow, M.G. Brattain, and J.I. Kreisberg, Separation and
characterization of epithelial cells from prostates and prostatic carcinomas: a review, Cancer Treatment Rep. 61:157 (1977).

19. K. Oishi, J.C. Romijn, and F.H. Schröder, Cell separation and
characterization of epithelial cells from human benign prostatic
hyperplasia. The prostate, In press, (1981).

20. M.M. Webber, Normal and benign human prostatic epithelium in
culture. I. Isolation. In vitro 15:967 (1979).

21. J.F. Lechner, M.S. Babcock, M. Marnell, K.S. Narayau, and
M.E. Kaighn, Normal human prostate epithelial cell cultures,
Methods in cell biology 21B:195 (1980).

22. D.S. Coffey, The biochemistry and physiology of the prostate and
seminal vesicles, in:"Campbells Urology," 4th edition,
H. Harrison, R.F. Gittes, A.D. Perlmutter, T.A Stamey, and
P.C. Walsh, eds., Saunders, Philadelphia, (1978), Vol.1, p. 161.

23. J.A. Serrano, W.A. Shannon, N.J. Sternberger, H.L. Wasserkrug,
A.A. Serrano, and A.A. Seligman, The cytochemical determination
of prostatic acid phosphatase using a new substrate:phosphoryl-
choline, J.Histochem Cytochem. 24:1046 (1976).

24. A.C. Jöbsis, G.P. de Vries, R.R.H. Anholt, and G.T.B. Sanders,
Demonstration of the prostatic origin of metastases. An
immunohistochemical method for formalin-fixed embedded tissue,
Cancer 41:1788 (1978).

25. H.R. Herschman, Prostatic acid phosphatase and cancer, T.I.B.S.
5:82 (1980).

26. R.W. Ban, J.F. Cooper, H. Imfeld, and A. Foti, Hormonal effects
on prostatic acid phosphatase synthesis in tissue culture,
Invest.Urol. 11:308 (1974).

27. M.M. Webber, In vitro models for prostatic cancer, in:"Models
for Prostatic Cancer," G.P. Murphy, ed., Progr.clin.biol.Res.
37, Alan R. Liss, New York, (1980), p. 133.

28. P. Chaisiri, M.E. Harper, R.W. Blaney, W.P. Peeling, and
K. Griffiths, Plasma spermidine concentrations in patients with
tumours of the breast or prostate or testis, Clin.Chem. Acta
104:367 (1980).

29. R.D. Williams, D.L. Bronson, A.Y. Elliott, G.W. Gehrke,
    K. Kuob, and E.E. Fraley, Biochemical markers of cultured human
    prostatic epithelium, J.Urol. 119:768 (1978).
30. J.C. Romijn, K. Oishi, and F.H. Schröder, Investigations on
    separated epithelium and stroma of human prostatic tissue,
    The Prostate 1:118 (1980).
31. M. Krieg, G. Klötzl, J. Kaufmann, and K.D. Voigt, Stroma of
    human benign prostatic hyperplasia: preferential tissue for
    androgen metabolism and oestrogen binding, Acta endocr. 96:422
    (1981).
32. F.K. Habib, A.L. Tesdale, G.D. Chisholm, and A. Busuttil,
    Prostatic retropubic and transurethral specimens. A comparison
    of androgen metabolism in the respective stromal and epithelial
    components,The Prostate 1:117 (1980).
33. N. Bruchovsky and G. Lieskovsky, Increased ratio of 5ʕ-
    reductase: 3ɑ(B)-hydroxysteroid dehydrogenase activities in the
    hyperplastic human prostate, J.Endocr. 80:289 (1979).
34. R.P. Wilkin, N. Bruchovsky, T.K. Shnitka, P.S. Rennie, and
    T.L. Comeau, Stromal 5ʕ-reductase activity is elevated in
    benign prostatic hyperplasia, Acta endocr. 94:284 (1980).
35. H.U. Schweikert, H.J. Hein, J.C. Romijn, and F.H. Schröder,
    Testosterone metabolism of fibroblasts grown from prostatic
    carcinoma, benign prostatic hyperplasia and skin fibroblasts.
    Invest. Urol. In Press (1981).
36. M. Krieg, I. Grobe, K.D. Voigt, E. Altenähr, and H. Klosterhalfen,
    Human prostatic carcinoma:significant differences in its androgen
    binding and metabolism compared to the human benign prostatic
    hypertrophy, Acta endocr. 88:397 (1978)
37. L.P. Pertschuk, E.H. Tobin, P. Tanapat, E. Gaetjens, A.C. Carter,
    N.D. Bloom, R.J. Macchia, and K.B. Eisenberg, Histochemical
    analysis of steroid hormone receptors in breast and prostatic
    carcinoma, J. Histochem. Cytochem. 28:799 (1980).
38. L.P. Pertschuk, D.T. Zava, E.H. Tobin, D.J. Brigati, E. Gaetjens,
    R.J. Macchia, G.J. Wise, H.S. Wax, and D.S. Kim, Histochemical
    detection of steroid hormone receptors in the human prostate,
    in:"Prostate Cancer and Hormone Receptors," G.P. Murphy and
    A.A. Sandberg, eds., Alan R. Liss, New York,(1980), p. 113.
39. G.C. Chamness, W.D. Mercer, and W.L. McGuire, Are histochemical
    methods for estrogen receptor valid?, J. Histochem. Cytochem.
    28:792 (1980).
40. J.B. Murphy, R.C. Emmott, L.L. Hicks, and P.C. Walsh, Estrogen
    receptors in the human prostate, seminal vesicle, epididymis,
    testis, and genital skin: a marker for estrogen-responsive
    tissues?, J.clin.Endocr. Metab. 50:938 (1980).
41. R.A. Cowan, S.K. Cowan, and J.K. Grant, Binding of methyl-
    trienolone (R 1881) to a progesterone receptor-like component
    of human prostatic cytosol, J.Endocr. 74:281 (1977).
42. E.J. Keenan, E.D. Kemp, E.E. Ramsey, L.B. Garrison, H.D. Pearse,
    and C.V. Hodges, Specific binding of prolactin by prostate gland
    of rat and man, J.Urol. 122:43 (1979).

GRADING OF PROSTATIC CARCINOMA — EVALUATION OF SINGLE

PARAMETERS AND CYTOMORPHOMETRY

J.H.M. Blom[1], F.J.W. ten Kate[2], F.K. Mostofi[3] and
F.H. Schröder[1].

The Institutes of Urology (1) and of Pathology (2)
Erasmus University
Rotterdam, Netherlands and
The Armed Forces Institute of Pathology (3)
Washington
U.S.A.

INTRODUCTION

Since Broders' first tumor grading system in 1926 many attempts
have been made to correlate various histologic features of a tumor
with the prognosis of the patient. Also for prostatic carcinoma
many grading systems have been developed (1), but only a few of them
have found wide acceptance. One of the reasons for this is the
tendency of many prostatic cancers to show varying degrees of
differentiation and structure within a single section and often within a single microscopic field. Another reason may be the lack of
reproducibility of most, if not all, grading systems. However, some
grading systems seem to be very promising. Among these the most
significant are those of Gleason (2) and of Mostofi (3).

Mostofi uses the term <u>differentiation</u> exclusively for the
tendency of the tumor to form glands, and the term <u>anaplasia</u> for the
variation from normal in size, shape, staining and chromatin
distribution of the nuclei in the tumor cells. His grading system
is built up with architectural criteria, such as the various tumor
formations (small, intermediate or large glands, cribriform tumor
and solid tumor), the amount of stroma and the amount of tumor, and
with cytological criteria such as size of cell, the aspect of the
cytoplasm, nuclear size, nuclear pleomorphism, presence of mitoses,
presence of nucleoli and the presence of nuclear vacuoles. With
these criteria he estimates an overall tumor grade.

Using Gleason's system Harada and associates (4) found a good reproducibility on repeat readings of this system, although there was less correlation between their readings and Gleason's readings of the same slides.   They also found, using Mostofi's system, that nuclear anaplasia and glandular differentiation correlated well with death rates.

MATERIAL AND METHODS

In a series of 484 patients on whom the late Dr Elmer Belt performed a radical perineal prostatectomy for cancer the patient charts were reviewed retrospectively and in 346 cases histological slides from the prostatectomy specimens were available for review. These tumors were all regraded by Mostofi without knowledge of the follow-up of the patients.   Most of the tumors consisted of a varying number of morphologically different formations.   As Table 1 shows their number varied from one to four per patient and a total of 668 tumor formations have been matched with the clinical data of 346 patients.

The survival curves were estimated according to Kaplan and Meier and have been corrected for intercurrent, tumor unrelated and unknown death causes.   For the calculations of P-values in the comparison of the survival curves the Logrank test was used.

In order to objectively evaluate nuclear variation in size and shape a semi-automatic computerized image analysing system was used (Videoplan, Kontron).   This consists of a graphic tablet, connected to a desk-computer, and a microscope with a drawing tube.   The graphic tablet is used for digitizing contour coordinates of figures drawn on the tablet with a cursor.   A light-emitting diode is mounted in the centre of the cursor, which is visible as a small, red spot together with the normal visual field of the microscope, via the

Table 1.   The Number of Tumor Formations and
           Their Relative Distribution in 346
           Patients with Prostatic Carcinoma.

No. of Tumor Formations	No. of Patients	%	No. of Formations
1	113	32.6	113
2	152	44.0	304
3	73	21.1	219
4	8	2.3	32
Total	346	100	668

drawing tube.   In this way contours of objects in the microscopic
image can easily be traced manually under visual control.   The
digitized contours are fed into the computer, which calculates the
preselected parameters.   The area and perimeter was calculated in
this case, together with two so-called form factors: a "form ellipse"
which is derived from the longest diameter of a structure and the
shortest diameter perpendicular to it in the following way:

$$\text{form}_{\text{ellipse}} = \frac{\text{shortest diameter}}{\text{longest diameter}}$$

As can easily be seen the largest value for "form ellipse" is one
for a circle and less than one in the case of other structures.   The
second factor we estimated was: "form pe" which is derived from area
and perimeter in the following way:

$$\text{form}_{\text{pe}} = \frac{4 \times \pi \times \text{area}}{(\text{perimeter})^2}$$

Here also the largest value for "form pe" is one in case of a
circle and is less than one in all other structures.   Reproducibility
of contour tracing was within 5%.   This is consistent with data
from the literature (6,7).

RESULTS

Figure 1 shows the tumor related survival rates for the various
tumor formations from tumors consisting of only one formation.
The survival probability is plotted against the time in months.
There is no difference in survival between patients with small glands,
intermediate glands or large glands in their tumors, but these three
differ significantly in survival from patients with cribriform or
solid tumors.   As Figure 2 shows, even the presence of cribriform
or solid tumor together with small, intermediate or large glands
makes prognosis significantly worse than in the case of small,
intermediate or large glands alone.   The amount of tumor (Figure 3)
has prognostic importance insofar that patients with small amounts
of tumor do better than those with medium or large amounts.   However,
one should not forget that all patients have had radical prostatectomy
and that especially the patients with small amounts of tumor might
have been cured by the operation.

The amount of stroma, the appearance of the cytoplasm, the
presence of nucleoli, the size of cell and the presence of nuclear
vacuoles, have all failed to identify groups of patients with
different survival rates.

On the other hand nuclear pleomorphism, i.e. the variation in
nuclear size and shape, identifies three groups of patients with

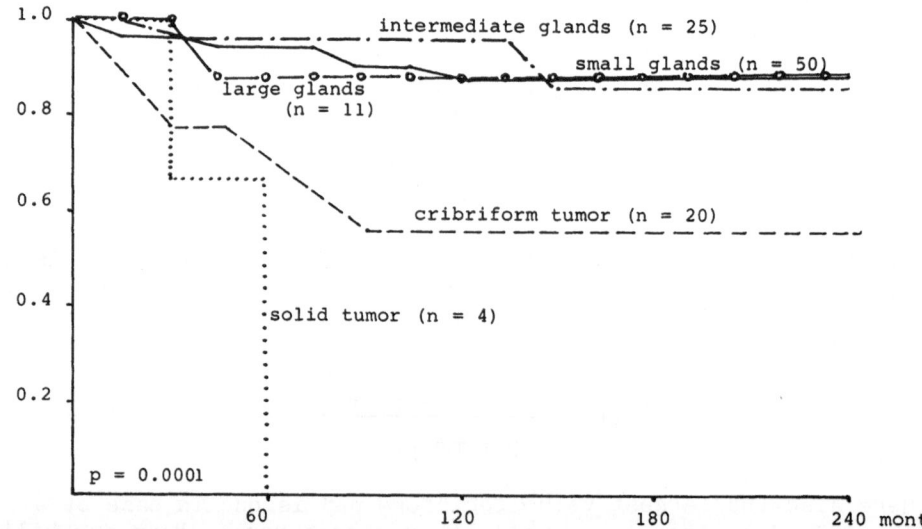

Fig. 1   Survival rates for 110 patients according to glandular
         differentiation.   In each tumor only one tumor formation
         is present.   (Mostofi's grading system).

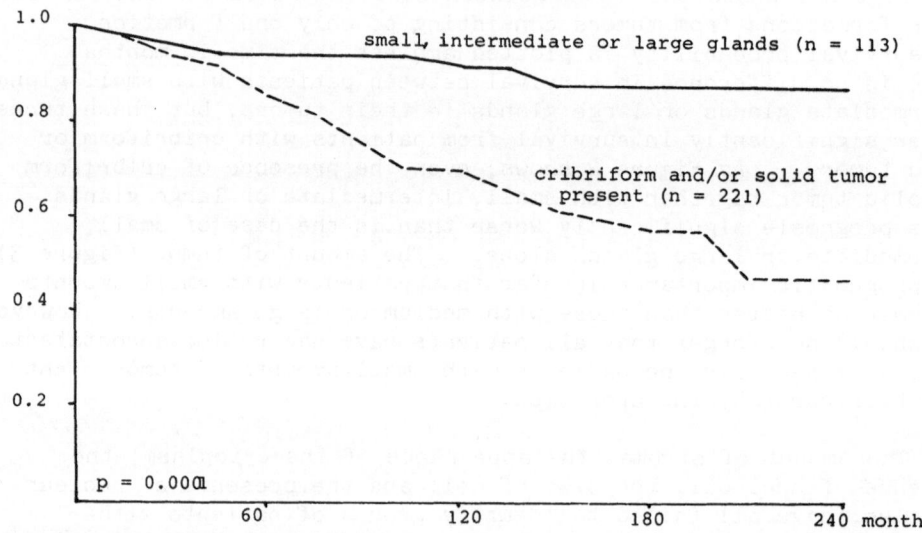

Fig. 2   Survival rates for 113 patients with only small, intermediate
         and/or large glands in their tumors vs. 221 patients who had
         glands and cribriform and/or solid parts in their tumors.
         (Mostofi's grading system).

Prostatic carcinoma
Survival according to amount of tumor.

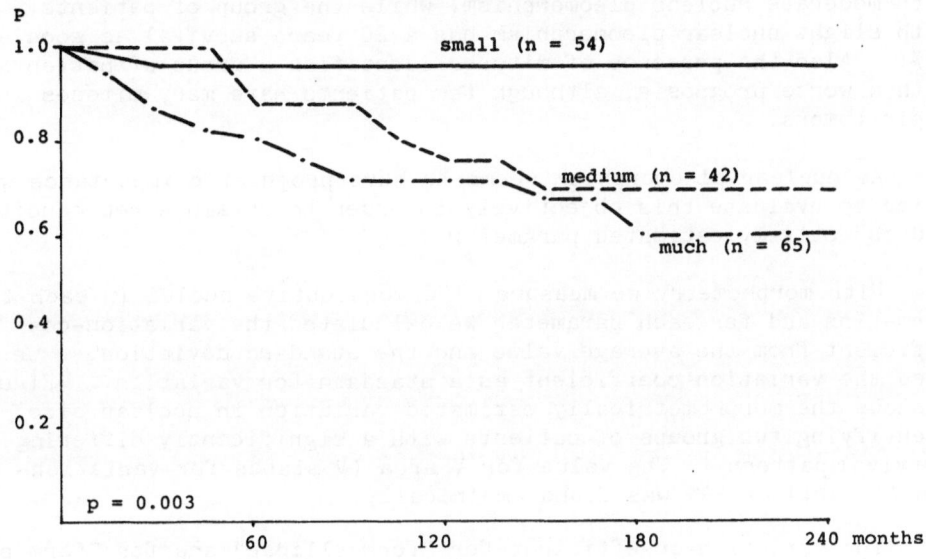

Fig. 3   Survival rates in 161 patients according to amount of tumor
        in their prostatectomy specimen (Mostofi's grading system).

Prostatic carcinoma
Survival according to nuclear pleomorphism.

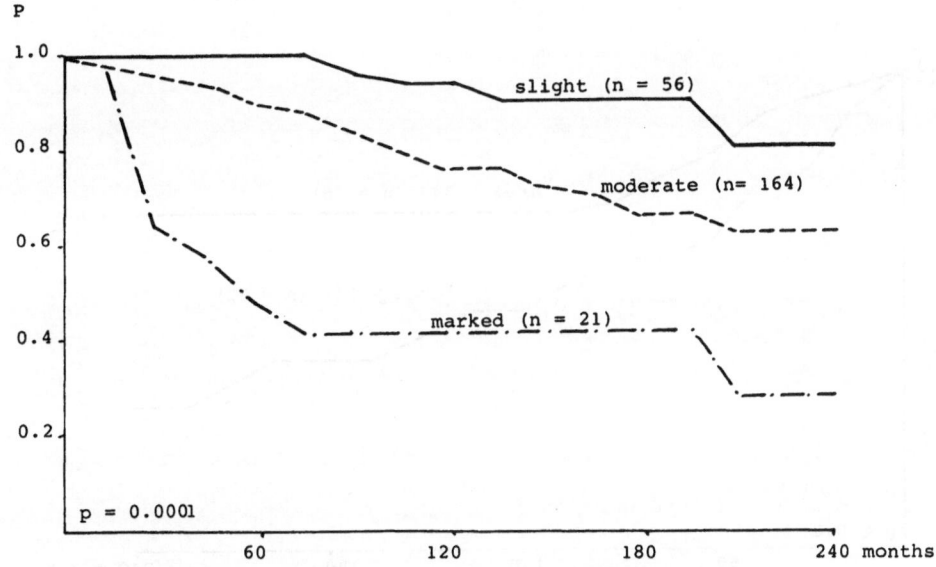

Fig. 4   Mostofi's grading system.   Survival in 241 patients
        according to nuclear pleomorphism.

significantly differing survival rates (Figure 4).   Patients with
marked pleomorphism of the nuclei do considerably worse than those
with moderate nuclear pleomorphism, while the group of patients
with slight nuclear pleomorphism has a 20 years survival as good as
80%.   Also the presence of mitoses identifies a group of patients
with a worse prognosis, although few patients have many mitoses in
their tumors.

    As nuclear pleomorphism seems to have prognostic importance we
tried to evaluate this objectively in order to obtain a reproducible
and objectively estimated parameter.

    With morphometry we measured 150 consecutive nuclei in each tumor
formation and for each parameter we calculated the variation-co-
efficient from the average value and the standard deviation.   We
used the variation coefficient as a standard for variation.   Figure
5 shows the morphometrically estimated variation in nuclear size
identifying two groups of patients with a significantly differing
survival pattern.   The value for V area (V stands for variation-
coefficient) of 34% was found empirically.

    The variation-co-efficient for "form ellipse" and for "form pe"
did not identify significantly in differing prognostic groups.

Prostatic carcinoma
Survival according to V area.

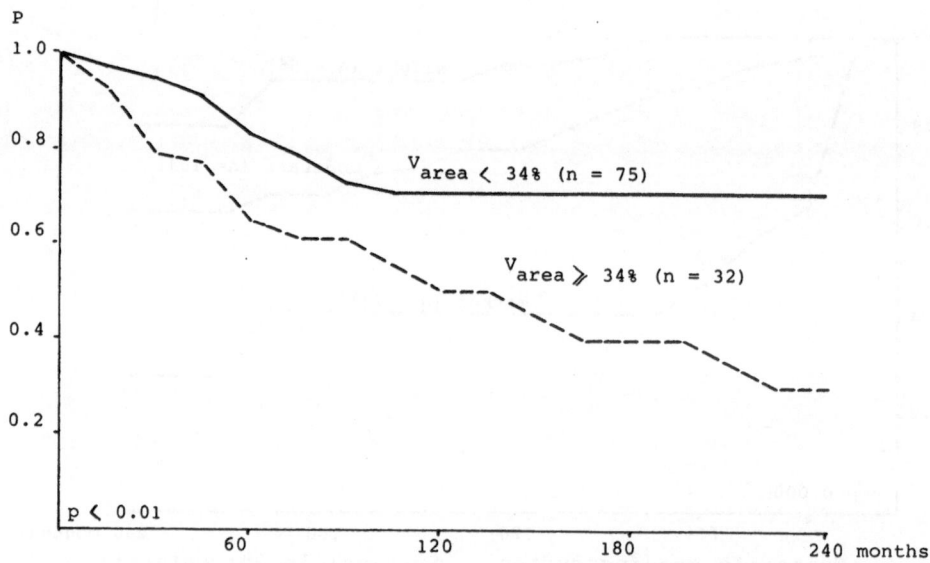

Fig. 5   Survival according to morphometrically estimated variation
          in nuclear size in 107 patients with prostate cancer.

DISCUSSION

As is shown, in Mostofi's grading system only a few parameters seem to have prognostic importance: glandular differentiation, whether the tumor forms only small, intermediate or large glands or whether it is growing in a cribriform or solid pattern.   Secondly anaplasia, and especially the variation in nuclear size and shape has prognostic importance.   The presence of mitoses may be of additional help, although most tumors show no mitoses.   This suggests that the Mostofi grading system could be made simpler than it now is.   With morphometry we were able to recognise two groups of patients with significantly differing survival patterns.   It seems that only variation in size might be of importance, as variation in shape failed to show prognostic significance.

Although preliminary, this study shows that there may be a role for morphometry in grading prostatic carcinoma.   It has the advantage of being objective and reproducible and is very easy to learn without special knowledge of grading.   Maybe morphometry can cast some light on the complex problem of grading prostatic carcinoma.   Until now we don't know the exact value of this technique in grading, but this will be a subject for further investigation.

ACKNOWLEDGMENTS

We are grateful to Dr W. Kern, who supplied us with the slides from the prostatectomy specimens and to the "Stichting Urologie 1973" and the Travel Fund "Professor Boerema" for their financial support.

REFERENCES

1.   F.K. Mostofi, Problems of Grading Carcinoma of the Prostate, Seminars in Oncology, 3:161 (1976).
2.   G.T. Mellinger, D. Gleason and J. Bailar, The Histology and Prognosis of Prostatic Cancer, J. Urol. 97:331 (1967)
3.   F.K. Mostofi, Grading of Prostatic Carcinoma, Cancer Chemother. Rep. 59:111 (1975).
4.   M. Harada, F.K. Mostofi, D.K. Corle, D.P. Byar and B.F. Trump, Preliminary Studies of Histologic Prognosis in Cancer of the Prostate, Cancer Treat. Rep. 61:223 (1977).
5.   R. Peto, M.C. Pike, P. Armitage, N.E. Breslow, D.R. Cox, S.V. Howard, N. Mantel, K. McPherson, J. Peto and P.G. Smith, Design and Analysis of Randomized Clinical Trials Requiring Prolonged Observation of Each Patient, Brit. J. Cancer, 34:585 (1976) and Brit. J. Cancer, 35:1 (1977).
6.   W.M. Cowan and D.F. Wann, A Computer System for the Measurement of Cell and Nuclear Sizes, J. Microscop. 99:331 (1973).
7.   C.J. Cornelisse, Real-Time Morphometric Analysis of Type I and Type II Fibers in Cryostat Sections of Human Muscle Biopsies. Path. Res. Pract. 166:218 (1980).

CARCINOMA OF THE PROSTATE: THE CLINICAL POTENTIAL OF BIOLOGICAL MARKERS OTHER THAN ACID PHOSPHATASE

M.R.G. Robinson, D. Daponte, A. Fryszman, and
C. Chandrasekaran

The General Infirmary
Pontefract
U.K.

INTRODUCTION

Carcinoma of the prostate is a slowly progressive disease which may be managed in many different ways. Treatment alternatives include no treatment, surgery, irradiation, endocrine therapy and cytotoxic chemotherapy. Diagnosis is easily achieved by rectal examination and biopsy, and scanning techniques are readily available for accurate clinical staging. The common osteosclerotic metastases are not, however, easily assessed for progression or regression and other marker lesions suitable for accurate measurement do not often occur, even in advanced progressive disease. Therefore a good biological tumour marker would be invaluable to aid the clinician monitor disease progression and the response to treatment and to assess new hormonal and chemotherapeutic regimes in phase II clinical trials. Although Huggins and Hodges (1) used plasma acid phosphatase as a marker for this tumour it has the disadvantage that it is rarely elevated in non-metastatic cancer and that in metastatic disease its sensitivity (percentage true positive elevations) as a marker is low. In addition during hormonal therapy disease progression is often not accompanied by rising plasma levels of this enzyme.

Many alternative specific and non-specific biological markers of potential value in the management of prostatic cancer have been investigated during the last decade. These include enzymes, antigens and acute phase reactant proteins.

Table 1.   Creatinine Kinase Levels in Patients
with Carcinoma of the Prostate

STAGE	ELEVATED CK-BB	
	(NO. ELEVATED/TOTAL PATIENTS)	
	FIELD et al 1980	SILVERMAN et al 1979
A	0/3	
B	1/26	3/4
C	0/35	2/2
D	11/46	10/11
D (with elevated acid phosphatase)	10/13	

POSSIBLE MARKERS

Creatinine Kinase

    Creatinine Kinase is a foeto-placental enzyme. Its BB isoenzyme
(SK-BB) is elevated in the serum of patients with metastatic carcinoma
of the prostate but not in normal adults (2). Table 1 reports the
experience of Silverman et al (3) and Field et al (4) in measuring
this isoenzyme in different clinical stages of prostatic carcinoma.
Homberger et al (2) found that it was elevated in 20 of 135 patients
with benign prostatic hyperplasia and in 10 of 35 patients with
bladder cancer. Therefore CK-BB does not have diagnostic value for
carcinoma of the prostate but may yet be of value in predicting the
development of metastases and in monitoring response to treatment.

Serum Lactic Dehydrogenase

    There has been much interest in serum lactic dehydrogenase
(SLDH) and its fifth isoenzyme SLDH-V as biological markers. Ishibi
(5) demonstrated that in 22 patients with prostatic cancer, low pretreatment plasma levels were associated with a 59% five year survival.
Only 28% of 29 patients with high pretreatment levels survived five
years. The prognostic significance of pre-treatment levels of total
LDH and SLDH-V were the same. Changes during therapy did not correlate with survival.

Fructose 1.6 Diphosphate Aldolase

This enzyme is associated with anaerobic glycolysis. Maganto-Pavon et al (6) found that in 43 patients plasma levels were elevated in 37% compared with 32% who had elevated prostatic acid phosphatase and 27% with elevated SLDH.

Bone Alkaline Phosphatase Isoenzyme

Wajsman et al (7) have measured plasma total and bone isoenzyme alkaline phosphatases in 105 patients with metastatic disease. Bone enzyme levels were elevated in 91%. The patients with higher pre-treatment levels of both phosphatases did not respond well to treatment. In patients with a partial remission there was a greater than 25% decrease in bone alkaline phosphatase levels. Therefore these enzymes have potential value in predicting prognosis and response to treatment.

Plasma Carcinoembryonic Antigen

Carcinoembryonic antigen has been extensively investigated in the management of many tumours. Kane and Paulson (8) in the study of 27 patients with carcinoma of the prostate found decreasing plasma levels in 19 patients responding to treatment and in eight with progressive disease. Increasing levels were found in only four responders and in 20 patients with progressive disease.

Hydroxyproline

Hydroxyproline is an amino acid constituent of the polypeptide chain in collagen. As such it is a marker of bone matrix turnover (9). Bishop and Fellows (10) found that whilst 24 hour urinary hydroxyproline excretion was normal in all of 14 patients with non-metastatic disease it was significantly elevated in all nine of their untreated patients with metastases. Urinary concentrations were high in only seven of 12 treated metastatic cases and reduction in the concentration during treatment corresponded with symptomatic improvement with little or no bone scan changes.

Urinary Fibronectin

Fibronectin is a high molecular weight glycoprotein. Episodic elevations have been observed in the early morning urine of patients with carcinoma of the prostate. Webb and Lin (11) found that it was not elevated in benign prostatic hyperplasia. Using a single assay there were 42% elevations in 32 patients with carcinoma of the prostate. In eight patients who had three sequential assays over a period of two to six months, elevations were found in 100%.

Serum Immunoglobulins

Serum Immunoglobulins reflect the host's humoral immune response to cancer and many other conditions. In 1972 Ablin and his colleagues (12) reported the remission of metastases after cryotherapy of the primary lesion in six patients. This phenomenon was associated with increased circulating antibodies. Gursel et al (13) confirmed that cryosurgery elevated circulating immunoglobulins IgG and IgM. They also found higher IgG levels in Stage II patients with untreated carcinoma of the prostate than in Stage IV patients. Lockwood et al (14) confirmed these results. In their series, in both treated and untreated patients, levels of IgG were higher in non-metastatic than in metastatic disease (Figure 1). In their series they were not able to show that oestrogen therapy like cryotherapy, produced elevations of immunoglobulins.

The immunoglobulin studies by Deture et al (15) give different results. They found significantly depressed levels of IgG in stage A and B disease compared with controls whilst the levels in patients with stages C and D disease were higher. The IgM levels were depressed in all stages of prostatic cancer and the IgA levels elevated in stages C and D disease.

The value of immunoglobulins in staging and monitoring prostatic cancer remains in doubt.

Acute Phase Reactant Proteins (APRP's)

APRP's are elevated in prostatic cancer as the total tumour mass increases (16,17). The levels of most APRP's are powerfully influenced by oestrogens making them unsuitable for monitoring Stilboestrol therapy (16,17,18). C-reactive protein (C-RP) and serum albumin concentrations, however remain independent of oestrogen control and Trautner and his colleagues (19) have shown that a chronic rise of C-RP, especially when preceded by normal levels for several months, strongly indicated disease progression. Albumin levels which fall with the development of metastases are a useful guide to overall biochemical status in a non-specific manner equivalent to performance status. Patients with high serum C-RP and low serum albumin levels have a poor prognosis.

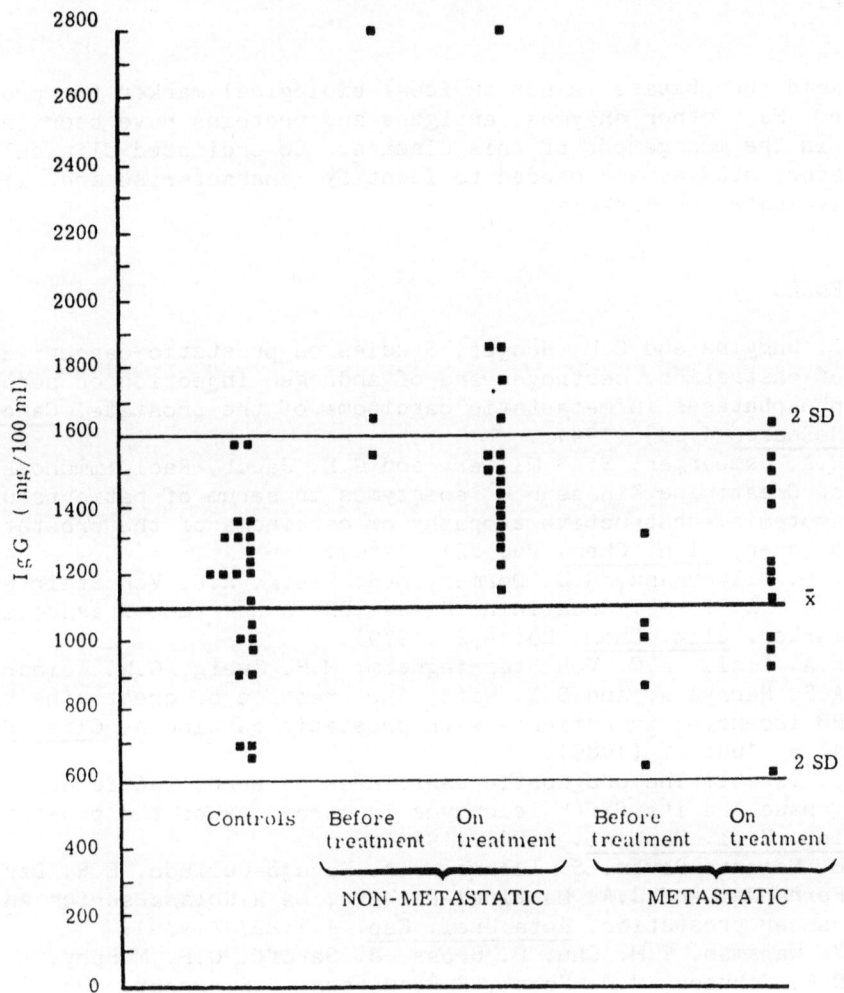

Fig. 1. Serum levels of IgG in patients with non-metastatic and
         with metastatic carcinoma of the prostate.

CONCLUSIONS

     This paper has reviewed some of the possible biochemical markers
of prostatic cancer alternative to acid phosphatase. An ideal marker
has not yet been found. Controlled clinical and laboratory studies
are required to identify and characterise all possible markers and
to explore their potential clinical use.

SUMMARY

    Acid phosphatase is not an ideal biological marker for prostatic
cancer. Many other enzymes, antigens and proteins have been investigated in the management of this disease. Co-ordinated clinical and
laboratory studies are needed to identify, characterise and clinically evaluate new markers.

REFERENCES

1. C. Huggins and C.U. Hodges, Studies on prostatic cancer: effect
    of castration, oestrogen and of androgen injection on serum
    phosphatases in metastatic carcinoma of the prostate, Cancer
    Research 1:293 (1941).
2. H.A. Homberger, S.A. Miller, and G.L. Jacob, Radioimmunoassay
    of Creatinine Kinase B - isoenzymes in serum of patients with
    azotemia, obstructive uropathy or carcinoma of the prostate or
    bladder, Clin. Chem. 26:1821 (1980).
3. L.M. Silvermann, G.B. Dormer, M.H. Zweig, A.C. Von Steirtegheim,
    and Z.A. Tokes, Creatinine Kinase BB: a new tumour associated
    marker, Clin. Chem. 25:1432 (1979).
4. R.A. Field, A.C. Von Steirtegheim, M.H. Zweig, G.W. Weinar,
    A.S. Narayana, and D.L. Witt, The presence of creatinine kinase
    BB isoenzyme in patients with prostatic carcinoma, Clin. Chem.
    Acta 100:267 (1980).
5. T. Ishibi, The prognostic usefulness of serum lactic dehydro-
    genase and its fifth isoenzyme in carcinoma of the prostate,
    Int. Urol. Nephrol. 8:221 (1976).
6. E. Maganto-Pavon, S. Isorna, J.A. Navajo-Guliudo, E.R. Darnial-
    Fernandez and J.A. Martinez-Pineiro, La aldolasa serica en el
    cancer prostatico, Acta Urol. Esp. 111:227 (1979).
7. Z. Wajsman, T.M. Chu, D. Bross, J. Saroff, G.P. Murphy,
    D.E. Johnson, W.W. Scott, R.P. Gibson, G.R. Prout, and
    J.D. Schmidt, Clinical significance of serum alkaline phosphat-
    ase isoenzyme levels in advanced prostatic carcinoma, J. Urol.
    119:244 (1978).
8. R.D. Kane and D.F. Paulson, Carcinoembryonic antigen as an
    adjunt to determination of clinical stage in prostatic cancer,
    Nat. Cancer. Inst. Mono. 49:231 (1978).
9. D.J. Prockop and K.I. Kivirikko, Relationship of hydroxyproline
    in urine to collagen metabolism, Ann. Int. Med. 66:1243 (1967).
10. M.C. Bishop and G.J. Fellows, Urinary hydroxyproline excretion -
    a marker of bone metastases in prostatic carcinoma, Brit. J.
    Urol. 49:711 (1977).
11. K.S. Webb and S.H. Lin, Urinary fibronectin, Invest. Urol.
    17:401 (1980).

12. R.J. Ablin, W.A. Soanes, and M.J. Gander, Alterations of serum proteins in patients with prostatic cancer following cryo-prostatectomy, Abstr. Clin. Res. 20:882 (1972).

13. E.O. Gursel, M.R. Megalli, M.S. Roberts, and R.J. Veenema, The effects of cryotherapy on serum immunoglobulins on patients with prostatic cancer, S.I.U. Proc. 16th Congress 2:256 (1973).

14. R. Lockwood, M. Sukhia, R.M. Basu, M.C. Stewardson, J. Sheard, and M.R.G. Robinson, Serum immunoglobulins before and during oestrogen treatment of carcinoma of the prostate, unpublished data.

15. F.A. Deture, L. Deardourff, A.G. Kauffman, and Y.M. Centifanto, A comparison of serum immunoglobulins from patients with non-neoplastic prostate and prostatic carcinoma, J. Urol. 120:435 (1978).

16. U.S. Seal, R.P. Doe, D.P. Byar, D.K. Corle, and the Veterans Administration Co-operative Urological Research Group, Response of plasma fibrinogen and plasminogen to hormone treatment and the relation of pre-treatment values to mortality in patients with prostatic cancer, Cancer 38:1108 (1976).

17. A. Milford-Ward, E.H. Cooper, and A.L. Haughton, Acute phase reactant proteins in prostatic cancer, Brit. J. Urol. 49:411 (1977).

18. C.B. Laurell, S. Kullander, and J. Thorell, Effect of combined estrogen-progestin contraceptive on the levels of individual plasma proteins, Scand. J. Clin. Lab. Invest. 21:337 (1968).

19. K. Trautner, E.H. Cooper, S. Howarth, and A. Milford Ward, An evaluation of serum protein profiles in the long term surveillance of prostatic cancer, Scand. J. Urol. Nephrol. 14:143 (1980).

THE PREDICTIVE VALUE OF SERUM C-REACTIVE PROTEIN (CRP) LEVELS IN UNTREATED PROSTATIC CANCER

A. Akdas, E.H. Cooper, P.H Smith and M.R.G. Robinson

Unit for Cancer Research
University of Leeds
U.K.

C-reactive protein (CRP) is an acute phase reactant protein (APRP). The APRP's are a group of mainly glycoproteins which alter their plasma concentrations in response to a variety of stimuli including tissue injury, acute and chronic inflammation, connective tissue disease and cancer (1-3). Most of them are also influenced by oestrogens, which are often employed therapeutically in the management of prostatic cancer. CRP differs from the others in this respect (4). Plasma concentrations are, however, elevated as tumour burden increases (5). This present study evaluates the pre-treatment levels of CRP and serum acid phosphatase (SAP) in patients with benign prostatic hyperplasia and carcinoma of the prostate to determine the prognostic value of these tumour markers in the management of malignant prostatic disease.

METHOD

Fifty patients with category T3 prostatic cancer were studied in the prostatic clinics of St James's University Hospital, Leeds, and Pontefract General Infirmary. Of these 19 had MO category cancer and 31 category M1 disease. An additional 15 patients with benign prostatic hyperplasia were also investigated. Pretreatment studies included clinical history and examination, digital examination of the prostatic gland, weight and haemoglobin measurements, histological confirmation of the diagnosis by transurethral resection or needle biopsy and isotopic bone scans for metastases with x-ray confirmation of hot spots. Minimal follow-up was at six-monthly intervals for the patients with malignant disease and included clinical history and examination, weight, haemoglobin estimation and bone scans.

Single radial immunodiffusion (6) was used to measure CRP (normal range 0-11 mg/l) and an enzymatic method (7) to estimate SAP (normal range 0-4 IU/l).

The 50 patients being treated for carcinoma of the prostate received different types of hormonal therapy.   Twenty-four of them (48%) had clinical progression during the period of follow-up.   Progression was defined as any increase in size of an existing marker lesion or the appearance of new lesions on a bone scan.   Subjective factors taken into consideration were loss of weight, pain, performance status and anaemia.

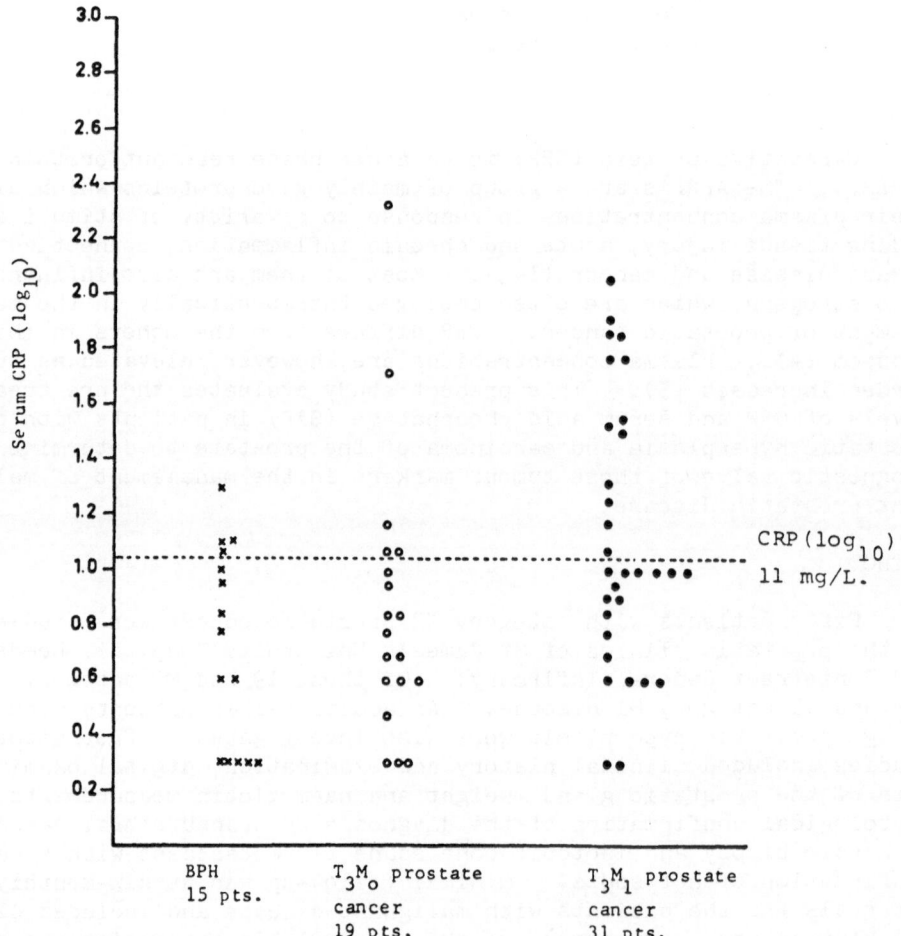

Fig 1.   Pretreatment serum CRP ($\log_{10}$) levels in BPH and prostate cancer.

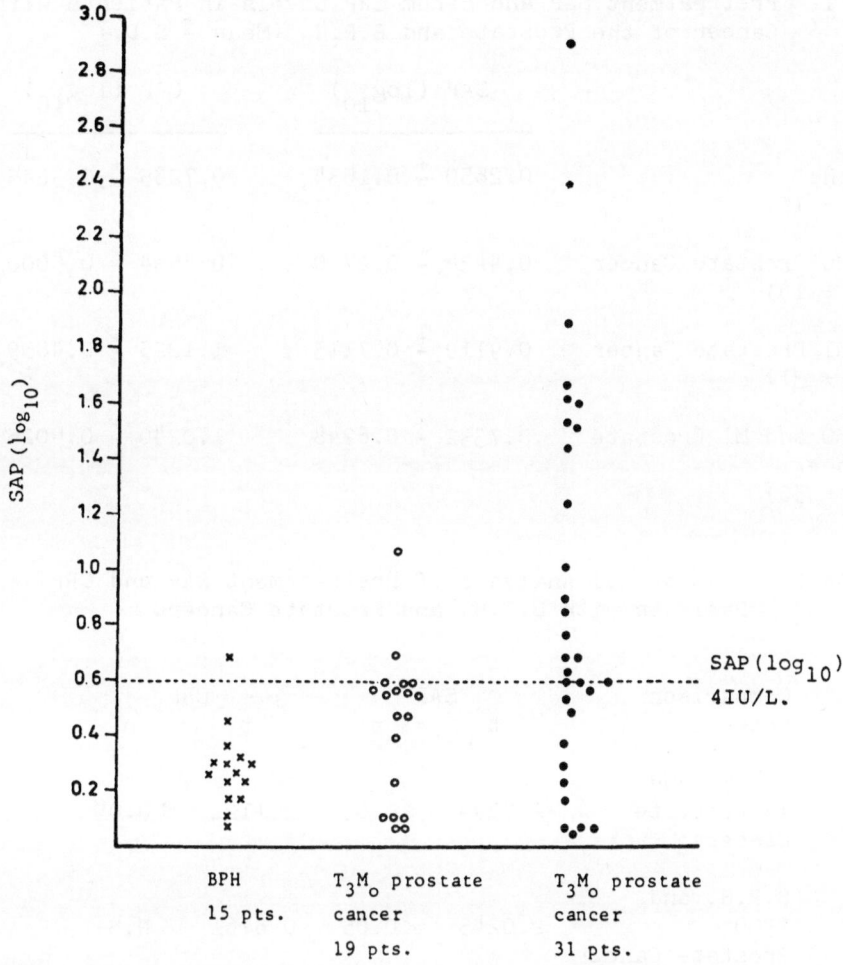

Fig 2. Pretreatment SAP levels in BPH and prostate cancer.

RESULTS

    Distribution of serum CRP levels are shown in figure 1 and the
SAP levels in figure 2.   In order to obtain a normal distribution
of this skewed data, the mean values of the results expressed as
logarithms are shown in table 1.   Statistical analyses employing
Student's t test and Gehan's test for censored data (8) show that
there is a significant difference between the CRP levels in patients
with BPH and both T3 M0 and T3 M1 disease (P <0.05) (Table 2).

Table 1.   Pretreatment SAP and Serum CRP Levels in Patients with
           Cancer of the Prostate and B.P.H. (Mean $\pm$ S.D.)

	SAP (log_{10})	CRP (log_{10})
B.P.H. (n = 15)	0.2850 $\pm$ 0.1534	0.7285 $\pm$ 0.3645
T3 M0 Prostate Cancer (n = 19)	0.4438 $\pm$ 0.2710	0.8634 $\pm$ 0.5000
T3 M1 Prostate Cancer (n = 31)	0.9119 $\pm$ 0.7113	1.1225 $\pm$ 0.4859
T3 M0 and M1 Prostate Cancer (n = 50)	0.7332 $\pm$ 0.6248	1.0240 $\pm$ 0.5025

Table 2.   Statistical Analysis of Pretreatment SAP and CRP in
           Patients with B.P.H. and Prostate Cancer.

Comparison Between	SAP		CRP	
	t	p	t	p
B.P.H. and T3 Prostate Cancer	2.7399	<0.05	2.1121	<0.05
B.P.H. and T3M0 Prostate Cancer	2.0245	<0.05	0.8761	N.S.
B.P.H. and T3M1 Prostate Cancer	3.3577	<0.05	2.7786	<0.05
T3M0 and T3M1 Prostate Cancer	2.7403	<0.05	1.8103	N.S.

The frequency of elevated levels of serum CRP (>11 mg/l) and
SAP (>4 IU/l) for benign hyperplasia and the different cancer categories are shown in Table 3.

Table 4 shows the relationship between elevated and non-elevated
SAP and CRP levels in patients with T3, M1 carcinoma of the prostate.
In 20 of them (64.5%) the SAP and/or CRP levels were elevated and

Table 3. Frequency of Elevated Levels of CRP (>11 mg/l)
and SAP (>4 IU/1) in Patients with Cancer of
the Prostate and B.P.H.

Disease	CRP No. (%)	SAP No. (%)	CRP and SAP No. (%)
B.P.H.	4/15 (26.7)	1/15 (6.7)	0/15 (0)
T3M0 Prostate Cancer	5/19 (26.3)	2/19 (10.5)	0/19 (0)
T3M1 Prostate Cancer	4/31 (12.9)	3/31 (25.8)	9/31 (29)

Table 4. The Relation of Pretreatment SAP and CRP Levels
in T3M1 Prostate Cancer.

Serum CRP Levels (mg/l)

SAP Levels (IU/L)	CRP $\leqslant$ 11	CRP > 11	Total
SAP $\leqslant$ 4	10	4	14
SAP > 4	8	9	17
Total	18	13	31

Table 5. Pretreatment SAP and CRP Levels in Patients Who Had
Progression as Clinical Response After Their Hormonal
Treatment.

	SAP $\leqslant$ 4IU/1 and CRP $\leqslant$ 11 mg/1	SAP > 4IU/1 CRP >11mg/1	SAP > 4IU/1 and CRP > 11 mg/1	Total
T3M0	1	–	2	–	3
T3M1	3	6	3	9	21
Total	4	6	5	9	24

of these 18 had progressive malignant disease within five months of
commencing endocrine therapy (Table 5).

DISCUSSION

The APRP's reflect tumour load in many cancers and are also
influenced by trauma and infection.   Therefore they have no place
as diagnostic tumour markers (4,9,10).   CRP levels are not influenced by oestrogens and urinary tract infections without fever but
they are powerfully stimulated by acute retention of urine (11).

Although SAP is a specific tumour marker in patients with T3, M1
disease, it is only elevated in 60% of those patients with demonstrable metastases (12).   CRP levels tend to rise with tumour progression and this study is unique in demonstrating that high pre-treatment levels of SAP and/or CRP predicted clinical progression within
five months in 18 of 21 patients.   If these findings are confirmed
in larger studies, there is a strong case for treating such patients
with a combination of hormones and chemotherapy from the time of
diagnosis.

REFERENCES

1.   C.L. Fischer and C.W. Gill, Acute Phase Proteins, in "Serum
      Abnormalities, Diagnostic and Clinical Aspects", E.S. Ritzman
      and J.C. Daniels (eds), Little Brown and Co, Boston (1975) p.331.
2.   A. Koj, Acute Phase Reactants, Their Synthesis, Turnover and
      Biological Significance, in "Structure and Function of Plasma
      Proteins", A.C. Allison (ed), Plenum Press, London (1974) p.73.
3.   J.A. Owen, Effect of Injury on Plasma Proteins, Advances in
      Clin. Chem. 9:1 (1967).
4.   A. Milford Ward, E.H. Cooper and A.L. Houghton, Acute Phase
      Reactant Proteins in Prostatic Cancer, Brit. J. Urol. 49:411
      (1977).
5.   J. Kohn, M. Hernandez and P.G. Riches, The Value of Acute Phase
      Reactants in the Management of the Disease, La Ricerca in Clin-
      ica e in Laboratorio, 8:61 (1978).
6.   G. Mancini, A.O. Carbonara and J.F. Heremans, Immunological
      Quantitation of Antigens by Single Radial Immunodiffusion,
      Immunochemistry, 2:235 (1965).
7.   M.A. Andersch and A.J. Szczypinski, Use of P-Nitrophenyl Phos-
      phate as the Substrate in Determination of Serum Acid Phospha-
      tase, Amer. J. Clin. Pathol. 17:571 (1947).
8.   B.W. Brown Jr. and M. Hollander, Censored Data, in "Statistics.
      A Biomedical Introduction", B.W. Brown Jr. and M. Hollander (eds)
      John Wiley and Sons, New York (1977) p. 341.
9.   J.A. Child, E.H. Cooper, S. Illingworth and T.S. Worthy, Bio-
      chemical Markers in Hodgkin's disease and Non-Hodgkin Lymphoma,
      Recent Results in Cancer Res. 64:180 (1978).

10. J.R.G. Bastable, B. Richards, S. Howarth and E.H. Cooper, Acute
     Phase Reactant Proteins in the Management of Carcinoma of the
     Bladder, <u>Brit. J. Urol</u>. 51:283 (1979).
11. E.H. Cooper, Personal Communication (1978).
12. H. Trautner, E.H. Cooper, S. Haworth and A. Milford Ward, An
     Evaluation of Serum Protein Profiles in the Long Term Surveil-
     lance of Prostatic Carcinoma, <u>Scand. J. Urol</u>. 14:143 (1980).

IMMUNOLOGICAL DETECTION OF PROSTATIC ACID PHOSPHATASE:

FIVE YEARS' EXPERIENCE

A.C. Jöbsis, G.T.B. Sanders, G.P. de Vries

The University Hospital
Amsterdam
The Netherlands

INTRODUCTION

In 1976, a rabbit antiserum was raised in Amsterdam against that isoenzyme of acid phosphatase (EC 3.1.3.2) which is usually designated prostatic acid phosphatase (PAP). The antigen used consisted of purified seminal plasma from vasectomized men. This antiserum has been extensively documented (1,2). The antiserum has been used principally in the field of histopathology and clinical chemistry.

PAP, a secretory glycoprotein, can be distinguished from most other acid phosphatase isoenzymes by, for example, inhibition tests (it is relatively insensitive to formaldehyde, but sensitive to L+tartrate (3,4) and by substrate specificity tests such as phosphorylcholine (5). These biochemical differences between prostatic and non-prostatic carcinomas enable the histopathologist to differentiate between them in cryostat sections using histochemical techniques (Fig. 1). But this method, which is so advantageous to the patient, cannot be applied once the tissue has been embedded in paraffin since ethanol irreversibly inhibits the PAP activity. This enzyme histochemical technique can therefore rarely be applied to small fragments of tissue such as needle biopsies or skeletal biopsies, which usually must be embedded completely for the pure morphological investigation. This is not only of importance in the differential diagnosis between bladder and prostatic carcinomas, but also in revealing the primary location of an otherwise occult prostatic carcinoma. The importance of the latter point is illustrated by the findings of Butler (6) that 18 out of 200 cases of prostatic carcinoma presented with a metastasis in the left supraclavicular lymph node. The limitations imposed by the inhibition

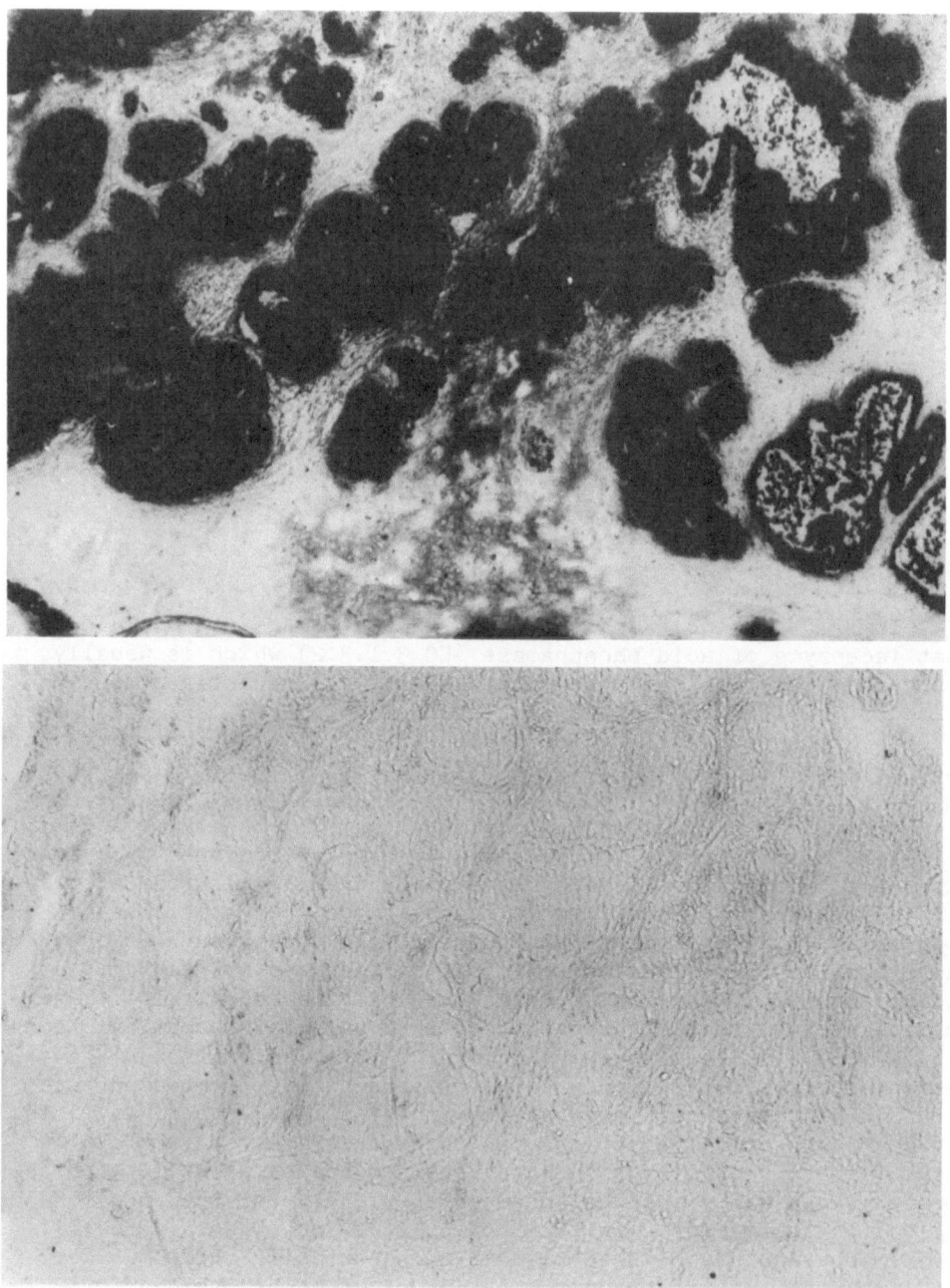

Fig. 1. Enzyme histochemical activity in two consecutive, formalin
         fixed cryostat sections of prostate with phosphorylcholine
         as substrate. The activity so strongly present in the
         epithelium (A) has been inhibited by L+tartrate (B).

of PAP activity by ethanol might be circumvented by the application
of immunohistochemical techniques for the antigenicity of a series
of secretory glycoproteins (alpha-1-antitrypsin, immunoglobulins,
thyroglobulin) is not essentially altered by the procedure of paraffin
embedding.

HISTOPATHOLOGY

     The Amsterdam antiserum was applied as the primary antiserum in
the indirect peroxidase technique (1) on paraffin sections of 300
cases of proven prostatic carcinoma (100 autopsies and 200 Surgicals)
and 350 cases of non-prostatic tumour. A tumour was considered to
be non-prostatic either on clinical grounds, histopathological grounds
and clinical chemical grounds or on autopsy grounds. The 350 non-
prostatic tumours came from 24 different organs amongst which were 70
bladder and/or urethral carcinomas, 10 kidney carcinomas, 10 testis
tumours and 10 seminal vesicle carcinomas. In several cases the
indirect fluorescence technique or the peroxidase-anti-peroxidase
technique (7) as post-primary antiserum methods was also applied,
either on paraffin sections or on cryostat sections. The results,
visually assessed, did not show essential differences between these
techniques except for a higher discriminative staining with the peroxidase-anti-peroxidase technique. Some cytological and haematological smears were also investigated. Control incubations were
performed each time (1). The results (Fig. 2, Table 1) show that
the immunological demonstration of PAP in paraffin sections circum-
vents the restrictions of the enzyme histochemical approach. The
prostatic epithelium in smears also gives a positive reaction for
PAP. The false negative percentage in the surgical material was
1.5% for the primary focus and 3% for the metastases. In the autopsy
material there were 3% overall false negative results (Table 1).
This is in agreement with the results in smaller series of other
groups (8,9,10). Apart from the prostatic tumours none of the 100
other urological tumours gave a positive reaction for PAP. This
may be of significance especially with regard to the differential
diagnosis of bladder versus prostatic carcinoma or in cases of a
metastasis as presenting symptom of a carcinoma (6). Only 7 positive
results were obtained in the 350 patients without prostatic cancer -
6 out of the 12 insulomas (11) and one out of the 10 carcinoids, and
do not detract from the practical application of this technique.

     The false negatives may result from several different causes:-

1.   The immunological staining of PAP in carcinoma may in general
not only be less intense than in benign epithelium but may also show
great variation within one section (Fig. 2). When a small tissue
fragment is used, for instance a needle biopsy, the pathologist
might only encounter the phosphatase negative part of the prostatic
carcinoma.

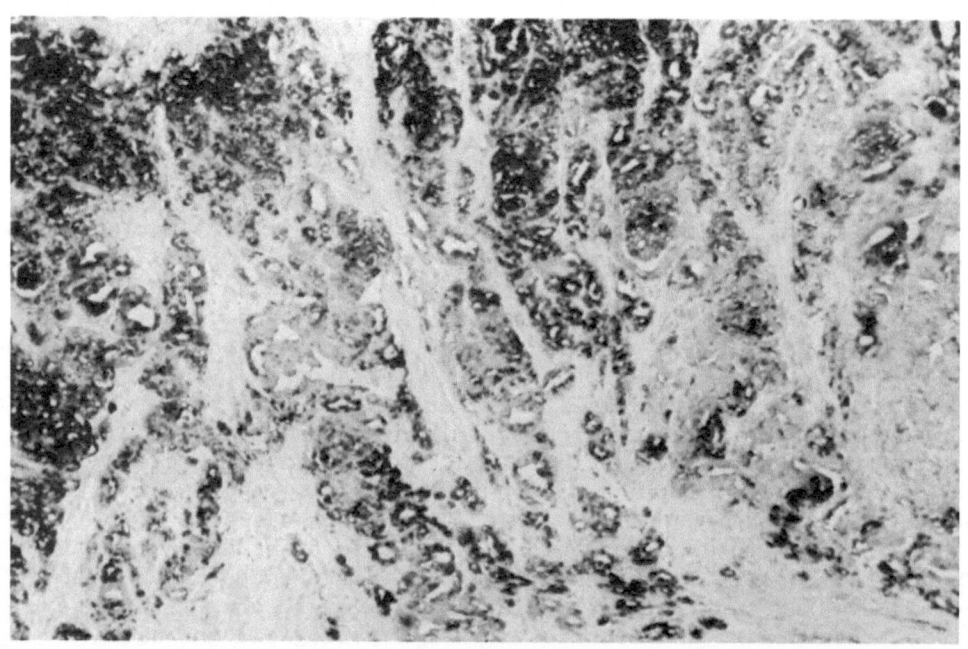

Fig. 2.   Immunologically demonstrated PAP in paraffin section of
          prostatic carcinoma. The great variation in intensity is
          clearly shown. Indirect peroxidase technique with diamino-
          benzidine as substrate. Weak counterstain with haematoxylin.

Table 1.   Intensity of Immunohistochemical Staining
           (300 cases, paraffin, indirect peroxidase)

	n	++	+[a]	(+)	-
Surgical material	200				
Carcinoma:					
Primary	200	5	81	111	3[c]
Metastasis	69[b]		20	47	2[d]
Benign epith.	172	172			
Autopsy material	107[e]				
Carcinoma:					
Primary	90[b]		29	59	2[f]
Metastasis	46		10	32	4[g]
Benign epith.	80	71	7	2	

Notes to Table 1

a. ++ strong, + moderate, (+) focally moderate or weakly positive,
    - negative.
b. in 69 of the surgical cases metastases could also be investigated;
    in 17 of the autopsy cases only the metastases could be inves-
    tigated.
c. Only tiny bits of carcinoma present in the needle biopsy.
d. Inappropriate decalcifying solution.
e. In 7 of the 200 cases in which surgical material was investigated
    an autopsy was subsequently performed.
f. Adenoid cystic carcinomas.
g. Only tiny bits of carcinoma present but in 3 cases the primary
    tumour showed focally moderate staining.

2.   Autolysis diminishes the antigenicity of PAP. In general, the
autopsy material and the inner parts of prostatectomy preparations
stain less intensely than biopsies or prostatic "chips".

3.   Some special fixatives, for instance Zenker's solution, or
inappropriate decalcification (by the almost obsolete nitric acid
procedure) diminish the antigenicity. Preparation of tissue for
paraffin sections will, in general, reduce the antigenicity slightly.
Granulocytes in smears show a weak positive reaction for PAP whereas
in paraffin sections no positive results could be obtained using our
technique.

4.   Hormonal treatment reduces the intensity of immunostaining of
PAP as could be shown in 13 cases (androgen deprivation or oestrogen
therapy).

5.   False negatives may also result from suboptimal circumstances
during the incubation procedure (10). For instance, in 12 cases a
positive reaction could only be established after application of the
more sensitive post-primary antiserum procedure (peroxidase-anti-
peroxidase technique). This again indicates the importance of
standardising the investigation in order to obtain comparable
results from different scientific groups.

     Table 2 shows the results of a comparison between the visually
assessed intensity of immunostaining in the dominant carcinoma field
and the grade of differentiation in the same field in the preceding
HE section (12). This short series clearly indicates the need for
objective quantification of both the intensity of immunostaining and
the parameters for morphological differentiation. In a pilot study,
we measured the staining intensity photometrically (13) in paraffin
sections of three positive carcinomas (grade II). The staining
intensity of the carcinomas was clearly less than that of the benign
epithelium in the same section. This may indicate the potential

Table 2.   Comparison of Grades and
           Immunostaining Intensity*

Grade	n	++	+	(+)	-
0	43	43			
I	2		2		
II	14	1	10	3	
III	24	1	20	2	1
IV	10		3	7	
Totals	50	2	35	12	1

*Indirect peroxidase, immunological staining of paraffin sections
(4u) of transurethral resected prostatic carcinomas (50 cases) of
which 43 also contained benign hyperplastic epithelium ("grade 0").
Visual assessment. Gaeta's grading system (1981).

value of the photometric technique in the differential diagnosis of
grade I adenocarcinomas and benign epithelial proliferation of the
prostate.

     The antiserum also has a more academic application in the field
of cell biology. For instance, the more precise localization of PAP
at the cell organelle level might shed some light on the background
of the hormonally influenced synthesis of PAP. Whereas acid phosphatases usually are localized in lysosomes for internal cell use,
PAP is a typical secretory product of the cell and might be localized
in the Golgi system. Until now we have only succeeded in developing
the technique of immunohistochemical demonstration of PAP at the
ultrastructural level. Work is in progress to collect the conclusive
data. The fact that human PAP is species specific (with the exception of the chimpanzee) presents difficulties in experimental studies.
We must therefore resort to fresh surgical material or to organ or
cell cultures.

CLINICAL CHEMISTRY

     The immunologically determined PAP serum level values were
compared with those obtained by means of the classical indirect
enzymatic procedure (4). The first mentioned one - usually called
enzyme immuno assay (EIA) or immuno fluorescent assay (IFA) depending
on the substrate and type of measurement used - consists of the
following procedure (Fig. 3): IgG is isolated from our antiserum
chromatographically and used to coat polystyrene tubes. Addition
of the serum sample results in a specific binding of PAP and the
enzymatic activity of the bound antigen (PAP) is measured either by

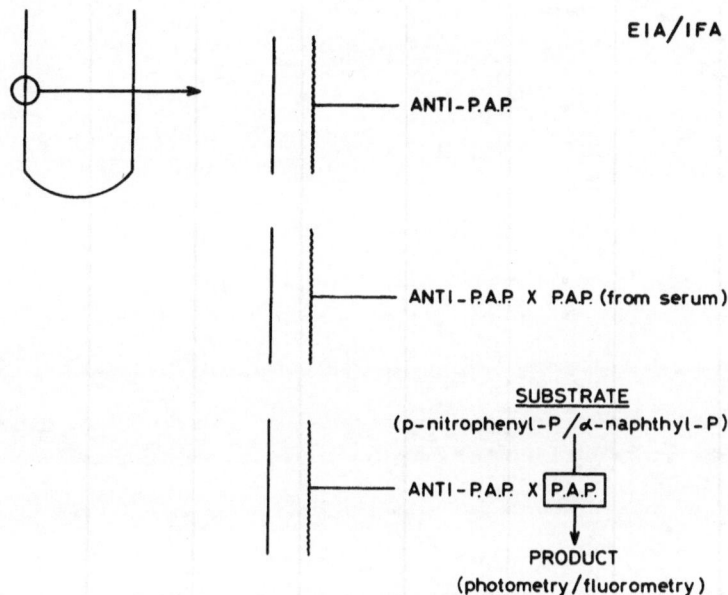

Fig. 3.   Schematic representation of the immunological method applied
for the determination of the PAP serum level.

spectrophotometry (paranitrophenylphosphate) or by fluorometry (alpha-
naphthylphosphate). Results of the EIA and IFA correspond. These
two immunoassays are of the same level of sensitivity as the radio-
immuno assay (RIA) (14) and the enzyme linked immunosorbent assay
(ELISA) now under development in our laboratory. The diagnostic
value of our immunological techniques has been established in a
number of patients (Fig. 4). The upper limit of normal is 1.0 U/l.
The diagnosis in all patients was made histopathologically. A prostatic carcinoma with metastases (P.Ca + m) had a raised PAP serum
level more often than a prostatic carcinoma without metastases (P.Ca).
Treatment reduces the PAP values (P.Ca tr.). As can be seen in Fig.
4, these three groups consisted of 56 cases. Patients with bladder
carcinoma (35 cases), bronchus carcinoma (17 cases) and other malignancies such as pancreatic (exocrine type) carcinomas (25 cases), were
used as controls. Benign prostatic hyperplasia (P. hyp.) showed an
elevated value in two out of 54 cases. It is especially in this
group of patients where sequential determination of PAP levels is
deemed necessary. Although the sensitivity of the immunological
method is inadequate for the early detection of a prostatic carcinoma
the specificity in the overall non-prostatic cancer patient group
(99%) and the sensitivity (7 out of 26 untreated cases; 73%) are an
improvement on the classical enzymatic method (specificity 85%). Our
sensitivity percentage corresponds with those recently reported by
other groups (15,16).

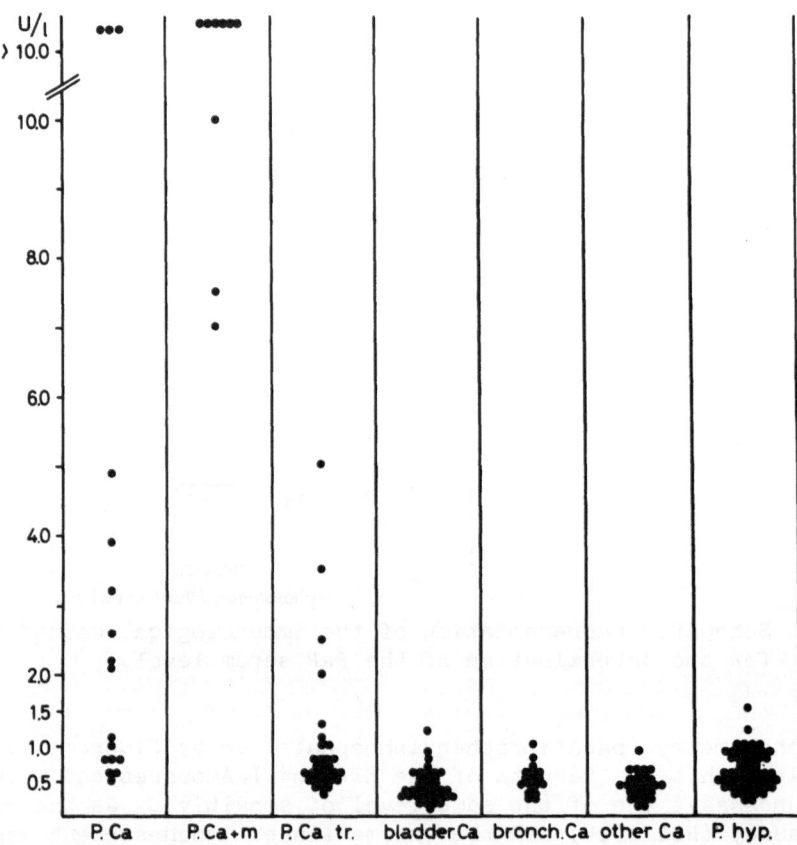

Fig. 4.   Results of the determination of PAP in the serum of the
         various patient groups. For explanation of the abbrev-
         iations see text. The upper limit of normal is 1.0 u/1.

CONCLUSION

    After five years of experience we may make the following obser-
vation: The application of the anti-PAP-serum tool has proved to be
a significant advantage in the field of histopathology, but the
sensitivity is less than we expected with regard to clinical chemistry. We cannot therefore speak of a screening test for prostatic
carcinoma in an early stage (16,17). A new prostate specific antigen demonstrable in serum has been announced (18). The chances that
this antigen will offer a screening test for prostatic carcinoma are
low for this recently discovered antigen is also demonstrable in
serum of normal males. The prime objective remains the demonstration
of a prostate specific antigen which can always be found in the serum
in the early stages of a carcinoma. The experiences with carcino-
embryonal antigen and foetal alkaline phosphatase in connection with

colon carcinoma, however, indicate that the chances of success within the near future are, at best, limited.

ACKNOWLEDGEMENTS

The authors are grateful to Dr. H. Barrowclough, who revised the English manuscript. The work was partially supported by grant GU-Path 79-4 from the "Koningin Wilhelmina Fonds" and by grant 28-510 from the "Praeventiefonds".

The excellent technical and administrative assistance of Mrs. M.Y. van Duuren, Mrs. B.C. Fortgens, Mrs. M.E. Gräber, Mrs. C.M. van Nieuwkoop and Mr. H.G. Lagerwey, Mr. W.P. Meun and Mr. A.J. Tigges is gratefully acknowledged.

REFERENCES

1. A.C. Jöbsis, G.P. de Vries, R.R.H. Anholt, and G.T.B. Sanders, Demonstration of the prostatic origin of metastases. An immuno-histochemical method for formalin-fixed embedded tissue, Cancer 41: 1788 (1978).

2. G.P. de Vries, A.W. Slob, A.C. Jöbsis, A.E.F.H. Meijer, and G.T.B. Sanders, Prostate-specific acid phosphatase. Purification and specific antibody production in rabbits, Am. J. Clin. Path. 72: 944 (1979).

3. M.A.M. Abdul-Fadl and E.J. King, Properties of the acid phos-phatases of erythrocytes and of the human prostate gland, Biochem. J. 45: 51 (1949).

4. C.P. Modder, Investigations on acid phosphatase activity in human plasma and serum, Clin. Chim. Acta. 43: 205 (1973).

5. J.A. Serrano, W.A. Shannon Jr., N.J. Sternberger, H.L. Wasser-krug, A.A. Serrano, and A.M. Seligman, The cytochemical demon-stration of prostatic acid phosphatase using a new substrate, phosphorylcholine, J. Histochem. Cytochem. 24: 1046 (1976).

6. J.J. Butler, C.D. Howe, and E.D. Johnson, Enlargement of the supra-calvicular lymph nodes as the initial sign of prostatic carcinoma, Cancer 27: 1055 (1971).

7. L.A. Sternberger, "Immunocytochemistry," 2nd Edition, John Wiley and Sons, New York (1979).

8. C.Y. Li, W.K.W. Lam, and L.T. Yam, Immunohistochemical diagnosis of prostatic cancer with metastasis, Cancer 46: 706 (1980).

9. M. Nadji, S.Z. Tabei, A. Castro, T. Ming Chu, and A.R. Morales, Prostatic origin of tumours. An immunohistochemical study, Am. J. Clin. Path. 73: 735 (1980).

10. G. Aumüller, C. Phol, R.L. van Etten, and J. Seitz, Immuno-histochemistry of acid phosphatase in the human prostate: Normal and pathologic, Virch. Arch. B 35: 249 (1981).

11. B.K. Choe, E.J. Pontes, N.R. Rose, and M.D. Henderson, Expression of human prostatic acid phosphatase in a pancreatic islet cell carcinoma. Invest. Urol. 15: 312 (1977).

12. J.F. Gaeta, Glandular profiles and cellular patterns in prostatic cancer grading, Urology (Suppl.) 17: 33 (1981).

13. J.S. Ploem, N. Verwoerd, J. Bonnet, and G. Koper, An automated microscope for quantative cytology combining television image analysis and stage scanning microphotometry, J. Histochem. & Cytochem. 27: 136 (1979).

14. C.L. Lee, C.S. Killian, G.P. Murphy, and T.M. Chu, A solid-phase immunoadsorbent assay for serum prostatic acid phosphatase, Clin. Chim. Acta 101: 209 (1980).

15. J.C. Griffiths, Prostate-specific acid phosphatase: Re-evaluation of radioimmunoassay in diagnosing prostatic disease, Clin. Chem. 26: 433 (1980).

16. R.A. Watson and D.B. Tang, The predictive value of prostatic acid phosphatase as a screening test for prostatic cancer, New Engl. J. Med. 303: 497 (1980).

17. R.A. Watson and D.B. Tang, Diagnosis of prostatic cancer, New Engl. J. Med. 304: 51 (1980).

18. M.C. Wang, L.D. Papsidero, L. Kuriyama, L.A. Valenzuela, G.P. Murphy, and T.M. Chu, Prostatic antigen: A new potential marker for prostatic cancer, The Prostate 2: 89 (1981).

IMMUNOLOGICAL ASSAYS FOR PROSTATIC

ACID PHOSPHATASE

N.A. Romas and M Tannenbaum

Columbia-Presbyterian Medical Center
New York
U.S.A.

ABSTRACT

Several immunological assays for the determination of prostatic acid phosphatase (PAP) in the diagnosis of prostate carcinoma have been developed since the demonstration of a specific antibody to PAP. Some of these assays have demonstrated increased specificity and a moderate degree of increased sensitivity over standard biochemical assays. The data presented should be used as routine screening tests for the early detection of prostatic carcinoma.

Acid Phosphatase (AP) was the first "tumor marker" to be measured in the blood and over 40 years have elapsed since an elevation of the serum AP level was observed in patients with prostatic carcinoma (1). However, significant elevations in the level of this enzyme have been observed in other diseases, as well as elevations of other tissue phosphatases. Many improvements in the biochemical technique have been introduced, but none have been used successfully to detect the tissue origin of this ubiquitous enzyme. The findings that prostatic acid phosphatase (PAP) is antigenically distinct from AP of other tissues opened a new horizon in the measurement of AP in prostatic cancer. On the basis of this immuno-chemical specificity, various immunological methods were developed.

Counterimmunoelectrophoresis (CIEP) is a rapid semi-quantitative method for measuring PAP. Romas et al (2) have compared a standard biochemical method with CIEP on a wide spectra of prostatic and non-prostatic diseases. Non-prostatic malignancies and other disorders associated with a raised acid phosphatase by the biochemical method were found to be non-reactive for PAP by CIEP.

Patients under treatment with various stages of prostatic carcinoma showed comparable elevations by both methods (35%). In untreated patients, the CIEP was statistically most sensitive in Stage A2 lesions (39% by CIEP versus 14% by chemical). Table 1 summarizes the CIEP findings in clinically staged prostatic carcinoma in two large series.

The initial report on radioimmunoassay (RIA) by Foti and associates (2), reported significant elevations of PAP not only with disseminated adenocarcinoma of the prostate but also in those with disease limited to the prostate. Subsequently, no other investigator has reported such encouraging results. Bruce et al (4) have recently attempted to define the role of RIA for PAP in prostatic carcinoma. These investigators compared three RIA assays and demonstrated marked similarity in results for the various stages of malignant disease and an increase in the percentage of elevation of PAP with increasing tumor burden. Significantly, the mean detection rate for localized prostatic carcinoma (Stage A and B) was only 22% (from 14 to 31%). However, this study not only showed relatively low sensitivity for intracapsular adenocarcinoma of the prostate, but also a false positive rate ranging from 3 to 27% in patients with benign prostatic hypertrophy. Other investigators, with the exception of Foti et al (2), have also failed to produce encouraging results in patients with

Table 1. Results of Acid Phosphtase by CIEP (% Positive)

	Stage			
Reference	A	B	C	D
Romas et al. (2)	39	22	46	97
Murphy et al. (5)	38	35	49	69

Table 2. Comparison of Immunological Assays for PAP (% Elevations)

Stage	Biochemical	RIA	CIEP	IEA
A(27)	7	26	0	26
B(12)	33	33	25	25
C(29)	55	72	52	62
D(18)	91	100	94	94
BPH(82)	9.1	17.1	1.2	8.5

localized prostatic carcinoma. These authors concluded that findings
of a low sensitivity for patients with early prostatic carcinoma and
the high falsely positive rate in patients with benign disease limit
severely the use of these assays in screening trials.

The present authors conducted a comparison study determining
PAP by four different methodologies (biochemical, CIEP, RIA, and
immunoenzyme IEA) on patients with various stages of untreated
prostate carcinoma (Table 2). The study indicates that RIA and IEA
were the most sensitive assays but RIA had the highest percentage of
false positives in BPH (17.1%).

REFERENCES

1. A. Gutman and E Gutman, An "acid" phosphatase occuring in the
    serum of patients with metastasizing carcinoma of the prostate
    gland, J. Clin. Invest. 17:473 (1938).
2. N. Romas, K. Hsu, P. Ng, M. Pitts, P. Tomashefsky, and
    M. Tannenbaum, Counterimmunoelectrophoretic studies of serum
    prostatic acid phosphatase, Prostate 1:451 (1980).
3. G. Andras, A.G. Foti, J. Fenimore Cooper, H. Herschman, and
    R.R. Malvaez, Detection of Prostatic Cancer by Solid Phase Radio-
    immunoassay of Serum Prostatic Acid Phosphatase, New Eng. J. Med.
    297:1357 (1977).
4. A. Bruce, D. Mahan, L. Sullivan, and L. Goldenberg, The signifi-
    cance of prostatic acid phosphatase in adenocarcinoma of the
    prostate, J. Urol. 125:357 (1981).
5. G. Murphy, T. Chu, and J. Karr, Prostatic acid phosphatase - the
    developing experience, Clin. Biochem. 12:226 (1979).

IS DETERMINATION OF PROSTATIC ACID PHOSPHATASE IN BONE MARROW BY RADIOIMMUNOASSAY (BM-PAP) USEFUL IN PATIENTS WITH PROSTATIC CANCER?

S.D. Fosså, A. Skinningsrud, O. Kaalhus, and A. Engeseth

The Norwegian Radium Hospital
Oslo
Norway

INTRODUCTION

Prostatic acid phosphatase (PAP) determined in serum and bone marrow, is claimed to be a useful tumour marker in prostatic carcinoma (1,2,3,4). The clinical significance of bone marrow PAP (BM-PAP) has, however, not been clearly defined, possibly due to methodological problems of BM-PAP analysis.

The aim of the present study is to analyse to what extent BM-PAP determinations by a specific radioimmunoassay (RIA) are of clinical significance in patients with cancer of the prostate.

MATERIAL AND METHODS

Sixty-one patients with histologically proven adenocarcinoma of the prostate were included in the study. Further details regarding the patients are given in Table 1. The stage distribution was performed according to the TNM system (5). Patients with serum PAP (Se-PAP) levels above 3.5 U/l, determined by the enzymatic method (6), were regarded as M1 patients. In general, M0 patients were treated by irradiation of the prostate and the regional lymph nodes (70 Gy). The treatment of M1 patients consisted of androgen-suppressive therapy (oestrogens, orchiectomy). Progressive disease was defined by the development of distant metastases (in M0 patients) or by death due to prostatic carcinoma (M1 patients).

Samples of bone marrow (1-3 ml) were aspirated from the posterior iliac crest as previously described (7). The aspirate was divided into two parts. One part was used for smear preparation and

147

Table 1. Details of 61 Patients with Prostatic Carcinoma

Age (Years) (At BM-PAP Determination)	Mean	64.9
	Range	41-83
Interval Between Initial Diagnosis and BM-PAP Determination (Months)	Median	7
	Range	0-105
No. of Patients With Androgen- Without Suppressive Treatment		29
		32
Stage Distribution (At BM-PAP Determination)	T1-2, N0/X, M0	10
	T3-4, N0/X, M0	13
	T1-4, N1-4, M0	2
	T1-4, N1-4/X, M1	36
Localisation of Metastases	Elevated Se-PAP* Only	4
	Bone $\pm$ Other Met.	27
	Lymphnode $\pm$ Soft Tissue Met.	7
No. of M0 Patients With Equivocal Findings	Se-PAP* Only	4
	X-ray/Bone Scan $\pm$ Se-PAP	8
Follow-up after BM-PAP Determination (Months)	Median	5.5
	Range	0-31

* Determined by the Enzymatic Method

for histological sections of the aspirated particles. The other part was allowed to coagulate for 30 to 60 minutes at room temperature before centrifugation. The serum was collected and stored at -20°C until final analysis.

At the same time as bone marrow was aspirated a blood sample was obtained from a peripheral arm vein for determination of Serum-PAP (Se-PAP).

The radioimmunoassay of PAP was performed by an analysis reported previously (8,9). A highly purified and immunochemically controlled enzyme preparation has been used that gave rise to a high affinity antiserum upon immunization on rabbits. The radioimmunoassay used has compared favourably with commercially available radioimmunoassays for PAP. (Upper reference limit for Se-PAP in healthy individuals: 3.0 ug/l) (8).

The present control group consisted of 45 cancer patients with diagnoses other than prostatic cancer. BM-PAP and Se-PAP samples were obtained and analysed by the same methods as used in the prostatic carcinoma group.

RESULTS

Figure 1 shows the frequency distribution of the BM-PAP and Se-PAP values in the control group. Based on the findings obtained, the upper reference limit of BM-PAP and Se-PAP was chosen at 28 μg/l and 4 μg/l, respectively. Two of the three patients with Se-PAP values above 4.0 μg/l had a pelvic recurrence of a rectal carcinoma. The third patient had a renal carcinoma.

In patients with M0 disease the median BM-PAP level was within the normal range for all T categories. The median Se-PAP, however, was pathological for the more advanced categories (Table 2a). Raised median BM-PAP and Se-PAP levels were found in hormonally untreated M1 patients (Table 2b). Androgen-suppressive treatment had only limited influence on the median BM-PAP and Se-PAP levels in M1 patients. In general, for the whole group of prostatic carcinoma patients the median BM-PAP was less often increased than the median Se-PAP (Table 2c).

There was no clear correlation between the Se-PAP and BM-PAP levels in the control group. (Correlation coefficient R=0.07, calculated by linear regression analysis in the log-log scale (Figure 2a). In M0 patients the correlation coefficient was R=0.39 (Figure 2b). In M1 patients a good correlation (R=0.86) was found between Se-PAP and BM-PAP, similarly for hormonally treated and untreated patients (Figure 2c). No clear relationship between BM-PAP/Se-PAP and future disease progression was noted.

Histological proof of metastases at the site of BM-PAP aspiration was obtained in six patients. The Se-PAP and BM-PAP levels were distributed over a wide range and were independent of hormonal treatment (Table 3).

Twelve M0 patients had equivocal findings, either regarding enzymatically analysed Se-PAP (>2.5 U/l up to 3.5 U/l) (four patients) or with regard to radiological examination and/or bone scan (eight patients). The Se-PAP and BM-PAP values, analyzed by RIA, are shown in Table 4a and 4b. Patient number four developed distant metastases nine months after the BM-PAP determinations. In this patient BM-PAP was within the normal range, whereas Se-PAP was elevated. The other patients were without evidence of progressive disease 1-24 months after the BM-PAP anlaysis.

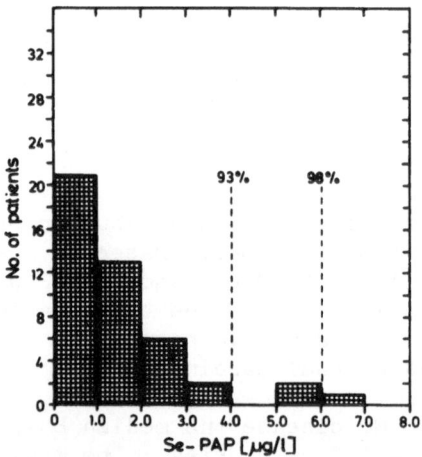

Fig. 1a.   Prostatic acid phosphatase in Serum (Se-PAP),
           determined by RIA, in 45 patients with non-prostatic
           carcinoma (control group).

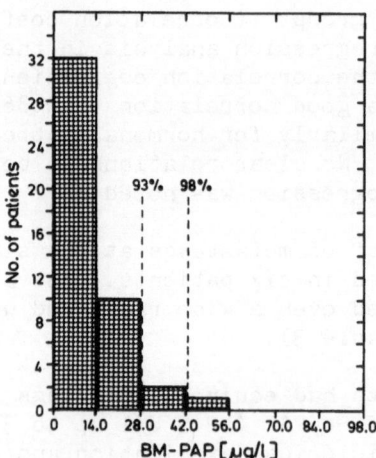

Fig. 1b.   Prostatic acid phosphatase in bone marrow (BM-PAP),
           determined by RIA, in 45 patients with non-prostatic
           carcinoma (control group).

Table 2a. Prostatic Acid Phosphatase in Serum (Se-PAP) and Bone Marrow (BM-PAP) in 23 M0 Patients with Prostatic Carcinoma

Category	Total No. of Patients	Patients with raised Se-PAP	Se-PAP (ug/l) Median	Range (Min-Max)	Patients with raised BP-PAP	BM-PAP (ug/l) Median	Range (Min-Max)
T1/2							
NX/0	10	2	1.3	0–14.2	2	13.0	0–279.0
M0							
T3/4							
NX/0	13	8	5.8	0–48.4	5	16.3	0– 73.7
M0							
T1–4							
NX/0	23	10	2.3	0–48.4	7	13.8	0–279.0
M0 (Total)							

Table 2b. Prostatic Acid Phosphatase in Serum (Se-PAP) and Bone Marrow (BM-PAP) in 38 M1 Patients with Prostatic Carcinoma

Category	Total No. of Patients	Patients with raised Se-PAP	Se-PAP (μg/l)		Patients with raised BP-PAP	BM-PAP (μg/l)	
			Median	Range (Min-Max)		Median	Range (Min-Max)
T1-4							
N0/1-4/X	13	12	20.3	0-129.8	7	30.3	3.0-313.5
M1 (Untreated)							
T1-4							
N0/1-4/X	25	16	14.7	0-310.0	11	23.5	2.2-1430.0
M1 (Treated)							
T1-4							
N0/1-4/X	38	28	17.9	0-310.0	18	25.0	3.0-1430.0
M1 (Total)							

Table 2c. Prostatic Acid Phosphatase in Serum (Se-PAP) and Bone Marrow (BM-PAP) in 61 Patients with Prostatic Carcinoma

Category	Total No. of Patients	Patients with raised Se-PAP	Se-PAP (ug/l)		Patients with raised BM-PAP	BM-PAP (ug/l)	
			Median	Range (Min-Max)		Median	Range (Min-Max)
Total No. of Patients with Prostatic Cancer	61	38	9.0	0-310.0	25	19.4	0-1430.0

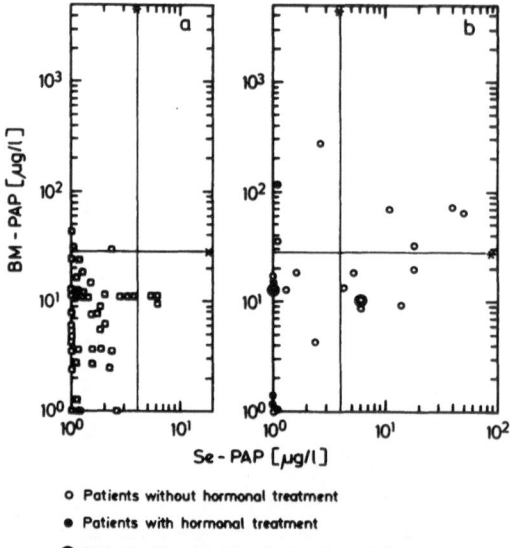

Figs 2a & 2b. Correlation between prostatic acid phosphatase in serum (Se-PAP) and bone marrow (BM-PAP), determined by RIA, in a control group of 45 patients with non-prostatic carcinoma and 23 patients with non-metastatic prostatic carcinoma.

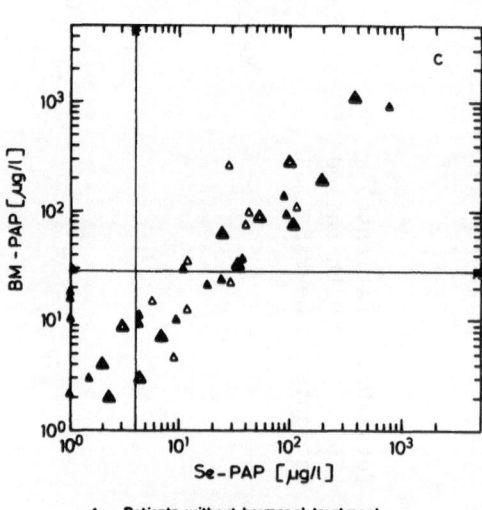

Fig. 2c. Correlation between prostatic acid phosphatase in serum (Se-PAP) bone marrow (BM-PAP), determined by RIA, in 38 patients with metastatic prostatic carcinoma.

Table 3. Prostatic Acid Phosphatase in Serum (Se-PAP) and
          Bone Marrow (BM-PAP) in 6 Patients with Prostatic
          Carcinoma and Histologically Proven Bone Marrow
          Infiltration at the site of Bone Marrow Aspiration

Identification		Androgen-Suppressive Treatment	Se-PAP (μg/l)	BM-PAP (μg/l)
No	26	No	3.0	7.7
	30	No	101.2	313.5
	32	No	27.1	176.0
	45	Yes	79.2	1199.0
	50	Yes	82.5	147.4
	53	Yes	42.9	95.7

Table 4a. Prostatic Acid Phosphatase in Serum (Se-PAP) and
           Bone Marrow (BM-PAP) Analyzed by RIA (μg/l) in
           M0 Patients with Prostatic Carcinoma and Slightly
           Elevated PAP in Serum ($\leqslant$ 3.5U/l). (Determined
           by the Enzymatic Method)

Identification		Androgen-Suppressive Treatment	Se-PAP (μg/l)	BM-PAP (μg/l)
No	1	No	48.4	64.9
	10	No	2.3	279.0
	16	No	14.2	9.4
	18	No	11.5	71.5

Table 4b.   Prostatic Acid Phosphatase in Serum (SE-PAP)
            and Bone Marrow (BM-PAP) in M0 Patients with
            Prostatic Carcinoma and Equivocal Findings on
            X-Ray/Bone Scan

Identification	Androgen-Suppressive Treatment	Se-PAP (ug/l)	BM-PAP (ug/l)
No 2	Yes	0	13.8
4*	No	6.4	11.8
6	No	5.4	17.2
8	No	18.2	33.0
9	No	39.6	73.7
11	Yes	0	12.1
13	Yes	1.1	144.0
23	No	2.2	4.4

*   Patient who developed bone metastases during follow-up

DISCUSSION

For the control group of this study the upper reference limit
of BM-PAP was found to be seven times higher than that of Se-PAP.
This may indicate that the specificity of the RIA used is not as high
as attempted. Acid phosphatases of non-prostatic origin, probably
from bone marrow cells, seem to be partially determined by the RIA
used. The amount of these phosphatases probably varies in the
different samples, mainly due to inter-patient variations in the
amount of peripheral blood in the bone marrow aspirate. Thus we
recognise some of the same problems as observed when using the
enzymatic method for BM-PAP analysis (7).

Treatment did not seem to have significant influence on BM-PAP
and Se-PAP levels. However, most of our hormonally treated patients
were patients whose disease had become hormone-resistant, after
primary response to hormonal manipulation. The BM-PAP and Se-PAP
levels may have risen again after an initial post-treatment decrease.

In symptomatic M1 patients the results of BM-PAP analysis correlated well with the serum values, but did not give any information to the clinician in addition to the information that was already obtained by the Se-PAP determination and the routine clinical/radiological examination of the patient. In particular, the BM-PAP levels, determined by RIA, did not seem to be of better prognostic value than the Se-PAP levels when survival curves were compared.

It was hoped that BM-PAP determination could indicate those M0 patients who had occult bone metastases and/or undetected lymph node metastases, especially in "borderline" cases with equivocal findings. Although the number of M0 patients examined is limited (only two M0 patients had progressive disease), the results of BM-PAP determinations so far do not seem to be correlated with the future development of bone metastases. Se-PAP analysis is probably more useful for indicating those high-risk patients (see patient no. 4, table 4b). Only by a longer follow-up period of M0 patients with known Se-PAP and BM-PAP values can the clinical significance of elevated BM-PAP and Se-PAP levels in M0 patients be determined definitely.

Bone metastases from an unknown primary tumour often present a diagnostic problem for the clinician. We had hoped that BM-PAP determinations from the metastatic area could indicate a possible prostatic origin in such patients. Indeed, five of six relevant BM-PAP analyses resulted in elevated levels. However, the Se-PAP levels were also significantly raised in these patients. Therefore the BM-PAP determination was in reality unnecessary for the diagnosis of prostatic cancer as it could have been considered on the basis of the raised Se-PAP level alone.

CONCLUSION

1.   The results of BM-PAP determinations in a control group of cancer patients with non-prostatic carcinoma have indicated that the specificity of RIA for PAP in bone marrow samples is less than expected.

2.   BM-PAP determinations by radioimmunoassay in M1 patients with prostatic carcinoma give no information in addition to that available from Se-PAP clinical/radiological examinations.

3.   Even in M0 patients with prostatic carcinoma the clinical significance of BM-PAP analysis is most probably very limited. Further studies are, however, needed to define the role of BM-PAP determinations in M0 patients.

REFERENCES

1. R.J. Veenema, E.O. Gursel, N. Romas, M. Wechsler, and
    J.K. Lattimer, Bone marrow acid phosphatase: Prognostic value
    in patients undergoing radical prostatectomy, J. Urol. 117:81
    (1977).
2. W.D. Belville, H.D. Cox, D.E. Mahan, J.P. Olmert, B.T. Mittemeyer,
    and A.W. Bruce, Bone marrow acid phosphatase by radioimmunoassay,
    Cancer 41:2286 (1978).
3. J.F. Cooper, A. Foti, and H. Herschman, Combined serum and bone
    marrow radioimmunoassays for prostatic acid phosphatase, J. Urol.
    122:498 (1979).
4. S. Beckley, T. Meng Chu, Z. Wajsman, A. Mittelman, N. Slack, and
    G.P. Murphy, Modern concepts of acid and alkaline phosphatase
    measurement, Scand. J. Urol. Nephrol. Suppl. 55:65 (1980).
5. UICC, TNM pre-treatment clinical classification. TNM classifi-
    cation of malignant tumours. Third edition, 119 (1978), Geneva.
6. P.B. Hudson, H. Brendler, and W.W. Scott, A simple method for
    determination of serum acid phosphatase, J. Urol. 58:89 (1947).
7. S.D. Fossa, J. Sokolowski, and L. Theodorsen, The significance
    of bone marrow acid phosphatase in patients with prostatic
    carcinoma, Brit. J. Urol. 50:185 (1978).
8. A. Skinningsrud, K. Nustad, S.D. Fossa, M. Aas and J.H.N.
    Syversen, Immunoassay of human prostatic acid phosphatase,
    Scand. J. clin. lab. Invest. 39:46 (1979).
9. A. Skinningsrud and K. Nustad, Prostatic acid phosphatase
    purification and iodination with iodogen, Clin. Chim. Acta.
    (1981) In press.

STUDIES OF ACID PHOSPHATASE IN PROSTATIC CANCER

D.P. Byar and D.K. Corle

National Cancer Institute
Bethesda, Maryland
U.S.A.

ABSTRACT

Various analyses of data gathered in the VACURG studies demonstrate that the extent of elevation of the pre-treatment acid phosphatase correlates with the probability of having detectable metastases and with survival.   Patients with increased acid phosphatase
but without evidence of metastases have a worse prognosis than
patients with normal acid phosphatase and no metastases.   For
patients in stages I and II treated with radical prostatectomy, even
values in the normal range were correlated with time until progression of tumor.   These findings suggest that increased acid phosphatase values probably represent undetected metastases.

Recent reports of more sensitive and specific immunologic methods
for measuring acid phosphatase (1-4) have stimulated new interest in
the diagnostic and prognostic importance of this serum enzyme.   For
this reason we decided to re-examine data collected in the large
randomized clinical trials of treatment of prostatic cancer conducted
by the Veterans Administration Cooperative Urological Research Group
(VACURG).   In all studies by that group, only newly diagnosed
patients were admitted.   The diagnostic work-up included digital
rectal examination, a skeletal survey using ordinary x-ray techniques
and a determination of the so called "prostatic fraction" of the
serum acid phosphatase as measured in King-Armstrong Units (KAU).
All acid phosphatase determinations were performed in a central
reference laboratory under the direction of Dr U.S. Seal.   Earlier
studies had established 1.0 KAU as the upper limit of normal for the
prostatic fraction determined by inhibition with L-tartrate, here-
after referred to simply as acid phosphatase.   Radioactive scans,

lymphangiograms, and laparotomies were not used in staging the patients. Stage I refers to patients who have no abnormal findings on rectal examination, and Stage II refers to those patients in whom palpable cancer confined to the prostate gland can be detected on rectal examination. In both stages the acid phosphatase values are normal and there is no evidence of distant metastases. Stage III refers to patients with tumors extended locally beyond the confines of the prostate gland but who have normal values of acid phosphatase and no x-ray or clinical evidence of distant metastases. Stage IV refers to patients who have either elevated acid phosphatase, evidence of distant metastases to bone or soft tissue, or both. Data reported in this article are taken from all three of the major clinical trials of the VACURG (5).

We first wanted to examine the relationship between the acid phosphatase at diagnosis and the presence of detectable metastases. For this purpose we tabulated the acid phosphatase into various categories and computed the percentage of patients with metastases in each category using data from patients in all four stages of Study 1. These data (Table 1) indicate that there is a strong correlation between the acid phosphatase value at diagnosis and the probability that metastases will be found. Note for example that in the top half of the normal range (0.6-1.0 KAU) only 7.6% of patients had metastases, but when the acid phosphatase rises slightly to values between 1.1 and 2.0 KAU, the probability of metastases rises dramatically to 17.6% and continues to increase thereafter reaching a value of 76% for patients whose initial acid phosphatase was between 50 and 100 KAU. From the data in Table 1 it can be calculated that the relative odds of having detectable metastases for patients whose initial acid phosphatase is elevated (>1.0 KAU) compared to those in the normal range (0-1.0 KAU) is 11.78. This can be interpreted as meaning that patients with elevated values of acid phosphatase are almost 12 times more likely to have detectable metastases. A similar calculation using 10.0 KAU as the cut-off value produced an odds ratio of 18.3.

Using data from the same study for stage III and IV patients, we examined the effects of endocrine treatment on the acid phosphatase measurements after six months of treatment. The treatments randomly assigned in that study for stage III and IV patients were placebo, 5.0 mg of diethylstilbestrol (DES), orchiectomy plus placebo, or orchiectomy plus 5.0 mg of DES. The placebo and estrogen treatments were administered daily by mouth as a single tablet. Changes in acid phosphatase values at six months were categorized by computing the percentage change between the initial and six month values, namely the six month value minus the initial value divided by initial value. These percentage changes were then classified as increased if the ratio just described was 0.5 (an increase of 50% or more), same if the value was between ± 0.5, and decreased if the ratio was -0.5 (50% or more decrease). These results (Table 2) show that endocrine

Table 1.   Relationship of Initial Acid Phosphatase
to Presence of Metastases in Study 1.

Initial Acid Phosphatase (KAU)	N	Percentage of Patients With Metastases
0.0 - 0.5	948	5.0%
0.6 - 1.0	527	7.6%
1.1 - 2.0	238	17.6%
2.1 - 5.0	185	29.2%
5.1 - 10.0	112	44.6%
10.1 - 20.0	80	62.5%
20.1 - 50.0	89	68.5%
50.1 - 100.0	50	76.0%
Greater than 100.0	70	78.6%

Table 2.   Effect of Treatment on Acid Phosphatase at
Six Months in Stage IV of Study 1.

Treatment	N	Acid Phosphatase		
		Increase	Same	Decrease
Placebo	148	35%	37%	28%
Estrogen	157	4%	13%	83%
Orchiectomy + Placebo	152	4%	12%	84%
Orchiectomy + Estrogen	161	1%	12%	86%

treatment produces a decrease of 50% or more in the initial acid
phosphatase in about 85% of the patients, whereas a decrease of this
magnitude was only seen in 28% of patients assigned to placebo.
These data dramatically demonstrate that endocrine therapy has a
direct effect on the prostatic cancer cells; the decreases in acid
phosphatase probably reflect a decreased rate of manufacture or secretion of the enzyme by the cancer cells, resulting from the lowered
cellular metabolism of the hormone-sensitive tumors following endocrine therapy (6).   Although the data presented in Table 2 are not
broken down by the levels of the pretreatment acid phosphatase, other
analyses not presented here revealed that endocrine treatment produced a 50% or greater fall in the acid phosphatase at six months
for about 85% of patients no matter what the initial value was.

The staging system used in the VACURG studies is based on the
assumption that elevated values of the acid phosphatase represent
undetected metastatic disease, and for that reason, patients having
such elevations were classified as stage IV.   This viewpoint, although it has been suggested in the literature by many authors, is
not universally accepted, especially since the advent of the new
immunological methods of measuring acid phosphatase.   Because these
newer methods find substantial percentages of patients with elevations in what appear to be clinical stages I, II and III, it was
hoped that these more sensitive assays could help in identifying
patients who might be suitable candidates for radical surgical treatment or curative x-ray therapy (7).   The data collected in the
VACURG studies allow us to examine the prognostic significance of
elevated acid phosphatase measurements in the absence of detectable
metastases, but it must be remembered that neither bone scans, lymphangiograms, nor laparotomies were used in staging the patients.
The reasons for being classified as stage IV in Study 3 are given
in Table 3.   Note that 62.4% of the patients in stage IV were so
classified because of elevated acid phosphatase alone.   By combining
categories in Table 3 we can compute that 85.6% of patients with
demonstrable metastases (bone, soft part, or both) had elevated
acid phosphatase.

The prognostic significance of acid phosphatase elevations with
or without demonstrable metastases is examined in Table 4 where death
rates for various categories of patients are displayed.   The death
rate is defined as the number of deaths per 1000 patient-months of
observation for all patients combined, whether they died or not.
Rates have been computed separately for all causes of death, for
deaths due to prostatic cancer, and for cardiovascular deaths.   In
the latter two analyses deaths from other causes are treated as withdrawals from observation at the time of death.   The determination
of the cause of death was made by a committee of clinicians who were
unaware of the treatment assignment.   The term "cardiovascular
deaths" includes deaths from myocardial infarcts, congestive heart
failure, pulmonary emboli, cerebrovascular accidents, and other

Table 3. Reasons For Classification
As Stage IV in Study 3.

Bone Mets	Soft Mets	Acid Phosphatase 1.0 KAU	N	Per Cent
X			19	4.1
	X		4	0.9
		X	289	62.4
X	X		2	0.4
X		X	116	25.1
	X	X	16	3.5
X	X	X	17	3.7
			463	100.1

Table 4. Death Rates for Patients in Stage III and
Various Categories of Stage IV in Study 3.

Category		Deaths per 1000 patient-months			
		N	All[1]	CAP[2]	CVD[3]
Stage III	Normal acid phosphatase and no metastases	531	11.8	2.1	5.1
	↑ Acid phosphatase only	289	19.7	8.8	5.0
Stage IV	Metastases only	25	19.5	9.0	4.5
	Both metastases and ↑ acid phosphatase	149	32.7	21.5	5.6

[1] All causes of death

[2] Deaths from prostatic cancer

[3] Deaths from cardiovascular causes

cardiovascular causes.   The data in Table 4 refer to the same
patients in stage IV as those shown in Table 3.   Examination of the
death rates for cardiovascular causes reveals no appreciable differences between the four groups.   However, both for all causes of
death combined and for deaths due to prostatic cancer, death rates
are increased when either the acid phosphatase is elevated or detectable metastases are present, and these rates are even higher when
both findings are present.   The increased death rates are much more
striking when we examine cancer deaths only because the results for
all causes of death are diluted by deaths from cardiovascular and
other causes.   These data clearly indicate that patients with elevated acid phosphatase alone have a worse prognosis than patients
in stage III, an important factor to keep in mind when reviewing
published treatment results for stage III patients from centers who
do not take the acid phosphatase into account in their staging
system.

Recent reports indicate that the more sensitive and specific
immunological methods for measuring acid phosphatase have detected
elevations in substantial numbers of stage I and II patients (1-4).
These findings stimulated us to analyze our data for patients whose
acid phosphatase values were in the normal range to see whether very
small elevations might possibly represent undetected metastases.
As mentioned earlier, the normal cut-off value in our studies was
1.0 KAU, but this figure, like any normal cut-off value, must be
regarded as arbitrary to some extent.   We decided to limit our
attention to patients who were treated by radical prostatectomy
because the operation would presumably have removed all the disease
if it were confined to the prostate gland.   In order to get large
enough numbers of patients, we combined data from all three VACURG
studies for patients in stages I and II who were treated by radical
prostatectomy.   We excluded patients who received estrogens as
initial therapy in addition to the prostatectomy.   Since there were
so few deaths due to prostatic cancer in stage I and II patients,
we decided to use a different end point in assessing the prognostic
significance of the acid phosphatase.   This was the rate of progression of the disease, expressed as the number of patients who progressed per 1000 patient-months of observation for all patients under
study whether they progressed or not.   Progression of disease was
defined at the first appearance of definite metastases, at the first
elevation of the acid phosphatase >2.0 KAU, or at death due to prostatic cancer.   In fact, all patients who died of prostatic cancer
had earlier had both an increase in acid phosphatase and the appearance of metastases.   The value 2.0 KAU was chosen after noting that
for some patients the acid phosphatase might hover in the range between 1.0 and 2.0 without a further rise later.   It was thought that
using a value below 2.0 KAU would result in a serious overestimation
of the proportion of patients progressing.   The results of this
analysis (Table 5) shows that, even in the normal range, initial acid
phosphatase values are correlated with the progression rate.   Even

Table 5.   Progression Rates by Categories of Acid Phosphatase
in the Normal Range for Patients in Stages I and II'
of Studies 1 and 2 Treated by Radical Prostatectomy.

Initial Acid Phosphatase	No. of Patients	No. Progressing	Progression Rate[1]
0.0-0.3	58	3	0.58
0.4-0.5	68	9	1.68
0.6-1.0	62	11	2.15

[1] Number progressing per 1000 patient-months of observation.

though the numbers progressing are relatively small, a statistical
test for trend for these three rates across the categories of acid
phosphatase was significant at $p = 0.02$ (one-tailed test).   If we
use first appearance of metastases alone as evidence of progression,
ignoring rises in acid phosphatase, the results are still significant
at $p = 0.04$ (one-tailed test).   Admitting that the fraction of the
acid phosphatase inhibited by L-tartrate is not precisely the same
as that detected by immunological methods, our data suggest that
slight rises in the acid phosphatase indicate patients in whom the
cancer has already spread, because all those patients had radical
prostatectomies.   If the tissue producing the acid phosphatase in
the serum had been confined to the prostate gland, then no prognostic
significance for the initial acid phosphatase measurements would have
been observed.   It appears then that rather than detecting patients
who might potentially be curable by surgery or other localized
modalities of treatment, even small elevations of the acid phosphatase may indicate that the disease has already spread.

REFERENCES

1.   A.G. Foti, J.F. Cooper, H. Herschman and R.R. Malvaez, Detection
of Prostatic Cancer by Solid-Phase Radioimmunoassay of Serum
Prostatic Acid Phosphatase, New Eng. J. Med. 297:1357 (1977).
2.   C.L. Lee, T.M. Chu, L.Z. Wajsman, N.H. Slack and G.P. Murphy,
Value of New Flourescent Immunoassay for Human Prostatic Acid
Phosphatase in Prostate Cancer, Urology 15:338 (1980).
3.   A.W. Bruce, D.E. Mahan, L.D. Sullivan and L. Goldenberg, The
Significance of Prostatic Acid Phosphatase in Adenocarcinoma
of the Prostate, J. Urol. 125:357 (1981).
4.   G.R. Quinones, T.J. Rohner Jr, J.R. Drago and L.M. Demers, Will
Prostatic Acid Phosphatase Determination by Radioimmunoassay
Increase the Diagnosis of Early Prostatic Cancer? J. Urol.
125:361 (1981).

5.   D.P. Byar, Contributions of the Veterans Administration Cooper-
      ative Urological Research Group Studies to our Understanding
      of Prostatic Cancer and its Treatment, in "Urologic Pathology:
      The Prostate, M. Tannenbaum (ed), Lea and Febiger, New York,
      (1977) p. 241.
6.   J.B. Goetsch, A Clinical and Histochemical Study of Acid and
      Alkaline Phosphatase in Normal and Abnormal Prostatic Tissue,
      J. Urol. 84:636 (1960).
7.   R. Gittes, Acid Phosphatase Reappraised, New Eng. J. Med.
      297:1398 (1977).

THE CLINICAL VALUE OF THE SERUM ACID PHOSPHATASE

IN CARCINOMA OF THE PROSTATE

B. Richards[1], R. Sylvester[2], M. de Pauw[2] and the

EORTC Urological Group

1. York District Hospital
    York, U.K.

2. EORTC Data Centre
    Brussels, Belgium

INTRODUCTION

A phosphatase which was particularly active at an acid pH was shown to be present in red blood cells in 1924 (1). Acid phosphatases are also present in leucocytes, platelets, osteoclasts, reticuloendothelial cells, and in liver, kidney, spleen and other organs. Their clinical importance derives from the fact that the concentration of the enzyme is far greater in the prostate than in any other human tissue (2).

The relevance of acid phosphatase to the patient first became obvious in 1936 when Gutman and his colleagues showed that it was found not only in normal prostatic epithelium but also in prostatic cancer (3), being present both in primary tumours and in secondary deposits. There is less activity in carcinomatous tissue than in normal prostate, and less still in metastases (4), loss of activity being correlated with de-differentiation.

The presence of acid phosphatase in the serum of some patients with metastasising adenocarcinoma of the prostate was first demonstrated in 1938 by Gutman and Gutman (5), and since that time a great deal of attention has been paid to its use in the diagnosis and management of prostatic cancer.

One problem which presented itself at once was the separation of acid phosphatases arising from various sources. Prostatic

167

acid phosphatase can be distinguished from that arising from blood
elements because it is inhibited by L-tartrate. Unfortunately
L-tartrate also inhibits the enzymes derived from spleen, liver and
kidney. Formadehyde, in contrast, inhibits the activity of red cell
acid phosphatase without affecting the prostatic enzyme (6). Despite
the introduction of these, and other inhibitants, enzymatic methods
for determination of acid phosphatase have not proved capable of
localising the prostatic enzyme precisely (7), and, in an attempt
to increase the specificity of the analysis, two further techniques
have been introduced.

MEASUREMENT OF ACID PHOSPHATASE IN BONE MARROW

     Elevation of the bone marrow acid phosphatase has been claimed
to be an early sign of metastatic spread of carcinoma to bone
(8-12). Initial reports suggested a good correlation between the
presence of metastases and an elevation of the bone marrow acid
phosphatase level. Gursel et al, for example, noted the development
of bone metastases in 5 of 16 patients in whom an elevated bone
marrow acid phosphatase was the only abnormal finding (9).
Unfortunately, there have been problems with false positives (13,
14), especially when enzymatic methods were employed (15), and at
the present time it seems clear that bone marrow acid phosphatase
determination by enzymatic techniques is of very little value (16,
17).

     The use of radio-immuno assay for the measurement of bone
marrow acid phosphatase may eliminate some of the false positive
results (15,18). The importance of detecting bony metastases in
patients whose prostatic lesions might be cured by radical therapy
is obvious, and the radio-immuno assay deserves further attention
(18). This subject will be reviewed by Fossa (19).

MEASUREMENT OF ACID PHOSPHATASE BY IMMUNOLOGICAL METHODS

     Prostatic acid phosphatase has been demonstrated to be anti-
genically distinct from acid phosphatase arising elsewhere (20),
and a specific antibody can be raised against it. The acid
phosphatase in tumour tissue appears to be antigenically similar to
that obtained from normal prostate (21) and similar also to that
obtained from expressed prostatic fluid and from semen, both of
which have been used as a source of antigen.

     Two techniques are available for measuring prostatic acid
phosphatase. In the first a radio-immuno assay (RIA) is used
which measures the total antigen (22). Foti and his colleagues
improved the procedure which they had originally used by changing
to a solid phase technique. The assay depends upon competition of
labelled and unlabelled antigen for antibody binding sites. The
second depends on counter immuno electrophoresis (CIEP) and was

developed by Chu and his colleagues (23). The antigen and antibody
move in opposite directions in an electrophoretic field, precipitat-
ing when they meet. The enzymatic activity of the precipitation
line can be determined. There is no doubt that these techniques
and their subsequent refinements (24,25) give rise to improved
sensitivity - the probability that the blood test will be positive
in patients with proved prostatic cancer - and specificity - the
probability that the test will be negative in men already known to
be free of disease - when compared with enzyme assays, and they have
led to a wave of enthusiasm suggesting that measurement of prostatic
acid phosphatase would detect cancer of the prostate before it had
given rise to metastases - while it was still curable by local
treatment. At first sight it seems very unlikely that this could be
the case. The level of acid phosphatase in prostatic cancer tissue
is considerably less than that in a normal prostate, and it would be
surprising if a small focus of tumour gave rise to a detectable
signal.

In the light of these expansive claims for the value of acid
phosphatase measurement, it seems appropriate to examine critically
the various uses to which it has been put. It may be employed in
one or more of three ways:

1. As a diagnostic tool
    (a) in screening for the disease
    (b) in staging

2. As an indicator of prognosis

3. As an indicator of response to therapy.

SERUM ACID PHOSPHATASE (SAP) IN THE DIAGNOSIS OF PROSTATIC CANCER

Its use in diagnosis is marred by the fact that it is rarely
elevated until metastases are present. Abnormalities occur when
the disease is still localised to the prostate with greater
frequency using radio-immuno assay than when enzymatic techniques
are employed; but this must, in part, be related to the range
which is accepted as normal. False positives (abnormal levels of
serum acid phosphase in the absence of carcinoma of the prostate)
are distinctly rare using enzymatic techniques, but were noted in
between 3 and 27% of cases using radio-immuno assay (26). The
incidence of abnormalities found in the various stages of the
disease in a number of series is listed in Table 1.

These figures, and especially the false positives, are
relevant to the enthusiastic claims for the use of serum prostatic
acid phosphase as a screening test for prostatic cancer (30,31,32).
It has been pointed out by Watson and Tang (33) and by Bruce and

Table 1:   The percentage incidence of raised serum acid phosphatase
           at different stages of the disease

	Radio-immuno assay				Enzymatic assa
Stage	Foti (22)	Murphy (27)	Griffiths (28)	Bruce (26)	Woodward (29)
A	33	38	12	14	)
B	79	35	32	29	)<10)
C	71	49	47	24	31
D	92	89	86	89	74

his colleagues (26) that the usefulness of a laboratory procedure
for screening depends not only on the sensitivity and specificity
of the test but also on the prevalence of the disease within the
population tested. Given this, one can calculate the positive predictive value, the probability that a person with a positive blood
test actually has the disease, and the negative predictive value,
the probability that a person with a negative blood test is in fact
free of disease. Combining the data of Foti and his colleagues (22)
with the prevalence of prostatic cancer of 35 per 100,000 in the
white male population of the United States, Watson and Tang calculated that only one in 244 subjects with a positive test would
actually have a carcinoma of the prostate, one in 526 if one excluded subjects with a prostatic cancer that could be felt digitally.

Estimation of the serum levels cannot be recommended for the
indiscriminate screening of men for prostatic cancer (26,33).
Nevertheless, selection factors may be combined with prostatic acid
phosphatase measurements to provide helpful information. Rectal
examination is the basic clinical procedure used to screen patients
for the possibility that they have prostatic carcinoma. Radio-
immuno assay of prostatic acid phosphatase has a much better predictive value here. Watson and Tang have calculated, again using
the sensitivity and specificity reported by Foti (22) that a
patient with a prostatic nodule and a positive test result would
have, at the time of detection, a 93% probability of carcinoma.
A patient with a nodule and a negative result would have an 84%
probability of having no tumour (33). Not everybody has been able
to match the sensitivity and specificity rates reported by Foti and
his colleagues. Even so, the technique appears to have much to
offer in the evaluation of such patients.

Paradoxically, the value of acid phosphatase determinations in
the diagnosis of metastatic disease has been reduced by the

increased sensitivity of the radio-immuno assay. Elevations of
the serum acid phosphatase have been reported while the cancer is
still confined within the prostatic capsule in 8% (15), 30% (23)
and even 79% (22) of patients. These differences reflect, in part,
the rigorousness of staging procedures (34), but it appears that
the radio-immuno assay is positive in at least 10% of locally operable cases even when the staging technique is rigorous and includes
pelvic lymphadenectomy (15). When this is considered together with
the fact that the acid phosphatase is not always raised, even when
the patient is known to have advanced disease (in 5% (15), 20% (23),
40% (25)), it can be seen that the test is too unreliable to be
used as a definitive guide to therapy (35). It remains useful as a
general guide, as most patients with a high acid phosphatase have
advanced disease. Hopes that the bone marrow acid phosphatase
would be more specific for the detection of early metastases to
bone (8) have not stood the test of time (14-17).

SERUM ACID PHOSPHATASE AS AN INDICATOR OF PROGNOSIS IN
PROSTATIC CANCER

    Since the serum acid phosphatase is more frequently elevated
when the disease is advanced, it would be hardly surprising if
patients who had a raised SAP at the time of diagnosis tended to
die sooner than those who did not, and this has been found to be
the case in several studies (36-39). Curiously, in a recent
EORTC study comparing the efficacy of Stilboestrol and Estramustine
Phosphate as primary treatments for patients with advanced
prostatic cancer, there was no prognostic advantage in having a
normal acid phosphatase (40).

SERUM ACID PHOSPHATASE AS AN INDICATOR OF RESPONSE TO THERAPY

    There remains the possibility that serum acid phosphatase may
be used as an indicator lesion in monitoring the course of the
disease and its response to therapy. It has been used in this
way in the past. Huggins and Hodges used it to demonstrate that
carcinoma of the prostate is hormonally responsive, regressing
after orchidectomy or oestrogen therapy and growing more rapidly
with testosterone (41). In their original paper, these workers
made the assumption that an elevation of acid phosphatase was
associated with advancing prostatic cancer, and that a fall in its
level indicated a remission. Various other authors have made the
same assumption, although the correlation is not always present.
For example, Franks noted progression of prostatic cancer in one
of seven patients having a fall of acid phosphatase. The others had
stable disease or responded to therapy (42).

    Assessment of the response of prostatic cancer to treatment is
notoriously difficult because measurement of the local disease is

Table 2:   Criteria of Evaluation of Response
in EORTC Protocol 30762

Evaluation of Local Response

1.   Complete Response.   The disappearance of any local
prostatic tumour.

2.   Partial Remission.   50% or more decrease in tumour
size (length x width).

3.   No Change.   Less than a 50% decrease or increase in
the size of the prostatic tumour.

4.   Progression.   A 50% or greater increase in tumour size
(length x width).

Evaluation of Response in Bony Metastases

1.   Complete Response.   Complete disappearance of all
lesions on X-ray and bone scan.

2.   Partial Response.   Disappearance of one or more lesions
seen on bone scan or X-ray with no increase in any
of the others and no new lesions.

3.   Progression.   The appearance of new lesions on
or X-ray at a site remote from known lesions.

4.   No change.   No new lesions and no disappearance of
known lesions.

inexact and because of uncertainty about evaluating changes in
bony metastases. All phase II trials require that the patient has
an indicator lesion. Acceptable indicator lesions are few in
prostatic cancer and it is very important to know whether the
acid phosphatase is one or not.

The EORTC has just completed a study (30762) in which Diethyl
Stilboestrol and Estramustine Phosphate are compared in previously
untreated patients with advanced prostatic cancer. Acid phosphatase
was measured each time the patient was examined but has not been
used in evaluating response, the criteria of which are listed in
Table 2. The acid phosphatase was measured in the local laboratory
of the centre submitting the case usually by enzymatic methods.
The upper limit of normal was that quoted by the local laboratory.
Repeated acid phosphatase results can be correlated with local
response in 172 cases, and with the response in metastatic disease
(as determined by an independent review of scans and X-rays) in 50.

Two groups are apparent, those with an elevated acid phosphatase at entry to the study, and those in whom it is normal. Of cases suitable for evaluation of the local response, 44 had a SAP more than twice the upper limit of normal at entry to the study. Table 3 compares the maximum changes in SAP with the response in these patients. It will be noted that progression of the local carcinoma was noted in four of 37 cases in which the serum acid phosphatase fell. Only 22 cases have been analysed from the point of view of the response of distant metastases. Once again, progression of the cancer is noted despite a falling SAP in about 10% of cases.

Table 4 shows the results in patients whose acid phosphatase was normal at entry to the study. In 108 cases suitable for evaluation of the local response, four progressed without a change in the normal acid phosphatase. In 13 cases there was an elevation of acid phosphatase. Of these, only one showed progression. Similar changes are seen for the 20 patients with metastases in bone. Again, the correlation is poor.

The data have been analysed so far with reference to the changes in SAP. If they are considered from the point of view of the clinical response to treatment, once again two groups of interest can be isolated, those that show remission on treatment and those that show progression on treatment.

In 57 cases there was remission of tumour within the prostate

Table 3: Correlation between SAP at the time of its greatest change and the clinical response - cases with SAP greater than twice normal at entry to study.

	Cases evaluable for response of the primary tumour (N = 44)		Cases evaluable for response of metastases in bone (N = 22)	
	SAP stayed elevated	SAP fell	SAP stayed elevated	SAP fell
Progression	0	4	1	2
No change	5	21	2	7
Remission	2	12	0	10
Total	7	37	3	19

Table 4:   Correlation between SAP at the time of its
greatest change and the clinical response - cases with
SAP normal at entry to the study

| | Primary Tumour (N = 108) | | Metastases in bone (N = 20) | |
	SAP stayed normal	SAP rose	SAP stayed normal	SAP rose
Progression	4	1	1	1
No change	59	9	11	2
Remission	32	3	5	0
Total	95	13	17	3

on treatment. Here the correlation with SAP was good. The SAP
was elevated in 22 (to above twice the normal figure in 15) and
fell to normal in all cases. In the remaining 35 it was normal
at entry to the study, stayed normal in 32 and rose to above twice
normal in only one patient. In nine patients progression of the
disease occured. The acid phosphatase rose in only one of these.
It fell to normal in four cases, despite progression, and stayed
normal in the other four.

It is clear that a fall in SAP correlated well with the
remission of the disease as determined by other parameters.
However, a fall in acid phsphatase does not mean that the patient
is in remission. In fact the SAP fell to normal in association
with progression of the local disease in all four cases in which
it was initially elevated.

The treatment (Stilboestrol or Estramustine Phosphate) given
in this study appears to reduce the acid phosphatase in the majority of cases. Changes in its level are largely independent of the
progression of the disease and it is clear that it cannot be
regarded as an indicator lesion by which the response of prostatic
cancer can be judged in phase II trials.

SUMMARY

The clinical significance of normal and abnormal serum acid
phosphatase levels is constantly being re-evaluated. Despite the
greater sensitivity of the newer techniques, it has a very limited
role as a screening test, and can give a rough guide only about
the presence of metastases. It is of very little value as an
indicator of tumour progression and its main value appears to be

the traditional one, that of screening patients with doubtful nodules, to assess the probability that the nodule is a primary or secondary prostatic cancer.

REFERENCES

1. M. Martland, F.S. Hansman and R. Robison, The phosphoric esterase of blood, Biochem. J. 18:115 (1924).
2. L.T. Yam, Clinical significance of the human acid phosphatase: a review, Am. J. Med. 56:604 (1974).
3. E.B. Gutman, E.E. Sproul and A.B. Gutman, Significance of increased phosphatase activity of bone at the site of osteoblastic metastases secondary to carcinoma of the prostate gland, Am. J. Cancer 28:485 (1936).
4. A.E. Reif, R.M. Schlesinger, C.A. Fish and C.M. Robinson, Acid phosphatase iso-enzymes in cancer of the prostate, Cancer 31:689 (1973).
5. A.B. Gutman and E.B. Gutman, An "acid" phosphatase occurring in the serum of patients with metastasising adenocarcinoma of the prostate gland, J. Clin. Invest. 17:473 (1938).
6. M.A. Abul-Fadl and E.J. King, Properties of the acid phosphatase of erythrocytes and of the human prostate gland, Biochem. J. 45:51 (1949).
7. T. M. Sodeman and J.G. Batsakis, Acid phosphatase, in: "Urologic Pathology: The Prostate," M. Tannenbaum, ed, Lea and Febiger, Philadelphia (1979) p 129.
8. D.T. Chua, R.J. Veenema, F. Muggia and A. Graff, Acid phosphatase levels in bone marrow: value in detecting early bone metastases from carcinoma of the prostate, J. Urol. 103:462 (1970).
9. E.O. Gursel, M. Rezvan, F.A. Sy and R.J. Veenema, Comparative evaluation of bone marrow acid phosphatase v. bone scanning in staging of prostatic cancer, J. Urol. 111:53 (1974).
10. J.E. Pontes, S.W. Alcorn, A.J. Thomas and J.M. Piercy, Bone marrow acid phosphatase in staging prostatic carcinoma, J. Urol. 114:422 (1975).
11. A.W. Bruce, F. O'Cleireachan, A. Morales and S.A. Owad, Carcinoma of the prostate: A critical look at staging, J. Urol. 117:319 (1977).
12. R.J. Veenema, E.O. Gursel, N. Romas, M. Wechsler and J.K. Lattimer, Bone marrow acid phosphatase: Prognostic value in patients undergoing radical prostatectomy, J. Urol. 117:81 (1977).
13. R. Kahn, B. Turner, M. Edson and M. Dolan, Bone marrow acid phosphatase: Another look, J. Urol. 117:79 (1977).
14. J.E. Pontes, B.K. Choe, N.R. Rose and J.M. Pierce, Bone marrow staging of prostatic cancer: How reliable is it? J. Urol. 119:772 (1978).
15. A. W. Bruce, D.E. Mahan, A. Morales, A.F. Clark and W.D. Belville, An objective look at acid phosphatase determinations, Brit. J. Urol. 51:213 (1979).

16. S.D. Fosså, J. Sokolowsi and L. Theodorsen, The significance of
     bone marrow acid phosphatase in patients with prostatic
     carcinoma, Br. J. Urol. 50:185 (1978).
17. W.M. Boehme, R.R. Augsburger, S.F. Wallner and R.E. Donohue,
     Lack of usefulness of bone marrow enzymes and calcium in
     staging patients with prostatic cancer, Cancer 41:1433 (1978).
18. A.N. Romas, R.J. Veenema, K.C. Shu, P. Tomashefszy,
     J.K. Lattimer and M. Tannenbaum, Bone marrow acid phosphatase
     in prostatic cancer. An assessment by immuno assay and bio-
     chemical methods, J. Urol. 123:392 (1980).
19. S.D. Fosså, A. Skinningsrud, O. Kaalhus and A. Engeseth, Is
     determination of prostatic acid phosphatase in bone marrow by
     radioimmunoassay (BM-PAP) useful in patients with prostatic
     cancer, in: "Cancer of the Prostate and Kidney," P.H. Smith
     and M. Pavone-Macaluso, eds., Plenum Press, London and New York
     (1982).
20. S. Shulman, L. Mamrod, M.J. Gonda and W.A. Soanes, The
     detection of prostatic acid phosphatase by antibody reactions in
     gel diffusion, J. Immunol. 93:474 (1964).
21. A.G Foti, H. Herschman and J.F. Cooper, Iso-enzymes of acid
     phosphatase in normal and cancerous human prostatic tissue,
     Cancer Res. 37:4120 (1977).
22. A.G. Foti, J.F. Cooper, H. Herschman and R.R. Malvaex,
     Detection of prostatic cancer by solid phase R.I.A. of serum
     prostatic acid phosphatase, N. Engl. J. Med. 297:1357 (1977)
23. T.M. Chu, M.C. Want, W.W. Scott, R.P. Gibbons, D.E. Johnson,
     J.D. Schmidt, S.A. Loening, G.R. Prout and G.P. Murphy, Immuno-
     chemical detection of serum prostatic acid phosphatase,
     Invest. Urol. 15:319 (1978).
24. B.K. Choe, E.J. Pontes, M.K. Morrison and N.R. Rose, Human
     prostatic acid phosphatases, 2: a double antibody radio-
     immuno assay, Arch. Androl. 1:227 (1978).
25. D.E. Mahan and B.P. Doctor, A radio-immune assay for human
     prostatic acid phosphatase levels in prostatic disease,
     Clin. Biochem. 12:10 (1979).
26. A.W. Bruce, D. Mahan and W.D. Melville, The role of radio-
     immuno assay for prostatic acid phosphatase in prostatic
     carcinoma, Urol. Clin. North Am. 12:226 (1979).
27. G.P. Murphy, T.M. Chu and J.P. Karr, Prostatic acid phosphatase:
     The developing experience, Clin. Biochem. 12:226 (1979).
28. J.C. Griffiths, Prostatic specific acid phosphatase, Re-
     evaluation of radio-immuno assay in diagnosing prostatic
     disease, Clin. Chem. 26:433 (1980).
29. K.Q. Woodward, Factors leading to elevation in serum and
     glycerophosphate, Cancer 5:236 (1952).
30. G.P. Murphy, J. Karr and T.M. Chu, Prostatic acid phosphatase:
     Where are we? Cancer 28:258 (1978).
31. Anonymous, New tests for prostatic cancer: Advisers routine,
     Med. World News 19:13 (1978).
32. R. Gittes, Acid phosphatase reappraised, New Engl. J. Med.
     297:1398 (1977).

33. R.A. Watson and D.B. Tang, The predictive value of prostatic
     acid phosphatase as a screening test for prostatic cancer,
     New Engl. J. Med. 303:497 (1980).
34. G.R. Lindholm, M.S. Stirton, R.J. Liedtke and J.D. Batjer,
     Prostatic acid phosphatase by radio-immuno assay, J.A.M.A.
     244:2071 (1980).
35. L.A. Klein, Prostatic carcinoma, New Engl. J. Med. 300:824
     (1979).
36. D.E. Johnson, W.W. Scott and R.P. Gibbons, Clinical significance
     of serum acid phosphatase levels in advanced prostatic carcinoma,
     Urology 8:123 (1976).
37. W.R. Berry, J. Laslo, E. Cox, A. Walker and D. Paulson,
     Prognostic factors in metastatic v. hormonally unresponsive
     carcinoma of the prostate, Cancer 44:763 (1979).
38. R.M. Nesbit and W.C. Baum, Serum phosphatase determination in
     diagnosis of prostatic cancer: A review of 1150 cases, J.A.M.A.
     145:1321 (1951).
39. V.A.C.U.R.G., Factors in the prognosis of carcinoma of the
     prostate: A cooperative study, J. Urol. 100:59 (1968).
40. M. de Pauw, S. Suciu, R. Sylvester, P.H. Smith,
     M. Pavone-Macaluso and the EORTC Urological Group, Preliminary
     results of two EORTC randomized trials in previously untreated
     patients with advanced T3 - T4 prostatic cancer, in: "Cancer
     of the Prostate and Kidney," P.H. Smith and M. Pavone-Macaluso,
     eds., Plenum Press, London and New York (1982).
41. C. Huggins and C.V. Hodges, Studies on prostatic cancer: 1.
     The effect of castration, of oestrogen and of androgen
     injection on serum phosphatases in metastatic carcinoma of
     the prostate, Cancer Res. 1:293 (1941).
42. C.R. Franks, Melphalan in metastatic cancer of the prostate,
     Cancer Treat. Reviews 6 (Suppl.):121 (1979).

PROSTATIC CANCER: ADVANCES IN DIAGNOSIS

L. Denis and A. Van Steirteghem

Academic Hospital
Free University of Brussels
A.Z. Middelheim (Antwerp) Belgium

Prostatic cancer constitutes one of the most commonly diagnosed cancers in older males (1). The accumulated information concerning this disease is enormous but we are still unable to diagnose the disease in the early stages, to assess the extent of disease in a non invasive way or to select treatment according to the lethal potential of the tumor. This paper brings data together that have or seem to have value in establishing answers to these three questions. Any of these problems, if answered, would represent a true advance in diagnosis. Physical examination, histological confirmation by biopsy, medical imaging techniques and prostatic tumor markers have been selected for presentation.

1. Physical Examination

Early prostatic cancer offers no symptoms suggestive of the disease and there is a general consensus that a careful rectal examination is required in all men over 50 years on a yearly basis. The first problem is that non neoplastic disorders such as inflammatory processes may mimic the induration which suggests prostatic carcinoma. However, induration presenting as a nodule has the probability of being neoplastic in about 50 per cent of the patients (2). This is a rather rare event and applies to a selective subpopulation of patients with prostatic cancer. We feel that any area of induration in the prostate felt on rectal examination should be biopsied. We apply this simple rule to our patient population presenting with urological symptoms; because of this the detection of unsuspected cancer at the time of surgery is a rare event. Out of 100 consecutive patients with prostatic cancer only two escaped preoperative diagnosis. Scientific support for this observation has been provided by Guinan et al (3) and Catalona (4)

who biopsied respectively 300 and 70 consecutive patients admitted
for a variety of urological conditions. In both series digital
rectal examination proved to be a most efficient test in the diagnosis of prostatic cancer.

The efficiency of the rectal examination in prostatic cancer
has also been evaluated in randomized prospective studies. In a
subpopulation of the VACURG study (5) rectal examination was
presented as 50 per cent correct in diagnosis in contrast to the
EORTC studies where this examination got better marks (6). It
should be noted that early cancers abound in the former series. The
score for the correlation between rectal examination and prostatic
cancer is even better in the famous Bowery series of Hudson et al
(7). Of 39 cases of prostatic cancer detected by open perineal
biopsy in a consecutive series of 300 symptomatic and asymptomatic
men only four did not show induration of the prostate on physical
examination. All four men had cancer limited to the prostate.

A second problem is the false negative prostatic needle
biopsies (with the exclusion of microcarcinoma which should not be
evaluated as a clinical cancer) (8). Repeat biopsy is advocated if
additional suggestive evidence for prostatic cancer is present or no
histological explanation for the induration is provided.

2. Histological Confirmation by Biopsy

Ever since Broders assigned a grading system to tumor differentiation we have been repeatedly warned by our pathologists about
the difficulty of classification in such a notoriously heterogeneous
tumor as prostatic cancer (9,10). A breakthrough in this respect is
the clinical application of the Gleason scale (11) in the prediction
of positive lymph nodes as demonstrated by Paulson et al (12). The
addition of nuclear morphology as a separate grading factor seems to
relate to the biological potential of the tumor (13). This correlates with our personal experience in 217 patients where tumor grade
based on histological and cellular differentiation predicted mortality rates in a reliable pattern (14).

An important aspect of the pathological evaluation concerning
the well differentiated cancers is the fact that perineural invasion
may occur in normal prostates (15). It is apparent from available
data that all biopsy material in a clinical situation should be
examined jointly by the pathologist and the urologist and that pathology material in randomized prospective studies should be reviewed
by a central pathology laboratory. The biopsy material is usually
obtained by needle biopsy but transurethral resection may serve the
purpose in selected instances. The division of the tissue according
to resected areas improves the overall accuracy and assessment of
the existing pathology (16). Repeated biopsies are necessary in
selected instances as only positive biopsies are valid; transrectal

aspiration biopsy submitted to an experienced cytologist may improve
on the diagnostic sensitivity.

Testing for detection of the blood group antigens (17) or
association to human leucocyte antigens (18) proved inconsistent in
predicting biologic aggressiveness. Pelvic lymphadenectomy on the
contrary has been demonstrated to give significant information on
the prognosis of the disease (19). It is of interest to note that
limited lymphadenectomy provides similar information without
considerable morbidity to the patient (20).

3. Medical Imaging

Two new non invasive techniques, ultrasonography (US) and
computerized axial tomography (CT), have been applied to the diagnosis and staging of prostatic cancer (21,22,23). The different
techniques and applications are reported elsewhere. Transrectal
ultrasonography in experienced hands provides better efficiency in
diagnosis and staging of prostatic cancer (24) and it is now well
established that transrectal ultrasonography as advocated by
Watanabe is the preferred technique for prostatic examination (25).

Ultrasound and CT constitute the only available cross-sectional
imaging in urological radiology. A comparison of different aspects
of the two techniques is given in Table 1. Basically CT scan
utilizes the penetration of x-ray photons and detects differences in
atomic composition. Its image resolution in a complete cross-
section of the abdomen is unsurpassed. One problem is that the
attenuation between tumoral and normal tissue is so small that
detection is difficult because of the isodensity. The presence of
fat or iodinated contrast agents helps to distinguish organ contours
or to detect unusual masses. Visulisation of ultrasound waves
reflects the elastic properties on a macromolecular structural level.
Echo texture differences are visible between tissues of different
composition and the main restriction in the abdomen is the presence
of gas, bone or obesity.

Our experience based on more than 1,500 US examinations with
five different improvements of technical material and on more than
200 CT examinations with three generations of CT scanners in
patients with lower urinary tract pathology allows us to draw the
following conclusions.

1. Both techniques cause minimal complications but radiation
   hazard and cost makes the CT scan less attractive for a routine
   work up.
2. The diagnostic criteria of prostatic tissue pathology are well
   established in transrectal ultrasonography (Table 2) and allow
   early diagnosis of prostatic cancer. This is impossible to
   diagnose on a CT scan. An example of a localized T2 tumor is

represented in Fig. 1. It should be clear that small well-differentiated carcinomas are easily missed and that areas of prostatic infection may mimic the echo pattern of prostatic cancer, especially in the newer real time technology. The echo pattern of prostatic cancer invites us to carry out a selective biopsy under visual control (26). The sensitivity in our hands oscillates around 80% without other information on the patient. This delays the possibility for mass screening by this technique though Watanabe reached a rate of sensitivity of 99.7% (27).

3. Tumor extent is appreciated in US by distortions of the prostatic capsule and by non-specific echo patterns in the seminal vesicles (Fig. 2). The mass of reflections is frequently continuous with a proven tumor in the prostate. This type of early infiltration or capsule distortion is difficult to visualize on CT.

4. Evaluation of prostatic mass is possible in both techniques by scanning at different levels to reach a tomographic reconstruction. These data are easy to obtain with US and were more reliable in our hands than with automated CT determination. For practical clinical purposes however where mass definition serves as a parameter in regression or progression of disease both methods are valid.

Table 1. Different Aspects of Ultrasound and Computerized Tomography in Prostatic Imaging

Transrectal U.S.	C.T. Scan
Sound (3.5 MH$_z$)	X-rays
Structural Elasticity	Electron Density
Gas, Bone, Obesity	Needs Contrast
No Side Effects	Radiation
Technical Skill	Automatic
Artifacts	Software
Available	Restricted
Minimal Cost	Expensive
Anatomy Good	Excellent
Histology Good	Fair

Table 2. Diagnostic Criteria. Transrectal Ultrasonography in Prostatic Pathology

	Normal Prostate	Peri-Urethral Adenoma	Prostatic Cancer
Transverse Section	Triangular Semilunar	Half/Full Circle	Deformations at Different Levels
Symmetry	Present	Usually Present	Absent
Capsule	Thin/Even	Thick/Regular/Even	Interrupted/Uneven Distorted
Sonic Density	Minimal	Present	Increased
Pattern	Regular	Regular	Irregular

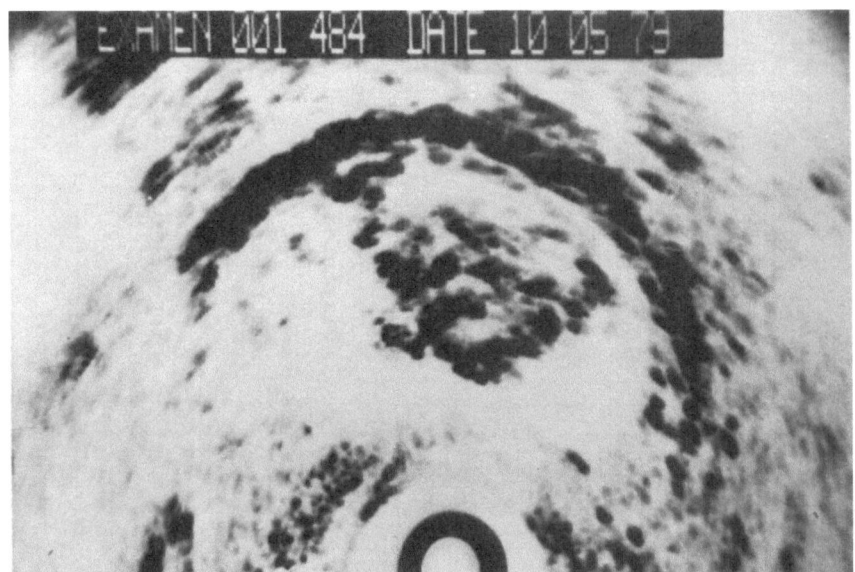

Fig. 1.   Strong internal mass echoes and unevenness in capsule
          thickness suggest prostatic cancer in this sonogram of
          a T2 prostatic cancer.

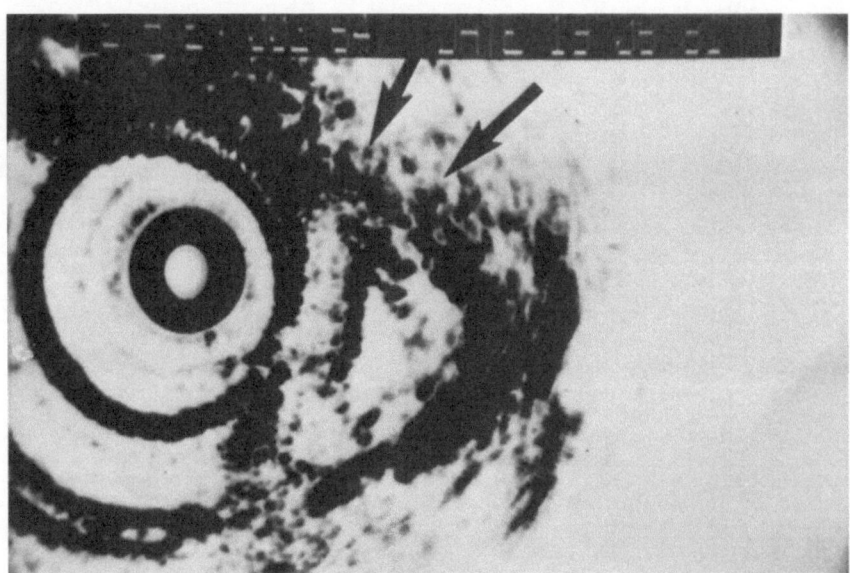

Fig. 2.   Discontinuity of capsular echoes and protrusion in the
          seminal vesicles is diagnostic of a T3 prostatic tumor.

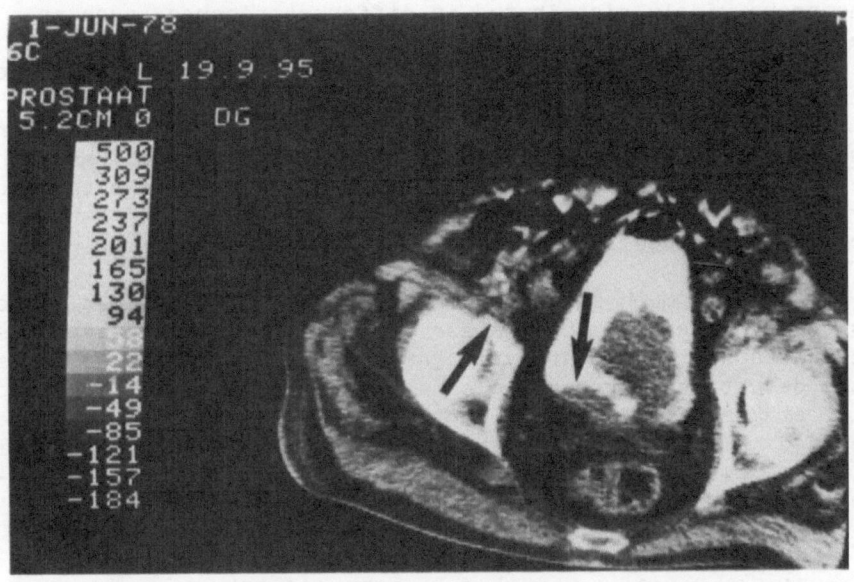

Fig. 3.   CT section of pelvis in a patient with advanced prostatic
          cancer demonstrates nodal obturator mass. Tumor invasion
          diagnosed by percutaneous fine needle biopsy.

5.   The diagnostic capacity of CT is remarkable in advanced tumor
     stages where the relationship to the surrounding organs or the
     pelvic bones are important with the additional benefit of the
     detection of nodal masses (Fig. 3) in the pelvis, in the retro-
     peritoneum and the detection of metastatic lesions to the liver
     or bone in selected instances.

     Constant refinements in both techniques will adjust their
     proper complementary role in clinical urology.

4.   Biochemical Markers

     Extensive research is going on to find biochemical markers for
prostatic cancer in easily accessible body fluids, especially in
blood and to a lesser extent in urine and in prostatic tissue.
Reliable blood markers could be useful for screening of populations
at risk, as well as for helping to determine if a patient is
responding to therapy and for the detection of recurrence in patients
in remission. Most emphasis here will be given to some of the serum
enzyme markers for prostatic cancer.

     As early as 1936 Gutman et al. described an association between
increased serum acid phosphatase activity and adenocarcinoma of the
prostate with metastases (28). Acid phosphatases belong to an

enzyme group widely distributed in different tissues, such as platelets, leucocytes, liver, spleen and kidneys. The highest concentration is found in prostatic tissue. Acid phosphatases exist as several molecular variants or isoenzymes, and even for the prostatic acid phosphatase (PAP), several isoenzymes exist. Current enzyme activity assay methods for PAP present some problems such as specificity of the substrates used for measuring their catalytic activity (29,30). The use of inhibitors of PAP such as L-tartrate are only partly specific.

Furthermore much attention should be paid to specimen collection and storage since acid phosphatase can deteriorate rapidly. Despite these drawbacks, serum catalytic PAP assays have proven to be useful for the detection of prostatic cancer with metastases. To detect earlier stages of the disease, more sensitive and specific methods are needed. Immunological methods, using specific antisera against PAP, became available recently. To date three different immunological procedures for measuring PAP have been described:

- radioimmunoassay - RIA (32,33,34,35)
- counterimmunoelectrophoresis - CIEP (36,37)
- Solid phase immunofluorescence - SPIF (37,38,39)

What are the advantages of these immunological methods compared to conventional catalytic activity assays? In terms of stability and accuracy, RIA and related procedures seem to be better since they are much less sensitive to storage conditions. To evaluate the different methodologies, the following factors need to be compared:

- Sensitivity i.e. percentage of patients in the disease group, who have positive tests;
- specificity i.e. percentage of individuals not having the disease who have negative results (40).

According to Griffiths, RIA has more diagnostic sensitivity than the conventional colorimetric method, while the change in specificity is less striking (41). Table 3 summarizes a comparison of reported diagnostic sensitivities for different clinical stages of prostatic cancer. The very high sensitivities described by Foti et al. (42) have not been confirmed by other workers, who found lower levels of sensitivity in the first three stages where these tests should be most useful. It seems therefore premature to accept this methodology as being able to diagnose localized prostatic carcinoma in a large percentage of patients.

Total alkaline phosphatase and its bone isoenzyme have some value in patients with metastatic prostatic cancer, especially for liver and bone metastases (43). It is useful to measure them together with PAP, which can be normal in some cases presenting a high serum alkaline phosphatase activity.

Table 3. Diagnostic Sensitivity of Immunological Procedures
for PAP as a Function of Disease Stage

		A (%)	B (%)	C (%)	D (%)
Foti et al.	(42)	33	79	71	92
Bruce et al.	(44)	8		35	
Wajsman et al.	(45)	38	35	49	69
Chu, T.M.	(37)	0	20	55	79
Mahan and Doctor	(46)	13	26	30	94
Griffiths, J.C.	(41)	12	32	47	86
Bruce et al.	(47)	14	29	24	89
Quinones et al.	(48)	25	8	46	52

Creatine kinase (CK) occurs as three isoenzymes, CK-MM, found
in skeletal and cardiac muscle, CK-MB, predominantly present in
cardiac muscle, and CK-BB, which is ubiquitous but in highest
concentration in the brain, the gastro-intestinal, and the genito-
urinary tract. Using conventional assay methods, CK-BB is rarely
found in human serum. By more sensitive methods, including RIA (49),
CK-BB has been found in abnormal amounts in the serum of patients
with a variety of malignant diseases. Feld and Witte (50) found
CK-BB by electrophoresis in nine out of 19 patients with stage D
cancer. Similar results were obtained when CK-BB was measured by
RIA (51). The possible role of BB isoenzyme as a tumor marker for
prostatic cancer was suggested by Silverman et al. (52) who found
elevated serum CK-BB concentrations in 15/17 stage D untreated
patients. The isoenzyme was not found in appropriate control
patients. When CK-BB was compared to PAP (both by RIA) as a tumor
marker for prostatic cancer in 23 patients with stage D carcinoma,
6/23 had elevated CK-BB while more than 60% of these patients had
increased PAP (53). The definitive value of CK-BB as a tumor marker
for cancer of the prostate needs further evaluation by long term
prospective study.

Besides serum enzyme markers there has been some recent work
concerning hormonal markers such as steroids, sex hormone or
testosterone binding globulin and prolactin. The data concerning
biochemical changes in prostatic tissue such as steroid oxido-

reductase enzymes and receptor and binding proteins were recently reviewed by Kirdani et al. (54).

DISCUSSION

A number of criteria are essential for a test to be useful in the clinical diagnosis and treatment of patients, and numerous tests and technological examinations await confirmation of clinical usefulness despite early claims. It is clear that one simply cannot multiply this diagnostic avalanche for ethical and economical reasons. Since 1975 the pace of discovery has accelerated dramatically and dozens of prostatic cancer markers look for clinical recognition (54). Apart from its scientific interest in a research setting a diagnostic test could have several uses; 1. for screening populations or high risk groups, 2. to confirm a diagnosis, 3. in the evaluation of a tumor, 4. to indicate prognosis, 5. for monitoring disease during treatment to indicate regression or progression, and 6. to assist in laboratory procedures as a comparison to other tests. In any one of these functions tests must be evaluated according to the three characteristics of sensitivity, specificity and the predictive value of the test (40). Where medical imaging, especially US, needs a certain tumor mass it is obvious that these tests should be reserved for screening selected populations. Patients with lower urinary tract obstruction or found coincidentally to have prostatic induration provide a good sub-set of patients at whom we might direct a battery of tests.

A biochemical marker specific for prostatic cancer is not yet available. The available markers help us to look for cancer in patients suspected of having the disease and allow us to monitor the biological behaviour of the tumor mass. Selectivity in the use of markers in a clinical setting is indicated since the use of a battery of assays will only add confusion. Extensive clinical research and exact recording of sensitivity and specificity may prepare the way for the addition of new markers to the routine clinical tests.

CONCLUSIONS

The diagnosis of clinical prostatic cancer starts with a careful rectal examination. Transrectal ultrasound and some biochemical markers are able to confirm the diagnosis with enough specificity to insist on repeated biopsy if the first biopsy is negative.

The tissue diagnosis coupled with the same diagnostic tests is able to predict prognosis in a reliable way. The tests should play a useful role as parameters in follow-up evaluations of the disease.

REFERENCES

1. C. Bouffioux, Le Cancer de la Prostate, <u>Acta Urol. Belg</u>. 47:190
    (1979).
2. H.J. Jewett, Significance of the palpable prostatic nodule,
    <u>JAMA</u> 160:838 (1956).
3. G. Guinan, I. Bush, V. Ray, R. Vieth, R. Rao, and R. Bhatti,
    The accuracy of the rectal examination in the diagnosis of
    prostate carcinoma, <u>New. Engl. J. Med</u>. 303:499 (1980).
4. W.J. Catalona, Yield from routine prostatic needle biopsy in
    patients more than 50 years old referred for urologic evaluat-
    ions: A preliminary report, <u>J. Urol</u>. 124:844 (1980).
5. D.P. Byar, F.K. Mostofi, and VACURG, Carcinoma of the prostate.
    Prognostic evaluation of certain pathological features in 208
    radical prostatectomies, <u>Cancer</u> 30:5 (1972).
6. M.R.G. Robinson, Personal Communication.
7. P.B. Hudson, A.L. Finkle, A.J. Hopkens, E.E. Sproul, and
    A.P. Stout, Prostatic cancer XI early prostatic cancer diagnosed
    by arbitrary open perineal biopsy among 300 unselected patients,
    <u>Cancer</u> 7:690 (1954).
8. D.P. Byar and VACURG, Survival of patients with incidentally
    found microscopic cancer of the prostate. Results of a clinical
    trial of conservative treatment, <u>J. Urol</u>. 108:908 (1972).
9. A.C. Broders, Grading of Carcinoma, <u>Minnesota Med</u>. 8:726 (1925).
10. F.K. Mostofi, Problems of grading carcinoma of the prostate,
    <u>Semin. Oncol</u>. 3:161 (1976).
11. D.F. Gleason, G.T. Mellinger, and VACURG, Prediction of
    prognosis for prostatic adenocarcinoma by combined histologic
    grading and clinical staging, <u>J. Urol</u>. 111:58 (1974).
12. D.F. Paulson, P.V. Piserchia, and W. Gardner, Predictors of
    lymphatic spread in prostatic adeno-carcinoma. Uro-oncology
    Research Group study, <u>J. Urol</u>. 123:697 (1980).
13. J.F. Gaeta, J.E. Asurwatham, G. Miller, and G.P. Murphy,
    Histologic grading of primary prostatic cancer. A new approach
    to an old problem, <u>J. Urol</u>. 123:689 (1980).
14. L. Denis, Clinical cancer of prostate. Influence of tumor
    stage and grade on five year survival, <u>Acta Urol. Belg</u>. 40:126
    (1972).
15. P.J.B. Carstens, Perineural glands in normal and hyperplastic
    prostates, <u>J. Urol</u>. 123:686 (1980).
16. N. O'Donoghue and R. Pugh, Early diagnosis of prostatic
    carcinoma: the role of trans-urethral resection, <u>Brit. J. Urol</u>.
    116:759 (1976).
17. W.J. Catalona and M. Menon, New screening and diagnostic tests
    for prostate cancer and immunologic assessment, Suppl. to
    <u>Urology</u> 17:61 (1981).
18. J.M. Barry, A. Goldstein, and M. Hubbard, Human leucocyte A
    and B antigens in patients with prostatic adenocarcinoma,
    <u>J. Urol</u>. 124:847 (1980).

19. G.R. Prout, Jr., P. Griffin, J.J. Daly, and W.U. Shipley,
     Nodal involvement as prognostic indicator in prostatic
     carcinoma, Suppl. to Urology 17:72 (1981).
20. C.B. Brendler, L.K. Cleeve, E. Anderson, and D.F. Paulson,
     Staging pelvic lymphadenectomy for carcinoma of the prostate:
     risk versus benefit, J. Urol. 124:849 (1980).
21. L. Denis, L. Appel, J. Broos, and G. Declercq, Evaluation of
     prostatic cancer by transrectal ultrasonography and CT scan,
     Acta Urol. Belg. 48:71 (1980).
22. M.I. Resnick, Non invasive techniques in evaluating patients
     with carcinoma of the prostate, Suppl. to Urology, 17:25 (1981).
23. J. Pradel, J.M. Duclos, M. Charton, and J.M. Brussel, La
     tomodensitometrie dans le bilan d'extension des cancers
     prostatiques, in:"Sem. D'Uro-Nephrologie," R. Kuss and
     M. Legrain, eds., Masson, Paris (1981), p.31.
24. G. Declercq, L. Denis, J. Broos, and L. Appel, Evaluation of
     lower urinary tract by computed tomography and transrectal
     ultrasonography, Comp. Tom. In Press.
25. H. Watanabe, S.H. Holmes, H.J. Holm, and B.B. Goldberg,
     "Diagnostic Ultrasound in Urology and Nephrology," Ingaku
     Shion Ltd., Tokyo (1981).
26. H.H. Holm and J. Gammelgaard, Ultrasonically guided precise
     needle placement in the prostate and the seminal vesicles,
     J. Urol. 125:385 (1981).
27. H. Watanabe, T. Mishina, and H. Ohe, Mass screening of prostatic
     diseases, in:"Prostatic Carcinoma and Biology and Diagnosis,"
     E.S.E. Hafez and E. Spring Mills, Martinus Nyhoff, The Hague
     (1981), p.71.
28. E.B. Gutman, E.E. Sproul, and A.B. Gutman, Increased phosphatase
     activity of bone at site of osteoplastic metastases secondary to
     carcinoma of prostate gland, Am. J. Cancer 28:485 (1936).
29. A.V. Roy, M.E. Brouwer, and J.E. Hayden, Sodium thymolphthalein
     monophosphate: a new acid phosphatase substrate with greater
     specificity for the prostate in serum, Clin. Chem. 17:1093
     (1971).
30. C.Y. Li, R.A. Chuda, W.K.W. Lam, and L.T. Yam, Acid phosphatases
     in human plasma, J. Lab. Clin. Med. 82:446 (1973).
31. W.H. Fishman and F. Lerner, A method for estimating serum acid
     phosphatase of prostatic origin, J. Biol. Chem. 200:89 (1953).
32. J.F. Cooper and A.G. Foti, A radioimmunoassay for prostatic
     acid phosphatase.I. Methodology and range of normal male
     serum values, Invest. Urol. 12:98 (1974).
33. J.F. Cooper and A.G. Foti, A radioimmunoassay for prostatic
     acid phosphatase, Nat. Can. Inst. Monograph 49:235 (1978).
34. J.F. Cooper, A.G. Foti, and P.W. Shank, Radioimmunochemical
     measurement of bone marrow prostatic acid phosphatase,
     J. Urol. 119:388 (1978).
35. P. Vihko, E. Sajanti, O. Jänne, L. Peltonen, and R. Vihko,
     Serum prostate-specific acid phosphatase: development and
     validation of a specific radioimmunoassay, Clin. Chem. 24:1915
     (1978).

36. T.M. Chu, M.C. Wang, R. Kajdasz, E.A. Barnard, P. Kucil, and
     G.P. Murphy, Prostate-specific acid phosphohydrolase in the
     diagnosis of prostate cancer, Proc. Am. Assoc. Cancer Res.
     17:191 (1976).

37. T.M. Chu, Serum acid phosphohydrolase (phosphatase) and ribo-
     nuclease in diagnosis of prostatic cancer, Antibiotics Chemo-
     therapy 22:98 (1978).

38. C.L. Lee, M.C. Wang, G.P. Murphy, and T.M. Chu, A solid phase
     fluorescent immunoassay for human prostatic acid phosphatase,
     Cancer Res. 38:2871 (1978).

39. C.L. Lee, C.S. Killian, G.P. Murphy, and T.M. Chu, A solid-
     phase immunoadsorbant assay for serum prostatic acid phosphatase,
     Clin. Chim. Acta 101:209 (1980).

40. R.S. Galen and S.R. Gambino, "Beyond Normality: The Predictive
     Value and Efficiency of Medical Diagnosis," Wiley, New York
     (1975).

41. J.C Griffiths, Prostate-specific acid phosphatase: re-evaluation
     of radioimmunoassay in diagnosing prostatic disease, Clin. Chem.
     26:433 (1980).

42. A.G. Foti, J.F. Cooper, H. Herschman, and R.R. Malvaez,
     Detection of prostate cancer by solid-phase radioimmunoassay
     of serum prostatic acid phosphatase, New Engl. J. Med. 297:1357
     (1977).

43. D.M. Goldberg and G. Ellis, An assessment of serum acid and
     alkaline phosphatase determination in prostatic cancer with a
     clinical validation of an acid phosphatase assay utilizing
     adenosine 3'-monophosphatate as substrate, J. Clin. Pathol.
     27:140 (1974).

44. A.W. Bruce, D.E. Mahan, A. Morales, A.F. Clark, and W.D.
     Belville, An objective look at acid phosphatase determinations.
     A comparison of biochemical and immunological methods, Brit.
     J. Urol 51:213 (1979).

45. A. Wajsman, T.M. Chu, J. Saroff, N. Slack, and G.P. Murphy,
     Two new, direct and specific methods of acid phosphatase
     determination, National field Trial. Urology 13:8 (1979).

46. D.E. Mahan and B.P. Doctor, A radioimmune assay for human
     prostatic acid phosphatase-levels in prostatic disease, Clin.
     Biochem. 12:10 (1979).

47. A.W. Bruce, D.E. Mahan, L.D. Sullivan, and L. Goldenberg,
     The significance of prostatic acid phosphatase in adeno-
     carcinoma of the prostate, J. Urol. 125:357 (1981).

48. G.R. Quinones, T.J. Rohnef, J.R. Drago, and L.M. Demers, Will
     prostatic acid phosphatase determination by radioimmunoassay
     increase the diagnosis of early prostatic cancer? J. Urol.
     125:361 (1981).

49. M.H. Zweig, A.C. Steirteghem, and A.N. Schechter, Radio-
     immunoassay of creatine kinase isoenzymes in human serum,
     Isoenzyme BB, Clin. Chem. 24:422 (1978).

50. P.D. Feld and D.L. Witte, Presence of creatine kinase BB iso-
     enzymes in some patients with prostatic carcinoma, Clin. Chem.
     23:1930 (1977).

51. R.D. Feld, A.C. Van Steirteghem, M.H. Zweig, G.W. Weimar,
     A.S. Narayana, and D.L. Witte, The presence of creatine kinase
     BB isoenzyme in patients with prostatic cancer, <u>Clin. Chim.
     Acta</u> 100:267 (1980).
52. L.M. Silverman, G.B. Demer, M.H. Zweig, A.C. Van Steirteghem,
     and Z.A. Tökés, Creatine kinase BB: a new tumor associated
     marker, <u>Clin. Chem.</u> 25:1432 (1979).
53. M.H. Zweig and A.C. Van Steirteghem, Serum creatine kinase BB
     (RIA) as a tumor marker: Studies in various cancers and a
     comparison to prostatic acid phosphatase, <u>J. Nat. Canc.
     Inst.</u> In Press.
54. R.Y. Kirdani, J.P. Karr, G.P. Murphy, and A.A. Sandberg,
     Clinical markers in prostatic cancer, <u>in</u>:"Prostatic Carcinoma
     - Biology and Diagnosis," E.S.E. Hafez and Spring - Mills,
     eds, Martinus Nyhoff, The Hague (1981), p.79.

FINE-NEEDLE ASPIRATION OF SOFT-TISSUE MASSES IN

PROSTATIC CANCER PATIENTS

J.D. Schmidt and J.J. Pollen

University of California Medical Center
San Diego
U.S.A.

INTRODUCTION

Fine-needle aspiration cytology of soft-tissue masses can play a major role in both staging and monitoring of therapy for patients with prostatic cancer. The procedure is safe, inexpensive and easy to perform in outpatients. Since the lesion itself is not removed, it serves as an indicator to gauge the response of either local or systemic therapy. An interested and skilled cytopathologist and cytotechnologist are essential for this technique to be useful.

In the United States most patients with prostatic cancer have their clinical diagnosis confirmed histologically via needle biopsy or transurethral prostatic resection (1). However fine-needle aspiration cytologic diagnosis of the primary tumor has not so far received the acceptance that it has in other countries (2,3). Yet its use in the evaluation of soft-tissue masses in many malignancies has recently been received with increasing enthusiasm (4). An example is the use of this technique to follow-up an abnormal finding at lymphangiography (5).

MATERIALS AND METHODS

In the last three years fine-needle aspirations have been attempted in 18 patients with 19 soft-tissue masses. These included 10 lymph nodes (both inguinal and supraclavicular, two skin nodules and seven intraabdominal masses). The latter category has variably consisted of combinations of local extensions of a large primary tumor and deep pelvic or retroperitoneal lymphadenopathy.

The technique is simple and fairly similar to that already

reported (1). Following the measuring of the mass, the overlying skin is prepared with Povidone iodine solution. Local anesthetic infiltration using 1% Lidocaine hydrochloride is optional since the small caliber needles are usually well tolerated and too much infiltration may distort the target. The lesion is stabilized with one gloved hand while the 20 or 22 gauge needle attached to a 6-12 cc syringe is passed into the mass. It is important to create a strong suction on the needle as it is passed back and forth through the lesion. In our urology clinic, we prefer to have a cytotechnologist present for the procedure. The technologist receives the needle and syringe and immediately prepares thin smears on slides and flushes the needle and syringe into fixative. The aspirate is often repeated with a second needle and syringe. Smears and cell washings are then submitted for routine staining and examination by both the cytotechnologist and cytopathologist. A small pressure dressing or band-aid over the puncture site suffices.

RESULTS

The results of our aspiration cytologies are listed in Table 1. Aspirates are reported as either diagnostic, i.e., positive or negative for malignant cells, or non-diagnostic, i.e., insufficient or unsatisfactory for any diagnosis. The latter report definitely needs to be followed up by another attempt at aspiration. Aspirates reported as negative are repeated if clinical suspicion of malignancy is high and a sampling error is likely.

Aspirates positive for malignant cells were found in 15 specimens. In many instances the material was sufficiently diagnostic for the reading of adenocarcinoma consistent with prostatic origin. One abdominal mass proved to be a full colonic segment. No complications occurred in this instance or in any of the other patients studied by this technique.

Table 1: Results of fine-needle aspirates of 19 soft-tissue masses (18 patients with prostatic cancer)

	Diagnostic		Non-diagnostic
	Positive	Negative	
Lymph nodes	9	1	---
Abdominal masses	4	1	2
Skin nodules	2	---	---
TOTAL	15	2	2

CASE REPORT

A 69-year old man had previously been treated with external beam irradiation to the prostate and pelvis for clinically localized prostatic carcinoma. Three years later because of right hip pain he was re-evaluated and found to have an elevated serum acid phosphatase activity and a positive bone scan. In spite of bilateral orchiectomy and intravenous diethylstilbestrol diphosphate (Honvan, Stilphostrol), the disease progressed as new lesions were identified on subsequent bone scans. At this time a 2 x 2 cm firm non-tender left supraclavicular mass was palpated. Fine-needle aspiration was performed without the need of local anesthetic. The aspirate was positive for malignant cells compatible with adenocarcinoma. With the confirmatory evidence that his prostatic cancer had indeed been documented as progressing on endocrine therapy, the patient was started on cytotoxic chemotherapy. The supraclavicular lymph node remains as an additional parameter by which to gauge his response to the new treatment.

DISCUSSION

Although soft-tissue metastases are uncommon in prostatic cancer, their identification can be critical in the accurate staging of individual patients. Benign lesions such as reactive lymphadenitis or hematoma must be distinguished from metastatic involvement or extensive local infiltration by the primary tumor.

Once the soft-tissue mass had been identified as malignant, the lesions serve as a marker for any response to therapy. Many of these masses are measurable; the remainder are at least evaluable regarding response to treatment. Thus, this does not require a minor or major surgical procedure to remove the mass which, in prostatic cancer, would rarely be an isolated metastasis.

The technique can be expanded to the cytologic diagnosis of masses detected by lymphangiography, computerized tomography or ultrasonography in the evaluation of a patient with prostatic cancer (5). In these situations, the fine-needle aspirate is performed by fluoroscopic or ultrasonic guidance as has been documented in other tumor systems.

The procedure is safe, easy to perform and relatively inexpensive considering the alternatives available. The accuracy of interpretation with well-preserved specimens should be over 90 percent (4). False-positive readings should not occur; a false-negative interpretation occurs in 10% of instances and can signify a sampling error. Non-diagnostic samples, whether due to poor aspirate technique or poor cytologic technique, should be repeated at an early date.

Complications of the fine-needle aspiration procedures are infrequent and bleeding is easily controlled by local pressure. We have not experienced any tumor seeding along the needle track and no infections have occurred.

REFERENCES

1. J.J. Pollen and J.D. Schmidt, Diagnostic fine-needle aspiration
    of soft-tissue metastases from cancer of the prostate, J. Urol.
    121:59 (1979).
2. P.L. Esposti, Cytologic malignancy grading of prostate
    carcinoma by transrectal aspiration biopsy. A five-year follow-
    up study of 469 hormone-treated patients, Scand. J. Urol. Nephrol.
    5:199 (1971).
3. F.P. Kohler, D.M. Kelsey, C.C. MacKinney and T.S. Kline, Needle
    aspiration of the prostate, J. Urol. 118:1012 (1977).
4. T.S. Kline and H.S. Neal, Needle aspiration biopsy: a critical
    appraisal - eight years and 3,267 specimens later, JAMA
    239:36 (1978).
5. S. Wallace, B.S. Jing and J. Zornoza, Lymphangiography in the
    determination of the extent of metastatic carcinoma: the
    potential value of percutaneous lymph node biopsy, Cancer
    39:706 (1977).

*   This work was supported in part by Public Health Service Grant
    CA 21438 through the National Prostatic Cancer Project, National
    Cancer Institute, National Institutes of Health, Department of
    Health and Human Services.

PROSTATIC CANCER STAGING - AN OVERVIEW

L. Andersson

Karolinska sjukhuset
Stockholm
Sweden

As in all malignant disease an accurate characterization of the tumour is mandatory to predict the prognosis and to guide the treatment. Most urologists and oncologists feel today that the malignancy grade is the most important parameter in the evaluation of tumour aggressiveness. Therapeutic decisions also imply assessment of the tumour extent.

In principle there are two kinds of system in use to describe tumour extent, staging systems which group the patients together according to a number of various characteristics, and a classification system which describes each parameter of the tumour disease separately.

The staging systems are variants or modifications of the system proposed by Whitmore in 1956 (1) (Fig. 1) and originally based on the pathological findings in specimens from radical surgery. In stage A the tumour is confined to the prostate and is not suspected clinically but an incidental finding on operation for obstructive disease, such as TUR or adenomectomy, or on postmortem examination.

Catalona and Scott (2), in 1978, proposed a more detailed subclassification of the Whitmore system where A1F denotes a focus of occult carcinoma, A1 a malignant lesion involving one lobe, and A2 a multifocal lesion or diffuse spread of the occult cancer. This subclassification was an improvement of the Whitmore system as widespread occult carcinoma is often of high grade and carries a much more sinister prognosis than does focal disease. Correa et al (3) reported a series of cases of carcinoma stage A, for the most part found on TUR. Forty-five patients were observed for more than a year up to a maximum of ten years. Of eight patients with diffuse

197

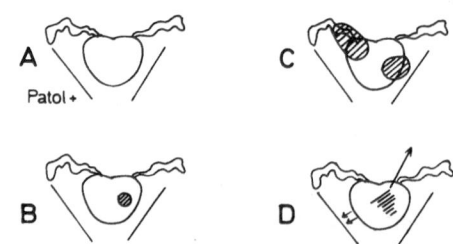

Fig. 1. Staging according to Whitmore

occult carcinoma, five had tumour recurrence. Two of these died
from their tumour and three further patients died with tumour present. Among the 37 patients with focal disease, tumour recurrence was
identified in three. No death from cancer occured in the latter
group within the observation period. There are also other investigations on record showing that average survival in A2 patients is
lower than in patients with localized stage B carcinoma.

Stage B indicates palpable tumour confined to the prostate. In
the subclassification according to Catalona and Scott (2), B1N
denotes a solitary nodule of estimated diameter 15 mm or less, B1
tumour involvement of an entire lobe or nearly entire lobe, and B2
diffuse involvement of the gland. The frequency of lymph node
deposits increases and the prognosis worsens with the extent of
tumour involvement.

In stage C there is tumour extension beyond the prostatic capsule but no evidence of distant metastases. Acid phosphatase
activity, as measured by enzymatic technique, is usually normal but
may be enhanced. Using radioimmunoassay, enhanced phosphatase
activity is recorded in about 70% of stage C cases. Lymph node
extension also occurs in a high percentage of stage C cases.

Stage D indicates cases where metastatic deposits are observed,
usually in the skeleton, lymph nodes or lungs. There may be any
local finding in the prostate from no palpable tumour to extensive
infiltration. Serum acid phosphatase activity is elevated in the
majority of stage D cases, 60% as measured by enzymatic techniques
and over 90% with radioimmunoassay.

The US Veterans Administration Co-Operative Urological Research
Group have used a staging system very similar to that of Whitmore,
except that the symbols A-D are changed for the roman numerals I-IV
(Fig. 2). The only difference of essential character is that in the
VACURG system an elevated acid phosphatase activity is accepted as
indication of tumour spread, and consequently stage IV, even in cases
where no metastases can be observed by other methods.

Stage	Rectal Examination	Prostatic Acid Phosphatase	X-ray Evidence of Metastases
I	No Induration	< 1.0 K.A.U.	0
II	Localized Nodule	< 1.0 K.A.U.	0
III	Extra Prostatic Extension	< 1.0 K.A.U.	0
IV	Equivocal Findings	> 1.0 K.A.U.	+

Fig. 2. Staging of prostatic cancer according to the U.S.
Veterans Administration co-operative Urological Research
Group.

With the increasing use of the sensitive radio-immunoassay
techniques with abnormal activity found in many cases of local disease
the definition can hardly be accepted today, even with the reservation
that our methods of identifying true local disease are still limited.

The TNM-system, originally described by Denoix in 1953 (4) and
adopted by the International Union Against Cancer, is a classification
system where the extent of the primary tumour, lymph node dissemination and distant metastases are indicated by separate symbols, T for
the local tumour, N for regional lymph nodes, and M for distant
metastases beyond the regional nodes. The TNM categorization is based
on clinical evaluation and not on pathological investigation except
for biopsy and thus involves the inexactitude of the clinical
evaluation. The pathological description is indicated by the symbol
pT which may supplement the T category but should never change it.

Fig. 3 represents the classification of the local tumour in
prostate cancer according to the TNM system. The rules were specified
in 1974 and it is now time to consider them for reevaluation. In T0
there is no palpable tumour but the cancer is an incidental finding
in an operative or biopsy specimen, analogous with stage A. In T1
the tumour is palpable but located within the gland and surrounded by
palpably normal gland tissue. In T2 the tumour is still confined to
the gland but the contour is deformed by the nodule. In borderline
cases it may be difficult to distinguish between T1 and T2 cases. In
T3 there is extension beyond the capsule or into the seminal vesicles
and T4 indicates extension to the pelvic wall or invasion into the
neighbouring organs other than the seminal vesicles.

In the TNM system there is no stage grouping but lymph node
dissemination is indicated by various N-symbols and distant
metastases by M-symbols.

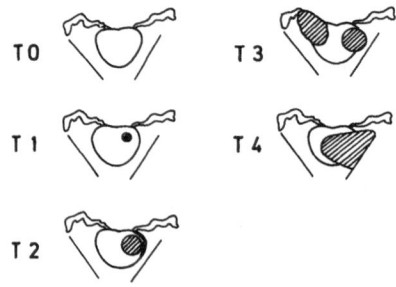

Fig. 3. TNM Classification

        Even with experienced examiners the intraprostatic extent of a
tumour and multifocal growth are difficult to assess. The accuracy
of digital examination increases with higher T category. Extracapsular infiltration is relatively easy to identify. In a review
of 103 malignant nodules, Jewett (5) noted that the extent of
carcinoma had been underestimated in 72% of the cases on rectal
examination. Hopefully modern imaging techniques, ultrasound
scanning in particular, will improve the accuracy of estimation of
the tumour extent, at least the local tumour. An exact recording of
tumour spread is especially important in those cases where radical
surgery or radical radiotherapy is aimed at. Assessment of the
biological activity, i.e. the aggressiveness of the tumour, as
reflected by the malignancy grade, DNA-pattern or some other
indicator, is also an indispensable part of the tumour characterization.

REFERENCES

1. W.F. Whitmore, Jr., Hormone therapy in prostatic cancer, Amer.
    J. Med. 21:697 (1956).
2. W.J. Catalona and W.W. Scott, Carcinoma of the prostate: A
    review, J. Urol. 119:1 (1978).
3. R.J. Correa, R.G Anderson, R.P. Gibbons, and J. Tate Mason,
    Latent carcinoma of the prostate - why the controversy?, J. Urol.
    111:644 (1974).
4. P.F. Denoix, Presentation d'une nomenclature classification des
    cancers basée sur un atlas, Acta Unio Internat. contra cancrum
    9:769 (1953).
5. H.J. Jewett, Significance of the palpable prostatic nodule,
    J.A.M.A. 160:838 (1956).

CARCINOMA OF THE PROSTATE - THE NEED FOR

A REVISION OF CATEGORY TO?

L.L. Beynon, G.D. Chisholm, A. Busuttil and
T.B. Hargreave

Western General Hospital
Edinburgh
U.K.

The survival of patients with carcinoma of the prostate is not always improved by commencing active treatment at the time of diagnosis. Byar (1) showed that the survival of a group of patients with unsuspected 'localised' carcinoma of the prostate was the same as that of an age-matched control population. Despite this finding it is not universal practice to defer treatment in this group of patients. Clinicians are undoubtedly influenced by the knowledge that in some cases, even with small well-differentiated tumours, metastases will develop (2). Attempts to predict those cases which will do badly have identified several prognostic factors including poor histological differentiation (3,4,5,6,7), age (8,9,10), tumour bulk (3,11) and the presence of a clear margin of resection (3).

A variety of definitions of 'local' disease have been introduced. In some the emphasis is on the extent of the tumour, in others the histological grade (12), the aim of each classification proposed being to improve prognostication and to allow the more logical selection of treatment in this group of patients.

We have reviewed a series of 34 cases of TO carcinoma of the prostate in an attempt to correlate their clinical progress with the histological features of the tumour at presentation. The aim of this study was to clarify the spectrum of disease represented by the TO category and to decide whether a revised category was indicated in the interests of appropriate treatment selection.

METHODS

In a series of 159 patients with carcinoma of the prostate
presenting consecutively at the prostate clinic, 34 were classified
as category TO. All patients had histologically proven carcinoma of
the prostate and pathology of the specimens obtained has been reviewed retrospectively. Grading has been carried out by a single
pathologist according to the Gleason system (13,14). This grading
is carried out at relatively low magnification, five patterns of
growth being assigned numbers in order of decreasing apparent histological differentiation. In order to allow for histological variation within the tumour two digits are recorded, first the predominant
pattern (by area), then the lesser pattern (by area). For example,
a well-differentiated tumour containing areas of poor differentiation
would be represented by the figures 2-4. In addition an attempt was
made, on the basis of the material available to the pathologist, to
assess the amount of tissue involved with tumour. Three categories
were chosen: $<$10% involved; 10-50% involved and $>$50% involved. This
does not correspond exactly to the American categories of A1$_f$ focal
microscopic tumour involvement, A1 microscopic involvement of one
lobe and A2 multifocal or diffuse involvement (15) but it was hoped
to get a reasonable measure of the extent of tumour involvement and
its relation to grading and prognosis.

At the time of diagnosis all patients had levels of blood urea,
creatinine, electrolytes, liver function tests and acid phosphatase
determined, together with isotopic bone scan. Out patient follow-up
was carried out at three-monthly intervals with clinical examination,
full blood count, and acid and alkaline phosphatase on each occasion.
In addition isotopic bone scans were repeated at six-monthly intervals or sooner if indicated by bone pain.

RESULTS

Of the 34 cases reviewed 26 were classified as category TO MO
and four as TO M1. Four patients who did not have an isotopic bone
scan were categorised as MX. The patients' ages ranged from 58-88
with a mean of 72.5 years. Follow-up varied from 1-138 months
(mean 22.2 months). During the course of this study eight patients
have died but only three of these deaths resulted from malignant
disease of the prostate. In six patients the diagnosis was made
following open prostatectomy and in one case histology was obtained
from a bone biopsy of a secondary deposit. In the remaining 27
patients the diagnosis was made following transurethral resection of
the prostate.

Treatment was deferred in 25 cases, primary radical radiotherapy
was given in three and six patients received hormonal treatment
initially. Of the six patients treated initially with hormonal

therapy, three had metastases at the time of presentation and one of
the other three has developed bony metastases during follow up. Of
the deferred treatment cases, four have developed metastases during
the course of follow-up and three have developed local progression
of their disease.

Table 1 shows the relationship between histological
differentiation expressed as the Gleason worst and summed score
means with a theoretical maximum of five and ten respectively, and
the presence or absence of metastases at presentation and during the
period of follow-up. One patient is excluded from this set of
results since he died before effective staging or follow-up could be
carried out. It will be clear that those presenting with metastases
have worse mean scores than either of the other groups, and that
those who developed metastases during follow-up had higher mean
Gleason scores than those patients without metastases. Sixteen of
the patients selected for deferred treatment have been followed for
longer than six months and these cases can be divided into two groups
(Table 2) - nine who have shown no disease progression, and seven
in whom local progression or metastatic disease has become evident.
Once again those with disease progression had worse mean scores than
those who have required no treatment intervention.

Comparison of histological scores with our assessment of
tumour extent at presentation (Table 3) show a definite tendency
to poorer histological differentiation in those patients with more
extensive infiltration of the gland. Despite this tendency it is

Table 1. Relationship between Gleason Score and Presence
          or Absence of Metastases at Presentation and during
          Follow-up.

	No metastases	Metastases developed	Metastases at presentation
Gleason mean worst score	2.25	2.6	4.5
Gleason mean summed score	3.83	4.4	8.25
No. of Patients	24	5	4

Table 2.   Relationship between Gleason Score and Subsequent
           Disease Progression.

	Deferred treatment No progression	Deferred treatment Disease progression
Gleason mean worst score	2.11	2.43
Gleason mean summed score	3.56	4.14
No. of Patients	9	7

Table 3.   Relationship between Gleason Score and Estimate
           of Extent of Infiltration of Prostate.

	Extent of Prostatic Infiltration		
	<10%	10 - 50%	>50%
Gleason mean worst score	2.25	2.62	3.2
Gleason mean summed score	4.0	4.32	5.5
No. of Patients	16	8	10

important to note that of the four patients presenting with
metastases, two had less than 10% of the gland involved and for these
cases the mean worst score was 4.5 and the mean summed score 8.5.

In this study no correlation was found between age and histological differentiation or between age and extent of gland involvement by tumour.

DISCUSSION

This study has emphasised again the heterogeneous nature of
patients falling into the TO category both in terms of tumour
histology and in the extent of the involvement of the prostate by
tumour.

Although patients with metastatic disease represent a distinct
group both in terms of treatment and prognosis, their inclusion in
this study is justified by the need to obtain an overall view of the
natural history of TO disease. The impression gained from this series
confirms the findings of other workers in that the poorer prognosis of
more extensive tumours is really a reflection of their poorer histological grade. This suggests that greater weight should be put on the
degree of tumour differentiation than upon the extent of tumour within
the prostate. Although we have found no relationship between age and
prognosis in this group of patients, we have relatively few aged 60
or below and it is quite possible that this younger age group form a
special category. The information collected in this study does not
allow us to draw any conclusions regarding the importance of a clear
margin of resection nor does it indicate the potential value of
assessing capsular involvement by a second resection or needle biopsy
of the posterior gland.

It is concluded that since our study has demonstrated a
relationship between clinical progress and histology of the tumour at
presentation, irrespective of the size of the primary lesion, a
decision for deferred treatment in category TO patients should be
related to histological grade rather than to any measure of extent of
local tumour and that the TO category should always be combined with
an indication of the histological grade of the tumour.

REFERENCES

1. D.P. Byar, VACURG studies on prostatic cancer and its treatment,
    in:"Urologic Pathology: the Prostate," M. Tannenbaum, ed., Lea
    and Febiger, New York, 241 (1977).
2. W.H. Kern, Well differentiated adenocarcinoma of the prostate,
    Cancer, 41:2046 (1978).

3. W.C. Bauer, M.H. McGravran, and M.R. Carlin, Unsuspected carcinoma of prostate in suprapubic prostatectomy specimens: A clinicopathological study of 55 consecutive cases, Cancer 13:370 (1960).

4. R.E. Wiederanders, R.V. Stuber, C. Mota, D. O'Connell, and G.J. Haslam, Prognostic value of grading prostatic carcinoma, J. Urol. 89:881 (1963).

5. J.N. Corriere Jr., J.L. Cornog, and J.J. Murphy, Prognosis in patients with carcinoma of the prostate, Cancer 25:911 (1970).

6. E. Belt and F.H. Schroeder, Total perineal prostatectomy for carcinoma of the prostate, J. Urol. 107:91 (1972).

7. H.J. Jewett, The present status of radical prostatectomy for stages A and B prostatic cancer, Urol. Clin. North America 2:105 (1975).

8. H.B. Tjadan, D.A. Culp, and R.H. Flocks, Clinical adenocarcinoma of the prostate in patients under 50 years of age, J. Urol. 93:618 (1965).

9. K.A. Hanash, D.C. Cook, W.F. Taylor, and J.L. Titus, Carcinoma of the prostate: A 15 year follow up, J. Urol. 107:450 (1972).

10. G.R. Ray, J.R. Cassidy and M.A. Bagshaw, Definitive radiation therapy of carcinoma of the prostate. A report of 15 years experience, Radiology 106:407 (1973).

11. R. de Vere White, D.F. Paulson, and J.F. Glenn, The clinical spectrum of prostate cancer, J. Urol. 117:323 (1977).

12. C.A. Sheldon, R.D. Williams, and E.E. Fraley, Incidental carcinoma of the prostate: A review of the literature and critical reappraisal of classification, J. Urol. 124:626 (1980).

13. D.F. Gleason and G.T. Mellinger, Prediction of prognosis for prostatic adenocarcinoma by combined histological grading and clinical staging, J. Urol. 11:58 (1974).

14. D.F. Gleason, Histologic grading and clinical staging of prostatic carcinoma, in:"Urologic Pathology: the Prostate," M. Tannenbaum, ed., Lea and Febiger, New York (1977).

15. W.J. Catalona and W.W. Scott, Carcinoma of the prostate, in: "Campbell's Urology," J.H. Harrison, R.F. Gittes, A.D. Perlmutter, T.A. Stamey and P.C. Walsh, eds., Saunders, Philadelphia (1979), Vol. 2, p. 1093.

LYMPH NODE METASTASES IN PROSTATIC CANCER

M. A. Bagshaw

Department of Radiology
Stanford University School of Medicine
California
U.S.A.

One of the first descriptions of the lymphatics of the prostate was that of Paolo Mascagni in his magnificent Vasorum Lymphaticorum Corporis Humani Historia et Iconographia, published in 1787 (1). A more modern work was that of Cuneo and Marcille, who completed the definitive dissections of the pelvic lymphatics at the turn of this century, and which later became the foundation for the definitive description of the pelvic lymphatics by Rouvière (2,3). According to Rouvière, the lymphatic drainage of the prostate consists of four main trunks. The first and most numerous lymphatic trunks emerge from the posterior surface of the prostatic capsule and go to the external iliac pedicle. The second group of lymphatics travels with branches of the hemorrhoidal artery to the hypogastric nodes. The third pedicle arises from the posterior surface, courses posteriorly to the pre-sacral region and encounters the first lymph node usually at the level of second sacral foramina. Other lymphatics in this group proceed to the region of the sacral promontory. The fourth pedicle descends from the anterior surface of the floor of the perineum going with the internal pudendal artery, and around the ischial spine into the pelvis, terminating in a hypogastric node.

The external iliac nodes are divided into three chains, the lateral, the middle and the medial. One of the nodes of the medial chain is placed opposite the pelvic aspect of the obturator canal and has been called "the node of the obturator foramen", and according to Rouvière, it is not be be confused with the "node of the obturator nerve."

Herman and co-authors who elegantly attempted to retrace the steps of Rouvière by modern lymphangiographic techniques appear to

believe that the "node of the obturator foramen" is the same as the
obturator node described by contemporary urologic surgeons (4). This
issue, however, remains in doubt because it seems that most urologists describe this node in relationship to the obturator nerve which
is separately described by Rouvière as "the node of the obturator
nerve." Whether or not this is important is an academic issue since
whichever node the urologist selects as the obturator appears to be
the one most frequently involved with prostatic cancer. It can be
identified by lymphangiography and contains lymphangiographic contrast
media in 100% of the obturator nodes resected by Merrin and in 94% of
the obturator nodes resected in the Stanford series (Table 1) (5,6).

The significance of the pelvic lymphatics appears to have
escaped serious surgical attention for many years, presumably because
radical perineal prostatectomy became the principal operative
procedure for the definitive surgical treatment of prostatic cancer.
Of course, in this operation the pelvic lymphatics were not exposed.
The fact that pelvic adenopathy was a serious problem, however, was
clearly appreciated, and radiotherapists in the mid 'twenties and
'thirties were known to use orthovoltage radiation in an effort to
palliate urethral, ureteral, and lymphatic obstruction secondary to
massive adenopathy. Surgeons who employed the retropubic approach to
the prostate were well aware of the significance of pelvic adenopathy.
Flocks, and also Arduino and Glucksman were among the first to call
attention to the importance of the lymphatic spread of prostatic
cancer and detailed the distribution of the adenopathy by regional
groupings (7,8). Recently the lymphatics of the prostate have been
the subject of more intense investigation, especially for the purpose
of mapping the distribution of lymphatic involvement prior to external
beam radiation therapy or, in some cases, the employment of definitive node dissection in an attempt to combine the surgical removal of
the lymph nodes with either radical resection of the prostate or
irradiation of the prostate by interstitial implant (9,10).

In the Stanford series of staged patients, 20% of those with
stage B (T1 and T2) and 59% with stage C (T3) had positive adenopathy. This incidence is consistent with that tabulated in Table 2.
In addition to the sites recorded in Table 1 Golimbu has sampled the
pre-sacral and pre-sciatic regions, finding involvement in about half
of the cases (11).

Lymphangiography has been considered by some to have merit in
the detection of lymph node metastases, especially when clearcut
positivity, either alone or proven by skinny needle biopsy, can save
the patient a useless extensive lymph node dissection (12). At
Stanford, after a feasibility study demonstrated that lymph node
metastases in prostatic cancer could be identified by lymphography
(Fig. 1) (13), a prospective study of consecutively surgically
staged cases demonstrated a sensitivity of 16/28 or 57% (true
positive), a specificity of 36/39 or 92% (true negative), and an

Table 1. Incidence of Lymph Node Involvement by Tumor (6)

(93 Patients)

Lymph Node Group	Number of Patients Biopsied	Number (%) With Tumor	Percent Opacified*
Para-Aortic	74	13 (18%)	93
Common Iliac	76	13 (17%)	95
External Iliac	74	16 (22%)	94
Internal Iliac	63	15 (24%)	87
Obturator	51	16 (31%)	94

*Percent opacified refers to histologic evidence of retained contrast material within the lymph node specimen.

Table 2. Histologically Proven Lymph Node Metastasis
in Prostatic Cancer

Series	Clinical Stage "B"		Clinical Stage "C"		Total	
Flocks et al. (1959)	2/29	(7%)	144/382	(38%)	146/411	(35%)
Arduino & Glucksman (1962)	19/71	(27%)	14/17	(82%)	19/71	(27%)
McCullough et al. (1974)	1/4	(25%)	27/46	(59%)	28/50	(56%)
Dahl et al. (1974)	3/25	(12%)	9/13	(69%)	12/38	(32%)
Hilaris et al. (1974)	6/29	(21%)	20/31	(65%)	26/60	(43%)
McLaughlin et al. (1976)	9/36	(25%)	12/24	(50%)	21/60	(35%)
Total	40/194	(21%)	226/513	(43%)	252/690	(37%)

Summary of surgical series in which pelvic lymphadenectomy was performed in patients with carcinoma of the prostate. In the Arduino and Glucksman series 17 of the 71 patients were found histologically to have tumor extending into peri-prostatic tissues and these are pathologically, not clinically, stage C tumors.

(Courtesy Spellman et al, 14)

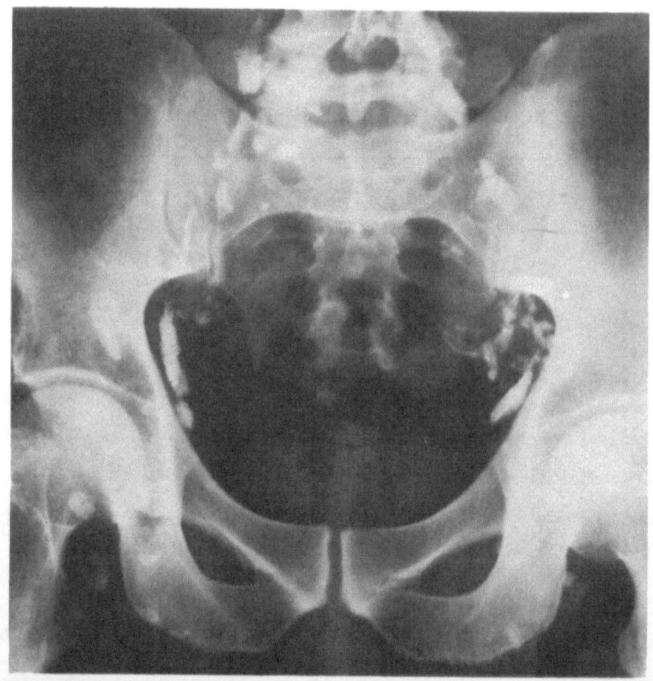

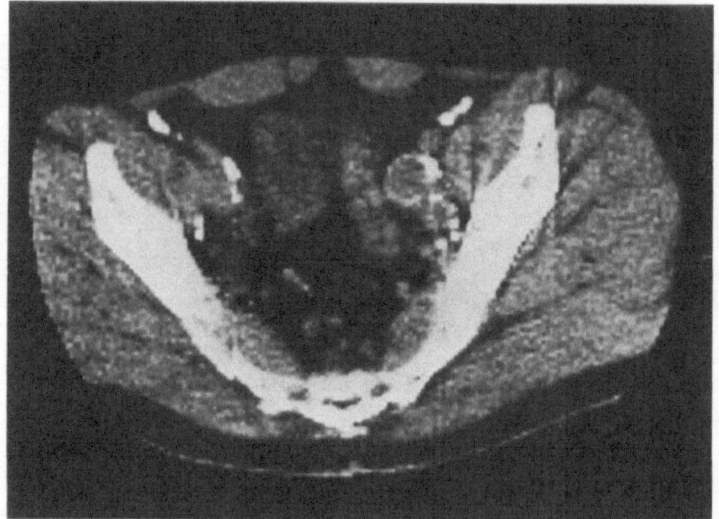

Fig 1.   Lymphogram showing an enlarged left external iliac node
          with an extensive filling defect and classical "egg shell"
          sign produced by contrast in the subcapsular sinus. The
          node is also shown on the CT scan. There is probably
          a right iliac node demonstrated by CT also.

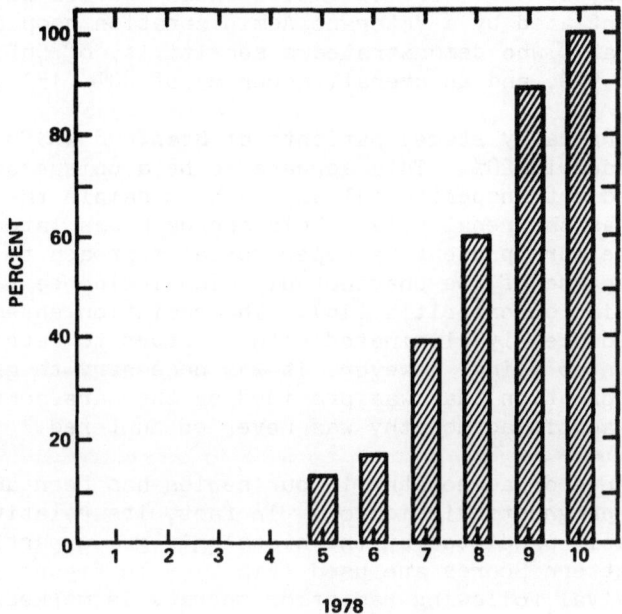

1978

Fig. 2. Correlation of 33 patients with biopsy-proven lymph node
metastases with the Gleason Pattern Scores among 93
consecutive protocol patients who were surgically staged.

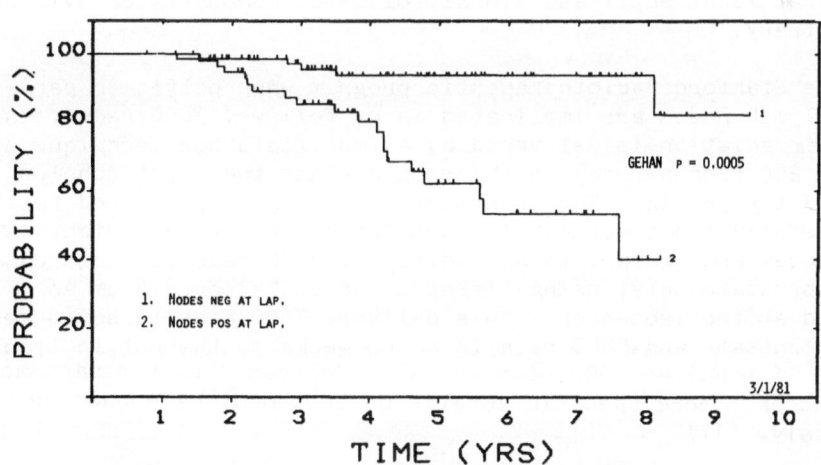

Fig. 3. Probability of surviving prostatic cancer. 151 patients
staged by pelvic laparotomy. 86 were histo-pathologically
negative, 65 were positive. These are disease specific
survival curves, i.e., patients dying of causes other than
prostatic cancer are withdrawn.

overall accuracy of 52/67 or 78% (14).   These results were almost
exactly substantiated by a Veterans Administration cooperative study
by Liebner et al., who demonstrated a sensitivity of 56%, a
specificity of 97%, and an overall accuracy of 80% (15).

In the surgically staged patients at Stanford we found positive
para-aortic nodes in 20%. This appears to be a unique observation
because we used a transperitoneal approach to sample the para-aortic
nodes as high as the renal hila. This approach was later abandoned
in favor of the more prudent retroperitoneal approach to the pelvic
lymph nodes because of the unacceptably high incidence (28%) of
subsequent radiation enteritis (16). The radiation enteritis was
subsequently completely eliminated with a return to retroperitoneal
dissection. In so doing, however, it was necessary to give up the
additional information that was provided by the para-aortic biopsies.
Isolated para-aortic adenopathy was never encountered.

The presence of adenopathy in our series has been an important
but unwelcome prognostic indicator. In fact, its relative incidence
can be reasonably predicted by the histologic grade particularly if
the Gleason Pattern Scores are used (Fig. 2). In Figure 3 it can be
seen that survival following radiation therapy is markedly adversely
influenced by positive lymph nodes. Even though the probability of
metastatic relapse is 80% at eight years (Fig. 4), still 9 of 59
patients with proven adenopathy are surviving without evident disease
for 26, 26, 41, 43, 48, 61, 62, 80, and 84 months. Thus although
the chances for long term disease-free survival are greatly reduced
when adenopathy is present, they are sufficiently high to warrant
therapy at least until additional follow-up demonstrates evidence to
the contrary.

The Stanford radiotherapeutic program when pelvic or para-
aortic lymph nodes are implicated is as follows. 2600 rads total
pelvic irradiation is delivered by a four field box technique at the
rate of 200 rads per day to the prostate and the first echelon lymph
nodes of the pelvis. The treatment volume is then reduced to the
prostate only and treatment is continued with left and right 120°
moving beam arc therapy to an additional 2000 rads in ten treatments
to the prostate only, using fields of about 7x7 or 8x8 cm as
measured at the isocenter. This delivers 7000 rads in seven weeks
to the prostate and 5000 rads in seven weeks to the pelvic lymph
nodes. If required 5000 rads are also delivered to the para-aortic
lymph nodes. More specific details on treatment have been presented
previously. (17)

SUMMARY

1. It has been recognized since at least the early '50s that
patients may have prostatic carcinoma metastatic to regional lymph
nodes without objective evidence of tumor in skeletal or other
metastatic sites.

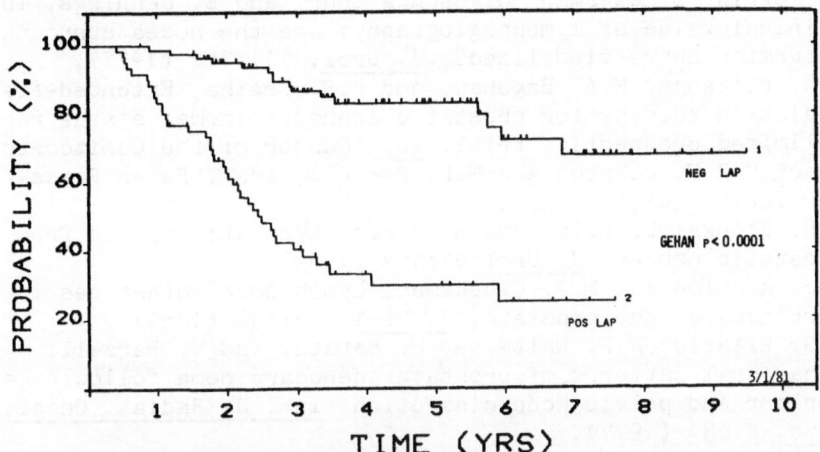

Fig. 4.   Same patients as noted in Fig. 3. In this case the
          calculation is based upon the probability of surviving
          without metastases. Osseous metastases dominated by a
          substantial margin.

2. More recent observations have shown that when the lymph
nodes are involved, however, subsequent development of osseous
metastases should be expected in 75-80% of cases.

3. A more thorough understanding of the true efficacy of the
irradiation of regional adenopathy must await a longer period of
follow-up.

4. Certainly patients with lymph node metastases and negative
bone scans are at high risk for the subsequent development of occult
bone metastases and are excellent candidates for effective adjuvant
therapy when such becomes available.

REFERENCES

1. P. Mascagni, "Vasorum lymphaticorum corporis humani historia et
    iconographia," P. Carli, Senis (Siena), (1787).
2. G. Delamere, The lymphatics. General anatomy of the lymphatics,
    in: "Special Study of the Lymphatics in Different Parts of the
    Body," P. Poirier and B. Cuneo, eds., English edition
    translated and edited by Cecil H. Leaf, W.T. Keener & Co.,
    Chicago, (1904), p.301.
3. H. Rouvière, "Anatomy of the Human Lymphatic System," Trans. by
    M.J. Tobias, Edwards Brothers, Inc. Ann Arbor, Mich., (1938).
4. P.G. Herman, D.L. Benninghoff, J.H. Nelson, and H.Z. Mellins,
    Roentgen anatomy of the ilio-pelvic-aortic lymphatic system,
    Radiology 80:182 (1963).

5. C. Merrin, Z. Wajsman, G. Baumgartner, and E. Jennings, The clinical value of lymphangiography: are the nodes surrounding the obturator nerve visualized?, J. Urol. 117:762 (1977).

6. D.A. Pistenma, M.A. Bagshaw, and F.S. Freiha, Extended-field radiation therapy for prostatic adenocarcinoma: status report of a limited prospective trial, in: "Cancer of the Genitourinary Tract," D.E. Johnson and M.L. Samuels, eds., Raven Press, New York, (1979), p.229.

7. R.H. Flocks, D. Culp, and R. Porto, Lymphatic spread from prostatic cancer, J. Urol 81:194 (1959).

8. L.J. Arduino and M.A. Glucksman, Lymph node metastases in early carcinoma of the prostate, J. Urol. 88:194 (1959).

9. B.S. Hilaris, W.F. Whitmore, M. Batata, and W. Barzell, Behavioral patterns of prostate adenocarcinoma following an ^{125}I implant and pelvic node dissection, Int. J. Radiat. Oncol. Biol. Phys. 2:631 (1977).

10. H. Zincke, T.R. Fleming, W.L. Furlow, R.P. Myers, and D.C. Utz, Radical retropubic prostatectomy and pelvic lymphadenectomy for high stage cancer of the prostate, Cancer 47:1901 (1981).

11. M. Golimbu, P. Morales, S. Al-Askari, and J. Brown, Extended pelvic lymphadenectomy for prostatic cancer, J. Urol. 121:617 (1979).

12. S.C. Efremidis, A. Pagliarulo, S.J. Dan, H.N. Weber, R.N. Dillon, H. Nieburgs, and H.A. Mitty, Post-lymphangiography fine needle aspiration lymph node biopsy in staging carcinoma of the prostate: preliminary report, J. Urol. 122:495 (1979).

13. W.R. Berry, J. Laszlo, E. Cox, A. Walker, and D. Paulson, Prognostic factors in metastatic and hormonally unresponsive carcinoma of the prostate, Cancer 44:763 (1979).

14. M.C. Spellman, R.A. Castellino, G.R. Ray, D.A. Pistenma, and M.A. Bagshaw, An evaluation of lymphography in localized carcinoma of the prostate, Radiology 125:637 (1977).

15. E.J. Liebner, S. Stefani and Uro-Oncology Research Group, An evaluation of lymphography with nodal biopsy in localized carcinoma of the prostate, Cancer 45:728 (1980).

16. F.S. Freiha and J. Salzman, Surgical staging of prostatic cancer: transperitoneal versus extraperitoneal lymphadenectomy, J. Urol. 118:616 (1977).

17. M.A. Bagshaw, External radiation therapy of carcinoma of the prostate, Cancer 45:1912 (1980).

LYMPH NODE DISSECTION IN THE MANAGEMENT OF PROSTATIC CARCINOMA

R.J. Macchia

Downstate Medical School
New York
U.S.A.

Lymph node dissection (LND) may be performed either for staging or for therapy. This discussion is limited to the former. LND has added considerable data to our clinical knowledge of prostatic cancer. At present it is the most accurate method of assessing nodal status. Utilizing LND the incidence of lymph node metastases has been related to the following parameters amongst others: size of the prostate, histologic grade (1), extent of intracapsular disease, extent of contiguous extra-capsular spread, especially to the seminal vesicles, and over-all clinical stage. LND has demonstrated that a percentage of patients felt to have disease limited to the prostate by clinical staging, in fact, have cancer metastatic to the lymph nodes. This information has had a significant impact on our concept of the percentage of patients in each stage at presentation. Patients with alleged localized clinical stage A1 disease have a 2-5% chance of having positive lymph nodes. The figure for A2 disease is 3-54%, for B1 disease is 10-40%, for B2 disease 39-45%, for C disease 50-80%. A recent review of the world literature (1) clearly documents the strong influence that histologic grade exerts on the likelihood of positive nodes.

Based on these data gained from LND, attempts are being made to develop a non-invasive system for predicting the probability of lymph node metastases. Perhaps the most widely used to date is the Gleason score (2). By assessing the clinical stage and histologic appearance, a number or score between three and 15 is assigned to each patient. Patients with elevated scores have a high probability of having lymph node metastases. The validity of the Gleason score for middle and lower values is less certain (3,4).

Lymphangiography (LAG) cannot detect micrometastases. False

negative results are in the range of 15-25%.   The true negative rate
runs between 80-95%.

What should be the extent of the LND?   A simple biopsy is
inaccurate unless the biopsy is positive (5).   If, on exploration,
the nodes look and feel negative, a systematic LND should be performed to detect micrometastases.   Serial sectioning of each node
by the pathologist increases the yield.   The most popular dissection
currently is a bilateral extraperitoneal one which removes the common,
external and internal iliac nodes and the obturator nodes.   Metastasis via the lymph system is usually orderly.   Combined pelvic and
retroperitoneal node dissection adds little to the yield and results
in a higher morbidity.   Both the extension of pelvic LND to include
the pre-sacral and pre-sciatic nodes (6) and the reduction of the
extent of pelvic LND have been proposed (7).

The impact of LND on the immunologic status of the patient
remains unsettled.

We are using the histochemical technique of Pertschuk (8) to
study the relationship of androgen binding in the primary site to
androgen binding in lymph node metastases.

Significant morbidity and occasional mortality is associated
with pelvic LND (9).   We suggest pelvic LND be limited to formal
study protocols with fully informed patients.   For individual
patients not involved in such a study, pelvic LND should be reserved
for those patients in whom the nodal status cannot be predicted with
high certainty by non-invasive methods and only if knowledge of the
nodal status will alter the management of the patient.

SUMMARY

1.   Bilateral systematic extraperitoneal pelvic LND has provided
excellent data and revised our thinking regarding the distribution
of stage at diagnosis.

2.   To my knowledge, no improvement in survival statistics has as
yet been demonstrated secondary to the acquisition of this new data.

3.   The simultaneous performance of a therapeutic procedure designed
to treat localized disease, e.g. total prostatectomy or I-125 implant
may be unwise.   A percentage of these patients will have positive
lymph nodes revealed only at permanent section and will have thus
been subjected to an invasive procedure with no proven likelihood of
success.

4.   Routine use of surgical staging is unwarranted unless a) the
patient is enrolled in a formal protocol designed to elicit new
information or b) in the case of a non-protocol patient, the selection

of therapy for that patient will be significantly modified.

5.   Finally, I speculate that non-invasive techniques will become increasingly reliable in predicting nodal status.   In those cases where such non-invasive techniques are not reliable, minimally traumatic procedures such as percutaneous "skinny needle" node biopsy will replace open surgical staging.   At that time open surgical staging will have outlived its usefulness and should be laid to an honorable and peaceful rest.

REFERENCES.

1.   R.E. Donohue, H.E. Fauver, J.A. Whitesel, R.R. Augspurger and R.R. Pfister, Prostatic Carcinoma: Influence of Tumor Grade on Results of Pelvic Lymphadenectomy, J. Urol. 17:435 (1981).
2.   D.F. Gleason, Histologic Grading and Clinical Staging Prostatic Cancer in "Urologic Pathology: The Prostate", M. Tannenbaum, ed., Lea and Febiger, Philadelphia (1977).
3.   S.A. Kramer, Esperience with Gleason Histopathological Grading in Prostatic Cancer, J. Urol. 124:223 (1980).
4.   Z. Wajsman, J. Gaeta, J.E. Pontes, L. Englander, S. Beckley and G.P. Murphy, Surgical Pathological Correlation of Pelvic Lymphadenectomy in Prostatic Cancer, Program of the Annual Meeting, American Urological Assn., p. 257, (1981).
5.   W.J. Catalona, Value of Frozen Section Examination of Pelvic Lymph Nodes at Pelvic Lymphadenectomy for Prostatic Cancer, Program of the Annual Meeting, American Urological Assn., p.137, (1981).
6.   M. Golimbu, P. Morales, S. Al-Askari and J. Brown, Extended Pelvic Lymphadenectomy for Prostatic Cancer, J. Urol. 121:617 (1979).
7.   C.B. Brendler, L.K. Cleeve, E.E. Anderson and D.F. Paulson, Staging Pelvic Lymphadenectomy for Carcinoma of the Prostate: Risk Versus Benefit, J. Urol. 124:849 (1980).
8.   L.P. Pertschuk, H.E. Rosenthal, R.J. Macchia, K.B. Eisenberg, J.G. Feldman, S.H. Wax, D.S. Kim, W.F. Whitmore Jr., J.I. Abrahams, E. Gaetjens, G.J. Wise, H.W. Herr, J.P. Karr, G.P. Murphy and A.A. Sandberg, Correlation of Histochemical and Biochemical Analyses of Androgen Binding in Prostatic Cancer: Relation to Therapeutic Response, Cancer (in press).
9.   H.W. Herr, Complications of Pelvic Lymphadenectomy and Retropubic Prostate I-125 Implantation, Urology, 14:226 (1979).

THE VALUE OF QUANTIFIED BONE SCANNING IN THE FOLLOW-UP OF PATIENTS WITH PROSTATE CANCER AND METASTATIC BONE LESIONS

J.C. Grob*, I. Carloz*, G. Methlin* and C. Bollack**

* Service de Médecine Nucléaire
**Service de Chirurgie Urologique du C.H.U.
  Strasbourg
  France

INTRODUCTION

Bone scanning is an essential technique in the diagnosis of metastatic lesions in bone seeking cancers and is particularly important in prostate cancer, in which up to 60% of patients develop bony metastases. The bone scan aims to confirm or exclude metastatic bone lesions at diagnosis, during the follow-up and to aid in evaluating the efficiency of hormonal treatment. We have paid particular attention to this last point using a quantitative method which has allowed us to determine the variations of isotope uptake in the metastases.

THE PHYSIOLOGICAL BASIS

Bone tissue presents a double structure -

a protein matrix framed with collagenous fibers and basic substance (polysaccharide and cells such as osteoblasts, osteocytes and osteoclasts, and

mineral substance made of hydroxyapatite crystals.

This bone tissue is constantly being reshaped: loss of calcium from the bone tissue is replaced by mineral salts from the blood. A percentage of the mineral substance is in equilibrium with the blood, the exchanges leading to a steady-state so that the calcium concentration in skeleton is constant. Areas of high uptake in abnormal scans result from any process that increases the bone turnover and/or the blood flow. A metastatic lesion in bone is such a process.

The growing tumor removes calcium while the bone reaction is to try to deposit mineral substance around the lesions. The calcium balance may be either positive or negative. For bone destruction to be demonstrable roentgenologically, a lesion must be 1 - 1.5 cm. in diameter and the mineral loss must be 30 - 50%.

By using bone seeking radioisotopes, it is not necessary to have net deposition of new bone mineral since areas of osteolytic and of osteoblastic activity are both visualized.

THE RADIOISOTOPES AVAILABLE

To be used as bone-scanning agents, the radioisotopes must have precise physical properties, a short half-life in order to reduce the radiation dose to bone, exclusive γ-ray emission, an energy detectable by γ-camera, sufficiently high concentration in normal bone tissue, a higher concentration in bone lesions, a low concentration in soft tissues including bone marrow, and rapid clearance from the body of the isotope not taken up in bone in order not to hide the pelvic area when the bladder is not empty.

There are three kinds of bone seekers, those which stay in the bloodstream, those which seek the protein matrix (rarely used), and those which seek the bone tissue itself.

Calcium would have been the most natural isotope but studies with the only clinically useful γ-emitting Ca isotope (Ca^{47}) have been limited by the difficulty of production with adequately high specific activity and the difficulty of collimation due to the high γ-energy (1,31 Mev). Ca^{45} also has too long a half-life (165 days).

Strontium follows calcium accurately in its participating in the formation of new bone. Sr^{85} as well as Sr^{87m} were used but neither was entirely satisfactory because of the long half-life of the former and very short half-life of the latter, and the unduly high γ-emitting energy of both.

There has been considerable interest in certain phosphate compounds labeled with Technetium^{99m} in the presence of the reducing agent stannous chloride. The physical characteristics of Technetium are ideal and it is produced from a simple generator.

The polyphosphates whose behaviour differs according to their molecular weight are little used because of the low labeling efficiency (about 70%). The background activity and thyroid uptake level are also high. However, Methyldiphosphonate (M.D.P.) is widely used because of its high labeling efficiency and its higher bone/blood and bone/soft tissue activity. Scans can be performed as soon as two hours after intravenous injection.

METHOD

The patients are given 15 mCi of Tc^{99m} M.D.P. intravenously. The scans are recorded on films using a Picker scinticamera equipped with a whole body system and connected to a computer.

A whole body scan is performed five minutes after injection in order to measure the whole body radioactivity immediately after injection. A second scan is recorded three hours after injection. In every case whole body retention is measured after the bladder has been completely emptied. The skeleton is clearly seen. The data are computerized and recorded. Bone images of the posterior aspect of the entire axial skeleton, skull, shoulder and pelvis are obtained. Images of clinically suspect regions are also included.

From the data recorded, the whole body scan is visualized. A region of interest (R.O.I.) selection program is used to delimit areas of high uptake levels as well as an area of normal bone tissue. As a reference area we always use the humerus, because it is seldom involved in metastatic lesions. The whole body retention measured at three hours is expressed as a percentage of whole body radio-activity measured immediately after injection and is called the general or global ratio (R.G.)

$$R.G. = \text{Percentage of skeletal uptake} = \frac{\text{Radioactivity at 3 hours}}{\text{Radioactivity at 5 minutes}}$$

The ratio of isotope activity in pathological areas relative to the isotope activity in normal bone is obtained:

$$R_1 = \frac{\text{Radioactivity in pathological area}}{\text{Radioactivity in humerus}}$$

An uptake index is computed:

$$R_2 = \frac{\text{Activity in pathological areas}}{\text{Activity in "normal" area}} \times \frac{\text{Activity at 3 hours}}{\text{Activity at 5 minutes}}$$

$$R_2 = R_1 \times R.G.$$

RESULTS

In 12 subjects with normal Tc^{99m} M.D.P. bone images, the global ratio (R.G.) was about 37%

$$R.G. = \frac{\text{Activity at 3 hours}}{\text{Activity at 5 minutes}} = 0.37$$

when the patients presented metastatic bone lesions, the ratio was about 58% (R.G. = 0.58).

The average of "area under test/humerus ratio" (R_1) calculated
for metastases in the spinal column was 17.8 and 9.3 for metastases
in the pelvis.   This ratio was respectively 7.1 and 6.6 in normal
subjects.   The average uptake index (R_2) was respectively 12.4 and
11.8 for the same areas where metastases were present and 2.5 and
2.4 in normal subjects.

This quantitative method allowed us to follow these patients
during the treatment and to evaluate the results of therapy.   We
compared these different ratios and the index calculated for each
patient before treatment and bimonthly thereafter.   We found three
groups of patients -

   those whose ratio and index were lower than before treatment,
      i.e. returning towards normal;

   those whose results did not change during the treatment, and

   those with increasing ratio and index in spite of the treatment.

We then compared these quantified data with the clinical data including lessening of the pain and normalization of the roentgenograms.

Of the five patients with numerous bone metastases showing
decreasing ratios, three were clinically better and two unchanged.
Increased ratios were seen in three patients; of these two had areas
of great pain and one showed deteriorating general health.   In the
group in which the ratios did not change we followed only two patients, both of whom noticed slight subjective improvement.

Although the numbers of patients are, as yet, small it seems
that quantified bone scanning is likely to prove to be a good method
for the assessment of changes in bone metastases and in evaluating
the effect of therapy.

PULMONARY AND OSSEOUS METASTASES IN PROSTATIC CANCER:

METHODS OF QUANTITATIVE ASSESSMENT

D.P. Byar[1] and J.A. Hovsepian[2]

1. National Cancer Institute
   Bethesda, U.S.A.

2. Stanford University School of Medicine
   California, U.S.A.

ABSTRACT

The extent of bone and lung metastases in each of eight sites was rated on a semi-quantitative scale using pretreatment films for 102 patients with known metastases at diagnosis. A statistical analysis revealed significant correlation between shortened patient survival and a combination of the number of sites involved and the extent of involvement in those sites. Correlations were also identified with acid phosphatase, pain and performance ratings, but not with tumor grade. Examination of several films for patients treated with endocrine therapy showed that some patients who ultimately show improvement may initially show pseudo-progression.

It is well recognised that for most cancers the prognosis is markedly different for patients having distant metastases at the time of diagnosis compared to that of patients clinically free of metastases. Generally the presence and absence of metastases define different stages of disease. However, because of difficulties of quantitation, little effort has been directed towards determing whether the extent of the metastasis, given that metastases are present, is a further prognostic variable. In order to study this question we examined the pretreatment x-ray films for 102 patients with bone metastases at diagnosis (1). The extent of metastatic involvement was recorded on a four point scale for each of eight major sites. The scale was simply based on the apparent percentage involvement in each site: no involvement, $<25\%$ involvement, 25-75% involvement, or $>75\%$ involvement. The eight sites studied (with the percentage of patients having metastases

at that site shown in parenthesis) were as follows: shoulder (39%),
rib (53%), lung (24%), thoracic spine (60%), lumbosacral spine (71%),
pubis-ischium (78%), ilium (83%), and femur (48%). "Femur" refers
to femoral heads and necks as seen on pelvic films. The patients
whose x-rays were examined were part of the first randomized
clinical trial of the Veterans Administration Cooperative Urological
Research Group (VACURG). They were selected simply because
metastases were present at one or more sites at diagnosis and the
films were available for study. In the VACURG system of staging,
all these patients would be classified as stage IV. The percentages
just given for each of the eight sites suggest that the most common
sites of metastases are those closest to the prostate, namely the
lumbo-sacral spine, the pubis-ischium, and the ileum, but an
appreciable number of patients had involvement at other sites as
well.

A statistical analysis using an exponential survival model
revealed significant correlation between shortened patient survival
and a combination of the number of sites involved and the extent
of involvement within each site. Because many patients have
involvement at multiple sites, the variables in the regression
equation were strongly correlated among themselves and therefore not
all were needed to predict survival. The variables found most useful
in the prediction equation were those representing extent of involvement in the pubis-ischium, femur, and lung. On the basis of these
variables, four risk groups were identified which showed marked
variation in death rates due to prostatic cancer (see Table 1).
Even in stage IV prostatic cancer, not all patients die of their
disease because of the strong competing risk of death due to cardiovascular or other causes in aged males. In the group with the
lowest risk (risk group 1) only 48% of the deaths were attributed
to prostatic cancer directly, while 87% of the deaths in risk group
4 were due to prostatic cancer. Risk group membership also correlated with the average initial acid phosphatase, the average pain
rating at diagnosis, and the average performance rating at diagnosis,
and there was some relationship between risk group membership and
the probability of having ureteral dilatation at the time of
diagnosis (2). This abnormality was found in only 10% of patients
in risk group 1, but it was present in 29-33% of patients in the
higher risk groups. Surprisingly, the risk group membership did
not correlate with the histological grade of the tumor as measured by
the Gleason system (3). A possible interpretation might be that the
histological grade of a tumor tells you how it might behave or what
its potential is, while the number and extent of metastases at
diagnosis tells you what the tumor has already done. For this
reason, in the design and analysis of studies confined to patients
with metastatic disease, it would be more important to stratify on
radiological risk group than on the histological grade.

Table 1: Relationship of various factors to radiologic
          risk groups

Risk Group

	1	2	3	4
Number of patients[1]	21	42	24	15
Death rate (CAP)[2]	17.2	21.8	34.9	59.9
Death rate (All)[3]	36.2	33.8	46.5	69.1
% Cancer deaths	48%	64%	75%	87%
% with Ureteral dilatation	10%	29%	30%	33%
Acid phosphatase (mean)[4]	17.6	23.9	70.2	72.6
Average pain rating[5]	1.38	1.81	1.92	2.00
Average performance rating[6]	1.38	1.69	1.75	2.40
Histologic grade (Gleason)	7.000	7.024	7.304	7.143

[1] One patient studied in the 1974 paper was omitted because
further study of his films suggested that he did not have
metastatic disease.

[2] Death rate for prostatic cancer only, treating other deaths
as withdrawals.

[3] Death rate for all causes combined.

[4] Measured in King-Armstrong units.

[5] Pain ratings were as follows: none=1, mild=2, moderate=3, and
severe=4.

[6] Performance ratings were as follows: normal activity=1, in bed
<50% of the time=2, in bed > 50% of the time=3, and confined
to bed=4.

Lung metastases have frequently been overlooked clinically in patients with prostatic carcinoma because they are usually lymph-angitic rather than nodular and may easily be confused with congestive heart failure, pneumonia, or fibrosis. However, histological examination of the lungs in 566 autopsies of patients from the first VACURG study revealed that 20% of stage III and IV patients had metastases in their lungs at death. Breaking down these results by the randomly assigned treatments, the results were 29% for placebo, 13% for estrogen, 22% for orchiectomy plus placebo, and 16% for orchiectomy plus estrogen. Despite the fact that many patients in these studies originally assigned to placebo were later changed to endocrine therapy because of progression of disease, these results suggest that estrogen is more effective than orchiectomy alone or placebo in preventing the spread of the tumor to the lungs. In the present study we have noted that 24% of the patients had lung metastases at the time of diagnosis, but these were identified by careful study and might easily have been overlooked in a more routine clinical setting.

CHANGES IN LUNG AND BONE METASTASES FOLLOWING ENDOCRINE TREATMENT

From the original set of 102 patients, 52 were selected for further study because serial x-rays were available (initial, three months, and every six months thereafter up to 78 months). Of these 52 patients, seven had lung metastases at the time of diagnosis. Two of these were originally assigned to placebo, and follow-up films revealed that the lung metastases remained stable in one and progressed in the other. Of the five patients with lung metastases assigned to endocrine therapy, complete disappearance was seen in four by three to twelve months and improvement in one at three and six months. These results suggest that lung metastases, when present, may be a valuable indicator of whether or not the metastatic tumor is responding to endocrine (or other) therapy.

The evaluation of changes in bone metastases are more difficult because for prostate cancer, unlike most other cancers, metastases are usually osteoblastic rather than osteolytic. Following endocrine therapy one must distinguish between early and late changes. Early changes may include both increased number and density of blastic lesions on standard x-ray examinations, increased activity on nuclear bone scans, decreased acid phosphatase, and increased values for that portion of alkaline phosphatase arising from bone. If a true response occurs, then late changes will show either decreased number and/or density of blastic lesions on x-ray, decreased activity on bone scan, a continued decrease in acid phosphatase, and a decrease in bone alkaline phosphatase. The difficulty is that the early increased bone density on x-ray (or increased activity on nuclear bone scans) may cause one to mis-diagnose the patient's condition as deteriorating rather than improving. For this reason the system of classification of changes

Table 2: System of classifying changes in appearance
          of bone metastases

X-ray patterns of bone metastasis change	Early	Late
Pseudo-progression	↑ Metastases	↓ Metastases
Regression	↓ Metastases	↓ Metastases
Stabilization	No change or slowed progression	No change
True progression	↑ Metastases	↑ Metastases

in the appearance of bone metastases on x-ray given in Table 2 was
used in our study, where increased or decreased metastases refer to
changes in number and/or density of blastic lesions. This system
can only be employed when serial films are available for
examination.

One of us (JH) examined serial films for all 52 patients without knowledge of the treatment to which they had been assigned and
rated the response to therapy at each examination by comparing films
with those from the preceding examination (4). The results of that
review are given in Table 3. Progression was observed in 9 of 12
patients (75%) originally assigned to placebo versus 7 of 40 (18%)
initially assigned to placebo showed pseudo-progression versus
26 of 40 (65%) of those assigned to endocrine therapy. It is very
important to distinguish between true progression and pseudo-
progression because failure to make this distinction could lead one

Table 3: Classification of x-ray response evaluated
          without knowledge of the assigned treatments

X-ray response	Placebo		Endocrine	
	N	%	N	%
Progression	9	75%	7	18%
Stable	1	8%	3	8%
Regression	0	0%	4	10%
Pseudo-progression	2	17%	26	65%

to conclude that endocrine therapy was not working when in fact it
was. Pseudo-progression can only be distinguished from true
progression by examining serial x-rays over considerable periods
of time, often as much as one year. For this reason the evaluation of response to endocrine therapy, and presumably chemotherapy,
cannot reliably be made by a simple examination of x-rays after
say, three months of treatment as is common in many phase II studies
of new agents. Nuclear bone scans were not generally available at
the time these patients were studied. In the last decade these
techniques of examination have become widely used and may provide
earlier indications of response to therapy. It is suggested that
researchers having data on serial changes in nuclear bone scans
undertake studies similar to those we have reported in order better
to define the usefulness of these methods in assessing prognostic
significance and response to therapy.

REFERENCES

1. J. Hovsepian and D. Byar, Carcinoma of prostate. Correlation
    between radiologic quantitation of metastases and patient
    survival, Urology 6:11-16 (1975).
2. J. Hovsepian and D. Byar, Quantitative radiology for staging
    and prognosis of patients with advanced prostatic carcinoma:
    Correlations with other pretreatment characteristics,
    Urology 14:145-150 (1979).
3. D. Gleason, Histologic grading and clinical staging of
    prostatic carcinoma, in: "Urologic Pathology: The Prostate,"
    M. Tannenbaum, ed., Lea and Febiger, Philadelphia (1977)
    p 171-198.
4. J. Hovsepian, D. Byar and the VACURG, Pseudo-progression and
    regression of bone metastases during endocrine therapy of
    prostatic adenocarcinoma, Proc. Amer. Soc. Clinical Oncology
    21:421 (Abstract) (1980).

THE PRESENT STATUS OF RECEPTOR STUDIES IN RELATION TO PROSTATIC CANCER

H. J. de Voogt

Free University Hospital
Amsterdam
The Netherlands

Research into androgen receptors in prostatic tissue started with the experimental work of Liao and Fang (1) and Bruchovsky and Wilson (2) in rats. They were able to identify the specific binding proteins for steroids, called receptors, in cytoplasm and nuclei of rat prostatic cells and they defined and confirmed their role in androgen metabolism of these cells.

For the physiological role of receptors three main models have been suggested:

1. that receptors act as storage and transport proteins protecting steroids against enzymatic attack and non-specific binding. In that philosophy steroids are the initiators of biological effects.

2. that receptors have a latent functional activity, that is activated by the steroid binding after which the steroid receptor-complex as a whole induces biosynthetic effects.

3. that receptors induce biological effects (such as transcription regulating). In this hypothesis steroids only amplify this action and thereby control the rate.

Whichever of these roles is considered to be true, there is no doubt that cytoplasmic as well as nuclear receptors play an important role in the metabolism of steroids in target cells. I should like to present here the first and the last scheme of Liao (1,3) and that of Ekman (4) for prostatic cells. The latter gives me the opportunity to show how it can be used to clarify the working mechanism of different hormonal treatments.

After the first successful attempts to determine androgen
receptors in human prostate (5-7), it soon became evident that many
technical (methodological) problems had to be solved. First of all,
the most common circulating androgen, testosterone, was not the
most potent and in fact not the one that is active within the
prostatic cell. It has to be reduced to 5 α-dihydrotestosterone
(DHT) in the cytoplasm by 5α-reductase and this is then in turn
bound to the specific receptor. But the most important difficulties
encountered were those listed in Table 1.

Gradually these problems have been surmounted in the last
10 years. Though it is still not easy to get normal prostatic
tissue, there are some contributions that deal with receptor content
in normal prostate (8,9). For benign prostatic hypertrophy (BPH)
receptor research and the whole picture of steroid metabolism has
largely solved the origin of this disease. But still prostatic
cancer (PCA) and BPH are usually compared to each other in consideration of receptor content.

The problem of endogenous androgens and SHBG-contamination has
been solved in different ways. Wagner (10) invented cold agar-gel-
electrophoresis to separate SHBG-bound and receptor-bound steroids
and Raynaud and co-workers (11) contributed largely to this by the
use of the artificial ligands of the Roussel-Laboratories (R-1881,
R-5020). Both methods found their (more or less fervent) supporters
and contributed to the solving of methodology. Others (12,13)
worked on exchange incubation techniques to determine nuclear
receptors and total receptors and so indirectly cytoplasmic
receptors, which in men are normally occupied by endogenous
androgens. Today the opinion is gaining ground that nuclear
receptors are probably more important than those in the cytoplasm
as far as the prognosis for hormonal therapy is concerned.

Table 1. Receptors in human prostate. Problems to be solved.

1. Normal prostatic tissue not usually available.

2. Therefore only tissue from patients with benign prostatic
    hypertrophy is available for comparison with neoplastic
    tissue.

3. Difficulties in obtaining enough suitable cancer tissue.

4. The endogenous androgens and plasma contaminants (SHBG).

5. The relation between stromal and epithelial elements in any
    given piece of prostatic tissue.

One must consider finally the relation between stromal and
epithelial elements in the usually very heterogeneous prostatic
tissue. The work of Bartsch and Röhr on stereology has to be
mentioned in the first place (14), but others by way of statistical
analysis (15) or by separation of stroma and epithelium (16) have
solved this and established that both stroma and epithelium have
their own steroid hormone metabolism. It is the interaction between
the two that plays such an important role in the embryonal development of the prostate as well as in BPH and perhaps in the lack of
inhibition of growth of prostatic cancer. Mc Neal's hypothesis (17)
that BPH is the induction of normal epithelium by an altered stroma,
while premalignant hyperplasia arises as an embryonic alteration of
epithelium that becomes unresponsive to a normal stroma, is worth
mentioning here. It probably also explains why oestrogen receptor,
E-r, can be found in prostatic tissue as well as those for DHT
(and also receptor for progesterone and corticosteroids).

Some difficulties still remain. Though there is increasing
evidence that a correlation exists between the occurrence of
receptors and the success of anti-androgenic therapy (4,18), we
have as yet no definite proof of it in such a way that it could be
used on a routine basis for the choice of treatment.

Also the problems of obtaining PCA tissue for biochemical assay
are not yet solved. Surgical excision or thick needle biopsy (5)
has to be used and there is increasing demand for micro-assays,
especially for those that could use the cell material obtained by
aspiration biopsy for cytologic diagnosis.

In my opinion the work of Nenci (19) and Pertschuk (20)
deserves our attention. They use steroid ligand conjugates, labeled
with fluoresceine isothiocyanate (FITC) to localize receptor sites
by way of fluorescence. They still need frozen sections of tissue-
biopsies to perform this histochemical receptor assay.

More promising is the use of the naturally fluorescent plant
estrogen coumestrol or the small molecule of dansyl-hexestrol as
fluorescent probes (21) that can be used in whole cells (for
instance by incubation of thin needle aspirates or cell cultures).
When these methods have been elaborated for all steroids and
developed into reliable and simple techniques we will have taken a
large step forward. In the same context should be mentioned the
attempts to purify receptor proteins in order to allow for immunological assays, as well as for better understanding of the mechanism
of action. Though much has been achieved in this respect for
oestrogen and progesterone-receptors, the purification of androgen
receptors has so far met with unsurmountable technical problems.
However the future prospects for investigation of the mode of action
of androgen receptors are favourable (22).

Finally, back to the experimental laboratory: I would like to end this paper by mentioning some very recent results of Rao and co-workers on the Dunning tumor in Copenhagen rats (23), one of the very few reliable animal models of prostatic cancer. Using a hormone-independent anaplastic (R 3327-AT) cell-line of this tumor they found neither DHT nor E_2 receptors. After continuous culturing of these cells in the presence of high concentration of estradiol an estrogen-adapted cell-line resulted. After a few passages E_2-R were detected in these cells and when they were injected to female rats tumors grew in 12 days. Androgens and anti-estrogens were cytotoxic to these cells.

This adaptation phenomenon, which resembles in many ways the work of Noble (24) could throw some new light on the problems which remain: First, as I mentioned earlier, it might explain the presence of receptors in non-target tissues, such as renal cell cancer. Secondly, it could explain the question of hormone-resistance at least partly, and thirdly it contradicts Coffey and Isaacs' hypothesis (25) of the survival of androgen-insensitive cells.

Though much work still has to be done to confirm this in human prostatic cancer cells, future prospects for receptor research are encouraging and this work is worthwhile pursuing.

REFERENCES

1. S. Liao and S. Fang, Receptor-proteins for androgens and the mode of action of androgens on gene transcription in rat ventral prostate, Vitam. Horm. 27:17 (1969).
2. N. Bruchovsky and J.D. Wilson, The intranuclear binding of testosterone and 5∝ DHT by rat prostate, J. Biol. Chem. 243:5953 (1968).
3. S. Liao, C. Chen, R. Loor and R.A. Hilpatka, Androgen-sensitive protein in rat ventral prostate: a specific intracellular protein and secretory protein, in: "Steroid Receptors, Metabolism and Prostatic Cancer," H.J. de Voogt and F.H. Schroeder, eds., Excerpta Medica, Amsterdam (1980).
4. P. Ekman, M. Snochowski, E. Dahlberg and J.A. Gustafsson, Steroid receptors in metastatic carcinoma of the human prostate, Eur. J. Cancer 15:257 (1979).
5. R.S. Hsu, R.G. Middleton and S. Fang, "Androgen Receptors in Human Prostate in Normal and Abnormal Growth of the Prostate," M. Goland, ed., Charles Thomas, Springfield p 663-675 (1975).
6. W.I.P. Mainwaring and E.J.G. Milroy, Characterization of the specific androgen receptors in the human prostatic gland, J. Endocrinol. 57:371 (1973).
7. K.J. Tveter, O. Unjhem, A. Attramadal, A. Aakvaag and V. Hansson, Androgenic receptors in rat and human prostate, Adv. Biosc. 7:193 (1981).

8. M. Krieg, W. Bartsch, W. Janssen and K.D. Voigt, A comparative
    study of binding, metabolism and endogenous levels of androgens
    in normal, hyperplastic, and carcinomatous human prostate,
    J. Steroid. Bioch. 11:615 (1979).

9. J.B. Murphy, R.C. Emmott, L.L. Hicks and P.C. Walsh, Estrogen
    receptors in the human prostate, seminal vesicle, epididymis,
    testis, and genital skin: A marker for estrogen-responsive
    tissues? J. Clin. Endocrinol. Metab. 50:938 (1980).

10. R.K. Wagner, Extracellular and intracellular steroid binding
    proteins, Acta Endocrinologica. Suppl. 218 (1978).

11. C. Bonne and J.P. Raynaud, Assay of androgen binding sites by
    exchange with R 1881, Steroids 26:227 (1975).

12. A.S. Shain and R.W. Boesel, Human prostate steroid hormone
    receptor quantitation, Invest. Urol. 16:169 (1978).

13. D.A.N. Sirrett and J.K. Grant, Androgen binding in cytosols and
    nuclei of human hyperplastic prostatic tissue, J. Endocrinol.
    77:101 (1978).

14. G. Bartsch and H.P. Rohr, Ultrastructural sterology: a new
    approach to the study of prostatic function, Invest. Urol.
    14:301 (1977).

15. H.J. de Voogt and P.G. Dingjan, Is there a place for assay of
    cytoplasmic steroid receptors in the endocrine treatment of
    prostatic cancer? in: "Steroid Receptors, Metabolism and
    Prostatic Cancer," H.J. de Voogt and F.H. Schroeder, eds.,
    Excerpta Medica, Amsterdam (1980).

16. F.H. Schroeder, K. Oishi and H.M. Schweikert, The application
    of cell culture techniques to human prostatic carcinoma,
    UICC Technical Report Series, 48:145 (1979).

17. J.E. McNeal, New morphologic findings relevant to the origin
    and evolution of carcinoma of the prostate and BPH, UICC
    Technical Report Series, 48:34 (1979).

18. A. Martelli, M. Soli, E. Bercovich, G. Prodi, S. Grilli,
    C. De Giovanni and M.C. Galli, Correlation between clinical
    response to antiandrogenic therapy and occurrence of receptors
    in human prostatic cancer, Urology 16:245 (1980).

19. I. Nenci, Cytochemistry of steroid-cell interactions, Abstract
    Internat. Symp. Perspectives in Steroid Receptor Research,
    Sorrento (1979).

20. L.P. Pertschuk, E.H. Tobin, P. Tanapat, E. Gaetjens, A.C. Carter,
    N.D. Bloom, R.J. Macchia and K. Byer Eisenberg, Histochemical
    analysis of steroid hormone receptors in breast and prostatic
    carcinoma, J. Histochem. and Cytochem. 28:799 (1980).

21. W.B. Dandliker, R.J. Brawn, M.L. Hsu, P.N. Brawn, J. Levin,
    C.Y. Meyers and V.M. Kolb, Investigation of hormone-receptor
    interaction by means of fluorescence labelling, Cancer Research
    38:4214 (1978).

22. W.I.P. Mainwaring, Steroid receptors and the regulation of
    transcriptional events in the prostate, UICC Technical Report
    Series 48:126 (1979).

23. B.R. Rao, G. Fry and M.J. Alsup, Prostatic tumor cells surviving estrogen treatment may become estrogen-adapted, Abstract Endocrine Society Meeting (and personal communication) (1981).

24. R.L. Noble, Sex steroids as a cause of adenocarcinoma of the dorsal prostate in Nb rats, and their influence on the growth of transplants, Oncology 34:138 (1977).

25. D.S. Coffey and J.T. Isaacs, Experimental concepts in the design of new treatments for human prostate cancer, UICC Technical Report Series 48:233 (1979).

METHODOLOGY AND PRINCIPLES OF IMMUNO-CYTOLOGICAL

ASSAYS OF STEROID RECEPTORS

D. Beccati[1] and I. Nenci[2]

1. St Mary's Hospital
   Ravenna, Italy

2. University of Ferrara
   Ferrara, Italy

Recent development in cytochemical techniques for steroid receptors may contribute to bridge the gap between molecular biology in vitro and cell biology in vivo, thus leading to significant progress in knowledge of cancer which can influence the treatment approach.

Since the first report (1) many generations of methods have rapidly followed.

To visualize steroid receptors under the microscope, the cytochemical techniques exploit the same binding properties of the receptor site as are used in biochemical assay.

The first generation belongs to immunocytochemistry; these methods utilize a specific anti-steroid antibody which is then traced by a second anti-immunoglobulin antibody labelled with a fluorescent or enzymatic tracer (2). By the antibody technique, the steroid molecules specifically retained by receptor sites in target tissues can be visualized under ultraviolet light and by electron microscopy.

The immunocytochemical techniques need accurate control tests of immunological specificity in addition to the tests of steroid binding specificity which are in common with other techniques.

The second generation methods, of labelled-ligand cytochemistry, involve steroid hormones coupled to a macromolecular protein carrier, such as bovine serum albumin, which is highly substituted with fluorescein or horse radish peroxidase (3,4). These labelled steroid derivatives may be applied only to the static evaluation of steroid binding on frozen tissue sections since they are prevented by their size from getting through the same plasma membrane.

The third generation of techniques is the use of affinity cytochemistry (5,6) allowed by the synthesis of steroid molecules directly labelled with a fluorescent tracer. These micromolecular derivatives bind to cytosolic receptor with a relative binding affinity higher than the macromolecular ones and interact with intact cells in a way similar to the native hormone. Therefore, these fluorescent hormonal probes can enter the cells, thus yielding information on the overall intracellular kinetics of steroid receptor complexes under appropriate experimental conditions (6). The latest technique, of affinity cytochemistry, exploits the intrinsic fluorescence of estrogen molecules such as Coumestrol, a blue fluorescing phytoestrogen whose relative binding affinity is within the range of that of physiologic E_1 and E_3 estrogens (7).

The fourth and last generation is now in gestation; these newer techniques attempt to exploit a specific anti-receptor raised in animals or hybridomas to trace the receptor protein itself (8). It is now possible to use this technique for glucocorticoid receptors and for estradiol receptors in breast cancer. In this way, a major breakthrough in the cytochemical approach to steroid receptors is being achieved. The demonstration of receptor through its binding capacity may be an advantage since not only the presence but also the primary function of the receptor can be assessed. The results of the various cytochemical techniques should be interpreted with strict attention to accurate control tests since the demonstration of binding site does not necessarily provide evidence for their receptor nature.

According to current concepts, the demonstration of finite binding capacity, high affinity, steroid and tissue specificity constitutes reasonably good evidence for the receptor nature of the displaced binding sites. Non specific binding would be, on the contrary, of limited capacity, rapidly dissociating, non steroid specific and ubiquitous. In cytochemical investigations the above criteria can be appropriately checked.

Some other data support the specificity of histochemical tracing of steroid binding sites; they are the consistency of the positivity by the same (intra-assay validation) or different (inter-assay validation) techniques when applied to tissue sections of the same specimen and chiefly the physiological validation since these techniques visualize specific binding sites which fulfil the intracellular requirement for steroid receptor sites.

In fact, the cytochemical techniques can display the site of steroid synthesis, the presence of binding sites in different cell compartments of target tissue and, of especial importance, the intracellular kinetics of steroid hormones. In this way, the precise identification of the structural expression of the mechanism of steroid action can be achieved, exploiting different experimental conditions.

Breast cancer has been the testing bench of all cytochemical approaches to steroid receptors, but the results can be applied to other tumors growing from steroid responsive tissue, such as the prostate.

The heterogeneity in hormone receptivity of tumor cells and the presence of several defects of the steroid action mechanism downstream to cytoplasmic uptake, such as impaired nuclear translocation and defective or absent nuclear retention, are responsible for the variable tumor hormone responsiveness and can be easily visualized by cytochemical procedures (9).

As far as the prostate is concerned, the above cytochemical techniques visualize a differential binding of estrogen and androgen with a very interesting dualism between the stroma and the epithelium (Fig. 1.).

While the androgen binding sites are predominantly located at the glandular level, the estrogen binding sites are chiefly distributed in the stroma. This result, besides confirming some recent results concerning cytosolic binding sites or separated epithelium and stroma of human prostatic hyperplasia (10), draws attention to the already suggested differential control of stromal and epithelial growth by sex steroid hormones at the prostatic level.

SUMMARY

Cytochemical techniques visualize steroid receptors under the microscope exploiting the same properties of the receptor site as do the techniques for biochemical assay.

Many generations of methods have followed in rapid succession including immunocytochemistry, labelled-ligand cytochemistry and affinity cytochemistry. These techniques, under different experimental conditions, can display the site of steroid synthesis, the presence of specific binding sites in target tissues and the intracellular kinetics of steroid hormones.

As far as the cancer is concerned, the cytochemical procedures easily visualize the heterogeneity in hormone receptivity of tumor cells and the presence of several defects of steroid action mechanism which are responsible for the variable tumor hormone responsiveness.

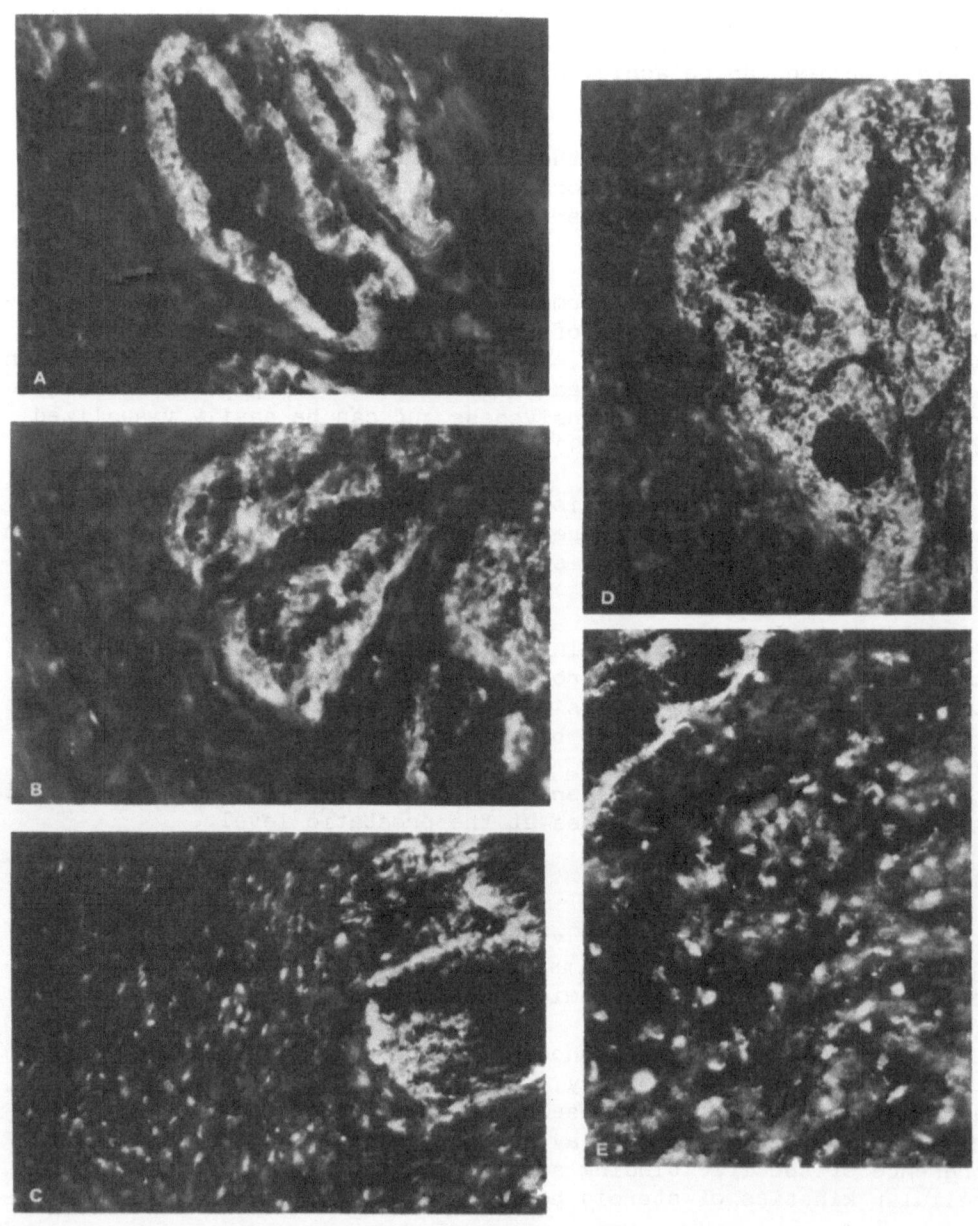

Fig. 1. Sex steroid binding sites detected in human prostate by
◄——————— cytochemical techniques.

A. <u>Normal gland</u>: Evident cytoplasmic uptake of labelled <u>androgen</u>
                   by epithelial cells; stroma is unstained.

B. <u>Benign hypertrophy</u>: Labelled <u>androgen</u> is taken up by hyper-
                        plastic epithelial glandular cells only; the
                        fibromuscular stromal cells are unstained.

C. <u>Benign hypertrophy</u>: Fluorescent <u>estrogen</u> shows specific
                        estrogen binding sites in both the epithelial
                        and the hyperplastic stromal cells.

D. <u>Cribriform carcinoma</u>: <u>Androgen</u> binding sites are clearly
                          displayed at the cytoplasmic level of neoplastic
                          epithelial cells.

E. <u>Infiltrating carcinoma</u>: Infiltrating neoplastic cells show a
                           predominantly nuclear localization of <u>androgen</u>
                           binding sites.

REFERENCES

1. D. Beccati, G. Lanza, I. Nenci, and A. Piffanelli, Microfluori-
    metric method to detect specific oestradiol receptors in
    different cell types on cell suspension from target tissues
    (Abstr.) <u>J. Steroid Biochem</u>. 6:Viii (1975).
2. I. Nenci, D. Beccati, A. Piffanella, and G. Lanza, Detection
    and dynamic localization of estradiol-receptor complexes in
    intact target cells by immunofluorescence technique,
    <u>J. Steroid Biochem</u>. 7:505-510 (1976).
3. G. Daxenbichler, H. Grill, R. Domanig, E. Moser, and O. Dapunt,
    Receptor binding of fluorescein labelled steroids, <u>J. Steroid
    Biochem</u>. 13:489-493 (1980).
4. E. Gaetjews, and L. Pertschuk, Synthesis of fluorescein-labelled
    steroid hormone-albumin conjugates for the fluorescent histo-
    chemical detection of hormone receptors, <u>J. Steroid Biochem</u>.
    13:1001-1003 (1980).
5. W. Dandliker, R. Brawn, and M. Hsu, Investigation of hormone
    receptor interactions by means of fluorescence labelling,
    <u>Cancer Res</u>. 38:4212-4224 (1978).
6. I. Nenci, W. Dandliker, C. Meyers, A. Marzola, E. Marchetti, and
    G. Fabris, Estrogen receptor cytochemistry by fluorescent
    estrogen, <u>J. Histochem. Cytochem</u>. 28:1081-1088 (1980).
7. Y. Lee, A. Notides, Y. Tsay, and A. Kende, Coumestrol, NBD-
    Norhexestrol, and Dausyl-Norhexestrol, fluorescent probes of
    estrogen binding proteins, <u>Biochemistry</u> 16:2896-2901 (1977).

8.   G. Greene, E. Jensen, C. Wolan, and J. Engler, Monoclonal
     antibodies to human estrogen receptor, Proc. Natl. Acad. Sci.
     USA, 77:5115-5119 (1980).
9.   I. Nenci, D. Beccati, C. Pagnini Arslan, Estrogen
     receptors and post-receptorial markers in human breast cancer:
     a reappraisal, Tumori 64:161-174 (1978).
10. M. Krieg, G. Klotzl, J. Kaufmann, and K. Voigt, Stroma of human
     benign prostatic hyperplasia: preferential tissue for androgen
     metabolism and oestrogen binding, Acta Endocrinologica 96:
     422-432 (1981).

HISTOCHEMICAL DETERMINATION OF ANDROGEN BINDING SITES

IN PROSTATIC ADENOCARCINOMA: CLINICAL CORRELATION

R.J. Macchia and L.P. Pertschuk and the New York
Prostate Binding Site Study Group*

Downstate Medical School
New York
U.S.A.

The figure of 80% is classically quoted as the percentage of
patients with advanced prostatic adenocarcinoma who respond at least
initially to hormonal manipulation. At the present time there is no
method of predicting whether a given patient will respond to such
therapy. It is not unreasonable to hypothesize that those patients
with androgen dependent tumors should have high levels of androgen
binding sites. A non-immunologic histochemical method has been
developed by Pertschuk (1,2,3,4,5) to measure androgen binding sites.
The principal purpose of this report is to update the clinical trial
we are currently conducting to determine whether or not the test can
be used to predict response to hormonal manipulation.

The clinical trial is being conducted as follows. Whenever
prostatic tissue is removed from a patient, a portion is reserved for
histochemical androgen binding site analysis and a portion for biochemical analysis. Each patient is entered into a computerized data
retrieval system together with all the clinical and pathological
facts pertinent to his case. The trial is double blind in that the
clinician is unaware of the histochemical and biochemical assay
results and the assayists are unaware of the clinical data. Response
to therapy is measured by the criteria of the National Prostate Cancer
Project (6).

The Pertschuk test has been completely described (1,2,3,4,5).
Briefly, a solution is prepared of testosterone linked to a fluorescein moiety (7). The specimen of prostatic cancer, which is
immediately frozen in liquid nitrogen after removal from the patient,
is subsequently sectioned (four microns thick) and placed on a glass
slide. After warming to room temperature, the section is covered

with the androgen fluorescein solution for two hours, then examined
under an ultraviolet light microscope. A step section of the frozen
specimen is taken and processed by the routine H & E technique. The
results of competitive and non-specific binding studies have been
published (1,2,3,4,5). To date 177 specimens of prostatic adenocarcinoma have been so studied.

   Specimens in which, by visual estimate, 0-8% of the cells
displayed fluorescence were designated as binding site poor, those
in which 9-14% were stained as borderline, and those with 15% or more
stained as positive. The predominant site of staining - cytoplastic,
nuclear or mixed - was noted.

RESULTS

   Of the first 107 cases the specimen was obtained by TURP in 45,
by needle biopsy in 41, by open prostatectomy in 11, by open biopsy
in 5 and by needle biopsy and TURP in 5.

   Histological grade was assigned using the Gleason system (8) and
clinical stage by the method of Whitmore (9). Tables 1 and 2 show
that neither estrogen nor testosterone binding correlated with
histologic grade or with clinical stage.

   The method of biochemical assay which we utilize has been
described (5). Table 3 demonstrates the agreement between biochemical testosterone (AR) assay and histochemical testosterone
binding. Our method of statistical analysis for this and subsequent
tables has been described (5). The agreement of qualitative histochemical androgen assay to biochemical androgen receptor assay is
indicated by the Kappa (K) statistic: K = .365 and p .0001.

Table 1. Histological Grade and Steroid Binding by Histochemistry
          in Prostatic Carcinoma (171 cases)

Tumor Grade	% E and T+	% E and T-	% E+ /T-	% E- /T+	Total
1 - 2	87	8	4	1	97
3	82	5	10	3	40
4 - 5	79	15	3	3	34

E = Estrogen binding,   T = Anrogen binding.

Table 2. Clinicopathologic Stage and Steroid Binding by Histochemistry in Prostatic Cancer (177 cases)

Stage	% E and T+	% E and T-	% E+/T-	%E-/T+	Total
A	86	14	0	0	29
B	87	7	2	4	45
C	92	8	0	0	15
D	83	7	6	4	88

E = Estrogen binding, T = Androgen binding

Table 3. Agreement Between Biochemical AR Assay and Histochemical
Androgen Binding Assays in Prostate Cancer (103 cases)

	Biochemical Assay		
Histochemical Assay	Positive	Negative	Total
Positive	77	9	86
Negative	9*	8	17
Total	86	17	103

* In three of these cases, histochemistry revealed the tumor to
be poor in androgen binding and adjacent benign glands to be
positive.

Table 4 further analyzes the histochemical to biochemical
agreement by examining the relationship with regard to subcellular
localization of binding sites. For this K = .546 and p .0001.

We have described a method for semi-quantitating the results of
histochemical assay (5). Table 5 related the quantitative biochemical assay to the semiquantitative histochemical assay. For this
K = .317 and p .0001.

Table 4. Agreement Between Histochemical and Biochemical Detection
          of Subcellular Androgen Binding Sites in Prostate
          Carcinoma (103 cases)

	Biochemical Assay				
Histochemical Assay	Cytoplasmic	Nuclear	Mixed	None	Total
Cytoplasmic predominant	38	3	7	6	54
Nuclear predominant	5	5	–	3	13
Mixed (circa 1:1 nuclear vs cytoplasmic)	3	1	21	–	25
None	1	1	1	8	11
Total	47	10	29	17	103

Includes correlations in histochemically processed tissue sections
designated as poor where <10% of cells were positive.

Table 5. Comparison of Quantitative Biochemical AR and Semi-
          quantitative Histochemical Androgen Binding Assay Results
          in Prostate Cancer (77 cases)

	Biochemical Assay			
Histochemical Assay	Zero-Trace	Low-Intermediate	High-Very High	Total
Zero-Trace	9	6	4	19
Low-Intermediate	10	15	7	32
High-Very High	5	3	18	26
Total	24	24	29	77

Biochemical designation of positive, non-quantifiable (+NQ), not
included as no comparative histochemical designation available.

Histochemistry (Semiquantified)	Biochemistry (fmoles/g tissue)
Zero-trace 0-<5	0- 150
Low-Intermediate >5-18	>150- 550
High-Very High >18->30	>550->950

Table 6. Comparison of Androgen Binding by Semiquantitative Histochemistry and Biochemistry to Clinical Response to Hormonal Therapy (38 cases)

	Histochemistry			Biochemistry				
Response	Z-T	L-I	H-VH	Z-T	L-I	H-VH	+NQ	NA*
Complete	0	0	3	0	2	1	0	0
Partial	0	8	8	1	5	5	2	3
Stable	2	5	0	0	0	0	2	5
Progressed	7	5	0	3	1	4	1	3

Histochemistry (Semiquantified)   Biochemistry (fmoles/g tissue)

Zero-trace (Z-T) 0-<5   0- 150
Low-Intermediate (L-I) >5-18   >150- 550
High-very high (H-VH) >18->30   >550->950
*NA - Not Suitable for Assay

Table 6 examines the ability of histochemical and biochemical analysis to predict response to hormonal manipulation. The clinical records of 38 men with stage C and D cancer where more than one year had elapsed since specimen acquisition were available. Both methods exhibit trends whereby patients with zero or trace androgen binding progress clinically and those with high binding have a response other than progression.

Statistical analysis indicates that treatment response was significantly associated (p .0001) with the histochemical result but not with the biochemical result (p .60).

COMMENTS

The histochemical technique has many advantages and few disadvantages when compared to biochemical techniques. It is simple, rapid and inexpensive. It can be performed in a simple community hospital laboratory by regular laboratory personnel. The technique allows for subcellular binding site localization (cytoplasmic vs nuclear). The test can be performed on minute pieces of tissue, even aspiration biopsy specimens. Binding capacity heterogeneity means that within a given specimen not all cells exhibit the same binding capacity. Variation of fluorescent intensity of a given specimen, we believe, represents this heterogeneity and is easily appreciated by

the histochemical method. Most specimens demonstrated significant
heterogeneity.

Of the first 108 patients known to have prostatic cancer, six
failed to have tumor on the particular specimen submitted for histochemical assay. Verification of the presence of tumor is an important
advantage of the histochemical technique.

In three specimens analyzed histochemically, the tumor was seen
to be poor in androgen binding while adjacent, non-malignant prostatic
glands were rich in binding sites. In all three cases, biochemical
assay was positive.

The histochemical technique allows for visual identification
of heat artifact in TUR specimens. Heat can destroy or alter androgen
binding sites and thus cause a falsely negative assay.

Do the biochemical and histochemical techniques measure the same
thing? At this point an answer cannot be given with certainty. The
ultimate test is not whether they agree but whether either can
accurately predict response to hormonal manipulation.

NEW YORK PROSTATE BINDING SITE STUDY GROUP - COLLABORATORS*

State University of New York Downstate Medical School, Brooklyn, N.Y.

        Louis P. Pertschuk, D.O.
        Richard J. Macchia, M.D.
        Karen B. Eisenberg, B.S.N., M.P.S.
        Virginia C. Leo, R.N.
        Eric Gaetjens, Ph.D.
        Joseph G. Feldman, D.P.H.

Roswell Park Memorial Institute, Buffalo, N.Y.

        Hanna E. Rosenthal, M.S.
        James P. Karr, Ph.D.
        Gerald P. Murphy, M.D., Ph.D.
        Avery A. Sandberg, M.D.

Brookdale Hospital Center, Brooklyn, N.Y.

        Sandor H. Wax M.D. (until January 1981)
        Dong S. Kim, M.D.

Veterans Administration Hospital, Brooklyn, N.Y.

        Jesse I. Abrahams, M.D.

Maimonides Medical Center, Brooklyn, N.Y.

Gilbert J. Wise

Memorial Sloan-Kettering Cancer Center, N.Y.

Willet F. Whitmore, Jr., M.D.
Harry W. Herr, M.D.

REFERENCES

1. L.P. Pertschuk, D.T. Zava, E. Gaetjens, R.J. Macchia, D.J. Brigati, and D.S. Kim, Detection of androgen and estrogen receptors in human prostatic carcinoma and hyperplasia by fluorescence micro-scopy, Res. Comm. Path. Pharmacol. 22:427 (1978).
2. L.P. Pertschuk, D.T. Zava, E. Gaetjens, R.J. Macchia, G.J. Wise, D.S. Kim, and D.J. Brigati, Histochemistry of steroid receptors in prostatic disease, Ann. Clin. Lab. Sci. 9:225 (1979).
3. L.P. Pertschuk, D.T. Zava, E.H. Tobin, D.J. Brigati, E. Gaetjens, R.J. Macchia, G.J. Wise, H.S. Wax, and D.S. Kim, Histochemical detection of steroid hormone receptors in the human prostate, in:"Prostate Cancer and Hormone Receptors," G.P. Murphy and A.A. Sandberg, eds., Alan R. Liss, Inc., New York (1979).
4. L.P. Pertschuk, E.H. Tobin, P. Tanapat, E. Gaetjens, A.C. Carter, N.D. Bloom, R.J. Macchia, and K.B. Eisenberg, Histochemical analyses of steroid hormone receptors in breast and prostatic carcinoma, J. Histochem. Cytochem. 28:799 (1980).
5. L.P. Pertschuk, H.E. Rosenthal, R.J. Macchia, K.B. Eisenberg, J.G. Feldman, S.H. Wax, D.S. Kim, W.F. Whitmore, Jr., J.I. Abrahams, E. Gaetjens, G.J. Wise, H.W. Herr, J.P. Karr, G.P. Murphy, and A.A. Sandberg, Correlation of histochemical and biochemical analyses of androgen binding in prostatic cancer: relation to therapeutic response, Cancer, in press.
6. J.D. Schmidt, D.E. Johnson, W.W. Scott, R.P. Gibbons, G.R. Prout, Jr., and G.P. Murphy, Chemotherapy of advanced prostatic cancer, evaluation of response parameters, Urology 7:602 (1976).
7. E. Gaetjens and L.P. Pertschuk, Synthesis of fluorescent labeled-steroid hormone albumin conjugates for the histochemical detection of hormone receptors, J. Steroid Biochem. 13:1121 (1980).
8. D.R. Gleason, Histologic grading and clinical staging of prostatic carcinoma, in:"Urologic Pathology: The Prostate," M. Tannenbaum, ed., Lea and Febiger, Philadelphia (1977).
9. R.J. Boxer, Adenocarcinoma of the prostate gland, Urol. Surv. 27:75 (1977).

PROSTATIC CANCER: CLINICAL SIGNIFICANCE

OF RECEPTOR STUDIES

G.D. Chisholm, T. Smith, and F.K. Habib

Western General Hospital
Edinburgh
Scotland

In recent years, there has been a substantial increase in our knowledge about the mechanism of action of sex steroids in hormone responsive target organs. It is now believed that the high concentration of hormones measured in cells of organs such as breast, uterus and prostate is due to a binding (receptor) protein in the cytoplasm; this protein binds the appropriate hormones specifically and with a high affinity. Following the binding, the receptor protein undergoes a process known as activation - permitting or causing its translocation to the nucleus. Activation and translocation occur within minutes of the hormone entering the cell and the whole process has been shown to be energy dependent. Once within the nucleus, the hormone receptor forms a complex with the chromatin. This final step induces several responses characteristic of the steroid sensitive tissue and it should be noted that these processes are not manifested before the hormonal stimulation. This is, however, an over-simplification - since in some target tissues hormones entering the cell may also be subjected to metabolism (1). Nonetheless, current theories attach major emphasis to the translocation of the steroid receptor complexes into the nucleus and with a few minor exceptions, hormonal responses are, on the whole, believed to be centred on the selective activation of nuclear processes in target cells (2).

Although receptor studies are now widely used for the identification of hormone responsive tissues in gynaecological and breast tumours (3), there is still little information on the relevance of these studies in the treatment and management of prostatic cancer (4). These attempts have been frustrated in part by the failure to characterise a specific receptor in the prostate and partly by the lack of a reliable assay for the measurement of these receptors.

Furthermore, the interpretation of biochemical data is complicated
by the heterogeneous nature of the prostate gland. Prostatic tissue
consists of a mixture of stromal and epithelial cells and the relative
proportion of these components in specimens removed at surgery
reveals considerable variation from patient to patient (5).

The most recent developments in prostate/steroid receptor
investigations and some of the more common pitfalls associated with
the measurement of these molecules are reviewed. The results of
studies on the distribution of hormonal binding proteins within the
separated prostatic tissue components are reported.

CYTOPLASMIC RECEPTORS

Most of the earlier receptor studies concentrated on the cytosol
fraction. Although androgens remain an important aspect of this type
of study, recent investigations have also established the presence of
oestrogen and progesterone receptors in the prostate.

Androgen Receptors

Androgen receptors have been demonstrated in normal prostate,
benign prostatic hyperplasia and carcinoma of the prostate (6,7,8,9,
10,11,12,13,14). The studies were characterised by a broad range of
receptor concentrations. Furthermore, preliminary correlation with
response to treatment has been mixed and inconclusive. Although
Mobbs et al, (12) and Ekman et al (7) observed partial responses to
hormonal manipulation, when the androgen binding capacity of cytosol
protein was between 0.3 and 2.0 fmol/per mg tissue, other workers
(6) were totally unsuccessful in demonstrating a consistent pattern
between a receptor concentration and clinical response.

There are many factors which may account for these reported
differences. Firstly, the contamination of tissue with sex hormone
binding globulin; this blood protein possesses similar properties to
the cytoplasmic receptor and it is more difficult to distinguish
between the two components. The second problem concerns the high
endogenous concentrations of dihydrotestosterone present in prostatic
tissue; although these steroids frequently mask the potential hormone
binding sites, reports on patients with low endogenous androgens
suggest that hormonal sensitivity of prostatic carcinoma is not
directly related to the concentration of androgen receptors (12).
Thirdly, the presence in the receptor of a protein with similar
characteristics to a progestin receptor which also binds to androgens
(15) may erroneously lead to higher estimates of androgen receptor
than is actually present in the tissue. Perhaps even more significant are our own recent observations revealing that the cytosolic
androgen receptor concentration per gm of tissue was higher in the

Table 1. The Relative Receptor Concentrations in the Cytosol
          of Stroma and Epithelial Components Obtained from
          Seven Patients with Benign Prostatic Hypertrophy.

Patients	Epithelium (fmol/gm wet tissue)	Stroma (fmol/gm wet tissue)
1	55*	23
2	56	62
3	12	9
4	56	31
5	47	58
6	86	58
7	146	120

* Mean of three separate readings

epithelial components than in the stroma (Table 1). This suggests
that the measurement of receptor concentrations in whole tissues is
probably related to the epithelial cell content in the analysed
specimens. Thus the stroma rich periurethral regions of the prostate
could maintain lower binding capacities than the predominantly
glandular peripheral sections of the gland. A recent study on various
lobes obtained from the same prostate have revealed that different
parts of the same tumour possess different degrees of hormone dependence (16). This further confirms the above hypothesis and underlines
the inherent danger of single sampling analysis in receptor studies.

Oestrogen Receptors

The extensive use of oestrogen therapy for the treatment of
prostatic cancer has led many investigators to examine the role and
function of the steroid in the prostate gland. Extensive studies on
the human prostate have revealed that oestrogens inhibit the binding
of dihydrotestosterone to the cytosol fraction; this may account for
some of the beneficial effects detected in carcinoma patients treated
with oestrogen based drugs. More important, however, are the reports
of a specific 17β oestradiol receptor in the cytosol of the human
benign hypertrophied prostate (17). Although the presence of
receptors has not been universally accepted, more recent investigations by Sidh et al. (18) have suggested that patients with

tumours deficient in oestrogen receptors but containing a full
measure of androgen receptors are less likely to respond to endocrine
manipulation.

Progesterone Receptors

There is increasing evidence that progesterone is important in
the development of benign prostatic hypertrophy. A number of studies
on the normal and pathological prostate demonstrated the presence of
progesterone receptors in most cases of B.P.H. (19) but they are less
common in normal prostatic tissue. It is possible that progesterone
receptors in B.P.H. are a phenomenon secondary to changes in androgen/
oestrogen blood levels and it may also be that progestational antiandrogens are more logical drugs to consider in the control and even
reduction of benign prostatic growth. Progesterone receptors were
also detected in prostatic carcinoma (7) and in view of the favourable
reports following progestin therapy, carcinoma patients with progesterone receptor rich tumours should possibly be considered for this
type of treatment.

NUCLEAR RECEPTORS

In view of the technical problems associated with the accurate
measurements of androgen receptors in the cytoplasm of the human
prostate, a number of attempts were made to quantify receptors
localised in the purified nuclear fraction (14,15,20). A high
affinity binding for androgens was demonstrated in all cases and it
is now believed that approximately 75% of the total measurable
androgen receptors in benign prostatic hypertrophy is located in the
nucleus. These results were further confirmed by our own studies
which also revealed that the bulk of these androgen binding proteins
was located in the stromal components of the nuclear extractions
(Table 2). The importance of these receptors as discriminant for
hormone responsiveness can not yet be determined but assuming that
nuclear receptor studies in malignant tissue will also yield a
correspondingly high localisation of binding sites in the nuclei, this
may prove a useful measure in assessing treatment of carcinoma of the
prostate. There are reports of patients with metastatic carcinoma of
the prostate who have a good response to hormone therapy despite poor
or negative levels of cytoplasmic receptors (21). It is possible
that nuclear receptor measurements might have identified these
patients as responders.

Preliminary studies on the nuclear components have also identified the presence of oestrogen and progesterone binding proteins, but
again as in the case of the androgen binding components the significance of these molecules has not yet been established.

Table 2. Variation in Nuclear and Cytosol Androgen Receptor Concentration in Tissue Components of Eight Patients with Benign Prostatic Hypertrophy.

	Cytosol fraction (fmol/gm tissue)	Nuclear fraction (fmol/mg tissue)
	Mean (range)	Mean (range)
Whole tissue	108 (71-209)	108 (62-385)
Epithelium	65 (12-146)	102 (43-326)
Stroma	51 (9-120)	128 (43-280)

Conclusions

The measurement of hormone receptors in human prostatic tissue has been greatly limited by many difficulties and until these have been resolved the success of the hormone receptor test in predicting the hormonal status of prostatic cancer will be of limited use in the management of this tumour. Several attempts have already been made to provide new methods for the measurement and the specific localisation of receptors in individual samples of human cancer. Perhaps the most promising of these new techniques are the immunocytochemical tests which will enable the direct identification of the specific binding proteins on the histology slides, thus allowing for a histological analysis and a biochemical test to be carried out on the same section of tissue. Another important approach will be the production of monoclonal antibodies which it is hoped will dramatically improve the sensitivity and specificity of the immunological procedures. At the same time, the possibility of alternative approaches for predicting clinical response, for example, the measurement of whole tissue concentrations of dihydrotestosterone, the assessment of androgen metabolism in subcellular fractions or further fundamental studies on receptor proteins, may still be necessary and should not be ignored.

Acknowledgement

The work described in this paper was generously supported by the Scottish Hospital Endowment Research Trust.

REFERENCES

1. F.K. Habib, A.L. Tesdale, G.D. Chisholm, and A. Busuttil,
    Metabolic patterns in the epithelial and stromal components of
    benign prostatic hypertrophy, J.Endocr. 91 (1981) (In Press).
2. W.I.P. Mainwaring, "The Mechanism of Action of Androgens.
    Monographs on Endocrinology," Springer Verlag, New York,
    Vol. 10 (1977).
3. E.V. Jensen and E.R. Desombre, The diagnostic implications of
    steroid binding in malignant tissues, Adv. Clin. Chem. 19:57
    (1977).
4. G.D. Chisholm and F.K. Habib, Prostatic cancer: experimental and
    clinical advances, in:"Recent Advances in Urology/Andrology No.
    3, W.F. Hendry, ed., Churchill Livingstone, Edinburgh (1981).
5. R.A. Cowan, B. Cook, S.K. Cowan, J.K. Grant, D.A.N Sirett, and
    A.M. Wallace, Testosterone 5α-reductase and the accumulation of
    dihydrotestosterone in benign prostatic hyperplasia, J.Steroid
    Biochem. 11:609 (1979).
6. H.J. de Voogt and P.G. Dingjan, Is there a place for the assay
    of cytoplasms dual receptors in the endocrine treatment for
    prostatic cancer?, in"Steroid Receptors, Metabolism and Prostatic
    Cancer, F.H. Schröder and H.J. de Voogt, eds., Excerpta Medica,
    Amsterdam 265 (1980).
7. P. Ekman, M. Snochowski, A. Zetterberg, B. Hogberg, and J.A.
    Gustafsson, Steroid receptor content in human prostatic
    carcinoma and response to endocrine therapy, Cancer 44:1173
    (1979).
8. R. Ghanadian, G. Auf, B.J. Chaloner, and G.D. Chisholm, The
    use of methyltrienolone and the measurement of the free and
    bound cytoplasmic receptors for dihydrotestosterone in benign
    hypertrophied human prostate, J.Steroid Biochem. 9:325 (1978).
9. M. Kreig, W. Bartsch, and K.D. Vogt, Binding metabolism and
    tissue level of androgens in human prostatic carcinoma, benign
    prostatic hyperplasia and normal prostate, in:"Steroid Receptors,
    Metabolism and Prostatic Cancer," F.H. Schröder and H.J. de Voogt,
    eds., Excerpta Medica, Amsterdam, 102 (1980).
10. G.N. Lieskovsky and N. Bruchovsky, Assay of nuclear androgen
    receptor in human prostate, J. Urol. 121:54 (1979).
11. M. Menon, C.E. Tananis, L.L. Hicks. E.F. Hawkins, M.G.
    McLoughlin, and B.C. Walsh, Characterisation of the binding of
    a potent synthetic androgen methyltrienolone to human tissues,
    J. Clin. Invest. 61:150 (1978).
12. B.G. Mobbs, I.E. Johnston, and J.G. Connolly, Androgen receptors
    and treatment of prostatic cancer, in:"Steroid Receptors,
    Metabolism and Prostatic Cancer," F.H. Schröder and H.J.
    de Voogt, eds., Excerpta Medica, Amsterdam, 225 (1980).
13. S.A. Shain, R.W. Boesel, D.L. Lamm, and H.M. Radwin, Cyto-
    plasmic and nuclear androgen receptor content of normal and
    neoplastic human prostates and lymph nodes metastases of human
    prostatic adenocarcinoma, J. Clin. Endocrinol. Metab. 50:704
    (1980).

14. D.A.N. Sirett and J.K. Grant, Androgen binding in cytosols
     and nuclei of human benign hyperplastic prostatic tissue,
     J. Endocr. 77:101 (1978).
15. L.L. Hicks and P.C. Walsh, A microassay for the measurement of
     androgen receptors in human prostatic tissue, Steroids 33:2390
     (1979).
16. J.G. Lehoux, B. Benard and Elhilali, Dihydrotestosterone
     receptors in the human prostate. I. Nuclear concentration in
     normal, benign, and malignant tissues, Arch. Androl. 5:237 (1980).
17. N. Bashirelahi, J.H. O'Toole, and J.D. Young, A specific 17
     B-estradiol receptor in human benign hypertrophic prostate,
     Biochem. Med. 15:254 (1976).
18. S.M. Sidh, J.D. Young, S.A. Karmi, J.R. Powder, and
     N. Bashirelahi, Adenocarcinoma of prostate: role of 17B-
     estradiol and 5α-dihydrotestosterone binding proteins,
     Urology 13:597 (1979).
19. W.D. Tilley, D.D. Keightley, and V.R. Marshall, Oestrogen and
     progesterone receptors in benign prostatic hyperplasia in humans,
     J. Steroid Biochem. 13:395 (1980).
20. N. Bruchovsky, P.S. Rennie, and P.R. Wilkin, New aspects of
     androgen action in prostatic cells: stromal localization of
     5α -reductase, nuclear abundance of androstanolone and binding of
     receptor to linker deoxyribonucleic acid, in:"Steroid Receptors,
     Metabolism and Prostatic Cancer," F.H. Schröder and H.J.
     de Voogt, eds., Excerpta Medica, Amsterdam, 57 (1980).
21. R.K. Wagner and K.H. Schultz, Clinical relevance of androgen
     receptor content in human prostatic carcinoma, Acta Endocrinol-
     ogica 87:139 (1978).

RADICAL PROSTATECTOMY

W.E. Goodwin

University of California at Los Angeles
School of Medicine
Los Angeles, California
U.S.A.

INTRODUCTION

Treatment of prostatic cancer is an interesting subject. One can expect cure from a radical prostatectomy providing there is no spread beyond the prostate gland. Radical perineal prostatectomy offers this cure without the advantage of sampling and testing the lymphatics which drain the prostate, staging only. Nonetheless, it is a time honored treatment which has excellent results and which is much less damaging to the patient than radical retropubic prostatectomy with node dissection. It is also less discomforting to the patient in the sense that the complications are much less and, in my opinion, the opportunity to do a direct anastomosis to the urethra under vision, allows for a better control and a decrease in the chance of urinary incontinence. There are no available figures that I know of to support my view, but I feel quite certain from watching the results of retropubic radical prostatectomy versus radical perineal prostatectomy, that the statements I have made are true.

When radical retropubic was a new operation, I tried to do it and subsequently tried to do a combination of radical retropubic and perineal, but I gave this up because it seemed to me that the patients fared much better with a radical perineal and I believe that when the figures are finally in, it will be seen that the idea of doing a radical node dissection, plus a radical retropubic prostatectomy does not justify the trauma to the patient.

PART I: RADICAL PERINEAL PROSTATECTOMY

My view is that a radical perineal prostatectomy is the surgery
of choice in A-2 and B-1 and B-2 lesions. There may also be a
particular place for it in stage C lesions, simply to relieve the
patient of any further difficulties with obstructive symptoms. I am
completely committed to this operation as the operation of choice
for early prostatic cancer. I would not do it in the presence of
known bony metastases or metastases elsewhere, but I believe that
some stage C lesions with lymphatic metastases are best handled in
this manner.

Radical perineal prostatectomy is one of the most intriguing and
exacting operations in the field of urological surgery. It requires
a perfect understanding of the anatomy and meticulous care whilst
trying to "sail 'twixt wind and water".*

There are many variants of technique, but the basic procedure
was described by Doctor Hugh Hampton Young. He describes the history
and genesis of this procedure in his classic article, "The cure of
cancer of the prostate by radical perineal prostatectomy (prostato-
seminovesiculectomy): History, literature, and statistics of Young's
operation" (1). In that article, he records his first operation note
in 1904 and the technique of his operation is beautifully illustrated
by William P. Didusch. It my view, it is impossible to improve on
Doctor Young's description. However, I am going to try to summarize
it.

In this discussion I wish to refer to figures 11 - 21 by
Didusch illustrating Hugh Young's operation (1) and to the illustrations in Elmer Belt's article (2). I will not attempt to reproduce
them because they are so numerous and because they are easily available to almost everyone with access to a library.

The first and most important step is to position the patient in
the exaggerated lithotomy position in such a way that the perineum
is parallel to the floor of the operating theatre. This allows the
rectum to drop backward and gives the surgeon the best access to the
prostate (3).

After meticulous cleansing of the penis, scrotum and perineum,
including the anal region, the anus is draped out of the field in
such a way as to give the operator access for a rectal examination
if he needs to do it during the operation. The important steps in
the operation are described on the following pages.

---

* "Young in heart; young in hand,
   Young is known throughout the land.
   Lord preserve us from the slaughter
   That he creates
   'Twixt wind and water."   (Keyes)

1.   The incision is an inverted "U" made, according to Young's plan, three scalpel handles anterior to the anal margin. A curved sound is inserted into the urethra to allow the prostate to be levered up- ward into the wound.

2.   After the skin has been opened, the ischiorectal fossa is devel- oped on each side of the central tendon by blunt dissection with the fingers and the handle of the scalpel.

3.   Young's bifid posterior tractor is used to pull the rectum back- ward which accentuates the central tendon which is then cut. This allows the rectum to drop backward and the transverse perineal muscles to go forward with the bulb and the urethral sphincter.

4.   Dissection is then carried downward bluntly until the fibers of the levator ani are found. Doctor Young identified the decussation of these fibers in the midline as the "rectourethralis muscle". The surgeon stays well posterior to the external urinary sphincter, which really should never enter into the field. The muscles of the levators, or the rectourethralis muscle as identified by Young, are either transected near the apex of the prostate, or pushed laterally until the fascia of Denonvilliers is encountered. It is a glistening white fascia which looks very much like peritoneum which, indeed, it was embryologically. There are two layers to it. Doctor Young used to describe this as "the pearly gates".

5.   The lateral fascia, together with the levator muscles, is pushed laterally to expose the lateral sides and the apex of the prostate. The prostate is pulled downward on traction to elongate the intra- sphincteric part of the urethra, and a very careful transverse in- cision is made just at the apex of the prostate without involving the urethral sphincter. The urethra is then completely divided and dissection is carried upward along the anterior surface of the pros- tate. Young's prostatic tractor is placed through the apex of the prostate into the bladder and used for traction to pull the prostate downward into the wound and identify the anterior portion. There is often excessive bleeding from the area of Santorini's plexus; and it is important, if possible, to secure these vessels with a good liga- ture before cutting the pubo-prostatic ligaments in that area. The endo-pelvic fascia is entered bluntly and dissected to free the pros- tate laterally on each side.

6.   The prostate is pulled downward into the wound with Young's prostatic tractor and the anterior fascia is pushed away from the bladder until one can see the junction between the prostate and the bladder. A knife is plunged through the bladder in the median line at its junction with the prostate to open the bladder anteriorly.

7.   The anterior bladder incision is then enlarged by cutting down- ward on each side exactly at the place where the prostate lies next

to the bladder neck. Young describes removing a small cuff of bladder
with the prostate. The trigone and ureteral orifices are visualized
and the incision is made distal to that point.

8.   The incision is carried all the way across to free the prostate
completely from the back of the bladder and this opens the retro-
vesical space to expose the anterior surface of the seminal vesicles.
The bladder is lifted off the seminal vesicles until the ampullae of
the vasa can be seen and the vasa are identified and transsected.
They may either be clipped or tied. The most difficult part of this
dissection now comes when the blood vessels leading into the tips of
the seminal vesicles have to be transsected between clamps, or, as
is now more usual, metal clips. The vascular pedicle of the prostate
and seminal vesicles is cross-clamped, cut and then ligated, usually
with a heavy chromic suture.

     This allows removal of the total prostate together with a cuff
of the bladder and the seminal vesicles with the anterior and posterior layers of Denonvilliers' fascia covering them, intact.
Didusch has made a perfectly beautiful drawing of one of these specimens which is demonstrated in Young's article.

9.   The closure is now performed after narrowing the neck of the
bladder. This can be done in several ways. I usually prefer to do
it by taking sutures at all four quadrants and simply bringing them
in closer and closer until the neck of the bladder is approximately
No. 20 French. It is then necessary to sew the neck of the bladder
to the severed urethra, usually with interrupted 3-0 chromic sutures.
The anterior sutures are placed first and then, working around the
circumference of the open bladder neck, other interrupted sutures
are placed. A No. 22 Foley catheter is inserted after the anterior
sutures are placed. Young's article illustrates the use of Vest's
suture which comes out through the urethra to pull the bladder neck
down. This is useful but not necessary when it is possible to obtain
an excellent direct anastomosis.

10.   After the careful anastomosis performed over a Foley catheter,
a search is made to be sure there are no bleeding areas deep in the
wound. Occasionally the artery that comes in near the seminal vesicle
can be a troublesome bleeding spot and difficult to find.

11.   Many perineal surgeons will, at this point, put on a new glove
over their already gloved hand and do a rectal examination to be sure
there has not been any rectal injury.

     Following this, a Penrose drain is placed and the levator
muscles are brought together with interrupted chromic sutures to
give further support. This also seems to help in the control of
urinary continence. Then the subcutaneous structures are brought
together with interrupted chromic sutures and the skin is closed

with interrupted nonabsorbable sutures, allowing the Penrose drain
to come out one side of the wound.

The drain is usually left in for 24 - 48 hours and then removed.
The urethral catheter is usually left in for approximately ten days.

A significant modification of the approach with a new anatomical
observation was described by Elmer Belt in 1942 (2). His contribution
was to show that it was anatomically feasible, and in his hands,
desirable, to approach the prostate by dissecting underneath the anal
sphincter and using the anterior wall of the rectum as a guide, to
expose the prostatic area. His perineal incision is a flatter inverted "U" shaped curve, a very short distance, perhaps half a centimeter, in front of the mucocutaneous junction of the anus.

As soon as the skin has been opened, the posterior flap is
turned downward to exclude the anus from the field to prevent contamination. One immediately encounters the anal sphincter, either
external or internal, and by blunt dissection with the scalpel handle,
lifts the anal sphincter off the rectum.

After identifying the levator ani muscles which Doctor Young
had called the rectourethralis they are separated from each other in
the midline and pushed laterally far enough to reveal the whole
posterior aspect of the prostate, which is apparent as the gleaming
fascia of Denonvilliers. The vertical fibers of the rectum are
pressed below the lower margin of the prostate.

After separating the lateral aspects of the prostate from the
surrounding fascia by blunt dissection the prostate is pulled
upward from behind to identify the vessels entering at the lateral
inferior border. These are isolated and either clamped and ligated
or they may be handled with metal clips.

At this point, his procedure differs from Doctor Young's in
that Denonvilliers' fascia which covers the back of the seminal
vesicles is opened by a transverse incision across the base of the
prostate and the vesicles are identified from behind while pulling
the rectum backward.

The seminal vesicles and their ampullae are then bluntly dissected from the fascia surrounding them and the large artery which
enters at the apex on each side is carefully ligated. The vas is
dissected free on each side and transsected and ligated, or it may
be clamped with a metal clip.

At this point, the operator turns his attention to the apex of
the prostate and Belt cuts across the gland "leaving a collar of
prostatic tissue to attach to the membranous urethra" to improve
urinary control. Hugh Young criticized this, saying that it was not

a true radical operation if some of the prostate was left behind.
The fact is that most patients would rather have residual cancer than
be incontinent of urine.

Traction is obtained on the apex of the prostate with two Lahey
type thyroid clamps, and the anterior surface is exposed by blunt
dissection. Santorini's plexus is pushed away from it in an attempt
to stay out of those veins.

This finally leaves the prostate attached to the bladder at the
bladder neck. This is cut across with scissors at a right angle so
that the prostate with its capsule and both seminal vesicles and
ampullae are removed as a single specimen.

The anastomosis is carried out under direct vision; usually 3-0
chromic is used. Two or three anterior sutures are placed under
direct vision and than a No. 22 Foley urethral catheter is introduced
and the rest of the anastomosis is carried out posteriorly with interrupted chromic sutures.

The posterior layer of Denonvilliers' fascia which has been
dissected in order to bring the seminal vesicles into the wound is
now seized and brought forward to cover the anastomosis and give added
support in that area.

The levator ani muscles, which instead of being transsected, as
in Young's procedure, have been separated laterally, are now brought
together with interrupted sutures in the midline to give further
support.

The edges of the rectal sphincter are picked up with a circular
suture which tends to pull the sphincter down and close the area that
has been opened between the sphincter and the rectum in the early
dissection. A Penrose drain is placed. This is brought out through
an angle of the wound and the skin is closed with a continuous sub-
cuticular stitch. The drain usually remains in place for 24 - 48
hours and is then removed. The urethral catheter usually remains in
place for approximately 8 - 10 days and is then removed, after which
the patient resumes his normal voiding.

If at any time during the procedure there is an injury to the
rectum, it is, of course, important to recognize and close it (3).
If such an injury should occur before the urinary tract is opened, it
has been my practice simply to get a biopsy to confirm the diagnosis
and then retreat after draining the wound and closing the opening in
the rectum. It is then possible to re-operate at a later date and
perform a radical procedure (4). If the injury to the rectum occurs
after the urinary tract is opened, one may as well go ahead with the
procedure, finish it, and then close the rectal injury in two layers
with a continuous chromic suture, inverting for the mucosal layer.

Then interrupted, nonabsorbable or Dexon sutures are used for the muscular layer of the rectum. Obviously the wound is contaminated and must be particularly well drained. It is probably a good idea under those circumstances to put in a suprapubic catheter as well, in order to ensure perfect urinary drainage, because if a fistula is going to develop, it usually occurs in relation to leakage of urine and abscess formation. In my opinion, it is not necessary to do a diverting colostomy (5).

Radical perineal prostatectomy is a difficult operation to learn and probably that is why it is not used more. In the hands of an expert, it is an exquisite experience and the patient has much less difficulty in the post-operative period. As far as I am concerned, it is the operation that should be one of choice in the treatment of early prostatic cancer.

PART II: RADICAL RETROPUBIC PROSTATECTOMY*

When I first accepted the assignment to speak about radical prostatectomy for cancer of the prostate, I had the illusion that I was to speak about my favorite method which is perineal prostatectomy; however, I learned later that I should cover all aspects of the field and regret that I had not done it in a more methodical fashion.

There is a great deal to be said about radical retropubic prostatectomy and I should like to include it here.

One of the most important things is to talk about the advantages and disadvantages concerning radical retropubic and total perineal prostatectomy, and this has been admirably summarized in the excellent article by Joseph D. Schmidt, "Indications and Surgical Approaches for Prostatic Cancer" (6).

On page 6, Schmidt has given us Table III, "Advantages and disadvantages of radical retropubic prostatectomy and total perineal prostatectomy". I am going to reproduce it here –

Prostatectomy	Advantages	Disadvantages
Radical retropubic	Direct assessment of regional nodes	Exposure poor for anastomosis
	Simultaneous prostato-seminal-vesiculectomy	Greater pelvic bleeding, lymphoceles
	Low urinary fistula rate	Increased cardiopulmonary complications
	Easier bladder reconstruction	Problem of frozen sections

*With the cooperation of J.B. deKernion.

Prostatectomy	Advantages	Disadvantages
Total perineal	Better patient selection	Unknown state of regional nodes
	Excellent exposure for anastomosis	Higher urinary fistula rate
	Easier control of vascular pedicle	Higher risk of rectal injury
	Decreased operating time	Need for special training in perineal surgical anatomy
	Decreased cardiopulmonary complications	

As I have already said in writing about radical perineal prostatectomy, I think it is the operation of choice, but there certainly is a place for radical retropubic prostatectomy. This is particularly true as concerns the staging that can be gained from lymph node biopsy. In my opinion, lymph node removal is not curative, and not therapeutic, but it does have a valuable prognostic function.

In our previous publication, we described 329 patients who had radical prostatectomy at UCLA, the majority of this work being undertaken by Dr. Boxer, then a resident. Unfortunately we missed the great opportunity to compare the results and the patients' reaction to the two different operations (7).

We stated "the perineal approach of Young, later modified by Belt, was chosen by the attending and resident staff in 265 cases (80.5%) and the retropubic approach with pelvic lymphadenectomy was performed in 64 cases (19.5%). The radical prostatectomy was not performed in two cases after frozen section analysis of lymph nodes proved metastases. This fact has been given as a reason for using the retropubic approach. Furthermore, because 80.5% of the cases had the perineal approach, accurate staging of the lymph nodes was not possible in those patients". It is a sorrow to me that we did not go on to compare the radical perineal in 80% versus the radical retropubic in 20%, but we did not seize that opportunity and I suppose it is lost unless some other more vigorous soul comes along to make the comparison. In my view, the radical perineal is kinder to the patient, and the radical retropubic, although it has its place, has only the advantage of the opportunity for staging with lymph node biopsy.

Having said that, I should like to go on to say something about technique. Probably the original article on this subject was written by Chute (8). The illustrations and the description of the operation are extremely clear. Although there have been many modifications since by numerous surgeons, the basic procedure is well described. If one would like to look further for a beautiful anatomical illustration of the procedure by Didusch, it can be found in the article by Memmelaar (9).

The operation is further described in some detail, without so many frills, in the excellent article by Kopecky et al (10).

When radical retropubic prostatectomy was a new procedure, I tried it in a number of cases and felt that it lacked the surgical finesse of allowing a careful and visible complete anatomic anastomosis of the bladder neck to the urethra. For this reason, I abandoned it because I thought that most patients would rather not know whether they had cancer in their lymph nodes, but would certainly rather be continent. Thus the radical perineal operation is my preference.

My colleague, Dr. Jean deKernion, also expresses support for perineal prostatectomy -

"Perineal prostatectomy, in my hands, is associated with much less blood loss and less post-operative morbidity than that accompanying retropubic prostatectomy. I, therefore, think it is still the treatment of choice in the poor risk patient with obesity or severe pulmonary disease, and in patients who are unlikely to have lymph node metastases (Stage B-1).

As we learn more about the implications of lymph node metastases, and develop new, more accurate methods of identifying tumor in lymph nodes, these indications may be further expanded. It would seem, therefore, that perineal prostatectomy is still an art worth learning and teaching."

Because of little recent personal experience with the radical retropubic operation, I asked Dr. deKernion to give some ammunition, and he did that with an operation report from June 1981, plus a special message, and I am going to include that here.

"Stage A-II cancer of the prostate. Bilateral pelvic lymphadenectomy, radical retropubic prostatectomy - 63 year old male, two months status post transurethral resection of the prostate. His metastatic workup was negative.

After adequate general anesthesia was obtained, the patient was placed in the supine position with some hyperextension at the sacrum. A catheter was placed in the bladder. An incision was made in the midline just below the umbilicus and carried through the abdominal fat and Scarpa's fascia down to the rectus fascia which was then incised in the midline. The rectus muscle bellies were dissected and retracted laterally, and the prevesical space was entered. The rectus muscles were taken down just very slightly at the symphysis pubis to gain adequate exposure. Blunt dissection was employed very carefully to dissect the perivesical fat and the peritoneum away from the pelvic sidewall on either side. The spermatic cords were identified on each side, and the iliac vessels were then gradually exposed. Dissection was begun by placing Harrington

retractors deep into the area surrounding the bladder to expose an
extremely tortuous external iliac artery. Pelvic lymphadenectomy was
performed from the ureter to the recurrent iliac circumflex vein on
the right."

I will not continue with that surgical note but will go on with
the special description which he gave me at my request. He said,
"I thought it might be helpful if I emphasized a few points".

"We perform the operation through a low midline incision. The
lymphadenectomy is done extraperitoneally and extends from the bifurcation of the common iliac vessels, distally to the inguinal
ligament. We no longer dissect the tissue on the lateral aspect of
the external iliac arteries since preservation of this lymphatic
drainage seems to decrease the incidence of lymphedema. Distally,
we make a big point of securing the large bundle of lymphatics that
enter the pelvis near the femoral canal, just medially and posteriorly to the external iliac vein. Gene Carlton brought this to my
attention six years ago, and I now assiduously clip these lymphatics
and have not had a single lymphatic leak or lymphocele since that
time. We then continue down into the obturator fossa. I do not
dissect any deeper than the obturator nerve which is, of course, well
dissected and visualized. The obturator vessels are only removed if
necessary, but they are often not in the way. I am also very cautious
about accessory obturator veins in a surprisingly large number of
patients. We then dissect the obturator fat pad upward as far as the
area of bifurcation of the iliac artery. Frozen sections are obtained
as each lymph node is removed. If the patient has more than one or
two microfoci of tumor, we abandon the plan for prostatectomy.

After lymphadenectomy, we begin the prostatectomy. A large
catheter is inserted into the urethra. The prostatectomy is begun
by incising the bladder neck fibers at the junction of the prostate
in the bladder. I like to put large figure of 8 hemostatic sutures
in each corner, both on the prostate and the bladder neck. These
serve both as retractors and hemostatic sutures. I identify the
ureteral orifices and then proceed directly across the posterior
bladder neck to expose and tie the vasa. We then isolate the seminal
vesicles and dissect them completely free. The vascular pedicle
then is obvious on each side, adjacent to the rectum. This is ligated
with large chromic sutures. (Note A).

I then lift up on the sutures to elevate the prostate gland
and develop the plane behind the prostate. This develops a nice
pedicle on each side of the prostate which extends between the
lateral aspect of the prostate and the rectum and contains much of
the prostatic blood supply. I then serially clip these pedicles
deep into the pelvis down toward the end of the pelvic fascia. At
this point, I narrow the bladder neck with a continuous running
2-0 chromic suture beginning in the midline posteriorly. This is

done with ureteral catheters in place to avoid ureteral obstruction. A vesical opening approximately one centimeter in diameter is left. (Note B).

I then like to remove a trapezoid of the pubis to facilitate the rest of the dissection and the incision of the urethra. We never take a full thickness of the pubis.

Dr. Charles Robson put me on to this idea, and I think it is a very good one. We do this very simply with an osteotome and a mallet and then apply bone wax to the raw area. I have never had a problem from this part of the procedure. Following the removal of this segment of bone, we are right down on the urethra. We then secure the dorsal vein with a 2-0 chromic tie; we never use clips in this area because they could occasionally erode into the anastomosis. I then gently incise the endopelvic fascia and the puboprostatic ligaments. There are large veins under them which I then secure by passing a curved clamp around and tie these vessels with chromic ties. (Note C).

At this point we have the prostate attached only by the urethra. Even if there is some bleeding from the pelvic veins, the operation is almost completed and one can quickly finish the final steps. I begin incising the urethra under direct vision, using a scalpel. I never leave a button of prostate and I never cut into the urogenital diaphragm. (Note D).

I like to divide the urethra part of the way and then insert the first 2-0 chromic anastomatic suture. Then, by rotating the prostate on the catheter, I can gradually incise the urethra and insert other sutures until finally the entire specimen is free on the catheter and I have inserted at least four or six sutures through the urethra only. We then quickly pass these through the bladder neck and the operation is completed. This is an excellent anastomosis which is done under more or less direct vision. Of course, a fresh catheter is inserted before tying the sutures.

I like to leave the catheter in for about 10 days and sometimes send the patient home with the catheter indwelling. I always use a drain, but almost never use a suprapubic tube."

Notes - W.E. Goodwin

A.   This is one of the advantages of the retropubic over the perineal approach. It is sometimes difficult to identify and secure these arteries which can be sources of considerable bleeding in the perineal approach.

B.   This is similar to the radical perineal approach where we narrow the neck of the bladder, usually from four quadrants, to make a vesical orifice of about 24 French.

C. In the perineal procedure, this is done, of course, from below
and the same maneuver is carried out more or less blindly by passing
a large curved clamp around the large veins and the puboprostatic
ligaments and making a tie just as he describes from above.

D. This should be compared with Belt's perineal approach which
leaves a small piece of the apex of the prostate in order to facilitate the anastomosis and prevent urinary incontinence.

        I believe that Dr. de'Kernion's description is as graphic as
any I could imagine, and putting it together with the excellent
illustrations of Chute and the recent contributions of Wettlaufer, I
believe this represents an adequate explanation of radical retropubic
prostatectomy which certainly has its place in the urologist's
armamentarium for dealing with prostatic cancer by radical surgery.

REFERENCES

1. H.H. Young, The cure of cancer of the prostate by radical peri-
    neal prostatectomy (prostatoseminovesiculectomy): History,
    literature and statistics of Young's operation, J. Urol. 53:
    188 (1945).
2. E. Belt, Radical perineal prostatectomy in early carcinoma of
    the prostate, J. Urol. 48: 287 (1942).
3. W.E. Goodwin, Complications of perineal prostatectomy, in:
    Complications of Urologic Surgery, Prevention and Management,"
    R.B. Smith and D.G. Skinner, eds., W.B. Saunders Co., Philadel-
    phia, London, Toronto (1976), p. 252.
4. W.E. Goodwin, Radical prostatectomy after previous prostatic
    surgery, JAMA 148: 799 (1952).
5. W.E. Goodwin, R.D. Turner, and C.C. Winter, Rectourinary fistula:
    principles of management and the technique of surgical closure,
    J. Urol. 80: 246 (1958).
6. J.D. Schmidt, Indications and surgical approaches for prostatic
    cancer, supplement to Urology 17: 4 (1981).
7. R.J. Boxer, J.J. Kaufman, and W.E. Goodwin, Radical prostatectomy
    for carcinoma of the prostate, review of 329 patients, J. Urol.
    117: 208 (1977).
8. R. Chute, Radical retropubic prostatectomy for cancer, J. Urol.
    71: 347 (1954).
9. J. Memmelaar, Total prostatovesiculectomy; retropubic approach,
    J. Urol. 62: 340 (1949).
10. A.A. Kopecky, T.Z. Laskowski, and Scott R. Jr., Radical retro-
    pubic prostatectomy in the treatment of prostatic carcinoma,
    J. Urol. 103: 641 (1970).

CRYOSURGERY OF PROSTATIC CARCINOMA

F.M.J. Debruyne and W.J. Kirkels

Radboud University Hospital
Nijmegen
The Netherlands

INTRODUCTION

Since the advent of cryosurgical equipment, first developed by Cooper and Lee in 1961 (1), much attention has been centered on the field of cryobiology and the destructive effect of cold on human tissues. In 1964 Gonder et al (2) first reported on experimental cryosurgery of the dog prostate. Two years later they introduced transurethral cryosurgery in the treatment of benign prostatic hyperplasia (3) and subsequently published their experience utilising the transurethral cryoprobe in 50 patients with prostatic carcinoma to produce local prostatic destruction (4).

The original purpose of this operation was to destroy obstructing prostatic tissue by freezing to provide an adequate urinary passage. Experience, after initial enthusiasm, has led to the conclusion that the procedure has a very limited field of application and is certainly not the panacea for prostatic obstruction as was originally hoped.

We decided to abandon this technique after an experience of over two years with more than 20 patients. We found that transurethral cryosurgery, as a blind procedure, was not without danger and had a large range of possible complications apart from the usual protracted course (Tables 1 and 2). In our opinion this technique has no advantage over transurethral resection or open prostatectomy, even in high risk patients, as the improvement of preoperative diagnostic procedures, anesthetic techniques and pre- and post-operative care makes it possible to treat older and poor risk patients by transurethral resection or, if necessary, by open prostatectomy.

Table 1.   Transurethral Cryosurgery of the Prostate.
           Immediate Postoperative Complications

- Haemorrhage

- Oligo-anuria (especially in lesion of the trigone and
  those involving the ureteric orifices)

- Acute pyelonephritis

- Epidydimitis and orchitis

- Periurethral abscesses

- Oedema of the penis

- Cardiopulmonary or cerebrovascular accidents

Table 2.   Transurethral Cryosurgery of the Prostate.
           Late postoperative Complications

- Urinary incontinence

- Secondary haemorrhage

- Retropubic infection

- Bladder calculi

- Protracted (severe) urinary tract infection

- Urethral (meatal) stenosis

In the last five years we have performed 679 prostatic operations, a substantial proportion of them in patients with cardiovascular or pulmonary disease. In this period hardly any patient was
excluded from transurethral resection. Despite this our peri-
operative mortality is less than one percent (Table 3).

We are therefore surprised by recent pulbications (5,6,7),
suggesting an indication for cryosurgery in 15 to 25% of patients
suffering from prostatic obstruction. A comparison of the worst
results of cryosurgery with those of transurethral resection (8)
suggests that this figure should be less than 5% as recently

Table 3. Prostatic Surgery

Radbound University Hospital Nijmegen, Department of
Urology

1975 - 1980

Transurethral Resection	482	(71%)
Open Prostatectomy	191	(29%)
Perioperative Mortality	3	(o.4%)

postulated by Groenteman and van Haga (9) in our country.

Refinements of transurethral cryosurgery by application of
"cryoresection" (transurethral resection after freezing of the
prostate) or "cryocautery" (the combination of freezing and subsequent
heating) do not seem to us to offer any improvement of the initial
technique.

CRYOSURGERY IN PROSTATIC CANCER

Control of the Primary Tumor

When Soanes and Gonder (3) introduced transurethral cryosurgery
it was a blind procedure and exact placement of the cryoprobe was
difficult unless it was used in combination with a suprapubic trocar
cystoscopy. Also, since at least 65% of the prostatic cancers develop
in the dorsolateral part of the gland, the lesion is difficult to
reach by transurethral freezing. Furthermore the bulk of prostatic
cancer in large lesions cannot be destroyed transurethrally. Therefore Flocks in 1972 (10) introduced cryosurgery via the perineal
route. With this approach, direct application of the cryoprobe to
the prostatic lesion is possible. The purpose of this method is
local destruction of the tumor while maintaining the integrity of
the adjacent bladder and urethra.

Crysurgery produces tissue death by intracellular dehydration
and toxic electrolyte concentration, crystallization with secondary
membrane rupture, denaturation of proteins, thermal shock and
vascular stasis. This degenerative phase, characterized by tissue
edema and necrosis, lasts one to 10 weeks and usually progresses to
a reparative phase between two and three months after treatment (11).
The depth of tissue destruction by freezing is difficult to assess.

This depends on many variables such as tissue sensitivity to
freezing, velocity of temperature reduction and subsequent thawing,
and the duration of the freezing period. Nowadays liquid nitrogen is
used as the cooling agent, reducing the temperature in the heat
exchanger tip of the probe to -180 to -190°C.

Perineal exposure provides excellent visualization of the
prostatic cancer and presents the least risk of cold injury to the
rectum. It also allows visualization of the seminal vesicles which
can be frozen to control extracapsular extension of the disease. The
freezing process can be repeated to ensure adequate tissue destruction. However one is never sure if all prostatic tissue in the center
of the gland is destroyed. Therefore Klosterhalfen et al (12) combined the perineal technique with transurethral freezing to control
centrally located tumors. Perineal cryosurgery and the combined
method are well tolerated by the patients. It seems clear that
prostatic cryosurgery can be effective in destroying the local
lesion. Rectal examination after three months shows striking changes
in the local prostatic lesion. Loening et al (13) found an empty
prostatic fossa with no clinical evidence of residual tumor in 161 of
215 patients (74.8%). In 32 patients (14.9%) no three months follow-
up or rectal examination was recorded and the remaining 22 patients
(10.2%) had incomplete destruction of the local prostatic lesion.
Klosterhalfen et al (12) and O'Donoghue et al (14) had identical
observations concerning local control of the prostatic lesion three
and six months after cryosurgery.

Loening et al (13) also noted that the cryosurgery patients had
a probability of survival equal to that seen in the total prostatectomy patients of each stage. The actuarial survival curves related
to clinical stage from their study gave a five year survival after
cryosurgery of about 75% for stage B lesions. This is almost identical with the five year survival rates reported by Boxer et al (15)
following radical prostatectomy for surgical stages A and B prostatic
cancer. For patients with stage C disease the results of radical
surgery as reported by Boxer et al (15) was 67% whilst Bagshaw et al
(16) found that external radiation therapy resulted in 73% five year
survival with stage B disease and 46% survival in patients with stage
C prostatic cancer. Again the results of cryosurgery as reported by
Loening et al (13) are comparable with these figures. Therefore to
those authors and to others, cryosurgery appears to be another
modality of treatment for local destruction of prostatic carcinoma.
Further they found that ablation of the primary site in locally
advanced disease avoided late urinary incontinence, decreased the
incidence of repeated transurethral resections and avoided late
complications such as ureteral obstruction or bladder neck infiltration by the neoplasm. In brief they favour perineal cryosurgery
for local tumour control.

Possible Immunological effect of Cryosurgery

The second reason to advocate cryosurgical therapy of the prostate is the possibility that cryosurgical destruction may elicit an immune response in the patient and, by immunologic means, may favourably influence distant metastases. Soanes et al (17) first postulated a cryo-immune response because two patients with metastatic disease had regression following this type of operation and Gursel et al (18) noted relief of pain from metastases following cryotherapy in eight of 11 patients. In only one patient was an objective response of bone metastases evident. Since then occasional remissions have been reported. Recently Gittes, in an editorial comment on a study of this subject by Milleman et al, in which the authors could not identify indirect evidence of an (humoral) immune response to cryosurgery, stated that cryosurgery in patients with prostatic carcinoma has not been shown to yield any proved immunological benefit.. However, the findings of Ablin and Fontana (20) contrast with the results of Milleman et al (19) as their data support the hypothesis of a systemic (humoral) immune response.

With respect to host cell-mediated immunologic activity there is now ample evidence that cellular immunity is depressed in many prostatic cancer patients. The aim of the clinical studies conducted by Ablin and the Cryoimmunotherapeutic Study Group was to prove an augmentation or inducement of host resistance as a result of in situ cryosurgical destruction. This would imply that cryosurgery may be effective as a means of immunotherapy. These studies are very difficult to conduct in man, since the antigenic properties of an individual prostatic carcinoma are not known and the humoral and cellular immune responses after cryosurgical treatment are difficult to assess and may be non-specific.

Therefore studies with an experimental animal model with known antigenic capacities are mandatory in the first instance. A suitable animal model seems now to be available in the Dunning R 3327 prostatic tumor system, induced in the Copenhagen rat, which is an appropriate model to use for studies of the immunobiology of prostatic carcinoma. Lubaroff and co-workers (21) developed a research program on the immunological responses after cryosurgery of this experimental animal tumor. The results to date demonstrate the production of humoral and cell-mediated immune responses. On the other hand other investigators (22,23) demonstrated the development of contradictory effects following cryostimulation including tumor enhancement. However all these data are still preliminary.

Many immunological problems still exist in the animal model and even greater questions remain in man. As long as these questions remain unanswered, we believe that certain favourable immunological effects on metastatic lesions are not sufficient indication for the general use of cryosurgery for prostatic carcinoma in man.

REFERENCES

1. I.S. Cooper and A.S.J. Lee, Cryothalamectomy - hypothermic
    congelation: a technical advance in basal ganglia surgery.
    Preliminary report, J. Am. Geriatr. Soc. 9:714 (1961).
2. M.J. Gonder, W.A. Soanes, and V. Smith, Experimental prostate
    cryosurgery, Invest. Urol. 1:610 (1964).
3. M.J. Gonder, W.A. Soanes, and S. Shulman, Cryosurgical
    treatment of the prostate, Invest. Urol. 3:372 (1966).
4. W.A. Soanes and M.J. Gonder, Use of cryosurgery in prostatic
    cancer, J. Urol. 99:793 (1968).
5. G. Rigondet, C. Barthe, and P. Dubernard, Résultats de la
    cryochirurgie prostatique (sept années de practique), J. Urol.
    Néphrol. 83 suppl. 2:393 (1977).
6. G. Sesia, Huits ans de cryotherapie pour adénomes prostatiques,
    J. Urol. Néphrol. 83 suppl. 2:415 (1977)
7. H.J. Reuter and M. Reuter, 20 Jahre Prostataoperationen.
    Senkung der Komplicationsrate durch eine neue Konzeption von
    TUR, Kryochirurgie und Chirurgische Operation, Z. Urol. u.
    Nephrol. 73:279 (1980).
8. K. Möhring, N. Pfitzmaier, and C. Panis-Hoffmann, Cryosurgery
    of the prostate and transurethral resection on poor surgical
    risk patients, Urol. Int. 30:414 (1979).
9. R.M. Groenteman and S.J.W. van Haga, Cryochirurgie van de
    prostaat, Ned. T.v.Geneesk. 125:731 (1981).
10. R.H. Flocks, C.M.K. Nelson, and D.L. Boatman, Perineal cryo-
    surgery for prostatic carcinoma, J. Urol. 108:933 (1972).
11. R.J. Hansen and J. Wanstrup, Cryoprostatectomy: histological
    changes elucidated by serial biopsies, Scand. J. Urol. Nephrol.
    7:100 (1973).
12. H. Klosterhalfen, M.W. Köllerman, H. Becker, W. Hupe, and
    G. Kessler, Kombinierte perineale und transurethrale Vereisung
    beim Prostatacarcinom im Stadium C. Urologe A 18:57 (1979).
13. S. Loening, C. Hawtrey, W. Bonney, A. Narayana, and D.A. Culp,
    Cryotherapy of prostate cancer, The Prostate 1:279 (1980).
14. E.P.N. O'Donoghue, L.A. Milleman, R.H. Flocks, D.A. Culp, and
    W.W. Bonney, Cryosurgery for carcinoma of the prostate, Urology
    8:308 (1978).
15. R.J. Boxer, J.J. Kaufman, and W.E. Goodwin, Radical prostat-
    ectomy for carcinoma of the prostate; 1951-1976. A review of
    329 patients, J. Urol. 117:208 (1977).
16. M.A. Bagshaw, D.A. Pistenma, G.R. Ray, F.S. Freiha, and
    R.L. Kempson, Evaluation of extended-field radiotherapy for
    prostatic neoplasm: 1976 progress report, Cancer Treat. Rep.
    61:297 (1977).
17. W.A. Soanes, M.J. Gonder, and R.J. Ablin, A possible immuno-
    cryothermic response in prostatic cancer, Clin. Radiol. 21:253
    (1970).

18. E.D. Gursel, M. Roberts, and R.J. Veenema, Regression of prostatic cancer following sequential cryotherapy to the prostate, J. Urol. 108:928 (1972).

19. L.A. Milleman, W.D. Weissman, and D.A. Culp, Serum protein, enzyme and immunoglobulin responses following perineal cryosurgery for carcinoma of the prostate, J. Urol. 123:710 (1980).   .

20. R.J. Ablin, G. Fontana, and the Cryoimmunotherapeutic Study Group, Cryoimmunotherapy: Continuing studies towards determining a rational approach for assessing the candidacy of the prostatic cancer patient for cryoimmunotherapy and post-operative responsiveness. An interim report, Eur. Surg. Res. 11:223 (1979).

21. D.M. Lubaroff, C.W. Reynolds, L. Canfield, D. McElligott, and T. Feldbush, Immunologic aspects of the prostate, The Prostate 2:233 (1981).

22. H. Kobayashi and T. Yamashita, Immunological enhancement of tumor metastases in rats by cryosurgery, Cryobiol.15:702 (1978).

23. T. Yamasaki, Immunological survey for endoscopic cryosurgery and its basic study, Cryobiol. 15:702 (1978).

CRYOSURGICAL AND CRYORESECTION TREATMENT OF PROSTATIC CANCER

M. Kralj

Clinical Centre
Ljubljana
Yugoslavia

SUMMARY

This paper reviews 160 cases of advanced prostatic cancer (category T3 and T4) treated by cryosurgery and cryoresection. In 52 patients cryosurgery only was undertaken, in 20 cases at first cryosurgery and then transurethral resection (TUR) was performed, and in 88 patients TUR was followed by cryosurgery. The last method yielded the best results.

PATIENTS AND METHODS

In the Urological Clinic of Ljubljana cryosurgery and cryoresection has been used since 1975 for the treatment of advanced prostatic cancer (category T3 and T4). From 1975 to 1980, 160 patients have been treated by this method (Table 1).

All the patients were older than 60 years, 53 (33%) aged 61 - 70, 90 (56%) aged 71 - 80, and 17 (11%) over 81 years of age. Before treatment all the patients were classified according to the TNM system. Of our patients, 66 were category T3 and 84 were category T4. The presenting symptoms before the cryosurgical treatment are listed in Table 2.

Before treatment we searched for metastases by biochemical examination, skeletal survey, chest X-ray and radioisotopic examination. The results are shown in Table III.

Histological or cytological evidence of tumour was available before cyrosurgical treatment in 142 patients (88%); in 18 patients

(12%) we were content to proceed, for various reasons, on the findings of rectal palpation. The results of histology and cytology in 160 patients are shown in Table 4.

Table 1. Number of patients treated by cryosurgery
(1976 - 1980)

1975	1
1976	30
1977	23
1978	31
1979	35
1980	40
Total	160

Table 2. Patients' symptoms prior to cryosurgical
treatment

Symptom	No. of patients	
Difficulty in micturition	142	(88%)
Retention of urine	66	(41%)
Haematuria	19	(12%)
Bone pain	42	(26%)
Other symptoms	51	(31%)

Table 3. Incidence of metastases in patients with
prostatic cancer

Site of metastases	No. of patients	
Skeleton	62	(38%)
Lungs	13	(8.6%)
Other organs (liver, palpable lymphatic glands)	6	(3.6%)
No metastasis demonstrable	79	(45.4%)

Table 4. Histological and cytological findings in
160 patients with prostatic cancer

Well differentiated	89	(55%)
Moderately differentiated	48	(31%)
Poorly differentiated	23	(14%)

In these five years we have used three methods of cryoprostatectomy. In the beginning cryosurgery only was practised, but soon
TUR was also carried out before or after cryosurgery. The duration
of freezing of the prostatic cancer was between three and eight
minutes, depending on the size of the prostate. After freezing the
phase of warming followed, the duration of which was equal to that
of freezing or about one minute longer. All these methods were
combined with bilateral subcapsular orchidectomy and a high dose
hormonal therapy - 1000 mg of Honvan daily for 10 days.

Cryosurgery alone was undertaken in 52 patients (32%). The
greatest problem of this method however was the elimination of necrotic tissue, which led to numerous complications including haematuria
and retention of urine. Post-operative catheterization was necessary
for up to six weeks.

In 1976 and 1977 TUR of frozen tissue was performed after cryosurgical treatment in 20 patients (12.4%). Because of changes in the
frozen tissue transurethral resection presented a greater risk
(especially towards the periphery) and control of haemostasis was
difficult.

RESULTS

The best results were obtained when TUR was performed first and
cryosurgery afterwards. In this way only the peripheral tissue is
frozen; 88 patients were treated by this method.

The advantages of this last method mentioned include -

1. lesser quantity of necrotic tissue than after cryosurgery alone,
2. easy elimination of necrotic tissue through the urethra (after
    the TUR),
3. obstructions after such treatment are less frequent,
4. the number of infections is minimal, and
5. the duration of use of the catheter and hospitalization is
    shorter.

Follow up examinations were made every three months. Among the
postoperative complications (Table 5) incontinence was the most
frequent (17 patients - 10.5%) because the malignant tissue spread

to the external sphincter. After cryosurgery alone, haematuria
occurred in nine patients (5.5%) and recurrent retention of urine in
eight (4.9%), associated with the elimination of necrotic tissue. In
115 patients (72.2%) no complications were observed.

In the postoperative period after cryosurgical treatment two
patients died (1.2%). In the first case perforation of the bladder
occurred and in the second case mortality was due to urosepsis.

At follow up examination 98 patients (61%) reported an improvement in general health. In 110 patients (69%) obstructive symptoms
were relieved and 28 patients (13%) mentioned a reduction of skeletal
pain. Twelve patients (7.4%) had no changes after cryosurgery and
25 patients (15.5%) were totally free of symptoms after treatment.

In 95 patients (59%) a large reduction of tumor mass was observed by repeated rectal examinations and only in 20 patients (12.4%)
was enlargement of the prostate found.

The amount of residual urine after cryosurgery is also of
interest, a great improvement being observed (Table 6). In four
patients skeletal metastases regressed and pulmonary metastases
resolved in one. The survival of our patients as recorded by the
central cancer register in the Institute of Oncology of Ljubljana
is shown in Table 7.

Table 5. Complications after cryosurgery

Symptom	No. of patients	
Incontinence	17	(10.5%)
Haematuria	9	(5.4%)
Recurrent retention of urine	8	(4.9%)
Stricture of urethra	5	(3.1%)
Epididymitis	3	(2%)
Perforation of bladder	1	(0.6%)
Urosepsis	2	(1.2%)
Without complications	115	(72.2%)

Table 6. Residual urine before and after treatment

Residual	No. of patients	
	Before	After
None	5	70
Up to 100 ml	14	84
From 100 - 200 ml	34	5
Above 200 ml	107	1

Table 7. Survival following treatment

Year of treatment	Patients surviving	
1976	12	(40%)
1977	16	(71%)
1978	24	(78%)
1979	30	(84%)
1980	36	(90%)

Editorial Note (P.H.S.)

Treatment in all patients included cryosurgery, bilateral sub-capsular orchiectomy and hormone therapy of ten days' duration. In addition, 108 of the 160 patients also had a transurethral resection. The procedure of cryosurgery is not without complications and the results of the combined therapy demonstrate no obvious benefit in terms of control of local symptoms, remission of distant metastases or survival which is directly attributable to the cryosurgery.

RADIOTHERAPY OF PROSTATIC CANCER

M.A. Bagshaw

Stanford University School of Medicine
Stanford
California

In the 1950's, new sources of deeply penetrating radiations, such as Cobalt-60 units, linear accelerators, and betatrons, became available and have become the standard for modern radiation therapy.

Clinical research has demonstrated that doses of 7,000 to 7,600 rads in 7 to 7-1/2 weeks can be delivered to the prostate and immediately adjacent tissues, and doses of 5,000 rads in 5 weeks can be absorbed in regional lymph nodes without undue morbidity. As the treatment techniques evolved, attention to tumor localization, individualized treatment planning, multi-portal treatment, daily fractionation, optimal radiation dose, and other therapeutic details have become relatively standardized.

In a recent review of over 1200 cases of prostatic cancer, five-year actuarial survivals ranged from 60% to 75%, while the 10-year actuarial survival was 40% (1). Updated reports of these series, along with new reports, further extend survival rates to nearly 80% at five years for patients with disease limited to the prostate (DLP), and to approximately 60% at five years for patients with extra-capsular extension (ECE) (2,3,4).

In spite of this evidence for the efficacy of the radiotherapy of prostatic cancer, one must interpret these statistics with caution, especially when comparing results between different institutions or between treatment by different modalities. For example, we will discuss in another presentation that among patients with no initial demonstrable hematogenous spread, the most important prognostic determinant for later metastases is the presence or absence of lymph node metastases at presentation and that lymph node metastases may be predicted with considerable accuracy by careful

clinical staging and histologic grading of the primary neoplasm (5).
Therefore, unless these prognostic indicators have been carefully
determined and analyzed, rigorous inter-comparison of survival
statistics is impossible. In recognition of these limitations, the
Stanford experience as reported here, which now extends over 20 years,
may be taken as a reasonable reflection of what might be achieved
with external beam radiation therapy in carcinoma of the prostate.

PRE-THERAPEUTIC PATIENT EVALUATION

1. Biopsy and Histopathologic Grading: Patients are usually
referred for radiotherapy after the biopsy has been obtained. This
is usually accomplished by trans-rectal or trans-perineal biopsy,
although transurethral resection is nearly equally as common.

   In our material, the close correlation between histologic grade
especially by the Gleason grading system and the degree of lymph
node involvement has been of inestimable value in predicting the
probability of lymphadenopathy (6).

2. History and Physical Examination: A simple diagram of the
prostate as perceived by digital examination, complete with metric
dimensions, should be mandatory. The physiologic sexual status of
the patient is often overlooked in the history. There is no way to
evaluate the influence of treatment on sexual potency without this
key information.

3. Acid Phosphatase Determination: Conventional acid phosphatase
determinations, using citrate or tartrate as a buffer, should be
carried out until the newer techniques such as radioimmune assay
have been more thoroughly evaluated.

4. Chest X-Ray: Although early pulmonary metastases are rare in
prostatic cancer, they should be ruled out before proceeding with
definitive therapy.

5. Intravenous Pyelogram: Ureteral obstruction occurs in about 15%
of patients with relatively early cancer and can be identified by an
IVP. Hydronephrosis, while a grave prognostic sign, is not
necessarily lethal.

6. Bone Scans: Currently Technetium-99m labeled methylene
disphosphonate is widely used for detection of osseous metastases.
Positive or equivocal findings should be confirmed by roentgenograms.

7. Special Examinations: Techniques for visualization of the
prostate include computerized tomography and ultrasound (7,8). These
methods are useful in establishing whether extracapsular extension
has occurred and should be used as an adjunct to the more

conventional localization procedures for the preparation of the
patient for radiation therapy.

8. Lymphangiogram (LAG): The lymphangiogram, although controversial
in prostate cancer, can be extremely useful. One careful efficacy
study correctly detected 30 of 54 patients with nodal metastases for
a sensitivity of 56%; and an independent study correctly detected 16
of 28 with nodal metastases for a sensitivity of 57% (9,10). Thus,
in many cases, the LAG combined with fine needle aspiration biopsy
offers an opportunity to prove the presence of lymph node metastases
without formal surgical intervention (11).

9. Surgical Staging of Lymph Nodes: Surgical mapping of lymph node
involvment in prostatic cancer has had a profound impact on understanding its natural history, especially as a predictor for disseminated disease (12,13).

RESULTS OF RADIOTHERAPY

    This treatment for prostatic cancer was started at Stanford in
1956. Since then 1293 patients have been referred. 382 were eliminated from this series because they were referred for consultation
only or because metastases were discovered. 226 patients have been
referred since 1 January 1977 and are not included because of short
follow-up. 24 patients were rejected from the analysis for miscellaneous reasons, leaving 661 for this analysis.

    This series has been updated recently. All patients at risk for
15 years or more and for 10 years or more were reviewed. The clinical
stage at the time of treatment was reevaluated and a TNM designation
was assigned. The original designations of disease limited to the
prostate (DLP) - 351 patients, and extracapsular extension (ECE) -
310 patients, were not modified. All patients had a histologic
diagnosis (Table 1).

    The current status of the patients was updated as of 1 March
1981. The cutoff date for patients entering this study was 31
December 1976, and therefore the minimum follow-up through 1 March
1981 is four years and three months.

Clinical Stage Versus Survival

    Figure 1 presents the overall survival of the 661 patients
divided between patients with disease limited to the prostate and
those with extracapsular extension. The same data at 5, 10, and 15
year intervals are presented in Table 1.

    Figure 2 displays the survival by T stage. The T1, T2, and T3

Table 1. Summary of Stanford Results in External
          Beam Radiotherapy of Carcinoma of the
          Prostate.

Actuarial Survival at Intervals of

Date of Report	Total No. of Cases	5 Years DLP	ECE	10 Years DLP	ECE	15 Years DLP	ECE	Follow-up
14 1965	73	All 54% cases combined						1-8 years
15 1973	160 DLP	72%		48%				2-15 years
	150 ECE		48%		30%			
1981 (March)	351 DLP	78% +4.8*		57% +6.4*		39% +8.4*		4-20 years
	310 ECE		59% +6*		39.5% +6.8*		30% +7.4	

DLP = Disease Limited to the Prostate, Nominal Stage B, or T1

ECE = Extracapsular Extension, Nominal Stage C, or T2 and T3

* 2 Standard errors

categories are essentially the same as those advocated by the UICC.
The lesser subdivisions within the T categories are unique to the
Stanford TNM system and have been described elsewhere (5). Without
going into the statistical differences between these curves, one can
see that there is clearly a difference between the T0 patients and
the rest. The T1 and T2 patients are not much different from each
other; however, they differ significantly from the T3 and the T4
patients.

    The differences in survival between T0 focal and T0 diffuse were
not significant. The large group of T1 patients were segregated
according to their respective subgroups, and substantial differences
in survival patterns between T1a, T1b, and T1c were observed (Fig. 3).
We then added the T1a and T1b patients together, because these
patients appear to be, by stage, the closest to those who are
regarded by Jewett, Culp, Walsh, and others as candidates for radical

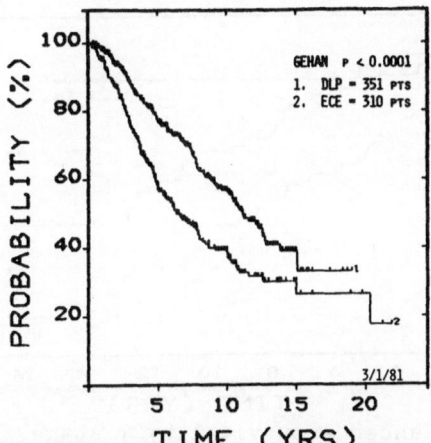

Fig. 1. Prostatic cancer survival – death due to all causes. Time 0
         is the first day of radiation therapy. The survival curves
         are after the method of Kaplan and Meier (16). In this
         instance we are plotting the probability of survival as a
         function of time from the first day of treatment. When a
         patient dies, the curve drops one unit, and each time a
         patient is withdrawn from the population – such as the end
         of the period of observation for that patient – there is a
         vertical tick. You can see with such large numbers as these
         that the curves are quite smooth and obviously quite differ-
         ent. Their difference can be quantified by the Gehan test,
         which shows that the probability of these two curves
         representing the same population is less than one chance in
         10,000.

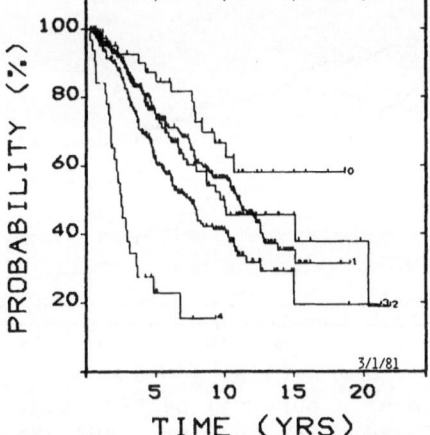

Fig. 2. Prostatic cancer – survival by T stage. Time 0 is the first
         day of radiation therapy. Curve 0 is limited to T0 patients,
         N=43. Curve 1 is limited to T1 patients, N=225. Curve 2 is
         limited to T2 patients, n=119. Curve 3 is limited to T3
         patients, N=242. Curve 4 is limited to T4 patients, N=32.

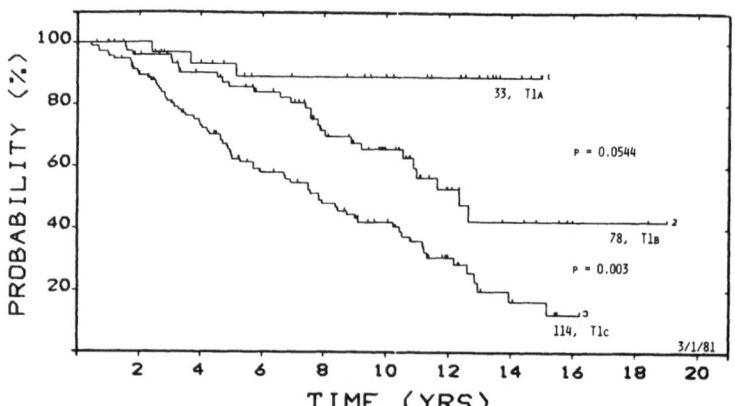

Fig. 3.   Prostatic cancer - survival by T stage.   Time 0 is the
          first day of radiation therapy.
          T1   Palpable tumor limited by the prostatic capsule without
               distortion of the superior or lateral anatomic
               boundaries.
          T1a Solitary nodule equal to or less than 1 cm in diameter
               with normal compressible prostatic tissue on 3 sides
               (the Jewett nodule, amenable to radical prostatectomy).
          T1b Palpable tumor greater than 1 cm occupying less than
               50% of a lobe.
          T1c Palpable tumor occupying greater than 50% of one lobe,
               multiple nodules limited to one lobe, or involvement
               of both lobes.

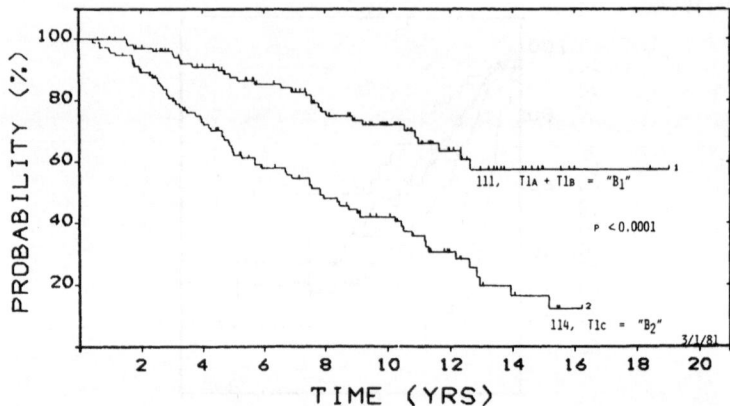

Fig. 4.   Prostatic cancer - survival by "B" stage.   Time 0 is the
          first day of radiation therapy.   "B" stage refers to the
          American Urological Staging system.   B1, or surgically
          resectable stage, corresponds to the Stanford T1a or T1b,
          whereas B2, considered by most authors to be too advanced
          for surgical resection, corresponds to the Stanford T1c
          group.

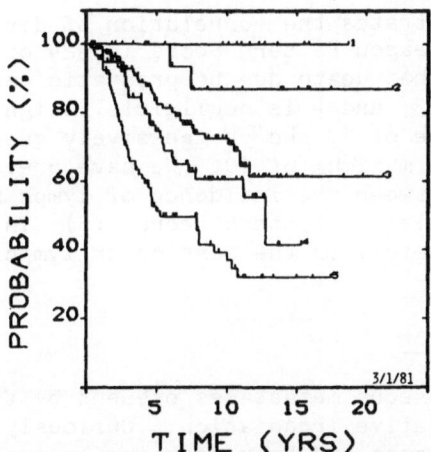

Fig. 5. Survival as a function of Gleason histopathologic pattern
         scores. Survival is calculated as a function of death due
         to prostatic cancer only, i.e., death due to intercurrent
         disease is withdrawn. The same patterns are seen when
         death due to all causes is calculated but the relationship
         is crisper in this presentation. Curve 1, Gleason 2,3,4;
         Curve 2, Gleason 5; Curve 3, Gleason 6; Curve 4, Gleason 7;
         Curve 5, Gleason 8,9,10.

prostatectomy (17,18,19). In other words, the Stanford T1a and T1b
appear equivalent to the American Urological Stage B1. A highly
significant difference in survival between these B1 patients and B2
patients was observed (Fig. 4). It is important to recall that the
B2 patients have been lumped togther with the B1 patients in the DLP,
(Disease limited to the Prostate) category, and therefore this group
as a whole is obviously more advanced than the patients subjected to
radical prostatectomy in the reports of Jewett, Culp, Walsh, and
others. Here we have tried to segregate a group of patients treated
by irradiation who are comparable by stage to those treated by radical
prostatectomy. We have been unable to stratify them by histologic
grade.

Histopathologic Grade Versus Survival

     Both Dr. Richard Kempson of Stanford Department of Pathology and
James Gleason have graded approximately one-half of the neoplams in
this series. The Gleason grading system is based upon microscopic
pattern recognition of the glandular elements at a relatively low
power. Gleason assigns an integer of 1 through to 5 to the major and
also the minor patterns recognized upon scanning the specimen. These
integers are added, giving a 9-step grading system, 2 through 9,
which is called the Gleason Pattern Score.

Figure 5 demonstrates the correlation of disease-specific survival with the Gleason Pattern Score in 324 of these patients. It is clearly evident that death due to prostatic cancer for Gleason Pattern Scores of 2,3, and 4 is negligible, slightly greater for a Gleason Pattern Score of 5, and progressively greater as the Pattern Score approaches the maximum of 10. We have previously reported a close correlation between the incidence of lymph node involvement and an increase in the Gleason Pattern Score. (5) This relationship will be covered in more detail in the session on lymph node metastases.

Palliative Irradiation

Disseminated osseous metastases present by far the most common indication for palliative irradiation. Curiously, although a patient may have many metastases and be responding generally well to hormonal management, only one or two metastatic sites become painful. Often these are near major joints, e.g., the acetabulum or within the spine. They usually respond promptly with pain relief. The dose should be relatively high and well fractionated, e.g., 4000 rads in 4 weeks, because the overall survival could be quite long and adverse sequelae should be avoided. Occasionally the dose is increased to 5000-5500 rads in 5-5 1/2 weeks when one is trying to prevent fracture of a weight bearing bone or prevent or relieve spinal cord compression.

SUMMARY

1. A substantial world experience in external beam irradiation of cancer of the prostate has been accumulated over the past 25 years.

2. Survival rates approaching 80% at 5 years, 60% at 10 years, and 40% at 15 years are being achieved for disease confined within the capsule. Comparable figures for extracapsular disease approach 60% at 5 years, 40% at 10 years, and 30% at 15 years, respectively.

3. The degree of aggressiveness of prostatic carcinoma is often telegraphed by the interrelationships between clinical stage, histopathologic grade, and lymphadenopathy. Unless these parameters are clearly described in any given series of patients, it is quite useless to try to compare treatment results.

4. Painful bone metastases are often alleviated by radiation therapy.

REFERENCES

1. M.A. Bagshaw, Perspectives on radiation treatment of prostate cancer: history and current focus, in:"Prostatic Cancer," G.P. Murphy, ed., PSG Publishing Co., Littleton (1979), p.151.

2. L. Harisiadis, R.J. Veenema, J.J. Senyszyn, P.J. Puchner, P. Tretter, N.A. Romas, C.H. Chang, J.K. Lattimer and M. Tannenbaum, Carcinoma of the prostate: treatment with external radiotherapy, Cancer 41:2131 (1978).

3. W.G. Guerriero, M.T. Barrett, T. Bartholomew, C.E. Carlton, Jr., and P.T. Hudgins, Combined interstitial and external radiotherapy in the definitive management of carcinoma of the prostate, in:"Cancer of the Genitourinary Tract," D.E. Johnson and M.L. Samuels, eds., Raven Press, New York (1979), p.207.

4. C.A. Perez, B.J. Walz, F.R. Zivnuska, M. Pilepich, K. Prasad, and W. Bauer, Irradiation of carcinoma of the prostate localized to the pelvis:analysis of tumor response and prognosis, Int. J. Radiat. Oncol. Biol. Phys. 6:555 (1980).

5. D.A. Pistenma, M.A. Bagshaw, and F.S. Freiha, Extended-field radiation therapy for prostatic adenocarcinoma: status report of a limited prospective trial, in:"Cancer of the Genitourinary Tract," D.E. Johnson and M.L. Samuels, eds., Raven Press, New York (1979), p.229.

6. D.F. Gleason and G.T. Mellinger, and the Veterans Administration Co-operative Urological Research Group, Prediction of prognosis for prostatic adenocarcinoma by combined histological grading and clinical staging, J. Urol. 111:58 (1974).

7. S.O. Asbell, B.A. Schlager, and A.S. Baker, Revision of treatment planning for carcinoma of the prostate, Int. J. Radiat. Oncol. Biol. Phys. 6:861 (1980).

8. D.J. Lee, S. Leibel, R. Shiels, R. Sanders, S. Siegelman, and S. Order, The value of ultrasonic imaging and CT scanning in planning the radiotherapy for prostatic carcinoma, Cancer 45:724 (1980).

9. E.J. Liebner, S. Stefani, and Uro-Oncology Research Group, An evaluation of lymphography with nodal biopsy in localized carcinoma of the prostate, Cancer 45:728 (1980).

10. M.C Spellman, R.A Castellino. G.R. Ray, D.A. Pistenma, and M.A. Bagshaw, An evaluation of lymphography in localized carcinoma of the prostate, Radiology 125:637 (1977).

11. S.C. Efremidis, A. Pagliarulo, S.J. Dan, H.N. Weber, R.N. Dillon, H. Nieburgs, and H.A Mitty, Post-lymphangiography fine needle aspiration lymph node biopsy in staging carcinoma of the prostate: preliminary report, J. Urol. 122:495 (1979).

12. B.S. Hilaris, W.F. Whitmore, M.A. Batata, and H. Grabstald, Radiation therapy and pelvic node dissection in the management of cancer of the prostate, Amer. J. Roentgenology, Radium Therapy and Nuclear Medicine 121:832 (1974).

13.   M.A. Batata, B.S. Hilaris, F.C.H. Chu, W.F. Whitmore, H.S. Song,
      Y. Kim, B. Horowitz, and K.S. Song, Radiation therapy in adeno-
      carcinoma of the prostate with pelvic lymph node involvement on
      lymphadenectomy, Int. J. Radiat. Oncol. Biol. Phys. 6:149 (1980).
14.   M.A. Bagshaw, H.S. Kaplan, and R.H. Sagerman, Linear accelerator
      supervoltage radiotherapy. VII. Carcinoma of the prostate,
      Radiology 85:121 (1965).
15.   G.R. Ray, J.R. Cassady, and M.A. Bagshaw, Definitive radiation
      therapy of carcinoma of the prostate, Radiology 106:407 (1973).
16.   E.L. Kaplan and P. Meier, Nonparametric estimation from
      incomplete observations, Am.Stat. Ass. J. 53:547 (1958).
17.   H.J. Jewett, R.W. Bridge, G.F. Gray, Jr., and W.M. Shelley,
      The palpable nodule of prostatic cancer. Results 15 years
      after radical excision, JAMA 203:403 (1968).
18.   O.S. Culp and J.J. Meyer, Radical prostatecomy in the treat-
      ment of prostatic cancer, Cancer 32:1113 (1973).
19.   P.C. Walsh and H.J. Jewett, Radical surgery for prostatic
      cancer, Cancer 45:1906 (1980).

Editorial Note -   Iridium 192 Wire Implantation in Prostatic
                   Carcinoma (C.C. Abbou).

     Since irradiation has been considered as the treatment of choice
for localised prostatic carcinoma, many attempts have been made to
replace tele-irradiation with interstitial irradiation. The latter
delivers a specific high radiation dose to the involved area only.

     Radium needles, colloidal radio-gold, radio-gold grains and
iridium 192 needles have been tried with variable success and
complications. Encapsulated iodine 125 has been used the most often.

     Iridium 192 wire has a half life of seventy four days, a low
energy gamma irradiation of 0.3 mev and a half attenuation constant
(HAC) of only 0.2 mm of lead. Because of these physical properties
and its low cost iridium 192 is used in our unit as the radio
active element of choice for interstitial irradiation. The active
zone is 1 cm broad (5 mm each side of the wire). The technique
of insertion is completely harmless to the surgeon's hand.

     Two techniques have been described:

     In Miller's Technique (1) a preoperative dose of 20 Gy in 10
fractions is given before operation after which a Pfannenstiel
incision is made and the retro pubic space opened. The lateral
surfaces of the prostate are exposed. Steel needles are inserted
into the prostate by perineal puncture and guided by rectal and
supra pubic palpation of the prostate. The needles are inserted
at one centimeter intervals. When in place they are replaced with
blind nylon tubes.

Postoperatively active iridium wires are loaded after dosimetry. The entire prostate is irradiated with a dose of 45 to 50 Gy for four to five days.

In the technique of Court and Chassagne (2) the patient is placed in a modified lithotomy position with the thighs flexed to approximately 30° - 45° on the trunk and abducted approximately to 30° - 45 from the central axis. A double abdominal and perineal operating field is prepared. A subumbilical transperitoneal approach permits one to proceed to a bilateral ilio-obturator node dissection for a frozen histologic section. Patients with metastatic nodes are excluded from the protocol.

The radiotherapist inserts the plastic tubes by means of stainless steel needles 15 cm long from the perineum towards the prostate. The needle is pushed by the left hand and guided by the right hand which also serves to palpate the prostatic nodule between the thumb and index finger. A loop is formed by means of an inter-mediate nylon obturator. The target volume includes the whole prostate. Two or three loops with a separation factor of 10 - 20 mm are implanted. These wires can be placed either in a frontal or a sagittal plane. During the operation non active lead wires are placed in the plastic tubes for radiologic control and to carry out dosimetric calculations.

Two or three days later, after obtaining precise dosimetry the lead wires are replaced with active iridium wires of 0.3 mm diameter. The technique allows a dose of 60 to 70 Gy to be given to a small volume at a low dose rate. Continuous irradiation is given for about six days.

This technique is suitable only for category T_1 and T_2 carcinoma of the prostate of the international UICC classification which are also NO and MO. NO, MO indicates that the patient must have had previously a normal bone scan and normal lymphangiogram. The absence of node metastases is confirmed by the ilio-obturator lymphadenectomy with frozen sections.

Miller used his protocol on 16 patients with major compli-cations in three (one pulmonary embolism, one proctitis, one anal ulceration). His series was too small and the follow up time too short to give a meaningful statement of survival experience. His minimum follow up was less than two years.

Court and Chassagne used their protocol on 13 patients. There was one post-operative death due to pulmonary embolism and one surgical infection with renal failure. The follow up was six months to six years with satisfactory control of the tumour.

As yet the place of this technique is not yet well defined

and the results of these small series are not significantly better
than those obtained by external irradiation.

REFERENCES

1. B.S. Hilaris et al, Radical radiation therapy of cancer of the
    prostate. A new approach using interstitial and external sources,
    Clin. Bull. Memorial Sloan Kettering Cancer Centre 2:94-99
    (1972).
2. B. Court and D. Chassagne, Interstitial radiation therapy of
    cancer of the prostate using iridium 192 wires, Cancer Treat.
    Rep. 61(2):329-30 (1977).

Editorial Note (M.P.M.)

    Interstitial irradiation of cancer localized to the prostate
has gained wide acceptance in the U.S.A. following the experience of
various workers who employed 1^{125} needles by open retropubic or by
perineal percutaneous implantation. Whitmore's experience is
particularly encouraging, but his results may be biased by case
selection. They are however very stimulating, especially as the
rate of secondary sexual impotence is negligible, if compared to
distant irradiation and, in particular, to radical prostatectomy.
Since 1^{125} needles are not readily available in Europe, iridium
may represent an alternative choice, as pointed out in Dr Abbou's
note. I wish to add that, in general, the addition of distant
irradiation to interstitial implantation of radioactive sources is
not advisable. The results are not improved, but the rate of untoward effects can be greatly increased, according to Shipley
(personal communication).

EXTERNAL IRRADIATION OF POORLY DIFFERENTIATED

PROSTATIC CARCINOMA

F. Edsmyr, L. Andersson, and P. Esposti

Karolinska Sjukhuset
Stockholm
Sweden

INTRODUCTION

Esposti (1) reported on 469 cases of prostatic carcinoma of all grades who were given hormone treatment at the Karolinska Sjukhuset in Stockholm. The survival rate up to five years in this series is given in Fig. 1. However in the patients with grade 3 carcinoma and without evidence of dissemination the five-year survival was only 14%.

Because of these depressing results in grade 3 tumors the therapy schedule was changed at the beginning of 1965 from hormone therapy to external irradiation.

MATERIAL AND METHOD

From the beginning of 1965 over 350 patients with poorly differentiated carcinoma of the prostate have received local irradiation of the primary tumor in our hospital. The majority had progressive disease after previous hormone therapy. Many were also given estrogens after the radiotherapy.

The evaluation comprises 107 patients treated between 1965 and 1973, initially free of clinical metastases and who were observed for at least five years or to death. The age varied between 47 and 81 years, average 66 years.

In all cases the diagnosis was verified by transrectal fine needle aspiration biopsy. Some patients had already had a histopathological diagnosis of poorly differentiated carcinoma but were

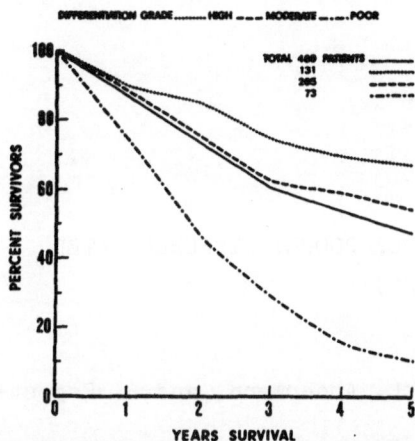

Fig 1. Histological grade and survival in 469 patients with
prostatic cancer treated with hormonal agents (1)

re-diagnosed with cytology. Skeletal x-ray and/or bone scans and
determination of the acid and alkaline phosphatase activity were
carried out. The tumors were categorized according to the TNM
system. The distribution by T category was T2-10 patients, T3-62
and T4-35 patients. Initially the treatment was given with a cobalt-
60 unit and thereafter by a 6 MV linear accelerator. The irradiation
was given with two oblique beams anteriorly and one open beam posteriorly. All treatment was individually planned. The tumor dose
including the volume of the true pelvis volume was a mean calculated
tumor dose of 5400 rad (54 Gy) given over six weeks.

RESULTS

     The five-year survival rate was 33% after correction for non-
cancer deaths. This figure is significantly higher than that for
the patients treated only with estrogens (Table 1). There was a
slight decrease in survival rate associated with a higher T category (Table 2).

     The five-year survival was approximately the same in those
patients who were given estrogens after irradiation as in the
group receiving no hormones (Table 3).

     In the majority of patients there was a slow regression of the
palpable tumor mass over the first three to six month period following irradiation. In 67% of cases there was no longer any tumor
palpable at the five-year review or at death (Table 4).

     In 33% of the patients no cancer cells were detectable on

Table 1. Survival in 107 Patients with no Detectable
          Dissemination Before Irradiation After
          Exclusion of Non-cancer Deaths

Survival (y)	No.	%
1	91/106	86
2	77/103	75
3	52/100	52
4	35/98	36
5	32/96	33

Table 2. Five Year Survival Related to T Category

	T2	T3	T4
Number of patients	10	62	35
Dead intercurrent disease	3	5	3
5-year survival	3	20	9
Corrected survival	43%	35%	28%

Table 3. Influence of Subsequent Estrogen Therapy on
          Five Year Survival After Irradiation

	No Hormone	Hormone
Number of patients	42	65
Dead intercurrent disease	4	7
5-year survival	13	19
Corrected Survival	34%	33%

Table 4. Local Tumor Response

	No.	%
Complete response	72	67
Partial response	18	17
Regression - progression	9	8
Unchanged	2	2
Progression	2	2
Not evaluated	4	4
Total	107	100

Table 5.   Cytologic Findings After Radiotherapy

	No.	%
Persisting cancer cells	44	41
No cancer cells found	35	33
Not evaluated	28	26
Total	107	100

repeated aspiration biopsies up to five years or more. In 41% the
smears contained malignant cells (Table 5). A number of these
patients had no palpable tumor. 26% of the patients were not evaluated because of early death within six months of irradiation, the
earliest time at which cytological evaluation can be carried out.

Side Effects

Proctitis, usually slight to moderate, occurred in many
patients, starting in mid-treatment. Bladder irritability was less
frequent and, as a rule, mild. Two patients had long-term intestinal
haemorrhage and persistent obstruction, necessitating surgery.

DISCUSSION

In the hormone treated patient with grade 3 carcinoma and without evidence of dissemination Esposti reported a 14% five-year survival rate. The 33% five-year survival rate in a comparable group in
the present study is significantly higher.

The finding of tumor regression, as judged by palpation, in 67%
of the patients was in good agreement with the experiences of Cantril
et al (2) and Mantyla (3) who reported local control of poorly
differentiated prostatic carcinoma in 79 and 64% respectively following radiotherapy. On the other hand, aspiration biopsy, when performed with an adequate technique, is no doubt a more sensitive
indicator of tumor existence than the digital examination.

The incidence of serious complications following radiotherapy
with this modern high voltage technique is low. A few years ago we
introduced an extended field technique, including the para-aortic
lymph nodes in the irradiated volume. The pelvic and para-aortic
nodes receive 5000 rad in seven weeks and the local tumour 7000 rad.

SUMMARY

At least in cases of poorly differentiated carcinoma of the
prostate, with no identified dissemination, it appears that radiotherapy may offer a chance of tumor control superior to hormone
treatment and with an acceptable incidence of side effects.

REFERENCES

1. P.L. Esposti, Cytologic malignancy grading of prostatic
    carcinoma by transrectal aspiration biopsy, Scand. J. Urol.
    Nephrol. 5:199 (1971).
2. S. Cantril, J. Vaeth, J. Green, and A. Schroeder, Radiation
    therapy for localised carcinoma of the prostate, Front Radiat.
    Ther. Oncol. 9:274 (1975).
3. M. Mantyla, Radiotherapy of carcinoma of the prostate,
    Strahlentherapie 154:542 (1978).

Editorial Note (M.P.M.)

According to the Stockholm workers, both estramustine phosphate
and irradiation are valid methods for treating high grade prostatic
cancer. In the paper by Andersson et al (this volume) of 90
patients with grade 3 cancer treated with estracyt, 42 had bony
metastases and 15 had soft tissue lesions. This leaves 33 patients
in whom the disease was apparently limited to the primary tumour.

The results are not given in detail and no survival figures are
presented, but it is stated that the local tumour regressed
objectively in 11 of 14 patients not previously treated with
oestrogens, which correpsonds to a 78.6% response rate. In this
article 62 patients had extensive local spread (62 T3 and 35 T4) with
an expected rate of lymph node metastases of 60% (see Bagshaw's
article on lymph node metastases, in this book), 80% of which will be
followed by bone metastases. One wonders, therefore, if an effective
systemic treatment such as estramustine, given alone or in combination with irradiation, might not prove to be superior to radiotherapy, at least in stage C patients.

IODINE-125 IMPLANTATION FOR PROSTATIC CARCINOMA

R.J. Macchia

Downstate Medical School
New York
U.S.A.

The technique and rationale for iodine 125 implantation for prostatic adenocarcinoma has been fully described by its originators (1). This article will be devoted to recent modifications and continuing controversies.

Clinical Stage

Whitmore and his colleagues had originally suggested that clinical stage B and the majority of clinical stage C patients were potential candidates for this procedure. Stage C patients are no longer considered amenable to implantation. Ill defined borders increase the probability that some tumor tissue will escape adequate irradiation. Because of their spongy nature the seminal vesicles cannot be implanted properly. Finally, the incidence of undetected metastases or metastases to the lymph nodes is high in stage C disease.

Tumor Grade

This is still not a factor in patient selection in most institutions. However, the incidence of early metastases, undetectable with current clinical staging techniques, is extraordinarily high. This is proven by the dismal survival statistics for very high grade tumors regardless of what modality of therapy is utilized. It is my practice to exclude very high grade tumors from iodine 125 implantation.

Lymph Node Metastases

The reader is referred to the article by this author elsewhere
in the book entitled "Lymph Node Dissection in the Management of
Prostatic Carcinoma". There has never been any solid evidence that
lymph node dissection for prostatic adenocarcinoma has any value as
a therapeutic maneuver. If a patient is known to have metastases,
it is difficult to imagine how any treatment confined to the primary
site can be of benefit. The pre-operative detection of lymph node
(or any other) metastases should exclude a patient from 1-125
implantation.

Let us imagine that a patient is thought from clinical and
pathological evidence to have disease limited to the prostate.
Suppose at exploration a positive lymph node is demonstrated. What
should be done? It has been the usual custom in some centers to
proceed to implant these patients. It is my practice, however, not
to implant. In my opinion iodine 125 implantation is of no proven
value in this setting. Some would argue that since the exploration
has exposed the prostate, one should proceed with the implant. My
retort is that even simple implantation without a full node dissection is not without complications (2).

Patient Selection

Our current practice is to divide patients into three groups
based on the Gleason score (3). Patients with low Gleason scores
have a very low likelihood of having lymph node metastases. We
suggest that these patients have an exploration. If no suspicious
lymph nodes are palpated, iodine 125 implant is performed without a
lymph node dissection. Patients with high Gleason scores are very
likely to have metastases. We offer these patients radiation therapy
with or without hormonal manipulation. Middle level Gleason scores
cannot predict lymph node status. We suggest an exploration. If
palpation at exploration does not reveal any suspicious nodes, we
proceed to modified systematic extra-peritoneal bilateral lymph node
dissection.

Seed Placement

The accurate placement of the iodine seeds is essential to
ensure adequate radiation of all cancerous tissue. Because of the
retropubic location of the prostate and the limited range of the
iodine 125 radiation, this has been a problem and the transcoccygeal
and percutaneous perineal approaches either alone or with retropubic
placement have been described.

Obstructing Glands

It has been common practice to perform a "conservative" TURP if a gland has produced retention or symptoms of severe obstruction to prevent a post-implant acute retention secondary to enlargement of the gland due to mechanical or radiation induced edema. Such a maneuver, while sometimes necessary, renders adequate implantation more difficult. Perhaps no more that 5% of the patients really need a pre-implant TURP. It is better to accept temporary post-operative retention, treating it with an indwelling catheter until the edema resolves.

Dosimetry

It is mandatory for any physician performing this procedure to have access to sophisticated computerized dosimetry techniques and to monitor that placement is accurate (4,5). If implant distribution has led to inadequate radiation, supplemental external radiation is essential.

Local Treatment Failure

As with other radiation techniques post-implant biopsies have documented the persistence of apparently viable tumor. The significance of this is not clear and the incidence decreases as the time between implantation and biopsy increases (6).

Sexual Function

An overall post-implant incidence of impotency of approximately 10% has been documented (7).

Complications

The significant complication rate has been discussed in the literature (2). It is my opinion that most of the morbidity is due to the lymph node dissection and not to the implant and it will be interesting to note the complication rate in patients treated with iodine 125 implantation without concomitant lymph node dissection.

Supplemental External Radiation Therapy (XRT)

Pelvic XRT following implantation and node dissection is associated with a high complication rate and pre-operative XRT has been proposed. However most patients with cancer-bearing lymph

nodes already have bony metastases (even if undetectable). One must
therefore question the use of XRT in this setting even if it is able
to sterilize lymph nodes as some claim.

Over all Cure of Cancer and Survival Statistics

Sufficiently long follow-up of patients is not currently
available. We are still debating the relative indications and merits
of total prostatectomy versus external radiation therapy despite the
fact that they have been with us for a long time. I fear the same
fate will befall iodine 125 implantation.

REFERENCES

1. W. Barzell, M.A. Bean, B.S. Hilaris, and W.F. Whitmore, Jr.
    Prostatic adenocarcinoma: Relationship of grade and local extent
    of metastases, J.Urol. 118:278 (1977).
2. J.E. Fowler, Jr., W. Barzell, B.S. Hilaris, and W.F. Whitmore,
    Jr., Complications of 125 iodine implantation and pelvic
    lymphadenectomy in the treatment of prostatic cancer, J.Urol.
    121:447 (1979), p.171.
3. D.F. Gleason, Histologic grading and clinical staging of
    prostatic carcinoma, in:"The Prostate," M. Tannenbaum, ed.,
    Lea and Febiger, Philadelphia (1977).
4. W.U. Shipley, G. Kopelson, D.H. Novack. C.C. Ling, S.P. Dretler
    and G.R. Prout, Jr., Preoperative irradiation, lymphadenectomy
    and 125 iodine implant for patients with localized prostatic
    carcinoma: A correlation of implant dosimetry with clinical
    results, J.Urol. 124:639 (1980).
5. B.S. Hilaris, W.F. Whitmore, Jr., M.A. Batata, W. Barzell, and
    N. Tokita, Iodine 125 implantation of the prostate: dose-response
    considerations, Front. Rad. Ther. 12:82 (1978).
6. B. Lytton, J.T. Collins, R.M. Weiss, M. Schiff, Jr., E.J McGuire,
    and V. Livolsi, Results of biopsy after early stage prostatic
    cancer treatment by implantation of iodine seeds, J.Urol. 121:
    306 (1979).
7. H.W. Herr, Preservation of sexual potency in prostatic cancer
    patients after pelvic lymphadenectomy and retropubic 125
    implantation, J.Urol. 121:621 (1979).

CONTROVERSIAL ASPECTS OF HORMONE MANIPULATION IN PROSTATIC CARCINOMA

J. Altwein

Bundeswehrkrankenhaus Ulm
Ulm
West Germany

INTRODUCTION

The biochemical similarity between the patient's normal and his cancerous prostatic tissue is one essential prerequisite for successful hormone manipulation basically directed at the deprivation of androgenic influences upon the prostate. In achieving this goal every therapeutic modality still relies on classical androgen control principles; however, new developments in the field of chemotherapeutic drugs and antihormones are being tested in multicenter phase II and III trials, e.g. under the auspices of the National Prostatic Cancer Project and the EORTC.

The aim of hormone manipulation may be achieved by the following basic mechanism described by Walsh (1),

1. Ablation of androgen sources,
2. Suppression of pituitary gonadotropin release,
3. Inhibition of androgen synthesis, and
4. Interference with androgen action at target tissues
    (= end organ antagonism).

INDICATIONS FOR HORMONE TREATMENT

Whether or not hormone treatment may be regarded as curative is far from clear, particularly when comparing the results of hormone therapy with those of radical surgery or irradiation. Thus at the present time those stages of carcinoma of the prostate (PCA) where a cure may be achieved should be excluded. A borderline situation is encountered in stage C tumors with few positive pelvic lymph nodes, i.e. T1-4 N1,2 MO. In the operable patient a thorough pelvic

Table 1. Metastatic PCA: Variety of Treatment Modalities

(67 pts. seen in one year: Murphy 1977)
(47)

Hormones	35.8%
Hormones + Surgery	19.4%
None	18.2%
Surgery	14.9%
Radiation + Hormones	2.9%
Radiation + Hormones + Surgery	2.9%
Hormones + Surgery + Chemotherapy	2.9%
Radiation	1.5%
Hormones + Chemotherapy	1.5%

lymphadenectomy with irradiation should precede attempts at hormone manipulation (2).   Progression despite local therapy with curative intent would leave the prostatic carcinoma still amenable to systemic treatment.   In patients with proof of metastases hormone therapy is usually indicated.

A special situation is created by ureteral obstruction due to seminal vesicle invasion or direct extension of the tumor to the bladder.   Michigan and Catalona (3) studied the charts of 1065 patients and found 10% with uni- or bilateral ureteral obstruction. Orchiectomy improved upper tract dilatation in 22 of 25 patients, whereas estrogen and antiandrogen were successful in only one of six patients.   Grade and stage did not correlate with response rate. This favourable effect of orchiectomy upon ureteral obstruction may even be encountered after long-term medical treatment.   Irradiation was far inferior in treating these patients.

Principal Methods of Hormone Manipulation

The variety of treatment modalities used in patients with metastatic prostatic carcinoma is remarkable and reflects the urologists dilemma in trying to cope with advanced disease (Table 1). Four controversial treatment categories evolve:

1.   Orchiectomy plus estrogens,
2.   Orchiectomy only.   Other hormonal therapy is withheld
       until symptoms arise,
3.   Hormones only.   Orchiectomy is postponed,
4.   Hormones plus chemotherapy.

Table 2. Androgen Control - Regimes Accepted as
          "Standard Treatment"

Subcapsular orchiectomy

Oral estrogens:
 3 mg DES or equivalent

Parenteral estrogens:
 80 mg polyestradiol phosphate

          or

100 mg estradiol undecylate

Pain:
Honvan-infusion 1.2 g q.d. over 10 days

Orchiectomy plus estrogens.   This is widely practiced in M1
prostatic carcinoma and may be considered a standard treatment (4,5),
(Table 2).   Once staging is completed, subcapsular orchiectomy is
carried out followed by a diethylstilbestrol diphosphate-infusion.
Maintenance therapy consists of four weekly injections of 80 mg.
polyestradiol phosphate or 100 mg. estradiol undecylate (6).   Some
advise additional intake of an oral estrogen, e.g. Tace^{TM} or diethylstilbestrol (DES) (4).   However, the drawback of all oral medication
in chronically ill patients is their poor compliance (7).

This treatment provides an excellent but transient palliation
in advanced disease.   There are also some long term survivors even
with prostatic carcinoma of this stage (8).   A recent retrospective
study revealed 40% (17/43 pts.) five-year and 12% (5/42 pts.) 10-year
survival following orchiectomy and estrogens (9).   The results of
the best known phase III trial (first VACURG study) showed that 5 mg.
DES was superior to placebo, orchiectomy plus placebo or orchiectomy
plus DES at the five-year follow up.   At nine years, orchiectomy
and placebo appeared to be the worst therapy.

In analyzing the causes of death (Table 3) in study I for stage
D prostatic cancer it is obvious that estrogens increase the non-
cancer mortality, but it is tempting to speculate that if these patients had lived long enough they would have succumbed to their cancer
(10).   This appears to be the case when taking into account the
results of VACURG II (11) comparing: placebo, 0.2, 1 and 5 mg. DES.
The two highest doses of estrogens slowed down the progression of
stage C and D prostatic cancer.

The widely discussed data of the VACURG I have been reconsidered
by Jordan et al (12) who arrived at the conclusion that estrogen is

Table 3. Causes of Death in First VACURG Study.

| | Cancer | | Cardiovascular | |
	Stage C	Stage D	Stage C	Stage D
Placebo	18%	47%	33%	24%
Placebo + Orchiectomy	13%	48%	35%	27%
Estrogen	6%	38%	42%	36%
Estrogen + Orchiectomy	9%	38%	42%	27%

more effective than orchiectomy in preventing deaths from prostatic
carcinoma and that the addition of orchiectomy to estrogen does not
offer any clear-cut advantage over estrogen therapy alone.   If
cancer symptoms necessitate treatment these authors prefer estrogens.
Orchiectomy should, according to these authors, be reserved for those
circumstances in which a patient is not reliable, cannot tolerate
estrogens or has severe cardiovascular disease.

    Orchiectomy only.   Other hormonal treatment is deferred.   This
concept is favored by Paulson (13) in the asymptomatic patient.
Likewise, Menon and Walsh (10) prefer orchiectomy alone with relapses
treated by chemotherapy.   However, two large-scale retrospective
studies have demonstrated the inferiority of orchiectomy vs estrogens
(14,15).   At the nine-year follow up even a phase III trial, VACURG
I, revealed a slight, but insignificant inferiority of castration vs
estrogens.   This trial clearly demonstrated that estrogens are more
effective than orchiectomy in preventing deaths from prostatic carcinoma (12).

    The main advantage of orchiectomy alone for distant prostatic
carcinoma - its excellent toleration by the patient - is more than
offset by Brendler and Prout's observation that patients resistant
to castration did not respond to later estrogen application (16).

    Hormones only.   Orchiectomy deferred.   Estrogens remain
the basis of all hormone preparations used for the palliation of
prostatic carcinoma.   A multitude of reports dealing with a variety
of estrogenic preparations have appeared in the literature.   Besides,
two large-scale retrospective studies (14,15) two phase III trials
(VACURG I and II) have exemplified the effectiveness of DES in comparison to orchiectomy plus placebo, placebo, and orchiectomy plus
estrogen.   The use of estrogens has been discredited, however, for
the following reasons: cardiovascular toxicity, hyperprolactinemia,
impairment of immune response, hepatic toxicity (17) and salt and
water retention (18).

    Gestagens.   The availability of well-tolerated 17α-hydroxy-

Table 4. Gestagens Used For The Treatment of Prostatic Carcinoma:
          17α - hydroxyprogesterone Derivatives.

Compound	Dose	Remarks
Hydroxyprogesterone caproate	1.5 g i.m./x 2 per week	---
Gestonorone caproate	400 mg/week i.m.	ineffective
Chlormadinone acetate	0.1 - 2.0 g q.d.	weak
Megestrol acetate	160 mg q.d.	active
Medroxyprogesterone acetate (MAP)	30 - 5000 mg/day	active

progesterone derivatives (Table 4) led Geller et al (19) to use these
compounds in patients with prostatic carcinoma. The rationale for
their use was the virtual lack of serious side-effects (20), even in
a phase II-study employing daily injections of 1500 mg medroxyprogesterone acetate (MAP) over 30 days (21) and despite the dopaminagonistic
action induced by gestagens with subsequent prolactin-suppression (22).
However, in a survey of the various phase II-trials conducted by
Bouffioux (23) none of the 17 -hydroxyprogesterone derivatives
appeared to be clearly effective. Another drug, gestonorone caproate,
was tested in a phase III-trial vs orchiectomy alone with negative
results (24).

     In the third VACURG study including 424 patients with stage IV
or D carcinoma of the prostate 30 mg.medroxyprogesterone acetate was
not worse than 1 mg DES (25) (Table 5). The EORTC compared cyproterone acetate, medroxyprogesterone acetate, and 3 mg DES in their
protocol no. 30761. At a preliminary evaluation the progression
rates were 33%, 41%, and 19% respectively. However, these differences did not reach the level of significance (26).

Table 5. Third VACURG Study for Stage D PCA (1969-1974)

No.	Treatment	
105	Premarin	2.5 mg
104	MAP	30.0 mg
105	MAP (30 mg) + DES	1.0 mg
110	DES	1.0 mg

Evaluation (1981): no significant difference in survival (36).

Table 6. Medroxyprogesterone Acetate (MAP) Versus
          Diethylstilbestrol (DES) (27)

	Number of Pts	1 year	Survival 2 years	3 years
DES (3 - 5 mg /day p.o.)	20	16/20	14/20	11/20 (55%)
MAP (1.0 - 2.0 g/week: then 0.1 g q.d.)	20	19/20	15/20	6/17 (35%)

The most recent randomized prospective trial was conducted by
Bouffioux (27) employing 500 mg medroxyprogesterone acetate 2-4 times
a week for one month, followed by an oral dose of 100 mg q.d. (Table
6). It turned out that the gestagen seemed less efficient than DES
in the treatment of advanced prostatic carcinoma with shorter periods
of remission; but the drug was well tolerated. The 60% impotence
rate was reversible after discontinuation of the medication. Gynecomastia or mastodynia did not occur.

Among the antiestrogens only tamoxifen has been tested, in a few
estrogen-resistent patients, resulting in some short term remissions
(28,29). A phase II-trial is expected.

Among the antiandrogens 3 compounds have been tested in patients
with carcinoma of the prostate: megestrol acetate, flutamide, and
cyproterone acetate.

1. Megestrol acetate was employed in a phase II-trial; four of
nine patients with prostatic tumor experienced a 12 month partial
remission (30). The "escape" of plasma testosterone-suppression
beginning at two to six months after use of the drug was embarrassing
and was possibly responsible for the development of resistance.

2. In a phase II-trial involving 13 men with previously untreated
stage D carcinoma of the prostate 750 mg flutamide was given over a
period of two to 20 months. Of the 13 patients seven showed an
objective response (31). Similarly 21 patients with stage D
prostatic carcinoma were treated by Sogani et al (32): eight of
ten patients with bone pain experienced relief from pain lasting
from three to 16 months. Remarkably, in three of four patients
with measurable lymph nodes the lesion disappeared. Altogether 19
patients responded with an average duration of 10-1/2 months. Although none of the 21 men enrolled into the trial had previous
hormonal therapy, 13 had had irradiation (Table 7).

Airhart et al (33) compared 1.5 mg DES plus 0.75 g flutamide with
1 mg DES in 20 patients with previously untreated stage D prostatic
carcinoma. Objective response was noted in 3/6 patients receiving

Table 7. Phase II Trials of Flutamide in M1-PCA:

	No	PR	Side Effects *	
Stoliar (48)	18	7	?	
Prout et al (31)	13	7	thromboembolism	2
			GI-tract	1
Airhart et al (33)	6	4	?	
Sogani + Whitmore (32)	21	19	cardiovascular	4
			hepatic	2
Total	58	37	(63%)	

* Gynecomastia regularly:
  Impotence rarely.

DES and 6/14 men on flutamide.   50% of the patients on flutamide survived one year and 43% two years.   A similar study comprising 15 patients was reported by Jacobo et al (34), who concluded that neither DES nor flutamide displayed significant superiority (Table 8).

In the light of these investigations, the side effects are crucial: Sogani et al (32) noticed gynecomastia in 18 of his 21 patients, two developed abnormal liver function tests, and four suffered from cardiovascular toxicity (with one death).   Fukushima et al (35) observed markedly altered cortisol metabolism in patients with prostatic carcinoma, presumably due to intrahepatic cholestasis or hepato-cellular damage.   In the continuation of this study reversible cirrhosis-like disturbances of steroid metabolism were found (36).   A positive effect of the drug is the apparent preservation of sexual potency (32).

Table 8. Phase III Trials of Flutamide in M1-PCA:

	Partial Remission		Total
	Jacobo et al (34)	Airhart et al (33)	
Flutamide 0.75-1.5 G	2/8	6/14	36%
vs.			
DES 1 mg	3/5	3/6	54%

3.   The classical antiandrogen cyproterone acetate has been tested
in more than 1000 patients with prostatic carcinoma (37,38).   The
literature contains reliable information of 101 patients treated with
cyproterone acetate who had no previous therapy; from these patients
the parameters best documented by Scott et al (39) and Wein et al (40)
are the decline of acid phosphatase in 14/23 patients, reduced local
tumor mass in 23/35 and relief of bone pain in 12/21 subjects.
Geller et al (41) noted an objective remission lasting from four to
14 months in all five patients with T3-4, MO-1 lesions.   The first
phase III-trial stems from Jacobi and Altwein (38): cyproterone
acetate (300 mg IM/week) was compared with estradiol undecylate (100
mg IM four-weekly).   The former drug proved to be more effective,
as the castration effect as judged by plasma testosterone was more
pronounced, the objective voiding pattern and tumor response was
superior and the side effects were fewer.

   Deferred Orchiectomy.   Whereas primary hormone therapy shows a
response rate of 83% (42), secondary endocrine manipulation is of
equivocal value.   Although the substitution of subcapsular orchiectomy for estrogens or cyproterone acetate after hormonal escape of
the tumor is common in urological practice, its effectiveness has
never been investigated properly.   In a retrospective study Stone
et al (42) evaluated the effectiveness of deferred orchiectomy in 21
patients with carcinoma of the prostate following the diagnosis of
estrogen escape.   Regression was seen in one patient and stabilization of disease in four.   Subjectively three patients improved and
six remained unchanged.   Biorn et al (43) in 29 patients with estrogen escape (defined differently however) noted a higher number of
subjective responses with regression in five of the 29 patients.
Denis et al (44) considered the testosterone level of critical value
in predicting which patient will benefit from deferred orchiectomy.
Further study of this topic appears to be desirable.

   Hormones plus Chemotherapy.   Primary chemotherapy would be the
ideal modality for the patients with carcinoma a priori resistant to
hormones; however, at the present time this cannot be reliably predicted.   Among the few primary chemotherapy trials reported, Merrin
(45) achieved a partial objective response to cis-platinum in 22/34
patients (64%).   However, in these patients orchiectomy and estrogens were administered at the same time (!)

SUMMARY AND CONCLUSION

   One is able to distinguish four therapeutic regimens for
metastatic prostatic carcinoma:

   1.   Orchiectomy plus estrogens,
   2.   Orchiectomy first; other hormonal treatment later,
   3.   Hormone application first; orchiectomy later, or
   4.   Hormones plus chemotherapy.

The employment of orchiectomy plus estrogens has been seriously questioned by the VACURG (Study I) and it appears that the addition of orchiectomy to estrogen-treatment does not give better results than estrogen alone. Some authors prefer orchiectomy alone in asymptomatic patients with stage D cancer and reserve estrogens until the disease progresses. However, evidence has been provided that patients whose prostatic carcinoma has progressed despite castration do not respond to estrogens. Furthermore, it has been shown that estrogens are superior to orchiectomy in preventing cancer deaths. The argument that the rate of lethal cardiovascular complications more than outweighs the anticancer activity has been refuted by Bennett et al (46) and De Vere White et al (9).

Thus, hormones evolve as the primary treatment of choice in metastatic prostatic carcinoma, independent of the patient's symptoms, as long as the prostatic carcinoma is "virginal". Taking into account the phase III-trials dealing with hormonal therapy only, one is surprised to find neither estrogen nor the non-estrogen compounds superior. Among the latter, cyproterone acetate is clearly the most effective drug among the available hormones. Since the estrogen side effects are lacking, one would favor cyproterone acetate as the first choice in patients with disseminated prostatic carcinoma and a good performance status. Progression while on cyproterone acetate requires a change of the primary treatment; it appears reasonable to use delayed orchiectomy, and possibly, as a secondary treatment, estrogen.

Adjunctive application of antiprolactins serve to suppress the estrogen and cyproterone acetate induced hyperprolactinemia. The latter phenomenon was found to be partly responsible for the development of gynecomastia, the increment of ACTH-like action upon the adrenal gland, and a rise of prolactin-binding to the prostate in the non-castrated individual. It is tempting to speculate that prolactin may contribute to the development of hormone resistance in the patient suffering from metastatic carcinoma of the prostate.

REFERENCES

1. P.C. Walsh, Physiologic Basis for Hormonal Therapy in Carcinoma of the Prostate, Urol. Clin. N Amer. 2:125 (1975).
2. C.E. Carlton, Combined Interstitial and External Radiotherapy in the Definitive Management of Carcinoma of the Prostate, Presented at The International Symposium on the Treatment of Carcinoma of the Prostate, Berlin, (1978).
3. S. Michigan and W.J. Catalona, Ureteral Obstruction from Prostatic Carcinoma: Response to Endocrine and Radiation Therapy, J. Urol. 118:733 (1977).
4. H. Gottinger and E. Schmiedt, Therapie des Prostatakarzinoms, Fortschr Med. 97:1881 (1979).

5. R. Hartung and W. Mauermayer, Therapie und Nachsorge des Prostat-
    akarzinoms, Ther Gegenwart 118:162 (1979).

6. G. Birke and L. Waldstrom, Progynon, A Depot Preparation with
    Oestrogenic Action in the Treatment of Prostate Carcinoma. Acta
    Chir. Scand 130:388 (1965).

7. R.M. Anikwe, Effect of Estrogen Therapy on Metastatic Carcinoma
    of the Prostate, Int. Surg 62:532 (1977).

8. W.S. Falkowski and V.J. O'Conor Jr, Long-term Survivor of Pros-
    tatic Carcinoma with Lung Metastases, J. Urol. 125:260 (1981).

9. R. De Vere White, D.F. Paulson and J.D. Glenn, The Clinical
    Spectrum of Prostatic Cancer, J. Urol. 117:23 (1977).

10. M. Menon and P.C. Walsh, Hormonal Therapy for Prostatic Cancer
    in "Prostatic Cancer", G.P. Murphy (ed), PSG Publishing Company,
    Littleton (1979) p. 175.

11. D.P. Byar, The Veterans Administration Cooperative Urological
    Research Group's Studies of Cancer of the Prostate, Cancer
    32:1126 (1973).

12. W.P. Jordan, C.E. Blackard and D.P. Byar, Reconsideration of
    Orchiectomy in the Treatment of Advanced Prostatic Carcinoma,
    South.Med. J. 70:1411 (1977).

13. D.F. Paulson, The Role of Endocrine Therapy in the Management of
    Prostatic Cancer, in "Genitourinary Cancer", D.G. Skinner and
    J.D. deKernion (eds), W.B. Saunders Company, Philadelphia, London
    and Toronto, (1978) p. 388.

14. J.L. Emmett, L.F. Greene and A. Papantoniou, Endocrine Therapy
    in Carcinoma of the Prostate Gland: 10-year Survival Studies,
    J. Urol. 83:471 (1960).

15. K. Ochiai and H. Takeuchi, Some Consideration on Rational for
    an Antiandrogenic Treatment of Advanced Prostatic Carcinoma,
    in "Proceedings of the 16th Congress of the International
    Society of Urology, Doin, Paris (1973) p. 256.

16. H. Brendler and G. Prout, A Cooperative Group Study of Prostatic
    Cancer: Stilbestrol Versus Placebo in Advanced Progressive
    Disease, Cancer Chemother. Rep. 16:323 (1962).

17. M. Kontturri and E. Sotaniemi, Effect of Estrogen on Liver
    Function of Prostatic Cancer Patients, Brit. Med. J. i:204 (1969)

18. U. Kunze and F. Orestano, Intra-und Extrazellulare Elektrolyt-
    konzentration Unter Oestrogen-Therapie bei Prostatacarcinompat-
    ienten, Urologa A 12:274 (1973).

19. J. Geller, B. Fruchtman, H. Newman, T. Roberts and R. Silva,
    Effect of Progestational Agents on Carcinoma of the Prostate,
    Cancer Chemother. Rep. 51:41 (1967).

20. S. Rafla and R. Johnson, The Treatment of Advanced Prostatic
    Carcinoma with Medroxyprogesterone, Curr. Ther. Res. 16:261
    (1974).

21. F. Pannuti, A.P. Rossi and E. Piana, Massive Doses of Medroxy-
    progesterone Acetate (MPA): Pilot Study in the Treatment of
    Advanced Prostate Cancer, IRCS Med. Sci. 5:375 (1977).

22. O.M. Cramer, C.R. Parker and J.C. Porter, Stimulation of Dopamine
    Release into Hypophyseal Portal Blood by Administration of
    Progesterone, Endocrinol. 105:929 (1979).

23. C.H. Bouffioux, Le Cancer de la Prostate, Acta Urol Belg 47:189 (1979).

24. S. Sander, R. Nissen-Meyer and A. Aakvaag, On Gestagen Treatment of Advanced Prostatic Carcinoma, Scand J Urol. Nephrol. 12:119 (1978).

25. D.P. Byar, VACURG Studies on Prostatic Cancer and Its Treatment, in "Urologic Pathology: The Prostate", M. Tannenbaum (ed), Lea & Febiger, Philadelphia (1977) p. 241.

26. M. Pavone-Macaluso, Phase III Studies of the EORTC: Treatment of Prostatic Carcinoma with Antihormones, Presented at Antihormones - Current Knowledge and Prospective Clinical Relevance in Urology, Innsbruck (1979).

27. C.H. Bouffioux, Treatment of Prostatic Cancer with Medroxyprogesterone-acetate (MPA), in "Bladder Tumors and Other Topics in Urological Oncology, M. Pavone-Macaluso, P.H. Smith and F. Edsmyr (eds), Plenum Publishing Corporation, New York (1980), p. 463.

28. A. Kocze and J. Szekely, Tamoxifen in Advanced Prostatic Carcinoma, Lancet i:539 (1980).

29. M Osama El-Arimi, Response to Tamoxifen in Drug-Reistant Prostatic Carcinoma, Lancet ii:588 (1979).

30. J. Geller, J. Albert and S.S.C. Yen, Treatment of Advanced Cancer of the Prostate with Megestrol Acetate, Urology 12:537 (1978).

31. G.R. Prout, R.J. Irwin, B. Kliman, J.J. Daly, R.A. McLaughlin and P.P. Griffin, Prostatic Cancer and Sch 13521: II. Histological Alterations and the Pituitary Gonadal Axis, J. Urol. 113:834 (1975).

32. P.C. Sogani and W.F. Whitmore, Experience with Flutamide in Previously Untreated Patients with Advanced Prostatic Cancer, J. Urol. 122:640 (1979).

33. R.A. Airhart, T.F. Barnett, J.W. Sullivan, R.L. Levine and J.U. Schlegel, Flutamide Therapy for Carcinoma of the Prostate, South Med. J. 71:798 (1978).

34. E. Jacobo, J. Schmidt, S. Weinstein and R. Flocks, Comparison of Flutamide (Schr 13521) and Diethylstilbestrol in Untreated Advanced Prostatic Cancer, Urology 8:231 (1976).

35. D.K. Fukushima, J. Levin, J. Kream, S.Z. Freed, W.F. Whitmore, L. Hellman and B. Zumoff, Effect of Flutamide on Cortisol Metabolism. J. Clin. Endocrinol. Metab. 47:788 (1978).

36. B. Zumoff, J. Fishman, S. Freed, J. Levin, W.F. Whitmore Jr, L. Hellman and D.K. Fukushima, Effect of Flutamide on Estradiol Metabolism, J. Clin. Endocrinol. Metab. 49:467 (1979).

37. U. Bracci, Antiandrogens in the Treatment of Prostatic Cancer, Eur. Urol. 5:303 (1979).

38. G.H. Jacobi, J.E. Altwein, K.H. Kurth, R. Basting and R. Hohenfellner, Treatment of Advanced Prostatic Cancer with Parenteral Cyproterone Acetate: A Phase III Randomised Trial, Brit. J. Urol. 52:208 (1980).

39. W.W. Scott and H.K.A. Schirmer, A New Progestational Steroid
     Effective in the Treatment of Prostatic Cancer, Trans Amer Assoc.
     GU Surg. 58:54 (1966).
40. A.J. Wein and J.J. Murphy, Experience in the Treatment of Pros-
     tatic Carcinoma with Cyproterone Acetate, J. Urol. 109:68 (1973).
41. J. Geller, G. Vazakas, B. Fruchtman, H. Newman, K. Nakao and
     A. Loh, The Effect of Cyproterone Acetate on Advanced Carcinoma
     of the Prostate, Surg. Gyn. Obst. 127:748 (1968).
42. A.R. Stone, T.B. Hargreave and G.D. Chisholm, The Diagnosis of
     Estrogen Escape and the Role of Secondary Orchiectomy in Pros-
     tatic Cancer, Brit. J. Urol. 52:535 (1980).
43. G.L. Biorn, C.P. Gray and E. Strauss, Orchiectomy After Presumed
     Estrogen Failure in Treatment of Carcinoma of the Prostate, West
     J. Med. 130:363 (1979).
44. L. Denis and P. Nowe, Bilateral Orchiectomy in Patients with
     Progressive Advanced Prostatic Cancer, Acta Urol. Belg 48:113
     (1980).
45. C.E. Merrin, Treatment of Previously Untreated (By Hormonal
     Manipulation) Stage D Adenocarcinoma of Prostate with Combined
     Orchiectomy, Estrogens and Cisdiamminedichloro-platinum, Urology
     15:123 (1980).
46. A.H. Bennett, J.B. Dowd and J.H. Harrison, Estrogen and Survival
     Data in Carcinoma of the Prostate, Surg. Gyn. Obst. 129:505 (1972)
47. G.P. Murphy, Current Status of Therapy in Prostatic Cancer, in
     "Urologic Pathology: The Prostate", M. Tannenbaum (ed), Lea &
     Febiger, Philadelphia (1977) p. 225.
48. B. Stoliar and D.J. Albert, SCH 13521 in the Treatment of
     Advanced Carcinoma of the Prostate, J. Urol. 111:803 (1974).

ESTROGENS IN THE TREATMENT OF PROSTATIC CANCER

J. Altwein

Bundeswehrkrankenhaus Ulm
Ulm
West Germany

INTRODUCTION

Treatment with estrogens is the most commonly used modality for the management of advanced prostatic carcinoma (PCA). Their major mode of action is thought to be by the suppression of Lutenising Hormone (LH) and Follicle Stimulating Hormone (FSH) release from the pituitary to control the output of testosterone (1). Only chlorotrianisene (Tace^TM) does not exert an antigonadotrophic action. The decrease of plasma testosterone and testicular atrophy result primarily from the central gonadotrophin suppression; however, a direct inhibition of testosterone synthesis is also involved (2) (Table 1). There is evidence that estrogens inhibit the testicular

Table 1. Estrogen* Inhibition of Androgen Synthesis

Enzyme	Lowered Precursor	Author
17.20 Desmolase	Dihydroepiandrosterone	Samuels 1964 (48)
	Androstenedione	
3 β OH Steroid dehydrogenase	Progesterone	Goldman 1968 (49)
	17 α Progesterone	Yanaihara 1972 (2)
	Testosterone	
17 α Hydroylase	17 α OH Pregnenolone	Samuels 1964 (48)
	17 α OH Progesterone	

* Estradiol - 17 β and DES

317

Table 2. Testosterone Levels (ng/dl) in PCA After Treatment
          With Orchiectomy and Estrogens

| Author | Orchiectomy | DES (mg q.d.) | | | |
		.2	1.0	3.0	5.0
Young 1968 (50)	50				50
Robinson 1971 (4)	30			10	
Mackler 1972 (51)	50 ± 50			80	190
Kent 1973 (5)		700 ±276	410 ±359		130 ±110
Shearer 1973 (6)	47 ± 23		66 -86	45 ±20	47 ±25

3β -hydroxysteroid dehydrogenase, thus blocking the degradation of
pregnenolone, one step in the formation of testosterone in vivo (3).
Since steroidogenesis inhibition requires a high dose of estrogen,
this mechanism may only be operative with chlorotrianisene.

The drop in plasma testosterone is dose dependent (Table 2):
1 mg. diethylstilbestrol does not cause uniform testosterone suppression whereas 3 mg. is generally regarded as effective as 30 mg. (4-6)
despite a recent study comparing testosterone levels in castrated
males and intact males receiving 1 mg. diethylstilbestrol for prostatic carcinoma (7) in which the results showed little change in
hormonal levels after six months in either group. The increase in
sex hormone binding globulin (SHBG) which reduces the percentage of
biologically active testosterone is a further beneficial effect of
estrogen therapy (8).

Table 3. Five-Year Survival After Estrogen Treatment for PCA.
          The Influence of the Degree of Differentiation

Grade	Schirmer et al. 1965 (52)	Esposti et al. 1971 (53)	Faul et al. 1977 (54)
I	90%	67.9%	59.6%
II	71%	54.7%	65.5%
III	65%	11.0%	35.8%
IV	52%	./.	32.1%

Besides their "extraprostatic" action estrogens exert some kind of end organ antagonism at the prostate itself.   In 1958 Franks (9) stated that estrogens will consistently produce cytologic damage to prostatic carcinoma cells, depending on the degree of differentiation (Table 3).   Cosgrove et al (10) treated nine patients with stage T3-4 prostatic carcinoma with estrogens only, and carried out a further biopsy after 12 months.   In four patients no tumor cells were found, confirmed by total prostatectomy in one patient. Furthermore, estrogens interfere with the 5α-reductase (11) and DNA polymerase (12) of the tumor cell.   This direct nuclear site of estrogen action, however, requires high doses which cannot be achieved in man.   Chronic estrogen treatment enhances the catabolism of the weak oxidized androgens (13).   Furthermore, estrogen can serve as an effective competitor for dihydrotestosterone binding to the high affinity androphile, an action which coincides with the ability of systemically administered estrogens to block the binding of H3-androgens to their receptors (14).

Recently specific estradiol receptor protein has been demonstrated in prostatic carcinoma (15), the presence of which is, according to Sidh et al (16), a guide to estrogen-sensitive tumors.

CLINICAL APPLICATION OF ESTROGENS IN PROSTATIC CARCINOMA

Since Strohm's attempts to ease pain with estrogens in patients with cancer of the prostate (17), a multitude of reports dealing with a variety of estrogenic preparations (Table 4) have appeared in the literature.   The experience accumulated to date may be summarized as follows:

Estrogens in Early Carcinoma of the Prostate

The five-year survival rates using different estrogens vary considerably but in retrospective studies a compound-related effect does not emerge.   More interestingly the 10 and 15-year survival rates are remarkably similar in patients with and without total prostatectomy (Table 5).

The prospective studies (Table 6) do not show a significant difference at five and 12 years.   Even though a word of caution is necessary, the effectiveness of estrogens in controlling intracapsular tumor is worth stating.   At any rate, one should realize that the response rate of the tumor to estrogen application is dependent upon the degree of differentiation (Table 3).   Recently, Sinha et al (18) have shown that the ultrastructural features of prostatic cancer cells permit the distinction of two basal cell types: type I (light) cells are estrogen-sensitive, whereas type II (dark) cells are refractory to hormones.

Table 4. Estrogens Used for the Treatment of Prostatic Carcinoma

Class	Drug	Dose	Remarks
Conjugated estrogens	Premarin	2.5 - 7.5 mg/d p.o.	used in VACURG III
Stilbene derivatives	DES	1 - 3 mg/d p.o.	reference estrogen
	Dienestrol	5 mg/d p.o.	very active
	Hexestrol	5 mg/d p.o.	somewhat less active
	Diethylstilbestrol diphosphate (Honvan)	360 mg/d p.o. 1.2 g/d i.v. (10 days)	active excellent palliation
	Chlorotrianisene (TACE)	12 - 24 mg/d p.o.	no LH suppression, no PRL release
Ester of estradiol	Ethinylestradiol	0.6 mg/d p.o.	very active; used in combination with a long acting estrogen
	Estradiol undecylate	100 mg/month i.m.	long acting
	Polyestradiol phosphate	40 - 80 mg/month i.m.	long acting
Combination with nitrogen mustard	Estramustine phosphate	560 mg/d p.o.	secondary treatment
Organosilicone	Cisobitan	900 mg/d p.o.	active, rather toxic

Table 5.   Estrogens in Early (T1-2 N0,x M0) PCA:
           Retrospective Studies

Author	No.	Treatment	Survival
Barnes, 1969 (55)	108	TUR + Stilbestrol and/or Orchiectomy	57% (10 years) 33% (15 years)
Belt, 1942 (56)	160	Stilbestrol + Prostatectomy	46% (10 years) 21% (15 years)
Bennett, 1970 (57)	30	Stilbestrol	56% (5 years)
	34	Tace	67% (5 years)
	37	Ethinyl estradiol	81% (5 years)
Belt and Schroeder, 1971 (58)	222	Stilbestrol + Prostatectomy	78.6% (5 years)

Estrogens in Advanced Carcinoma of the Prostate

The first convincing evidence of the efficacy of estrogens was provided by Nesbit and Baum in 1950 employing historical controls for comparison (19).   Further proof has been obtained by two large-scale retrospective studies in which classical "androgen control" therapy (orchiectomy plus estrogens) led to a 15.5% five-year and 3.9% 10-year survival rate (20).   Results of orchiectomy alone were somewhat inferior (five-year survival 11.6%) and estrogens alone slightly superior (five-year survival 21.4%).   These retrospective findings were confirmed by a prospective trial conducted by the Veterans Administration Cooperative Urological Research Group (VACURG) in patients with locally advanced and disseminated prostatic carcinoma (21), from which the following facts emerged:

1.   placebo as initial therapy was the worst treatment in terms of nine-year survival,

2.   estrogen alone was superior, and

3.   survival with orchiectomy plus estrogens was slightly better than with orchiectomy plus placebo (comparable to orchiectomy alone in Emmett's (20) retrospective study).

Thus, two independent trials demonstrated that estrogens are

Table 6. Estrogens in Early (T0-2 NO/NX,MO) PCA:
           Prospective Studies

Author	No.	Treatment	Survival	P	Remarks
Byar, 1972 (59)	148	Placebo	46% (5 years)		no cancer deaths
		Stilbestrol	59% (5 years)		
		Orchiectomy + Placebo	52% (5 years)		
		Orchiectomy + Stilbestrol	31% (5 years)	n.s.	
Madsen, 1980 (60)	120 Stage I	Stilbestrol + Prostatectomy	31% (12 years)		19 cardio-vasc. deaths
		Placebo + Prostatectomy	35% (12 years)		17 "
	179 Stage II	Stilbestrol + Prostatectomy	35% (12 years)		29 "
		Placebo + Prostatectomy	32% (12 years)	n.s.	26 "

somewhat effective in retarding the course of prostatic carcinoma.
The first VACURG study, however, indicated that lethal cardiovascular
side effects more than offset the retardation of tumor growth.   The
second VACURG study revealed a strong influence of the estrogen dose
in stage III disease (patients with potential longevity) and a weak
influence in stage IV prostatic carcinoma (21).

    Even though, the action of "androgen control" treatment is
cancerostatic rather than cancerocidal (22) it apparently prolongs
life (23) and provides excellent palliation in advanced disease.
There are some long term survivors even with prostatic carcinoma at
this stage (24).   A recent retrospective study by de Vere White et
al (25) revealed a 40% (17/42 patients) five-year and 12% (5/42)
10-year survival following orchiectomy and estrogen therapy.   Recently Lepor et al (26) have shown in a non-concurrent prospective
study that estrogen treatment reduced the tumor death rate by 45%
(62 patients without endocrine treatment vs 54 patients with estrogen
treatment - p < .004).

DOSAGE OF ESTROGENS

The recommended dose of the standard estrogen diethylstilbestrol has ranged from .25 mg. q.d. (27) to 100 mg. q.d. (28). Occasionally even 1000 mg. q.d. has been given (29). Whether or not it is useful to start with doses between 30-100 mg. reducing to a maintenance dose between 1-3 mg. is not clear. In metastatic disease the optimal dose was investigated in the VACURG study II where 1 mg. diethylstilbestrol daily was found clinically sufficient and produced only a few adverse side effects. This also holds true for 3 mg. diethylstilbestrol daily (30). This appears to be the critical estrogen dose (31) to which the equieffective daily dose of other estrogen compounds is: 0.2 mg. ethinylestradiol, 360 mg. diethylstilbestrol diphosphate (Honvan[TM]), 24 mg. chlorotrianisene (Tace[TM]), and 7.5 mg. Premarin[TM], a natural conjugated water-soluble estrogen.

SIDE EFFECTS OF ESTROGENS

Although of great value in prostatic cancer estrogen therapy may also be accompanied by undesirable side effects. The most common include reversal of the normal masculine characteristics, decreased libido, impotence, gynecomastia, mastodynia, salt and water retention, and disturbance of the coagulation mechanism and of lipid metabolism. However, the use of estrogens has been particularly questioned in recent years for the following reasons:

Cardiovascular toxicity (myocardial infarction, cerebrovascular accidents, arteriosclerotic heart disease, pulmonary embolism) is a phenomenon to which Blanchot et al had already directed attention in 1952 (32). This observation passed more or less unnoticed until the famous first VACURG study (33) proved that the estrogen arms had a cardiovascular death rate of 42% each vs 33% and 35%, respectively in the non-estrogen arms for stage III (C) cancer and 36% and 27% vs 24% and 27%, respectively for stage IV (D) cancer. It is noteworthy that these differences are obvious only when comparing the estrogen with the arm in which placebo was given as the initial therapy. Further investigation on this subject has made it clear that patients with pre-existing cardiovascular disease are particularly at risk and that the cardiovascular side effects are dose-related. This toxicity was particularly distressing for patients with potential longevity, e.g. stage III (C) tumors, where 5 mg. diethylstilbestrol led to an excess of non-cancer deaths as compared to 1 mg. which still seemed to produce equal survival rates. The risk may be further reduced if those patients with elevated triglyceride- and plasminogen levels (34,35) are excluded or receive an inhibitor of platelet aggregation.

Hyperprolactinemia. Ratner et al in 1963 were the first to demonstrate the ability of estrogens to stimulate release of prolactin from the pituitary (37). Boyns et al in 1974 found a dose and drug-related effect (38) and Jacobi (39) has summarized all the evidence regarding the positive influence of prolactin on the testis, adrenal gland and the prostate itself. Hanafy et al (40) brought up the point that the hyperprolactinemia may be responsible for the development of estrogen resistance of the tumor.

Impairment of the immune response. Estrogen and prolactin are active in this regard (41).

Hepatic toxicity and salt and water-retention.

Psychic alterations requiring psychiatric treatment have been observed in 40% of the patients (44).

SUMMARY AND CONCLUSION

Estrogens are active concerostatic drugs in early prostatic cancer producing survival rates which can match far more radical means of treatment. Their use in patients with low-stage cancer and potential longevity has been discredited mainly due to serious adverse side effects. However long term survivors have been reported even in metastatic tumors. In addition estrogens have been recognized as providing excellent palliation.

Simultaneous castration has not been proven to be superior to estrogen treatment alone. The value of delayed castration in estrogenized men is not yet clear (45). Delayed estrogen treatment in patients subjected to castration only as suggested by Menon et al (46) does not slow down the progression of cancer (47).

In the EORTC Urological Group studies (reported in this volume) none of the alternative treatments has yet been shown to be superior to Stilbestrol, though some may have less cardiovascular toxicity. Therefore it seems reasonable to replace estrogen treatment for metastatic disease in asymptomatic patients by other compounds, e.g. cyproterone acetate, and to reserve the palliative effect of estrogens for those patients presenting with serious symptoms related to their prostatic carcinoma.

REFERENCES

1. H.W.G. Baker, H.G. Burger, D.M. DeKretser, B. Hudson and W.G. Straffon, Effects of Synthetic Oral Estrogens in Normal Men and Patients with Prostatic Carcinoma: Lack of Gonadotrophin Suppression by Chlorotrianisene, Clin. Endocrinol, 2:297 (1973).

2. T. Yanaihara and P. Troen, Studies of the Human Testis. III. Effect of Estrogen on Testosterone Formation in Human Testis in vitro, J. Clin. Endocrinol. Metab. 34:968 (1972)

3. P.C. Walsh, Physiological Basis for Hormonal Therapy in Carcinoma of the Prostate, Urol. Clin. N Amer. 2:125 (1975).

4. M.R.G. Robinson and B.S. Thomas, Effect of Hormonal Therapy on Plasma Testosterone Levels in Prostate Carcinoma, B.M.J. 4:391 (1971).

5. J.R. Kent, A.J. Bischoft, L.J. Arduino, G.T. Mellinger, D.P. Byar, M. Hill and X. Kozbor, Estrogen Dosage and Suppression of Testosterone Levels in Patients with Prostatic Carcinoma, J. Urol, 109:858 (1973).

6. R.T. Shearer, W.F. Hendry, I.F. Sommerville and J.D. Fergusson, Plasma Testosterone: An Accurate Monitor of Hormone Treatment in Prostatic Cancer, Brit. J. Urol. 45:668 (1973).

7. H.H. Beck, H. McAninch, J.W. Goebel and R.E. Stutzman, Plasma Testosterone in Patients Receiving Diethylstilbestrol. Urology, 11:157 (1978).

8. A.L. Houghton, R. Turner and E.H. Cooper, Sex Hormone Binding Globulin in Carcinoma of the Prostate, Brit. J. Urol. 49:227 (1977).

9. L.M. Franks, Some Comments on the Long-Term Results of Endocrine Treatment of Prostatic Cancer, Brit. J. Urol. 30:383 (1958).

10. M.D. Cosgrove, F.W. George III and R. Terry, The Effects of Treatment on the Local Lesion of Carcinoma of the Prostate, J. Urol, 109:861 (1973).

11. J. Shimazaki, T. Horaguchi and Y. Ohki, Properties of Testosterone 5 Alpha-Reductase of Purified Nuclear Fraction from Ventral Prostate of Rats, Endocr. Japan 18:179 (1971).

12. M.E. Harper, A.R. Fahmy, C.G. Pierrepoint and K. Griffiths, The Effect of Some Stilbestrol Compounds on DNA Polymerase from Human Prostatic Tissues, Steroids 15:89 (1970).

13. J.S. Jenkins and V.M. McCafferty, Effect of Estradiol 17β and Progesterone on the Metabolism of Testosterone by Human Prostatic Tissue, J. Endocrinol. 63:517 (1974).

14. P. Rennie and N. Bruchovsky, Studies on the Relationship Between Androgen Receptors and the Transport of Androgens in Rat Prostate, J. Biol. Chem. 248:3288 (1973).

15. E.F. Hawkins, M. Nijs and C. Brassinne, Steroid Receptors in Human Prostate. 2. Some Properties of the Estrophilic Molecule of Benign Prostatic Hypertrophy. Biochem. Biophys. Res. Commun. 70:854 (1976).

16. S.M. Sidh, J.D. Young, S.A. Karmi, J.R. Powder and N. Bashirelahi, Adenocarcinoma of Prostate: Role of 17 -Beta Estradiol and 5 Alpha-Dihydrotestosterone Binding Proteins, Urology. 13:597 (1979).

17. J.G. Strohm, Carcinoma of the Prostate, Urol. Cutan. Rev. 45:770 (1935).

18. A.A. Sinha, C.E. Blackard and U.S. Seal, A Critical Analysis of Tumor Morphology and Hormone Treatments in the Untreated and Estrogen-Treated Responsive and Refractory Human Prostatic Carcinoma, Cancer 49:2836 (1977).

19. R. Nesbit and W. Baum, Endocrine Control of Prostatic Carcinoma, J.A.M.A. 143:1317 (1950).
20. J.L. Emmett, L.F. Greene and A. Papantoniou, Endocrine Therapy in Carcinoma of the Prostate Gland: 10-Year Survival Studies, J. Urol. 83:471 (1960).
21. D.P. Byar, The VACURG Studies of Cancer of the Prostate, Cancer, 32:1126 (1973).
22. C. Bouffioux, Le Cancer de la Prostate, Acta. Urol. Belg. 47:189 (1979).
23. W.G. Reiner, W.W. Scott, J.C. Eggleston and P.C. Walsh, Long-Term Survival After Hormonal Therapy for Stage D Prostatic Cancer, J. Urol. 122:183 (1979).
24. W.S. Falkowski and V.J. O'Conor Jr., Long-Term Survivor of Prostatic Carcinoma with Lung Metastases, J. Urol. 125:260 (1981)
25. R. De Vere White, D.F. Paulson and J.F. Glenn, The Clinical Spectrum of Prostatic Cancer, J. Urol. 117:323 (1977).
26. H. Lepor, A. Ross and P.C. Walsh, Hormonal Therapy Prolongs Survival in Advanced Prostatic Cancer, AUA Abstract, May 1980.
27. R. Baker, Studied on Cancer Prevention in Urology. I. Prostate, Ann. Surg. 137:29 (1953).
28. J.D. Fergusson, Prostatic Cancer - Endocrine Therapy, in "Malignant Disease", B.A. Stoll (ed), W.B. Saunders, London, (1972) p. 237.
29. G. Jönsson and T. Nilsson, Pharmacology of Drug Therapy, in "Scientific Foundations of Urology", D.I. Williams and G.D. Chisholm (eds), William Heinemann Medical Books, London, (1976) p. 347.
30. M. Pavone-Macaluso, F. Lund, J.H. Mulder, P.H. Smith, M. De Pauw, R. Sylvester and EORTC GU Group, EORTC Protocols in Prostatic Cancer. An Interim Report, Scand J. Urol. Nephrol. Suppl. 55:163 (1980).
31. J.E. Altwein, Hormontherapie des Prostatakarzinoms, in "Chemotherapie Urologischer Malignome", G.H. Jacobi and J.E. Altwein (eds), Karger, München, (1979) p. 78.
32. H. Blanchot and F. Laporte, Traitement Hormonal des Neoformations Prostatiques, Rapport 46me Session, AFU. Imprimérie Saints Peres, Paris (1952) p. 5.
33. VACURG, Treatment and Survival of Patients with Cancer of the Prostate, Surg. Gynecol. Obstet, 124:1011 (1967).
34. U.S. Seal, R.P. Doe, D.P. Byar, D.K. Corle and VACURG, Response of Serum Cholesterol and Triglycerides to Hormone Treatment and the Relation of Pretreatment Values to Mortality in Patients with Prostatic Cancer, Cancer 38:1095 (1976).
35. U.S. Seal, R.P. Doe, D.P. Byar, D.K. Corle and VACURG, Response of Plasma Fibrinogen and Plasminogen to Hormone Treatment and the Relation of Pretreatment Values to Mortality in Patients with Prostatic Cancer, Cancer 38:1108 (1976).
36. M. Eisen, H.E. Napp and R. Vock, Inhibition of Platelet Aggregation Caused by Estrogen Treatment in Patients with Carcinoma of the Prostate, J. Urol. 114:93 (1975).

37. A. Ratner, P.K. Talwalker and J. Meiter, Effect of Estrogen Administration in vivo on Prolactin Release by Rat Pituitary in vitro, Proc. Soc. Exp. Biol. Med. 112:12 (1963).

38. A.R. Boyns, E.N. Cole, M.E.A. Philips, S.G. Hillier, E.H.D. Cameron, K. Griffiths, M. Shahmanesh, R.C.L. Feneley and M. Hartog, Plasma Prolactin, GH, LH, FSH, TSH and Testosterone During Treatment of Prostatic Carcinoma with Estrogen, Eur. J. Cancer 10:445 (1974).

39. G.H. Jacobi, Palliativtherapie des Prostatkarzinoms, Zuckschwerdt Verlag, München (1980).

40. H.M. Hanafy, E. Gursel and R.J. Veenema, A Possible Role of Sertoli Cells in Prostatic Cancer Refractory to Estrogen: A Preliminary Report, J. Urol. 108:914 (1972).

41. R.A. Karmali, I. Lauder and D.F. Horrobin, Prolactin and the Immune Response, Lancet ii:106 (1974).

42. M. Kontturri and E. Sotaniemi, Effect of Estrogen on Liver Function of Prostatic Cancer Patients, B.M.J. i:204 (1969).

43. U. Kunze and F. Orestano, Intra- und Estrazelluläre Elektrolyt-konzentration unter Ostrogen-Therapie bei Prostatakarzinom-Patienten, Urologe A 12:274 (1973).

44. H. Köhler, Zur Behandlung des Prostatkarzinoms mit Polyestra-diolphosphat (Estradurin™), Inaugural-Disseration, Würzburg (1978).

45. L. Denis and P. Nowe, Bilateral Orchiectomy in Patients with Progressive Advanced Prostatic Cancer, Acta Urol. Belg. 48:113 (1980).

46. M. Menon and P.C. Walsh, Hormonal Therapy for Prostatic Cancer, in "Prostatic Cancer", G.P. Murphy (ed), P.S.G. Publishing Co., Littleton (Mass.), (1979) p. 175.

47. H. Brendler and G. Prout, A Cooperative Group Study of Prostatic Cancer: Stilbestrol vs. Placebo in Advanced Progressive Disease, Cancer Chemother. Rep. 16:323 (1962).

48. L.T. Samuels, J.G. Shirt and R.A. Huseby, The Effect of Diethyl-stilbestrol on Testicular 17 Alpha-Hydroxylase and 17-Desmolase Activities in BALB/C Mice, Acta Endocrinol. 45:487 (1964).

49. A.S. Goldman, Further Studies of Steroidal Inhibitors of Delta-5-3 Beta-Hydroxysteroid Dehydrogenase and Delta 5 - Delta 4, 3 Beta-Ketosteroid Isomerase in Pseudomonas Testosteroni and in Bovine Adrenals, J. Clin. Endocrinol. 28:1539 (1968).

50. H.H. Young and J.R. Kent, Plasma Testosterone Levels in Patients with Prostatic Carcinoma Before and After Treatment, J. Urol. 99:788 (1968).

51. M.A. Mackler, J.P. Liberti, M.J.V. Smith, W.W. Koontz and G.R. Prout, The Effect of Orchiectomy and Various Doses of Stilbestrol on Plasma Testosterone Levels in Patients with Carcinoma of the Prostate, Invest. Urol. 9:423 (1972).

52. H.K.A. Schirmer, G.P. Murphy and W.W. Scott, Hormonal Therapy of Prostatic Cancer: A Correlation Between Histologic Differ-entiation of Prostatic Cancer and the Clinical Course of the Disease, Urol. Digest 3:15 (1965).

53. P.L. Esposti, Cytologic Malignancy Grading of Prostatic Carcinoma by Transrectal Aspiration Biopsy. A Five-Year Follow-Up Study of 469 Hormone-Treated Patients, Scand. J. Urol. Nephrol. 5:198 (1971).

54. P. Faul, E. Schmiedt and R. Kern, Die Prognostische Bedeutung des Zytologischen Differenzierungsgrades beim Ostrogenbehandelten Prostata-Carcinom, Urologe A 17:377 (1978).

55. R.W. Barnes, R.T. Bergman, H.L. Hadley and A.L. Dick, Early Prostatic Cancer: Long-Term Results with Conservative Treatment, J. Urol. 102:88 (1969).

56. E. Belt, Radical Perineal Prostatectomy in Early Carcinoma of the Prostate, J. Urol. 48:287 (1942).

57. A.H. Bennett, J.B. Dowd and J.H. Harrison, Estrogen and Survival Data in Carcinoma of the Prostate, Surg. Gyn. Obst. 129:505 (1970).

58. E. Belt and F.H. Schroeder, Östrogenbehandlung des Prostata-karzinoms nach Totaler Prostatektomie: Uberlebensraten und Cardiovasculäre Komplikationen in den serien von Mellinger und Belt, Urologe A 10:56 (1971).

59. D.P. Byar, Treatment of Prostatic Cancer: Studies by the VACURG, Bull. N.Y. Acad. Med. 48:751 (1972).

60. P.O. Madsen, S. Maigaard, D.K. Corle and D.P. Byar, Radical Prostatectomy for Carcinoma of the Prostate, Stages I and II, in "Proceedings. II. International Symposium on the Treatment of Carcinoma of the Prostate, Rost & Fiedler, Berlin (1978) p.46.

TREATMENT OF PROSTATIC CANCER WITH DIETHYLSTILBOESTROL –

DETECTION AND EVALUATION OF THE VASCULAR RISK

C.C. Abbou, V. Beaumont, D. Chopin, J.P. Deburge,
J.L. Beaumont and J. Auvert

Hôpital Henri-Mondor
Creteil
France

SUMMARY

A retrospective study of patients suffering from prostatic cancer and treated with estrogens has allowed us to develop a test to discriminate a population with a high risk of thrombotic complications due to estrogens from a population that can benefit without danger from this form of hormonal therapy. The so-called "estrogen tolerance test" relies on the presence of circulating immune complexes which can be precipitated from serum by 25% saturated ammonium sulphate.

In the group of patients in which immune complexes exceeded 700 μg/ml, 41% developed thrombo-embolic complications including embolism and arterial thrombosis. The group of patients in whom the values were under 300 μg/ml had a lower risk of arterial thrombosis (2.5%) and the observed incidents were benign and mostly venous thrombosis.

Test values above 700 μg/ml should preclude treatment with diethylstilboestrol.

INTRODUCTION

The treatment of prostatic carcinoma by estrogens is associated with an elevated risk of venous and arterial thrombosis (1). In women, oral contraception using combined therapy with estrogens and progestogens is also responsible for an increase in the incidence of vascular thrombosis (2,3,4).

The discovery of circulating immune complexes (C.I.C.) containing
a monoclonal IgG with anti-ethinyl estradiol activity (5) which could
be precipitated by ammonium sulphate at 25% saturation in the serum
of a woman who had suffered a pulmonary embolism whilst taking the
pill, led to the development of a simple test of serum precipitation
which was shown to precipitate almost exclusively immunoglobulins and
complement fractions, a finding consistent with precipitation of
C.I.C. (6). These C.I.C. were later shown to contain anti-ethinyl
estradiol antibodies in several cases (7).

The test was used to detect the vascular risk in women on oral
contraceptives.

The immune complex precipitation test was positive in 95% of
women who had suffered vascular thrombosis while using the pill. In
those who had not experienced such a complication, there were two
different groups, one in which the test was found to be negative,
even after years of use and a second group in which the test was positive. The latter group could be considered "at risk" (8). This paper
presents the results of this test applied to patients suffering from
prostatic cancer who were or were not treated by estrogens.

MATERIAL AND METHOD

Three groups of patients were selected for this study, a group
of 65 patients with prostatic cancer treated with varying doses of
diethylstilboestrol (D.E.S.) ranging from 1 - 25 mgs per day, a
second group of 19 patients with untreated prostatic cancer, and
a third group of 25 men of about the same age, in apparently good
health and with no evidence of any cancer.

The detection of circulating immune complexes was achieved by
precipitation of serum in 25% saturated ammonium sulphate. The proteins were measured by the method of Lowry and expressed in μg/ml
(6,8).

RESULTS

Thrombosis

Thrombotic complications were found in 12 of 84 patients (14.2%)
before treatment with D.E.S., and in 18 of 65 (22.7%) patients
treated with D.E.S. The difference is significant (p < 0.05).

In patients treated with D.E.S. the observed venous thrombotic
complications were nine cases of venous thrombosis and two cases of
pulmonary embolism. In addition, seven cases of arterial thrombosis
occurred including four cases of coronary thrombosis and one cerebral
thrombosis and two patients with thrombosis in a limb.

The influence of D.E.S. dosage in the 57 cases in which dosages are known with precision is shown in Figure 1. Of the patients, seven were treated with 1 mg per day. In this group one case of venous thrombosis was observed, the incidence of complications being similar to the group without estrogens. Twenty-seven patients received doses of 2 - 3 mg. of D.E.S. per day. In this group eight cases of thrombosis were seen (30%) of which four were venous thrombosis, two were pulmonary embolism or pulmonary artery thrombosis and two developed systemic arterial thromboses. Twenty-three patients received at least 5 mg. of D.E.S. per day. In this group eight cases of thrombosis were seen (35%), three cases of venous thrombosis and five of systemic arterial thrombosis. The mean duration of estrogenic treatment was no different in patients with and without thrombosis, being 17.6 ± 33.1 months during the first group and 16 ± 13.9 months in the second ($p > 0.1$). The thrombosis appeared at the earliest 12 dyas and at the latest 12 years after starting treatment.

Immune complex precipitation test

The average quantity of proteins precipitated in 25% saturated ammonium sulphate expressed in μg of protein per ml of serum was the same in the control group and in the group with untreated prostatic cancer (Table 1). These values were 387 ± 197 μg and 396 ± 294 μg respectively, with extreme values between 0 and 800 μg. The distribution curve was unimodal (Fig. 2A).

In the group treated with D.E.S., the mean quantity of precipitated proteins was 746 ± 698 μg/ml with extreme values ranging from 94 to 2,400 μg. The distribution was bimodal with two subpopulations as shown in Figure 2B - a subgroup similar to the control group and a further group above the normal values. This second subgroup represented 27 of the 65 patients treated by D.E.S.

These two sub populations did not differ statistically with regard to mean age (71 and 75 years respectively), length of treatment (12.1 and 17.3 months), or dosage (4.7 and 4.6 mg of D.E.S. per day).

Relation between increase in immune complexes and thrombosis

Among the 65 treated subjects, 47 suffered no thrombosis on treatment. In this group the mean value of precipitated immune complexes was 687.9 ± 676 ug/ml. In the 18 patients who suffered thrombosis the mean value was 839.2 ± 716 ug/ml. This is not significantly different from the above group.

The distribution of the values in these two groups however is not homogeneous as the distribution was bimodal, as it was in the group suffering thrombosis (Fig. 3). However, when the frequency of

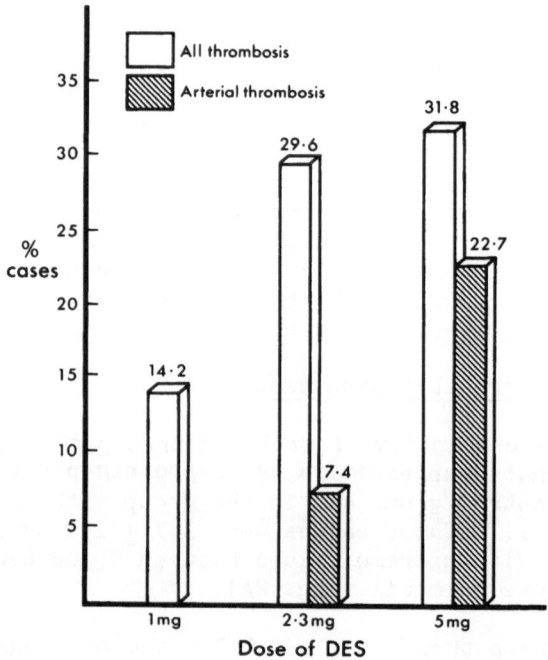

Fig. 1. Frequency of vascular thromboses in relation to the
dose of D.E.S.

Table 1. Precipitation test of serum proteins
in 25% saturated $(NH_4)_2SO_4$ solution

Group	No. of patients	Proteins ug/ml	T
Controls	24	387.7	197.7
Untreated cancers	19	396.6	294.0
Treated cancers	65	746.1	698.0

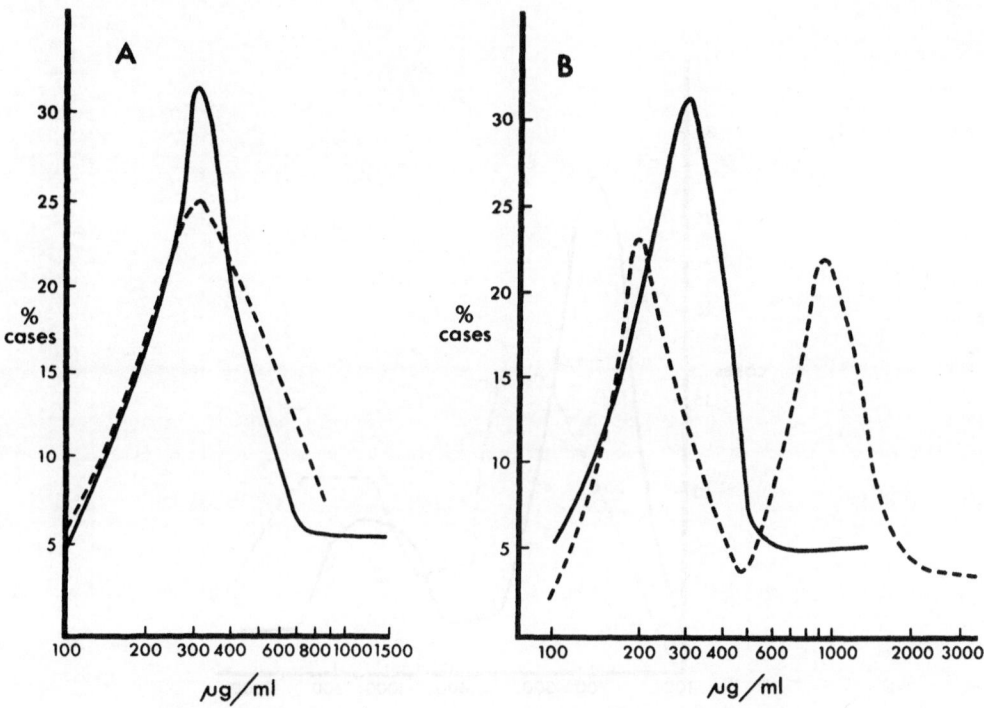

Fig. 2. Distribution of patients based on the quantity of immuno-
         globulins precipitated by 25% ammonium sulphate solution.
         A: dotted line - controls. solid line - patients with un-
            treated prostatic cancer. The distribution is normal for
            these two populations.
         B: solid line - patients with an untreated prostatic cancer.
            dotted line - patients with prostatic cancer treated with
            D.E.S. The treated patients exhibit a bimodal distri-
            bution.

thrombosis in the total treated population was analysed as a function
of the critical value of 700 μg/ml, it may be seen from Table 2 that
thrombotic complications were more frequent in the group with high
values (nine of 27 patients) than in the group with low values (nine
of 38 patients), and that they were of a different type, nearly all
venous thrombosis occuring in the group with low values (eight out of
nine cases, $p < 0.05$) whereas arterial thrombosis (six out of seven
cases, $p < 0.02$) were seen in the group with high values.

The two cases of pulmonary embolism which also had high values
were classified separately. The lack of signs suggesting either pelvic or lower extremity phlebitis in these two cases suggests the possibility that they were due to pulmonary arterial thrombosis and not
to embolism.

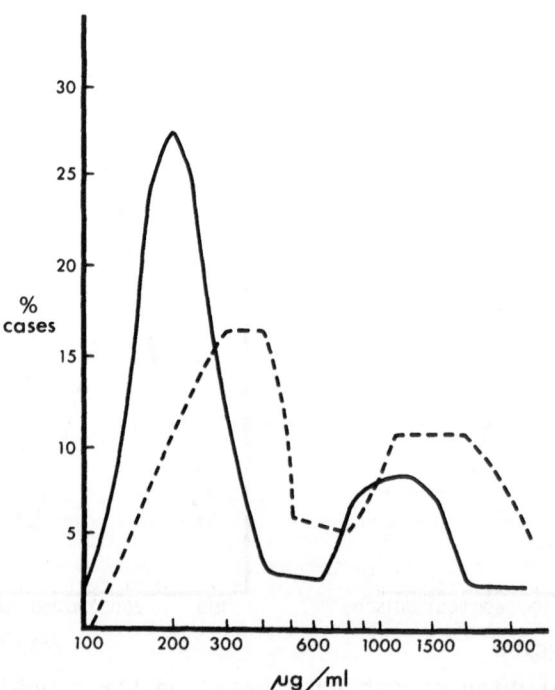

Fig. 3. Distribution of patients treated with D.E.S., based on the
         values of precipitated immunoglobulins. solid line -
         patients without, and dotted line - patients with
         vascular thromboses.

Table 2. Thromboses and precipitation test of serum
          proteins in 25% saturated $(NH_4)_2SO_4$ solution

Protein precipitates in $\mu g/ml$ of serum	< 700	>700	p
No. of patients	38	27	
No. of thromboses	9 (23.6%)	9 (33.3%)	
- venous thrombosis	8	1	<0.05
- arterial thrombosis	1	6	<0.02
- pulmonary embolus or pulmonary artery thrombosis	0	2	

DISCUSSION

     After reviewing the pertinent literature one is inclined to
revise the classical notion of the benignity of estrogen treatment of
prostatic cancer. In TO cancers, the global mortality rate is greater
in the group treated with D.E.S. as a result of thrombo-embolic accidents. In cases where the tumor is clinically perceptible and metastases are present, treatment with D.E.S. does not significantly modify
the survival rate, for the increased mortality due to thrombo-embolic
complications more than compensates for the decreased mortality due
to the drug's anti-cancer effect (1,9.10).

     If it became possible to identify patients in whom the estrogen
related thrombo-embolic risk was minimal, it would be tempting to
continue to offer them the opportunity of treatment with D.E.S.,
whose anti-tumoral effectiveness has been clearly established (11-16).

     The test that has been used here relies on the detection of cir-
culating immune complexes containing antibodies to estrogens. It was
developed to study the vascular risk in women using oral contraceptives and has been responsible for the discrimination of a group of
women at special risk, evaluated as being about 30% of users. This
test is positive in 95% of women who have suffered a thrombosis.

     In prostatic cancer, the same test used in patients treated with
D.E.S. allows one to distinguish two populations, (i) a group with
values less than 300 μg/ml in which the probability of arterial thrombosis is small (2.5%) and the observed cardiovascular complications
are those of venous thrombosis and (ii) a group with values above
700 μg/ml in which the thrombo-embolic risk is probably above 30%
with serious complications such as pulmonary embolism and arterial
thrombosis. In our study this group represents 41% of treated subjects.

     These findings are the basis for an argument in favor of a ther-
apeutic attitude based upon the evaluation of the tumoral risk, the
iatrogenic risk of D.E.S. and the eventual benefits that the patient
may gain from such treatment. Small doses of D.E.S. 2 mg per day or
less should be recommended, while, at the same time, monitoring
C.I.C. and plasma testosterone values (17). Patients treated with
D.E.S. for three months, whose C.I.C. levels are above 300 μg/ml,
should ideally be treated by other means. However, when other forms
of therapy are impractical and the C.I.C. levels are between 300 and
700 μg/ml, continuing treatment with D.E.S. is probably acceptable.

     A test value above 700 μg/ml should exclude D.E.S. treatment no
matter what the observed tumoral situation is. Moreover, therapeutic
safety could possibly be enhanced through study of the blood coagulation factors.

In fact, the physiopathologic mechanisms responsible for the arterial and venous thrombosis seen in prostatic cancers treated with D.E.S. may not be univocal.

As we have seen, a number of thromboses, essentially those due to arterial thrombosis, appear to be associated with the presence of circulating immune complexes. In one case it was demonstrated that these complexes contained an immunoglobulin that reacted specifically with D.E.S. (18) in the same way that immunoglobulins found in women using oral contraception reacted with ethinyl-estradiol (7). These estrogen-antiestrogen complexes could be a cause of endothelial alteration, leading to thromboses (19) and may be compared to the experimental vasculitis due to immune complexes (20). In these cases the lesions increase with the quantity of foreign proteins injected. Even though a dose related effect was observed in our study, it must be stressed that immune complexes appear even for small doses of D.E.S. and that vascular thromboses are also seen in women taking low dose oral contraceptives.

Concerning the fact observed in our study that venous thromboses do not seem to be correlated with the presence of immune complexes, it may be due to the fact that many other factors predisposing to venous thrombosis exist in these aged men suffering from a disease which is thrombogenic in itself.

REFERENCES

1.   D.P. Byar, Treatment of prostatic cancer : studies by the Veterans Administration Cooperative Urological Research Group, Bull. N.Y. Acad. Med. 48: 751 (1972).
2.   Collaborative Group for the Study of Stroke in Young Women, Oral contraception and increased risk of cerebral ischemia or thrombosis, N. Engl. J. Med. 288: 871 (1973).
3.   J.I. Mann, M.C. Vessey, M. Thorogood, and A. Doll, Myocardial infarction in young women with special reference to oral contraceptive practice, Br. Med. J. 2: 241 (1975).
4.   Report from the Boston Collaborative Drug Surveillance Program, Oral contraceptives and venous thrombo-embolic diseases, surgically confirmed gall-bladder disease and breast tumors, Lancet 1: 1399 (1973).
5.   J.L. Beaumont and N. Lemort, Oral contraceptives, pulmonary artery thrombosis and anti-ethinyl-oestradiol monoclonal IgG, Clin. Exper. Immunol. 24: 455 (1976).
6.   V. Beaumont, L. Lorenzelli-Edouard, N. Lemort, and J.L. Beaumont, Composition of circulating immune complexes induced by oral contraceptives, Biomedicine 30: 256 (1979).
7.   J.L. Beaumont, N. Lemort, L. Lorenzelli, B. Delplanque, and V. Beaumont, Antiethinylestradiol antibody activities in oral contraceptive users, Clin. Exper. Immunol. 38: 445 (1979).

8. V. Beaumont, N. Lemort, L. Lorenzelli, A. Mosser, and V. Beau-
    mont, Hormones contraceptives, risque vasculaire et précipit-
    abilité anormale des gamma-globulines sériques, Pathol. Biol.
    26: 531 (1978).

9. R.P. Doe and C.E. Blackard, Incidence of cardiovascular disease
    and death in patients receiving diethyl-stilbestrol for carcinoma
    of the prostate, Cancer 26: 249 (1970).

10. J.A. Heaney and H.C. Chang, Prognosis of clinically undiagnosed
    prostatic carcinoma and the influence of endocrine therapy,
    J. Urol. 118: 283 (1977).

11. E.F. Hawkins and M. Nijs, Steroid receptors in the human pros-
    tate. Detection of tissue-specific androgen binding in prostate
    cancer, Clin. Chim Acta 75: 303 (1977).

12. C. Huggins and C.V. Hodges, Studies on prostatic cancer, Cancer
    Res. 1: 293 (1941).

13. A.C. Jackson and M. Tenniswood, Effects of androgen and estradiol
    administration on the weights of the central prostate, seminal
    vesicles and testes of immature rats, Invest. Urol. 14:
    351 (1977).

14. M.W. Woodruff, The effect of estrogen and androgen on the rat
    prostate gland and testes, J. Urol. 84: 162 (1960).

15. M.W. Woodruff, The effect of hormonal modification on prostatic
    morphology, J. Urol. 88: 273 (1962).

16. J.D. Young and N. Bashirelahi, Specific binding protein for 17-
    beta-estradiol in prostate with adenocarcinoma, Urology 8:
    553 (1976).

17. P.H. Beck and W.J. McAninch, Plasma testosterone in patients
    receiving diethylstilbestrol, Urology 11: 157 (1978).

18. R.K. Kanis, G. Lasry, D. Melliere, V. Beaumont, and H. Botto,
    Thrombose aigue artérielle sévère sous oestrogénothérapie à
    forte dose, Nouv. Presse Méd. 7: 2396 (1978).

19. L. Irey, W.C. Havion, and H.B. Taylor, Vascular lesions in women
    taking oral contraceptives, Arch. Pathol. 89: 1 (1970).

20. F.J. Dixon, J.D. Feldman, and J.J. Vasquez, Experimental glom-
    erulonephritis. The pathogenesis of a laboratory model resem-
    bling the spectrum of human glomerulonephritis, J. Exper. Med.
    113: 899 (1961).

PROGESTINS IN PROSTATIC CANCER

L. Denis[1] and C. Bouffioux[2]

1. A.Z. Middelheim
   Antwerp
   Belgium

2. Hôpital de Bavière
   University of Liège
   Belgium

Progestins are synthetic compounds with progestational activity. One group of these compounds related to 17-alpha-hydroxyprogesterone has mainly progestational effects while another group exerts more anti-androgenic activity. This paper reviews the effect of treatment of the first group of compounds in patients with advanced prostatic cancer.

The first favourable and preliminary results with the then available progesterone compounds were reported more than thirty years ago (1,2). Subsequent reports in a small number of patients utilizing a series of progesterone derivatives - hydroxyprogesterone caproate (3), chlormadinone acetate (4) and megestrol acetate (5), have also yielded favourable results. The synthesis of a new semi-synthetic compound, medroxyprogesterone acetate (MAP), in 1958 (6,7) with high progestational activity and active by the oral route brought a well tolerated drug that has been widely used in clinical oncology especially in endocrine related tumors (8).

REPORTED RESULTS

MAP was used in low doses for long periods in two studies. Ferulano et al (9) treated thirty-four patients with locally advanced tumor of whom eleven also had metastases. Roughly half of the patients were previously treated by estrogens. The treatment scheme provided a total dose of MAP of 900 mg IM every five months with an interval rest of two months. Good objective and subjective results

were reported with no side effects over a period of twenty months
in all patients.

Kondo and Saito (10) treated ten patients with advanced tumor
and no previous therapy with oral doses of MAP of 15 to 50 mg/day
for one to eleven months. Objective improvement based on prostatic
size was noted in all patients. All patients had subjective improvement. No side effects were noted.

In the VACURG study III, MAP in low doses was compared to
Stilboestrol (DES), conjugated equine estrogens and the combination
MAP-DES. No significant differences in survival were noted in
patients with advanced prostatic cancer (11). Higher doses were
used by Rafla and Johnson (12). They treated twelve evaluable
patients with 300 mg/day orally. A satisfactory response was noted
in nine out of twelve patients with an average duration of four
months.

Bouffioux (13) reported on the response of forty untreated
prostatic cancers which were randomly given MAP or estrogens. MAP
was given at a dose of 500 mg IM 2 - 4 times a week for one month,
followed by 100 mg/day orally. A 40% objective remission rate was
observed with a mean duration of thirteen months. The results with
estrogens were somewhat better. Twelve patients in relapse on
estrogens were also treated with MAP. A good subjective result
was obtained in seven and an objective response in two.

Our own experience goes back to 1961 when we treated nine intact patients with advanced prostatic cancer in a pilot trial with
1 g/day orally for one month. No objective responses according to
the protocol were noted but three patients showed subjective response.
Seven cases were interrupted by a switch to bilateral orchiectomy in
the third week of the study (14). Another schedule was applied in
a second trial (15) where MAP was given in a loading dose of 3 x 500
mg IM weekly for two weeks, followed by an oral dose of 3 x 100 mg
for two weeks and a maintenance of a daily oral dose of 2 x 100 mg
for two months. In eleven patients with clinically advanced previously untreated prostatic cancer a partial remission was obtained
in six patients with a fair subjective response. In nine patients
with prostatic cancer in relapse only three patients showed some
subjective response and no objective response was noted.

DISCUSSION

It is difficult to give a clear view on the activity of MAP as
a single agent in patients with prostatic carcinoma due to the contradiction of data and the variability of the patients. It is however
safe to say that MAP treatment in new untreated cases of prostatic
cancer will bring objective partial and/or subjective remission in
some patients. However few subjective remissions have been noted in

patients with prostatic cancer in relapse and almost no objective
remissions.

In a preliminary study where the activity of MAP was compared
to diethylstilboestrol (DES) Bouffioux was able to conclude that MAP
seems less efficient than DES expressed in terms of duration of
remissions and survival (16). The decrease in plasma levels of
testosterone is notably slower than with bilateral orchiectomy or
DES treatment (15,16).

This decrease is a reflection of the pituitary inhibitory
activity of MAP which has been reported (17). The overall net benefit could however be attributed to a variety of pharmacological
actions demonstrated by MAP: interactions with circulating hormones,
competitive binding to 5 alpha-reductase, competitive binding to the
androgenic receptor sites and a direct toxic effect on tumor cells
(8). The role of progestins in prostatic cancer will relate to the
net result on the metabolic pathway of the androgens which is obtained
by a FSH-LH blockade, a competitive binding to 5 alpha-reductase and
the enhanced catabolism of circulating androgens (18) (Fig. 1). This
may explain the varied effects of progestins in selected cases.
Concerning its activity on prostatic cancer we hope that the EORTC
Urological Group's Protocol 30761 comparing the effect of cyproterone
acetate, medroxyprogesterone acetate and stilboestrol in patients
with advanced prostatic cancer stage T3 and T4 will allow a final
conclusion on the effect of MAP in prostatic cancer as a single
agent.

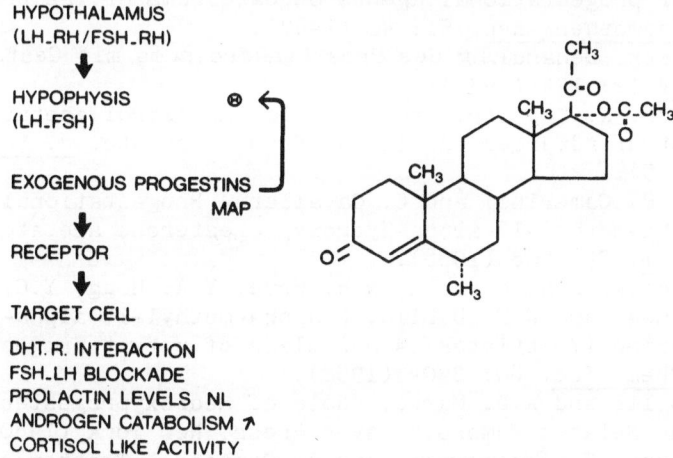

Fig. 1. Pathways of progestin activity in patients with
         prostatic cancer.

The rationale for the use of progestins in prostatic cancer has already been outlined by Scott in 1973 (19). At the moment we know that androgen, estrogen, progestin and prolactin receptors have been demonstrated in prostatic tissue with collateral activity of other hormones (20). It is possible that overall results will be improved by combination hormonal therapy eventually coupled to chemotherapy in earlier stages of the diseases (21). Combination hormonal treatment will be studied in a randomized way by the EORTC Urological Group in its protocol 30805 in which bilateral orchiectomy versus stilboestrol versus bilateral orchiectomy plus cyproterone acetate is to be evaluated in patients with metastatic prostatic cancer.

CONCLUSIONS

From the published data and our own clinical experience we conclude that MAP teatment as a single agent in patients with advanced prostatic cancer may show objective and subjective responses mainly in untreated cases.

The results obtained are probably inferior to those of standard treatment and future application of this drug may be in combination with other hormonal treatment.

REFERENCES

1. R. Gutierrez, New horizons in surgical management of carcinoma of the prostate gland, Amer. J. Surg. 78: 147 (1949).
2. J. Trunnel and B. Dubby, Influence of certain steroids on behaviour of human prostatic cancer, Trans. N.Y. Acad. Sci. 12: 238 (1950).
3. J. Geller, B. Fruchtman, H. Newman, J. Roberts, and R. Silva, Effect of progestational agents on carcinoma of the prostate, Cancer Chemother. Rep. 51: 41 (1967).
4. G. Popelier, Behandlung des Prostatakarcinoms mit Gestagenen, Urologe A 12: 134 (1973).
5. D. Johnson, K. Keasler, and A. Ayala, Megestrol acetate for treatment of advanced carcinoma of the prostate, J. Surg. Oncol. 7: 9 (1975).
6. G. Sala, B. Camerino, and C. Cavallero, Progestational activity of 6 alpha-methyl-17-alpha-hydroxyprogesterone acetate, Acta Endocrinol. 29: 508 (1958).
7. Y.C. Babcock, E.S. Gutsell, N.H. Heve, Y.A. Hogg, Y.C. Stucky, W.E. Barnes, and W.E. Dublin, 6 alpha-methyl-17 alpha-hydroxyprogesterone-17-acylates: A new class of potent progestins, J. Am. Chem. Soc. 80: 2904 (1958).
8. S. Iacobelli and A.D. Marco, "Role of Medroxyprogesterone in Endocrine Related Tumors," Raven Press, New York (1980), p.29.
9. O. Ferulano, F. Petrarola, and A. Castaldo, Trattamento del cancro della prostata con il controllo dell'arco dienfalo-ipofisario, Minerva Urologica 24: 274 (1972).

10. A. Kondo and Y. Saito, Gestagen Therapy of Benign Prostatic
    Hyperplasia and Prostatic Carcinoma, Jap. J. Urol. 36: 730
    (1974).

11. D.P. Byar, VACURG Studies on Prostatic Cancer and its Treatment,
    in: "Urologic Pathology: The Prostate," M. Tannenbaum, ed.,
    Lea & Febiger, Philadelphia (1977), p. 241.

12. S. Rafla and R. Johnson, The treatment of advanced prostatic
    carcinoma with medroxyprogesterone, Current Therapy Research,
    16: 261 (1974).

13. C. Bouffioux, Le Cancer de la Prostate, Acta Urol. Belg. 47:
    189 (1979).

14. G. Prout Jr. and L. Denis, Unpublished Data on Pilot Trial,
    Prostate StudyGroup, 1962 Grant GYP 5631.

15. L. Denis and G. Declercq, Progestagens in Prostatic Cancer,
    Eur. Urol. 4: 162 (1978).

16. C. Bouffioux, Treatment of Prostatic Cancer with Medroxyprog-
    esterone Acetate (MAP), in: "Bladder Tumors and Other Topics
    in Urological Oncology," M. Pavone-Macaluso, P.H. Smith, and
    F. Edsmyr, eds., Plenum Press, London and New York (1980), p.463.

17. A. Rifkind, H. Kulin, C. Cargille, P. Rayford, and G. Ross,
    Suppression of urinary excretion of luteinizing hormone (LH)
    and follicle stimulating hormone (FSH) by medroxyprogesterone
    acetate, J. Clin. Endocr. 29: 506 (1969).

18. C.W. Bardin and J.F. Catterall, Testosterone: A Major Determinant
    of extragenital Sexual Dimorphism, Science 211: 1285 (1981).

19. W.W. Scott, Rationale and results of primary endocrine therapy
    in patients with prostatic cancer, Cancer, 32: 1119 (1973).

20. D.S. Coffey and J.T. Isaacs, Prostate Tumor Biology and Cell
    Kinetics Theory, Urology Suppl. 17: 40 ·(1981).

21. J.F. Altwein and G.H. Jacobi, Hormontherapie des Prostatak-
    arzinoms, Der Urologe A: 19: 350 (1980).

NOLVADEX (TAMOXIFEN) AN ANTIOESTROGEN OF POTENTIAL USE IN THE MANAGEMENT OF CARCINOMA OF THE PROSTATE

M.R.G. Robinson

The General Infirmary
Pontefract
U.K.

Well-differentiated prostatic cancer cells, like normal prostatic cells, remain for a time, androgen-dependent. Oestrogens in sufficient dosage reduce circulating androgens, and this has been the rationale for conventional oestrogen therapy. At least 3 mg. daily of Stilboestrol, in divided doses, are needed to suppress plasma testosterone levels throughout 24 hours (1,2), but clinically 1 mg. per day is as effective in controlling the disease (3). This therapeutic evidence for an additional direct action of oestrogens upon the prostate is supported by the classical animal experiments of Huggins and Clark in 1940 (4) and by the tissue culture studies of Earnsworth (5).

Oestrogen receptors occur in normal, hyperplastic and malignant prostatic tissue (6,7) and if these receptors are functional it can be postulated that antioestrogens will also influence prostatic metabolism and growth. There is increasing experimental and clinical evidence to support this concept.

Nolvadex (Tamoxifen) is an active antioestrogen which is a nonsteroidal derivative of triphenylethylene. It specifically binds to oestrogen receptors in target tissues and is effective in the management of post-menopausal women with hormone dependent breast cancer (8-10). Animal and in vitro studies demonstrate that this drug also influences the growth and metabolism of prostatic cancer.

Using male Copenhagen X Fischer Fl rats bearing the androgen dependent well-differentiated R3327 Dunning rat carcinoma, Ip, Milholland and Rasen (11) have shown that 0.5 mg/Kg Nolvadex given five times a week suppresses tumour growth in 91% of rats. Plasma testosterone levels in the rats are also reduced. However, in young

human males treated with Nolvadex for oligospermia, continual administration of the antioestrogen results in an elevation of gonadotrophins and a secondary rise of plasma testosterone (12).

Habib et al (13) have shown in vitro that Nolvadex displaces
plasma androgens from sex hormone binding globulin.   In the tissue
it inhibits 5 α-reductase and 17-β-hydroxysteroid dehydrogenase
activity with a corresponding reduction of 5α-dihydrotestosterone
(to 13% of total metabolites) and androstenediol totally.   3 α(β)
hydroxysteroid dehydrogenase activity is markedly increased with a
large increase (75%) of androstendione levels.

This experimental data suggests that the reduction of 5α-reduc-
tase activity and the diminished conversion of testosterone to its
most active metabolite dihydrotestosterone, by Nolvadex, may be beneficial in the treatment of human prostatic cancer.   This is supported by the objective response observed in antioestrogen treated rat
prostatic carcinoma.   The displacement of bound testosterone from
sex hormone binding globulin and the secondary rise of plasma testosterone levels could, however, be detrimental and may explain the
exacerbations of bone pain which have been observed in patients with
prostatic cancer and bony metastases treated with Nolvadex (14).

The results reported from two clinical studies of Nolvadex in
the management of advanced progressive disease are encouraging.
Morgan et al (15) noted seven "responders" and eight "disease stabilisation" in 28 patients.   In a phase II trial, reported by Glick (16)
which recruited 31 patients and used National Prostatic Cancer Project
criteria of response, three patients showed objective partial response
and four objectively stable disease, an overall response rate of 23%.
In this series no patient experienced exacerbation of bone pain.
These results suggest that Nolvadex has some activity and that it
deserves further study.

Nolvadex is not excessively toxic.   Although major untoward
effects which have been reported include nausea and vomiting, hot
flushes, mild thrombocytopenia and leukopenia, skin rashes, retino-
pathy and corneal opacities, and hypercalcaemia, all are rare when
this agent is used in the management of breast cancer (17).   In a
personal toxicity study of 11 patients with non-metastatic prostatic
cancer and one with metastases treated with Nolvadex 10 mg. b.d. for
a mean period of 26 months, no toxicity was observed.   It is clear
that further phase II studies and controlled clinical trials are
needed to establish the possible role of Nolvadex in the management
of carcinoma of the prostate.

SUMMARY

Experimental and clinical evidence suggests that the antioestrogen Nolvadex directly influences prostatic metabolism.   Clinical
trials are needed to evaluate its role in the management of prostatic
cancer.

REFERENCES

1. M.R.G. Robinson and B.G. Thomas, Effect of Hormone Therapy and Plasma Testosterone Levels in Prostatic Cancer, B.M.J. 4:391 (1971).

2. R.J. Shearer, W.F. Hendry, I.F. Sommerville and J.D. Fergusson, Plasma Testosterone: An Accurate Monitor of Hormone Treatment in Prostatic Cancer, Brit. J. Urol. 45:668 (1973).

3. D.P. Byar, The Veterans Administrators Co-operative Urological Group's Studies of Cancer of the Prostate: A Preliminary Report, Cancer 32:1126 (1973).

4. C. Huggins and P.J. Clark, The Effects of Castration and Estrogen Injections on the Normal and Hyperplastic Prostate Gland of Dogs, J. Exp. Med. 72:747 (1941).

5. W.E. Farnsworth, The Normal Prostate and Its Endocrine Control, in "The Third Tenovus Workshop - Some Aspects of the Aetiology and Biochemistry of Prostatic Cancer", K. Griffith and C.G. Pierrpoint (eds), Alpha Omega Ltd., Cardiff (1970) p. 3.

6. E.F. Hawkins et al, Steroid Receptors in the Human Prostate, Steroids, 26:458 (1975).

7. J.R. Murphy, R.C. Emmott, L.L. Hicks and P.C. Walsh, Estrogen Receptors in the Human Prostate, Seminal Vesicle, Testes and Genital Skin: A Marker for Estrogen - Responsive Tissues? J. Clin. Endocrinol. and Metab. 50:938 (1980).

8. T.T. Kiang and B.J. Kennedy, Tamoxifen (Antioestrogen) Therapy in Advanced Breast Cancer, Ann. Intern. Med. 87:687 (1977).

9. S. Legha and F.M. Muggia, Antiestrogens in the Treatment of Cancer, Ann. Intern. Med. 84:751 (1976).

10. R.C. Heel, R.C. Brogden, T.M. Speight and G.S. Avery, Tamoxifen; A Review of its Pharmacological Properties and Their Therapeutic Use in the Treatment of Breast Cancer, Drugs. 16:1 (1968).

11. M.M. Ip, R.J. Milholland and F. Rosen, Functionality of Estrogen Receptor and Tamoxifen Treatment of R3327 Dunning Rat Prostate Adenocarcinoma, Cancer Res. 40:2188 (1980).

12. F. Comhaire, Hormone Effect of an Antioestrogen, Tamoxifen, in Normal and Oligospermic Men, Fertility and Sterility, 29:320 (1978).

13. F.K. Habib, G. Rafat, M.R.G. Robinson and S.R. Stitch, Effects of Tamoxifen on the Binding and Metabolism of Testosterone by Human Prostatic Tissue and Plasma in Vitro, J. Endocrinol. 83:369 (1979).

14. J.L. Williams, Personal Communication (1980).

15. L.R. Morgan, L.E. Posey and J. Lanasa, Therapeutic Use of Nolvadex (Tamoxifen ICI 46, 4741) in Advanced Prostatic Cancer, Proc. of 12. Int. Cancer Congress, Beunos Aires, 5-11 October 1978, W51 page 111, Abstract 17.

16. J.H. Glick, A. Wein, K. Padavic, W. Negendamk, D. Harris and H. Brodovsky, Tamoxifen in Refractory Metastatic Carcinoma of the Prostate, Cancer Treat. Rep. 64:813 (1980).

17. W.B. Pratt and R.W. Ruddon, "The Anticancer Drugs, Oxford University Press, (1979) p. 212.

CARCINOMA OF THE PROSTATE: ADRENAL INHIBITORS

M.R.G. Robinson

The General Infirmary
Pontefract
U.K.

SUMMARY

Adrenal androgens may continue to stimulate prostatic carcinoma after the suppression of testicular function by orchidectomy or oestrogen therapy. The production of adrenal androgens may be prevented by adrenalectomy, pituitary ablation or adrenal inhibitors. This paper discusses the therapeutic potential and complications of these techniques with special reference to the adrenal inhibitors.

Until recently, primary conventional endocrine therapy for carcinoma of the prostate gland has been orchidectomy or oestrogen administration. The principle objective of both methods has been to suppress the major androgen, testosterone, which stimulates this hormone dependent tumour. Oestrogens may have an additional direct action on the gland. Treatment failure may be because cancer cells which remain hormone dependent are secondarily stimulated by adrenal androgens or because clones of non-hormone dependent cells develop and cause tumour progression. Non-hormone dependent cells will only respond to cytotoxic chemotherapy whereas hormone dependent cells may respond to secondary hormonal therapy.

There is evidence for increased androgen production by the adrenal gland following conventional endocrine therapy. During oestrogen treatment there may be a small rise in plasma testosterone levels (1,2). This may be due in part to increased adrenal cortical activity and in part due to increased binding of testosterone by sex hormone binding globulin. Oestrogens do stimulate adrenal cortical activity. Doe et al (3) found that serum non-protein bound cortisol levels were higher in untreated carcinoma of the prostate patients

at 9 a.m. and 9 p.m. The 9 p.m. levels were again significantly
higher in oestrogen treated patients. Peeling and Griffiths (2) found
that the stimulation of the adrenal gland with Tetracosactrin does
not significantly elevate plasma testosterone levels in untreated
carcinoma of the prostate, but may do so after several months of
oestrogen treatment.

Following orchidectomy Sciarra et al (4) found that in 17 of 28
patients with carcinoma of the prostate plasma testosterone fell to
very low levels. In 10, however, they did not fall below 100 ng/
100 ml. Dexamethasone treatment reduced these higher levels. Inadequate reduction of plasma testosterone by orchidectomy in their experience was not associated with clinical improvement.

The principal androgens produced by the adrenal cortex are Androstenedione and dehydroepiandrosterone (Fig. 1). Compared with testosterone and dihydrotestosterone, they only weakly stimulate the
prostate (5). They are, however, converted in peripheral target
organs, including the prostate, to testosterone and dihydrotestosterone. Adrenal androgen production is stimulated by adrenocortico-
trophic hormone (ACTH) but the adrenal androgens do not themselves
suppress ACTH production by a feedback mechanism.

The rationale for secondary endocrine therapy is to suppress
the adrenal androgens. This may be achieved by pituitary ablation
or by surgical or medical adrenalectomy. The pituitary may be ablated
by surgery, irradiation (6) or alcohol injection (7). By removing
the source of ACTH, there is secondary hypoplasia of the adrenal
cortex.

As long ago as 1945, before the advent of corticosteroid replacement therapy, Huggins and Scott (8) reported a series of patients
subjected to bilateral total adrenalectomy. Adrenalectomy, even after
replacement steroids became available, has not been widely practised.
This is because the best results achieved have only been a temporary
subjective improvement in 50% of patients (9) and in addition there
are major surgical complications of adrenalectomy in elderly men with
advanced malignant disease.

Pituitary ablation is less traumatic and also results in a 50%
subjective response (10).

For many years alternative methods of suppressing adrenal cortical activity without subjecting the patients to surgery or irradiation have been suggested. In 1950 Sprague et al (11) observed that
corticosteroid without adrenalectomy, reduced adrenocortical activity
by suppressing ACTH production. Several workers have reported various
response rates to corticosteroid therapy (12,13,14). In general
there is temporary subjective improvement manifest by less metastatic
pain, improved appetite and increased weight. Only occasional

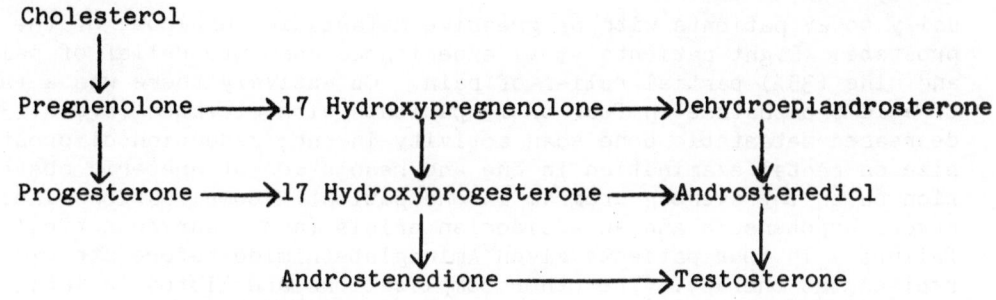

Fig. 1. Production of Androgens by the Adrenal Cortex.

objective responses have been claimed. Complications include fluid
and sodium retention, potassium loss, hypertension, gastro-intestinal
irritation and peptic ulcer, glycosuria and osteoporosis.

Drugs which specifically inhibit adrenal androgen synthesis
include Aminoglutethimide, Spironolactone, Cyproterone acetate,
Cyanoketone, Estradiol 17β, Hydroxymethylene and Medrogesterone (5).
Cyproterone acetate is currently being investigated by the EORTC and
other clinical groups because of its direct antiandrogen activity on
the prostate gland, but it also acts on the adrenal gland by inhibiting the enzyme 17,20 desmolase (responsible for the conversion of 17
hydroxypregnenolone to dehydroepiandrosterone) and 17β hydroxy steroid
dehydrogenase (responsible for conversion of Pregnenolone to Progesterone and 17 Hydroxypregnenolone to 17 hydroxyprogesterone - see
figure 1). Two other adrenal inhibitors have been investigated.
These are Aminoglutethimide which inhibits 20,21 desmolase and suppresses the conversion of cholesterol to pregnenolone, and Spironolactone (an aldosterone inhibitor) which suppresses 17,20 desmolase
activity and the conversion of 17 Hydroxypregnenolone to dehydroepiandrosterone.

Walsh and Siiteri (15) reported that spironolactone produced a
subjective remission in three of seven orchidectomised patients with
progressive prostatic cancer. Plasma levels of testosterone, androstenedione and dehydroepiandrosterone were significantly reduced.

Aminoglutethimide is a derivative of glutarimide which was used
in the USA as an anticonvulsant until it was withdrawn because of its
endocrine side effects. It inhibits adrenal production of aldosterone, cortisol and androgens (16) by inhibiting the conversion of
cholesterol to delta 5-pregnenolone (17). There is no evidence to
indicate that it inhibits testicular function (18). In a personal
series reported in 1974 (19) we administered Aminoglutethimide 500-
1000 mg in divided doses daily, together with Stilboestrol 1 mg three
times a day, cortisone 20-25 mgs daily and Fludrocortisone 0.1 mg

daily to 27 patients with progressive metastatic carcinoma of the
prostate. Eight patients (30%) experienced complete relief of pain
and nine (35%) partial relief of pain. Objectively there was a fall
of acid phosphatase in four of 13 patients with elevated levels (31%),
decreased metastatic bone scan activity in one, reduction of prostatic
size on rectal examination in one and resolution of ureteric obstruction on an intravenous urogram in one patient. Complications included
severe hypotension and an Addisonian crisis (acute adrenocortical
failure) in four patients given Aminoglutethimide before steroid
replacement therapy. The other complications are listed in Table 1.

Sanford et al (20) gave Aminoglutethimide with steroid replacement therapy to seven patients. They reported three responses (two
reductions of acid phosphatase and one regression of bone metastasis).
They observed that rising ACTH levels can reverse the effect of
Aminoglutethimide unless suppressed by dexamethasone or hydrocortisone.

It would seem, therefore, that Aminoglutethimide may be of some
value in the management of advanced prostatic cancer. This claim,
however, can only be confirmed by a controlled Phase II trial using
modern criteria of response. A second Phase II trial is also probably needed to determine the true objective response to the steroid
"replacement" therapy given without the Aminoglutethimide, as this
also suppresses adrenal cortical activity.

Table 1. Aminoglutethimide
Side Effects in 27 patients (19)

Side Effects	No. of patients
1. Before Steroid Replacement	
Hypotension, "Addisonian Crisis"	4
2. With Steroid Replacement	
Nausea and vomiting	8
Lassitude	11
Depression	5
Oedema	3
Skin rash	1

CONCLUSIONS

This paper has discussed the concept of adrenal inhibitors as a form of secondary hormonal therapy. Evidence has been given for increased production of androgens by the adrenal cortex during conventional endocrine therapy. Three clinical questions need to be answered:-

1. Is pituitary ablation as effective as adrenal ablation and inhibition with fewer complications?

2. Has the advent of cytotoxic chemotherapy obviated the need for further consideration of secondary endocrine therapy?

3. Should adrenal inhibitors ever be combined with conventional endocrine therapy as primary treatment (e.g. orchidectomy and cyproterone acetate as proposed by Bracci in 1975) (21)?

REFERENCES

1. M.R.G. Robinson and B.S. Thomas, Effect of Hormone Therapy on Plasma Testosterone Levels in Prostatic Cancer, BMJ 45: 556 (1971).
2. W.B. Peeling and K. Griffiths, The Adrenal Cortex and Prostatic Cancer, Proc. Roy. Soc. Med. 67: 42 (1973).
3. R.P. Doe, P. Dickenson, H.H. Zinnerman, and U.S. Seal, Elevated Non-protein Bound Cortisol (NPD) in Pregnancy during Oestrogen Administration and in Carcinoma of the Prostate, J. Clin. Endocrinol. 29: 757 (1969).
4. F. Sciarra, G. Sorcini, F. Di Silverio, and V. Gagliardi, Plasma Testosterone and Androstenediol after Orchidectomy in Prostatic Carcinoma, Clin. Endocrinol. 2: 101 (1973).
5. P.C. Walsh, Physiologic Basis for Hormonal Therapy in Carcinoma of the Prostate, Urol. Clin. N. Am. 2: 125 (1975).
6. J.D. Fergusson and W.F. Hendry, Pituitary Radiation in Advanced Carcinoma of the Prostate: Analysis of 100 Cases, Br. J. Urol. 43: 514 (1971).
7. A.B. Levin, R.C. Benson, and T. Nielsson, Chemical Hypophysectomy for Relief of Bone Pain in Carcinoma of the Prostate, J. Urol. 119: 517 (1978).
8. C. Huggins and W.W. Scott, Bilateral Adrenalectomy in Prostatic Cancer, Clinical Features and Urinary Excretion of 17 Ketosteroids and Oestrogen, Ann. Surg. 122: 1031 (1945).
9. M.I. Resnick and J.T. Greyhack, Treatment of Stage IV Carcinoma of the Prostate, Urol. Clin. N. Am. 2: 141 (1975).
10. C.R. West and G.P. Murphy, Pituitary Ablation and Disseminated Prostatic Carcinoma, JAMA 225: 253 (1973).
11. R.G. Sprague, M.H. Power, H.L. Mason, A. Albert, D.R. Mathieson, P.S. Hench, E.C. Kendall, C.H. Slocomb, and H.F. Polley, Observations on the Physiological Effect of Cortisone and ACTH in Man, Arch. Intern. Med. 85: 199 (1950).

12. G.M. Muller and F. Hinman, Cortisone Treatment in Advanced
     Carcinoma of the Prostate, J. Urol. 72: 485 (1954).
13. J.T. Greyhack, Hormonal Treatment of Prostatic Cancer, Surg.
     Clin. N. Am. 39: 13 (1959).
14. J.D. Fergusson, Secondary endocrine therapy, in: "Endocrine
     Therapy in Malignant Disease," B.A. Stoll, ed., W.B. Saunders
     and Co. (1972), p. 264.
15. P.C. Walsh and P.K. Siiteri, Suppression of Plasma Androgens by
     Spironolactone in Castrated Men with Carcinoma of the Prostate,
     J. Urol. 114: 254 (1978).
16. R.N. Dexter, I.M. Fishman, R.L. Ney, and G.W. Liddle, Inhibition
     of Adrenal Corticosteroid synthesis by Aminoglutethimide: studies
     of mechanism of action, J. Clin. Endocrinol. Metab. 27:
     473 (1967).
17. R. Cash, A.J. Brough, M.N.P. Cohen, and P.S. Satah, Aminoglut-
     ethimide (Elipten-Ciba) as an inhibitor of adrenal steroido-
     genesis: mechanism of action and therapeutic trial, J. Clin.
     Endocrinol. Metab. 27: 1239 (1967).
18. R. Gaunt, B.G. Steinitz, and J.J. Chart, Pharmacologic alter-
     ation of steroid hormone functions, Clin. Pharmacol. Ther. 9:
     657 (1968).
19. M.R.G. Robinson, R.J. Shearer, and J.D. Fergusson, Adrenal
     Suppression in the Treatment of Carcinoma of the Prostate,
     Br. J. Urol. 46: 555 (1974).
20. E.J. Sanford, J.R. Drago, T.J. Rohner, R. Santon, and A. Lipton,
     Aminoglutethimide Medical Adrenalectomy for Advanced Prostatic
     Carcinoma, J. Urol. 115: 170 (1980).
21. U. Bracci, Our present procedures in the treatment of prostatic
     cancer, in: "Hormonal Therapy of Prostatic Cancer," U. Bracci
     and F. Di Silverio, eds., COFESE, Palermo (1975), p. 177.

CARCINOMA OF THE PROSTATE - ADRENALECTOMY AND HYPOPHYSECTOMY

J. P. Blandy

The London Hospital and Institute
    of Urology
London

Today we must ask ourselves whatever happened to adrenalectomy and hypophysectomy for carcinoma of the prostate. Those of us who are old enough, will remember the busy days, 20 years ago, when we took adrenals out for carcinoma of the breast and prostate, and when that did not work, we would refer the patient for removal of the pituitary by one method or another. Today, we have altogether stopped taking out the adrenals, and we refer the patient for hypophysectomy less and less often. But it is timely to think why, especially since there appears to be a new vogue of treatment by 'medical adrenalectomy' about to be launched upon us.

Adrenalectomy was introduced by Huggins and Scott in 1945 (1) with the intention of removing the extratesticular androgens that were thought to be keeping the prostate cancer cells stimulated. It was found that relapse of the disease was mirrored by the rise in urinary 17-ketosteroids and that this could be diminished by bilateral adrenalectomy (2). Occasionally there were quite remarkable cures. Most of us can remember cases such as:-

M.J. aged 61. Relapse of carcinoma of prostate after previous stilboestrol and orchidectomy 1958. Bilateral adrenalectomy 1958. Complete relief of pain. Equivocal changes in x-rays. Back at work until 1967. Readmitted with carcinoma of sigmoid colon. Anterior resection, liver found full of metastases. Died 1968.

Equally, when the operation was performed on a large scale, all surgeons agreed in the finding that about 50% had a subjective relief of pain - often quite dramatic. In Murphy's review (3) of his own experience and that from the literature, he noted subjective improve-

ment that was "good" or was maintained for longer than 3 months in 58
out of 126 patients (46%).   But the snag was that the objective
response was seldom so convincing: indeed in the same series only
6 (5%) were thought to have objective evidence of healing of metastases.   Moreover the improvement in symptoms, however subjective, and
however suspect to objective criteria - was never long-lived.   In
Murphy's experience (3) the survival in 26 such patients was, on
average, between 6.8 and 20.8 months.

The failure of adrenalectomy in practice to produce a lasting
result made us turn away from an operation that was not without
morbidity in the old men who had to undergo it.   It seemed as if we
could obtain just as good results by giving them cortisone, without
the discomfort and morbidity of surgery.   We were reinforced in our
reluctance to undertake the operation when laboratory workers discovered that after castration the adrenal glands only produced a tiny
fraction, some 0 - 3%,of the normal testosterone production.   It
hardly seemed worth while removing the adrenals to remove this tiny
additional source of stimulation to the cancer which had probably in
any event escaped from hormonal control.

And so we turned to hypophysectomy.   This seemed more promising,
once our colleagues in neurosurgery had developed a technique for
removing the hypophysis either by transnasal introduction of Yttrium
rods, or the cryosurgical probe, or with the combined transethmoid-
transsphenoid approach.   Hypophysectomy would remove the source of
adrenal stimulation and decrease the supply of prolactin which was
believed to assist the prostate in its handling of androgen.   The
procedure was introduced for the prostate by Scott in 1952 (4) and at
first the operative and post operative complications were so great as
to make the procedure unjustifiable.   When techniques were simplified,
and as a method for measuring whether or not the hypophysectomy had
been completely done was developed - the measurement of the rise in
growth hormone output to a hypoglycaemic challenge - the operation
won itself an established position as a useful measure.   It was
specially useful in controlling pain: here it was quite remarkable.
Most series, whatever the technique used to ablate the pituitary,
claimed a 70% incidence of pain relief.   At the same time, it was
disappointingly short-lived;   survival after hypophysectomy being
measured in months, not in years.   The mean survival reported by
Murphy in 27 patients (3) was 4.8 months and the longest survival
was 13.6 months.

In our hospital such patients have been referred to A.W.
Morrison, an otorhinolaryngologist, who uses the combined transnasal
transethmoid approach and has allowed me to quote his unpublished
figures from a much larger series of hypophysectomy, most of which
were performed for carcinoma of the breast.   There were 21 patients.
There was no operative mortality.   All experienced subjective relief
of pain, and there were no cases of blindness.   Three patients

needed treatment for meningitis and in 2 there were persistent CSF
leaks that required a second operation.   There was however no
suggestion in his series that life was prolonged, even though the
relief of pain often lasted for up to a year.   The pain relief was
so striking that one patient at least rose from his bed in his
euphoria only to sustain a pathological fracture.

In my own practice hypophysectomy is still requested for the
occasional patient, otherwise reasonably well, and with a reasonable
life-expectancy, who is in uncontrollable pain despite appropriate
radiotherapy and orchidectomy.   Given a trustworthy technique, relief
of pain is almost certain even if it may not last very long.   Other
methods of obtaining pituitary ablation, such as the transnasal
introduction of Yttrium, have been equally successful (5).

As with adrenalectomy, so with ablation of the pituitary
experience forces us to ask the question - why do these patients
experience such striking, and often such sudden relief of pain?   And
in the context of adrenalectomy more specially, we must ask why the
occasional patient has experienced a prolongation of life.   If we
could find out more about the answers to these 2 questions we might
find it easier to be enthusiastic about techniques that offer medical
adrenalectomy with newer agents that try to improve upon the effects
of cortisone and aminoglutethimide.

We must not forget these 2 procedures, obsolete though they may
have become, for they hold out a hope for the future.   It is possible
(and laboratory studies already suggest that it may be feasible) that
we may be able to re-educate those wild clones that have abandoned
their responsiveness to oestrogens and their dependence upon androgens.   If this proves to be so, then we may need to look again at
the timing of the use of chemotherapy and hormone treatment: if
chemotherapy can convert anaplastic clones back towards their parent
tissue - and it seems that it sometimes can - then perhaps in the
future we shall reverse the order of battle, start off with chemotherapy, and follow with stilboestrol, orchidectomy and perhaps - who
can say - even with adrenalectomy and hypophysectomy again.

REFERENCES

1.   C. Huggins and W.W. Scott, Bilateral Adrenalectomy in Prostatic
     Cancer, Annals of Surgery, 122:1031 (1945).
2.   T. Bhanalaph, M.J. Varkarakis and G.P. Murphy, Current Status
     of Bilateral Adrenalectomy for Advanced Prostatic Carcinoma,
     Annals of Surgery, 179:17 (1974).
3.   G.P. Murphy, Management of Advanced Cancer of the Prostate, in
     "Genitourinary Cancer", D.G. Skinner and J.B. deKernion, eds.,
     W.B. Saunders Co., Philadelphia (1978), p. 397.

4.   W.W. Scott, Endocrine Management of Disseminated Prostatic
      Cancer, Including Bilateral Adrenalectomy and Hypophysectomy,
      <u>Transactions of the American Association of Genitourinary
      Surgeons</u>, 44:101 (1953).
5.   J.M. Fitzpatrick, R.A. Gardiner, J.P. Williams, P.R. Riddle
      and E.P.N. O'Donoghue, Pituitary Ablation in the Relief of Pain
      in Advanced Prostatic Carcinoma, <u>Brit. J. Urol</u>. 52:301 (1980).

ESTRAMUSTINE AND PREDNIMUSTINE

L. Andersson, F. Edsmyr and I. Könyves

Karolinska Sjukhuset
Hälsingborg
Sweden

Estramustine and prednimustine are both hormone-cytostatic agents where a steroid hormone compound known to have antitumour effect has been linked to an alkylating agent.

ESTRAMUSTINE

The intention with estramustine was to carry the cytostatic agent to the target organ where the drug is accumulated due to the action of specific receptors. Originally estramustine was considered for the treatment of mammary carcinoma but its main use has been in cancer of the prostate. Estramustine phosphate or estracyt is an estradiol phosphate which is esterified with a nor nitrogen mustard derivative in the form of a carbamate. In recent years there has been much discussion of estramustine. This presentation will not report details but will give an updated review.

Estramustine strongly inhibits the pituitary production of gonadotrophic hormones and in vitro studies have shown that it also has a local effect on the prostate. Høisaeter (1) demonstrated that estramustine phosphate inhibits DNA synthesis in the ventral rat prostate in vitro and induces cell degeneration of the ventral rat prostate in organ culture. He also showed that conversion of testosterone to dihydrotestosterone by 5α- reductase is inhibited by estramustine phosphate (2).

Recently Hartley-Asp and Gunnarsson (3) studied in tissue culture the effect of estramustine on a cell line of human prostate cancer that was lacking androgen and estrogen receptor and unresponsive to hormone stimulation either by testosterone or estradiol. Exposure of the cells to estramustine caused inhibition of cell

growth and cell destruction which was dependent on dose and on
exposure time.   The inhibitor effect of estramustine was higher
than that of the nor nitrogen mustard moiety indicating that the
unmetabolized compound has the strongest cytotoxic effect.   It could
also be shown that the effect of estramustine is due to interactions
between estramustine and intracellular cell components.

A direct cytotoxic effect of estramustine on human prostate
cancer in vivo was reported by Osafune et al in 1978 (4) who treated
a 46 year old man with poorly differentiated prostatic cancer with
estramustine and subsequently performed a total prostatectomy.   The
tumour was found to be necrotic.   In the remaining part of the
prostate there were hormonally induced changes but no necrosis.

Initially estramustine was mainly used in advanced prostate
cancer, resistant to ordinary hormone therapy but in recent years
it has been evaluated even in other patient categories.   Table 1
gives a survey of the effect of estramustine phosphate therapy in
868 patients reported in the literature.   Of 597 patients resistant
to previous hormone therapy, 48% responded favourably.   In those 271
cases where estramustine was given as the initial treatment there was
a good effect in 84%.

Since estramustine has a good effect even in a number of cases
resistant to ordinary hormone treatment we decided to investigate
whether the drug, when given as initial therapy, would be more
effective than the ordinary estrogenic regime.   We performed a
prospective randomized multi-centre trial in the Stockholm area in
which all patients with well and moderately well differentiated
prostate carcinoma and needing treatment were given either estramustine or our conventional estrogenic regimen, polyestradiol
phosphate + ethinyl estradiol.   Patients with poorly differentiated
tumours were excluded from this trial as they were involved in
another study.

Table 1. Clinical Results of Estracyt in Prostatic Carcinoma.

Route of Administration	Previous Estrogen Therapy		Previously Untreated		Total	
	No. of Patients	Positive Responses	No. of Patients	Positive Responses	No. of Patients	Positive Responses
Intravenous	252)		45)		297)	
	)	288	)	228	)	516
Oral	345)		226)		571)	
Total	597	48%	271	84%	868	59%

Of 182 patients observed for two years or more, 88 received estramustine and 94 the standard hormonal regimen.   In both groups reduction of the local tumour occurred in about 80% of the cases and elevated acid phosphatase activity as a rule was reduced to normal.   There was no significant difference between the two groups with respect to the duration of remission, incidence of cytologic remission and the frequency of cardiovascular and other complications.

Patients with advanced and poorly differentiated prostatic carcinoma were treated with estramustine phosphate in a non-randomized trial.   Of 90 patients, 76 had verified metastases.   In 73 cases the disease was progressive in spite of previous hormone and/or irradiation therapy and in 17 cases estramustine phosphate was given as primary therapy (Table 2).   In Table 3 it is seen that the treatment had better effect in those patients given no previous hormone therapy.   However, even some estrogen-resistant cases had benefit from estramustine.

Leistenschneider and Nagel (5) performed a randomized study of estramustine in poorly differentiated prostate carcinoma, previously untreated.   Ten patients were given estramustine and ten ordinary estrogenic hormones.   Following 3-6 months observation, cytologic remission was observed in seven of ten cases on estramustine and one of ten cases on conventional estrogen medication.

From the findings mentioned above we have concluded that in the primary treatment of well and moderately well differentiated prostate carcinoma, estramustine has no advantage over ordinary hormone therapy. On the other hand the drug has a favourable effect in a number of hormone resistant cases.   There is also evidence that estramustine is superior to conventional estrogen therapy in disseminated poorly differentiated prostate cancer and should probably be the treatment of first choice in this category of patients.

Table 2.   Estramustine Therapy in 90 Cases of Poorly
           Differentiated Prostate Carcinoma.

           Previous estrogenic therapy   64
              (estrogen + irradiation 39)

           Previous irradiation   9

           Previously untreated   17

Table 3.   Effect of Estramustine Phosphate in Patients With Poorly
           Differentiated Prostate Carcinoma Who Had Previous
           Estrogen Therapy, Compared With the Effect in Patients
           Given No Previous Hormone Therapy (Improved/Number of
           Cases Observed).

	Previous Estrogen	No Previous Estrogen
Regression of local tumour	8/16	11/14
Cytologic remission	12/22	5/8
Reduction of soft tissue lesions	5/8	5/7
Reduction of bone tissue lesions	3/28	2/14
Reduction of elevated acid phosphatase activity	10/29	8/14

(This table only includes those cases with evaluation of the
respective parameter both before and after treatment)

PREDNIMUSTINE

     Prednimustine is another antitumour drug where a steroid hormone
group is linked with a nitrogen mustard derivative.   In 1954 Valk
and Owens (6) reported that high dose corticosteroid therapy provides
palliation in many cases of advanced prostate carcinoma and such
therapy has since been frequently used in the treatment of this
disease.   The antitumour effect of corticosteroid compounds is
incompletely elucidated but it is believed that they affect cell
division by inhibiting the number of cells entering the S-phase.

     Prednimustine is a chlorambucil ester of prednisolone.   In
experimental tumour systems the drug was found to have a high therapeutic index.   The drug has been used mainly in hematological
diseases, mammary carcinoma and carcinoma of the ovary but has also
been evaluated in carcinoma of the prostate in the United States by
members of the National Prostatic Cancer Project (NPCP).

     In NPCP protocol 400 patients who were progressing despite
hormonal therapy and pelvic irradiation were randomized to receive
either the combination of estramustine and prednimustine or to
prednimustine alone.   If prednimustine was ineffective they were
crossed over to estramustine.   Although objective response was
minimal and approximately equal in both groups there was a relatively
good subjective response in each group with pain relief in 34% and
improved performance status in 39% (7).

Prednimustine has a certain antitumour effect but does not appear to be superior to estramustine.   It may be worth trying in cases where the tumour does not respond to estramustine.   Its main indication, however, is in malignant disease of the hematopoietic system.

SUMMARY

Estramustine and prednimustine are hormone-cytostatic agents with antitumour properties.   Both drugs have a low myelotoxic effect. Estramustine phosphate has two-fold effect in prostate cancer, inhibition of gonadotropin production and, at least in certain cases, a local effect in the prostate by inhibiting cell growth.   A number of hormone resistant patients have responded favourably to estramustine therapy.   The drug has also been found useful in disseminated and poorly differentiated prostate cancer.   So far there is limited experience of prednimustine therapy in prostate cancer. The main indication of the latter drug is malignant disease of the hematopoietic system.

REFERENCES

1.   P.A. Høisaeter, Incorporation of 3 H-thymidine Into Rat Ventral Prostate in Organ Culture.   Influence of Hormone-cytostatic Complexes, Invest. Urol. 12:479 (1975).

2.   P.A. Høisaeter, The Effect of Oestradiol - 3N - bis - (2 - Chlorethyl) Carbonate - 17β - Phosphate (Estracyt[R]) On The 5α- Reductase in the Rat Ventral Prostate, Acta. Endocrinol. 18:188 (1975).

3.   B. Hartley-Asp and P.O. Gunnarsson, Growth of Cell Survival Following Treatment with Estramustine, Nor-nitrogen Mustard, Estradiol and Testosterone of a Human Prostatic Cancer Cell Line (DU 145), in press (1981).

4.   M. Osafune, H. Seike, M. Ishibashi, M. Matsuda and T. Kotake, Histologic Observation on Influences of Estracyt[R] on Prostatic Cancer.   A Case of Oral Estramustine Phosphate Administration Followed by Total Prostatectomy, Acta. Urol. Japan, 24:429 (1978).

5.   W. Leistenschneider and R. Nagel, Estracyt Therapy of Advanced Prostatic Cancer with Special Reference to Control of Therapy with Cytology and DNA - Cytophotometry, Eur. Urol. 6:111 (1980).

6.   W.L. Valk and R.H. Owens, Endocrine Inhibition as Related to Carcinoma of the Prostate, J. Urol. 72:516 (1954).

7.   S. Beckley, Z. Wajsman, N. Slack, A. Mittelman and G.P. Murphy, The Chemotherapy of Prostatic Carcinoma, Scand. J. Urol. Nephrol. Suppl. 55:151 (1980).

Editorial Note (P.H.S.)

The 868 patients mentioned in Table 1 represent cumulative figures from the literature and as Professor Andersson has observed 48% previously treated with estrogens responded favourably.

Unfortunately the criteria of response in the 51 publications from
which these patients come are not always clearly defined and in the
absence of the accompanying references it is difficult to draw firm
conclusions.   The data in Table 3 refer to the 90 patients with
poorly differentiated cancer treated in a non-randomized study.
Unfortunately not all patients were evaluated with respect to all
parameters before and after treatment.   This accounts for the
relatively small numbers for which observations are available.

PEPLEOMYCIN, INTERFERON AND ESTRACYT IN THE TREATMENT OF

POORLY DIFFERENTIATED PROSTATIC CARCINOMA

F. Edsmyr, L. Andersson, P. Esposti, and P.O. Hedlund

Karolinska Institute
Stockholm
Sweden

PEPLEOMYCIN

An investigation using Pepleomycin in the treatment of prostatic carcinoma was reported at the WHO centre meeting on prostatic carcinoma in March 1979 in Stockholm (1). Some degree of objective and subjective improvement was observed in a series of six patients with stage C and D tumors. Side effects including gastro-intestinal disturbances, fever and dermatological symptoms were noted.

A pilot study has also been performed in Stockholm, including 12 patients with poorly differentiated prostatic carcinomas, initially treated by a full course of irradiation to the local tumor. In seven patients hormone therapy had been given after the finding of persistent cancer cells in the local tumor. When this therapy failed, Pepleomycin was given in a dose of 5 mg i.m., three times weekly to a total dose of 90 - 200 mg. In the remaining five patients Pepleomycin was given immediately after the irradiation therapy failed, without any hormone therapy.

RESULTS

In eight patients the serum acid phosphatases levels were raised before Pepleomycin was given. In four of these, they returned to normal, in one the acid phosphatases level remained high and in the other three patients the levels increased markedly. A decrease in the size of the prostate was observed in four patients, no change in three and an increase in size in one. In three patients who received 200 mg of Pepleomycin, the cytological smear showed regressive cells compared with the smear prior to therapy.

The duration of remissions was from two to ten months (mean five months) but most of the patients have ongoing therapy.

Subjective response with pain relief was observed in four of five patients with pain before the therapy. The remaining patient had increasing pain during treatment.

The side effects of Pepleomycin included loss of hair and skin changes in all and fever after the injections in six patients. No lung toxicity was observed.

INTERFERON

Interferon has been given to three patients with disseminated poorly differentiated prostatic carcinomas. All were previously untreated.

Daily doses of 3 million I.U. of Interferon were given and treatment has now continued for 6, 7, and 9 months.

The preliminary results indicate a stabilization of the disease with no progression of the bone metastases. All have had total pain relief and no infection of any kind has been observed during the treatment.

Cytological smears taken after 1, 3, 6 and 9 months are unchanged. The serum acid phosphatase levels are all above normal.

One patient with a bulky tumor of the head had an almost complete remission (nine months), his neurological symptoms have disappeared, his weight has increased and he feels better in himself.

RANDOMIZED TRIAL WITH INTERFERON, PEPLEOMYCIN AND ESTRACYT

In patients with poorly differentiated prostatic carcinoma, verified with fine needle aspiration biopsy, a phase III study has been started to compare Interferon vs Pepleomycin vs Estracyt. All patients have disseminated tumors, verified with scintigraphy, skeletal X-rays and computerized tomography. An increased serum acid phosphatase is not regarded as an indication of tumor spread. Immunological tests are performed during the treatment.

TREATMENT

Pepleomycin is given at a dose of 5 mg i.m. three times weekly to a total dose of 150 mg. Interferon is given in daily doses of 3 million I.U. for at least three months and Estracyt 280 mg is given orally twice daily for an unlimited time period.

So far only 12 patients have been randomized - five to Estracyt, four to Pepleomycin and three to Interferon.

In this preliminary report it is only possible to observe that the serum acid phosphatase level has become normal in the group of patients treated with Estracyt but is unchanged in the other two groups and that prostatic size has decreased slightly in patients receiving Pepleomycin and Interferon but markedly in those receiving Estracyt. Pain relief has been observed in all three groups.

REFERENCES

1. T. Niijima and K. Koiso, Effect of Pepleomycin in Prostatic Carcinoma. A Preliminary Report. Scand. J. Urol. Nephrol. Suppl. 177 (1980).

Editorial Note - P.H.S.

The information on the activity of Pepleomycin in prostatic cancer is limited and that on Interferon is even more so. The introduction of a randomized study at this time seems premature. Treatment is limited to three months in those receiving Pepleomycin. This is a very short period of time in a patient with cancer of the prostate and will make assessment of objective response a difficult task.

CHEMOTHERAPY OF PROSTATE CANCER: THE NATIONAL PROSTATIC CANCER PROJECT EXPERIENCE

J.D. Schmidt

University of California Medical Center
San Diego
USA

ABSTRACT

Since 1972 the Treatment Subgroup of the National Prostatic Cancer Project has accessioned 1748 patients with various stages of prostatic cancer to 13 different treatment protocols. Seven of these protocols have been closed and the results in the initial studies have been published. Six protocols are active and continue to accrue patients. Principal investigators have a prominent role in protocol design as well as in the evaluation and publication of data emanating from these protocols. Active agents identified to date include cyclophosphamide, 5-fluorouracil, methyl-CCNU, imidazole-carboxamide, estramustine phosphate and streptozotocin. Agents chosen for their presumed activity, but currently under investigation, include methotrexate and cis-platinum.

ORGANIZATION AND RESPONSIBILITIES

The Treatment Subgroup of the National Prostatic Cancer Project was organized in 1972. The original membership consisted of five institutions (M.D. Anderson Hospital and Tumor Clinic, University of Iowa, the Virginia Mason Clinic, Massachusetts General Hospital and the Johns Hopkins Hospital) whose representatives agreed to design protocols directed at the treatment of specified groups of patients with prostatic cancer, accession patients into such protocols as well as share the results of such clinical evaluations. In the nine years since its inception, the Treatment Subgroup has been expanded by the addition of several institutions either on active or provisional status. Only one institution is no longer active in the Subgroup.

Table 1. United States National Prostatic Cancer Project
Director - Gerald P. Murphy, M.D., D. Sc.

Treatment Subgroup Members

Institution	Principal Investigator
M.D. Anderson*	Douglas Johnson, M.D.
University of Iowa	Stefan Loening, M.D.
Mason Clinic	Robert Gibbons, M.D.
Massachusetts General Hospital	George Prout, Jr., M.D.
Johns Hopkins	William Scott, Ph.D., M.D.
University of Tennessee	Mark Soloway, M.D.
University of California, San Diego	Joseph Schmidt, M.D.
Tulane University	Stuart Bergman, M.D.
Wayne State University	James Pierce, M.D.
Roswell Park	Sunmolu Beckley, M.D.
Baylor College of Medicine	Peter Scardino, M.D.
Walter Reed**	David McLeod, M.D.
Rush-Presbyterian-St. Luke's**	Charles McKiel, Jr., M.D.
University of California, Los Angeles**	Jean De Kernion, M.D.

* No longer active member

** Provisional status

Table 2. United States National Prostatic Cancer Project

Protocol Chairmen

Protocol Number	Principal Investigator
100	Dr. William W. Scott
200	Dr. William W. Scott
300	Dr. Joseph D. Schmidt
400	Dr. Gerald P. Murphy
500	Dr. Joseph D. Schmidt
600	Dr. Robert P. Gibbons
700	Dr. Stefan A. Loening
800	Dr. Mark S. Soloway
900	Dr. Joseph D. Schmidt
1000	Dr. Robert P. Gibbons
1100	Dr. Stefan A. Loening
1200	Dr. Mark S. Soloway
1300	Dr. J. Edson Pontes

The professional and scientific activities of each member
institution's participation in the clinical trials is the responsibility of the principal investigator (Table 1). Each principal
investigator heads his institutional team for screening, accession,
treatment and evaluation of patients with prostatic cancer. Although
there is some variation among institutions, this team consists of
the principal investigator, one or more co-investigators, a research
assistant or project coordinator, an oncology nurse and either a
urology fellow or resident.

Again starting in 1972, responsibility for each specific protocol was assigned to one individual generally from among the
principal investigators (Table 2). Each Protocol chairman has
responsibility not only for the design of the protocol but for
evaluation of data collected regarding efficacy and toxicity of
agents, presentation of such data at national meetings and eventual

publication of the data in urology or cancer-related journals.

SPECIFIC PROTOCOLS

The initial studies executed by the Treatment Subgroup were protocols 100 and 200 (Figures 1 and 2). Protocol 100 was designed to study two single agents, cyclophosphamide and 5-fluorouracil, compared to standard or conventional treatment in patients with relapsing advanced prostatic cancer who had not had excessive prior radiotherapy to the lumbosacral spine and/or pelvis (1). On the other hand, Protocol 200 was designed to study two single agents, estramustine phosphate and streptozotocin, each with minimal myelo-suppression, compared to standard therapy in patients with stage D prostatic cancer who also had relapsed to endocrine manipulation but who had extensive irradiation therapy (2).

As data on toxicity and response rates were accumulated, active agents were selected from existing protocols and then used as indicator agents for successive protocols. Thus Protocol 100 was succeeded first by Protocol 300 (figure 3) which in turn was followed by protocols 700 and 1100 (Figures 7 and 11) (3,4). Again, the common denominator for these clinical trials has been the patients with metastatic prostatic cancer who have not had extensive irrad-iation therapy but who have failed endocrine manipulation.

Similarly, Protocol 200 was succeeded by Protocol 400 (Figure 4) which in turn was succeeded by Protocol 800 and later Protocol 1200 (Figures 8 and 12) (5,6). All patients entered into this sequence of studies had relapsed to endocrine manipulation and had had extensive irradiation.

In 1976 because of the results in the protocols extant, the Treatment Subgroup initiated a study of chemotherapy and conventional endocrine manipulation in newly diagnosed patients with stage D disease (7). These patients had a common background of having had no prior hormonal manipulation. Protocol 500 (Figure 5) was the prototype. This study has recently been closed to patient entry and has been succeeded by Protocol 1300 (Figure 13). At about the same time, the Treatment Subgroup initiated a study of hormonal therapy and chemotherapy in patients with stage D prostatic cancer who had been considered stable on diethylstilbestrol (DES) therapy, 1 mg t.i.d. for a minimum of three months. Protocol 600 (Figure 6) is still open.

In 1978 the Treatment Subgroup, again based on the efficacy and acceptable toxicities of agents used in patients with advanced disease, embarked on studies evaluating adjuvant chemotherapy, either with cyclophosphamide or estramustine phosphate, in patients with earlier and potentially curable prostatic cancer. Protocol 900

(Figure 9) has been designed for patients having their primary
disease treated either with radical surgery alone, with radionuclide
implantation or with cryosurgery. Protocol 1000 (Figure 10) employs
the same chemotherapeutic agents but in patients who have been

A COMPARISON OF 5-FLUOROURACIL (NSC 19893) AND
CYCLOPHOSPHAMIDE (26271) IN PATIENTS WITH ADVANCED
CARCINOMA OF THE PROSTATE

Schema

5-FU, 600 mgm/M^2 I.V. given weekly

vs

Cytoxan, 1 gm/M^2 I.V. every three weeks

vs

Standard treatment

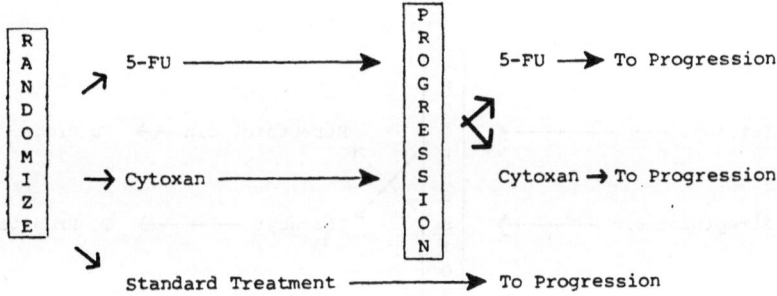

Fig. 1. National Prostatic Cancer Project. Protocol 100.

treated primarily with external beam radiotherapy either to the
prostate alone or to the prostate and the pelvis as based on either
preliminary pelvic lymphadenectomy or lymphangiogram followed by
needle aspiration biopsy. Both protocols 900 and 1000 continue
to accession patients.

A COMPARISON OF ESTRACYT AND STREPTOZOTOCIN (NSC 85998)
IN PATIENTS WITH ADVANCED CARCINOMA OF THE PROSTATE
WHO HAVE HAD EXTENSIVE IRRADIATION

Schema

Estracyt, 600 mg/M^2 p.o. daily in
three divided doses

vs

Streptozotocin 500 mg/M^2 I.V. daily
for five days every six weeks

vs

Standard therapy

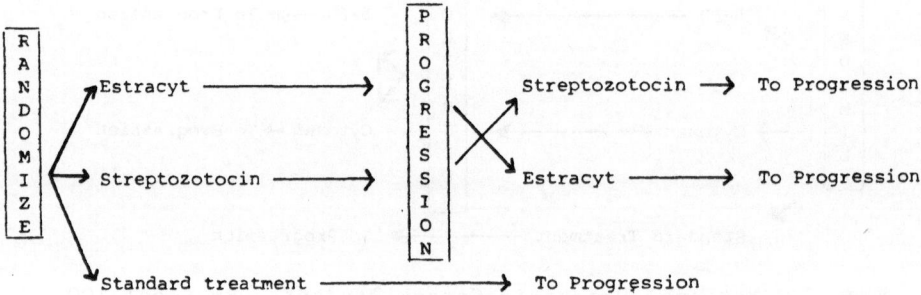

Fig. 2.   National Prostatic Cancer Project.   Protocol 200.

A COMPARISON OF PROCARBAZINE (NSC 77213),
DTIC (5- (3,3 DIMETHYL-1-TRIAZENO) IMIDAZOLE-4-CARBOXAMIDE)
(NSC 45388) AND CYCLOPHOSPHAMIDE (NSC 26271) IN PATIENTS WITH
ADVANCED CARCINOMA OF THE PROSTATE

Schema

DTIC, 200 mg/M^2 I.V. days 1-5, 21 days rest, then repeat the cycle

vs

Procarbazine, 100 mg/M^2 p.o. daily days 1-22, 3 weeks rest. Rx days 44-65, 3 weeks rest, etc.

vs

Cytoxan, 1 gm/M^2 I.V. every three weeks

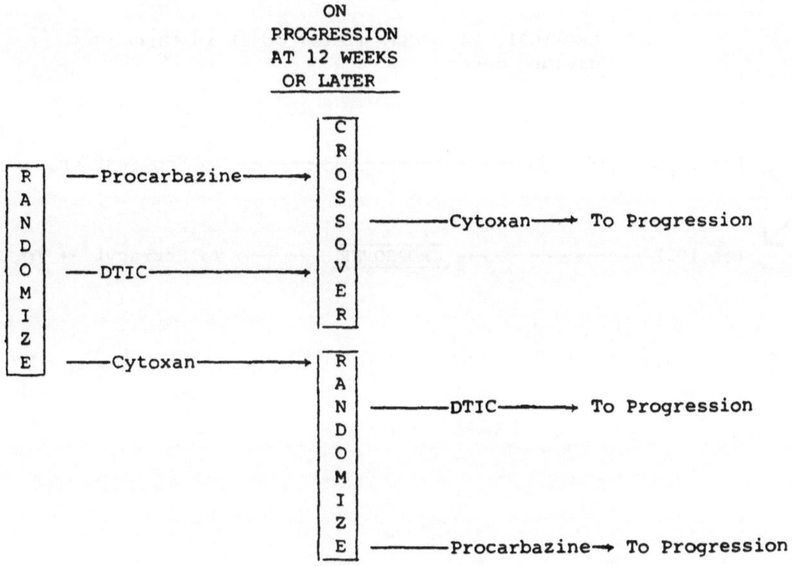
ON PROGRESSION AT 12 WEEKS OR LATER
RANDOMIZE
Procarbazine
DTIC
Cytoxan
CROSSOVER
Cytoxan
To Progression
RANDOMIZE
DTIC
To Progression
Procarbazine
To Progression

Fig. 3. National Prostatic Cancer Project. Protocol 300.

A COMPARISON OF ESTRACYT PLUS LEO 1031 (NSC-134087)
AND LEO 1031 ALONE IN PATIENTS WITH ADVANCED CARCINOMA
OF THE PROSTATE WHO HAVE HAD EXTENSIVE IRRADIATION

Schema

Estracyt, 600 mg/M^2 p.o. daily in three
divided doses + LEO 1031, 24 mg/day (total
dose) p.o. in three divided doses

vs

LEO 1031, 24 mg/day (total dose) in three
divided doses

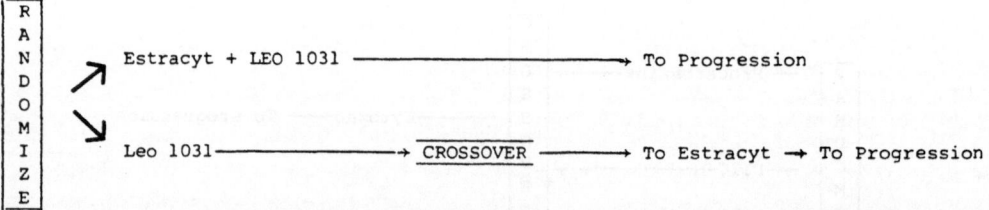

Fig. 4.   National Prostatic Cancer Project.   Protocol 400.

A COMPARISON OF CYCLOPHOSPHAMIDE (NSC-26271) PLUS
ESTRACYT (NSC-89199) VS CYCLOPHOSPHAMIDE (NSC-26271)
PLUS DIETHYLSTILBESTROL VS DIETHYLSTILBESTROL OR
ORCHIECTOMY IN NEWLY DIAGNOSED PATIENTS WITH CLINICAL
STAGE D CANCER OF THE PROSTATE WHO HAVE NOT HAD PRIOR
HORMONAL THERAPY

Schema

Cytoxan, 1 gm/M^2 I.V. every three weeks
plus
Estracyt, 600 mg/M^2 p.o. daily in three
divided doses

vs

Cytoxan, 1 gm/M^2 I.V. every three weeks
plus
Diethylstilbestrol, 1 mg t.i.d. p.o.

vs

Diethylstilbestrol, 1 mg t.i.d. p.o.
or
Orchiectomy
(Investigator's Option)

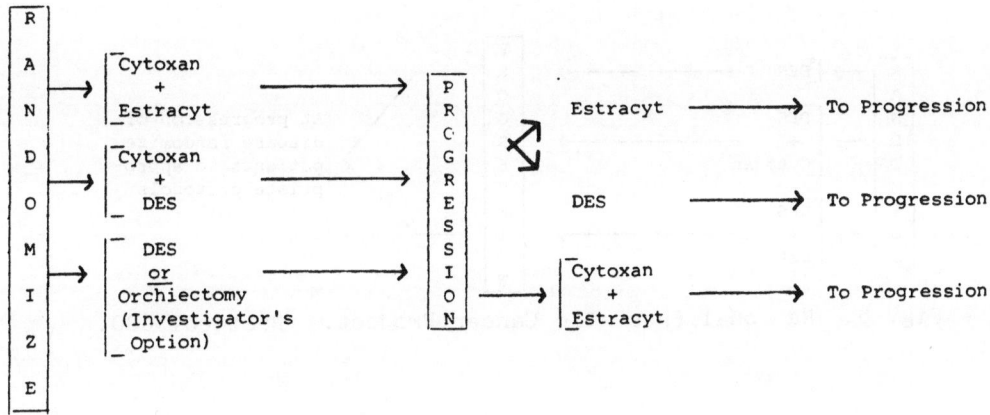

Fig. 5. National Prostatic Cancer Project. Protocol 500.

A COMPARISON OF COMBINATION CHEMOTHERAPY-HORMONAL
THERAPY WITH HORMONAL THERAPY ALONE IN PATIENTS WITH
CLINICAL STAGE D PROSTATIC CARCINOMA

Schema

Diethylstilbestrol, 1 mg t.i.d. p.o.

vs

Diethylstilbestrol, 1 mg t.i.d. p.o.
plus
Cytoxan, 1 gm/M^2 I.V. every three weeks

vs

Diethylstilbestrol, 1 mg t.i.d. p.o.
plus
Estracyt, 600 mg/M^2 p.o. daily in three
divided doses

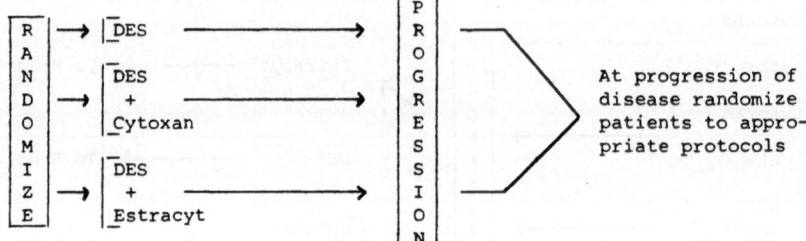

Fig. 6.   National Prostatic Cancer Project.   Protocol 600.

A COMPARISON OF HYDROXYUREA (NSC 32065),
METHYLCCNU (NSC 95441), AND CYCLOPHOSPHAMIDE
(NSC 26271) IN PATIENTS WITH ADVANCED
CARCINOMA OF THE PROSTATE

Schema

Hydroxyurea, 3 mg/M^2 p.o. every three
days in three divided doses

vs

MECCNU, 175 mg/M^2 p.o. every six weeks

vs

Cytoxan, 1 gm/M^2 I.V. every three weeks

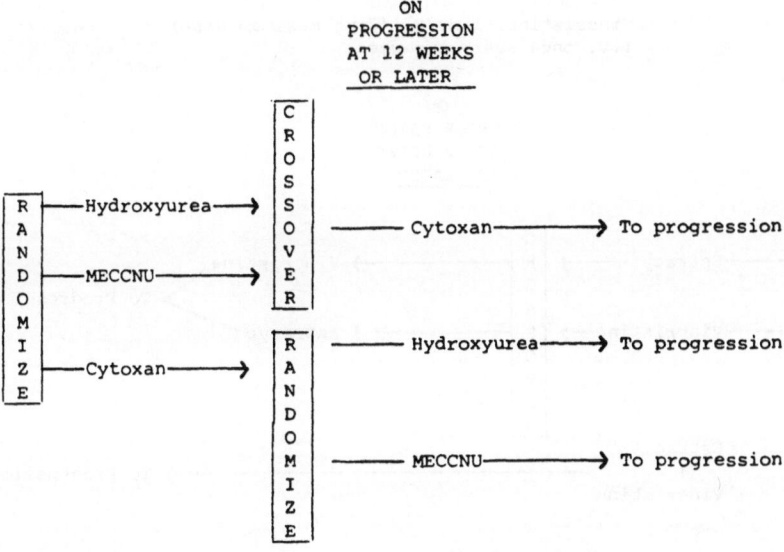

Fig. 7. National Prostatic Cancer Project. Protocol 700.

A COMPARISON OF ESTRACYT (NSC 89199), VINCRISTINE (NSC 67574)
AND ESTRACYT PLUS VINCRISTINE IN PATIENTS WITH
ADVANCED CARCINOMA OF THE PROSTATE WHO HAVE HAD EXTENSIVE IRRADIATION

Schema

Estracyt, 600 mg/M^2 p.o. daily in three
divided doses

vs

Vincristine, 1 mg/M^2 (2 mg maximum dose)
I.V. once every two weeks

vs

Estracyt, 600 mg/M^2 p.o. daily in three
divided doses

plus

Vincristine, 1 mg/M^2 (2 mg maximum dose)
I.V. once every two weeks

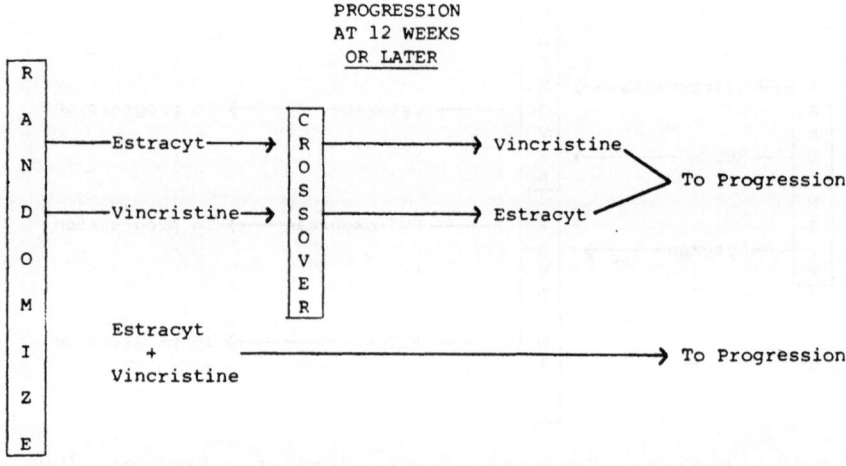

Fig. 8. National Prostatic Cancer Project.   Protocol 800.

A COMPARISON OF LONG-TERM ADJUVANT CHEMOTHERAPY WITH CYCLOPHOSPHAMIDE
(NSC 26271), ESTRACYT (NSC 89199), OR NO-ADDITIONAL-TREATMENT
IN PATIENTS WITH DEFINITIVE SURGICAL TREATMENT
FOR ADENOCARCINOMA OF THE PROSTATE

Schema

Prior total prostatectomy alone or with
^{198}Au seed implants or cryosurgery and lymph
node evaluation by pelvic lymph node dissection
or lymphangiogram with fine needle biopsy
followed by randomization for adjuvant chemotherapy to receive either:

Estracyt, 600 mg/M^2 p.o. daily in three
divided doses

or

Cyclophosphamide, 1 gm/M^2 I.V. every three
weeks

or

No treatment

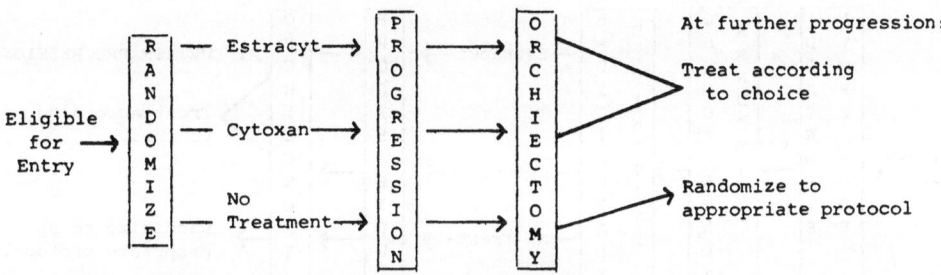

Fig. 9. National Prostatic Cancer Project. Protocol 900.

A COMPARISON OF LONG-TERM ADJUVANT CHEMOTHERAPY WITH
CYCLOPHOSPHAMIDE (NSC 26271), ESTRACYT (NSC 89199)
OR NO-ADDITIONAL-TREATMENT IN PATIENTS WHO HAVE HAD
DEFINITIVE EXTERNAL BEAM OR INTERSTITIAL RADIOTHERAPY
FOR ADENOCARCINOMA OF THE PROSTATE

Schema

Prior definitive radiotherapy and lymph
node evaluation by pelvic lymph node dissection or lymphangiogram with fine needle
biopsy, followed by the randomized adjuvant
chemotherapy to be either:

Estracyt, 600 mg/M^2 p.o. daily in three
divided doses

or

Cyclophosphamide, 1 gm/M^2 I.V. every
three weeks

or

No treatment

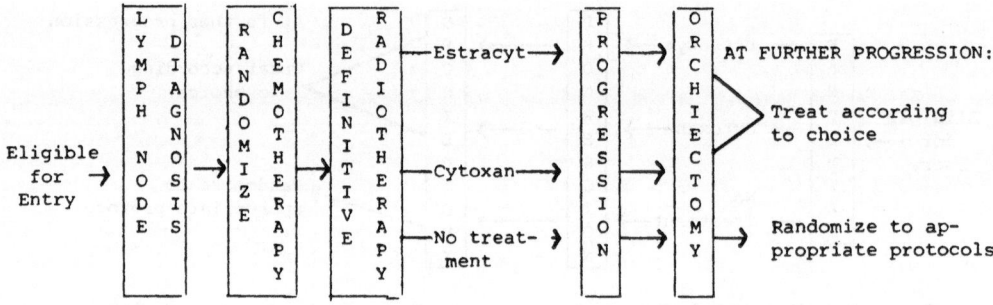

Fig. 10.   National Prostatic Cancer Project.   Protocol 1000.

A COMPARISON OF METHOTREXATE (NSC-740),
CIS-DIAMMINEDICHLOROPLATINUM (II-NSC-119875), AND
ESTRACYT (NSC-89199) IN PATIENTS WITH ADVANCED
CARCINOMA OF THE PROSTATE

Schema

Methotrexate, 40 mg/M^2 I.V. on day 1,
60 mg/M^2 I.V. on day 8, q 7 days thereafter

vs

DDP - prehydrate the patient over 60 minutes prior to DDP with 500 ml of
5% dextrose/½ normal saline (D5/½NS). Place 60 mg/M^2 of DDP in 100 ml
D5/½NS for I.V. infusion over 15 minutes. Follow the DDP with 3 hours of
I.V. infusion with 1000 ml of D5/½NS + 40 meq KCl + 37.5 gm mannitol. Give
Compazine at 10 mg I.M. q 4 hours around the clock on the day of DDP therapy
then q 4 hours PRN. DDP will be given on days 1, 4, 21, 24, and then once
every month. Prevent exposure of DDP to light and do not bring DDP into
direct contact with equipment containing aluminum.

vs

Estracyt, 600 mg/M^2 p.o. daily in three
divided doses.

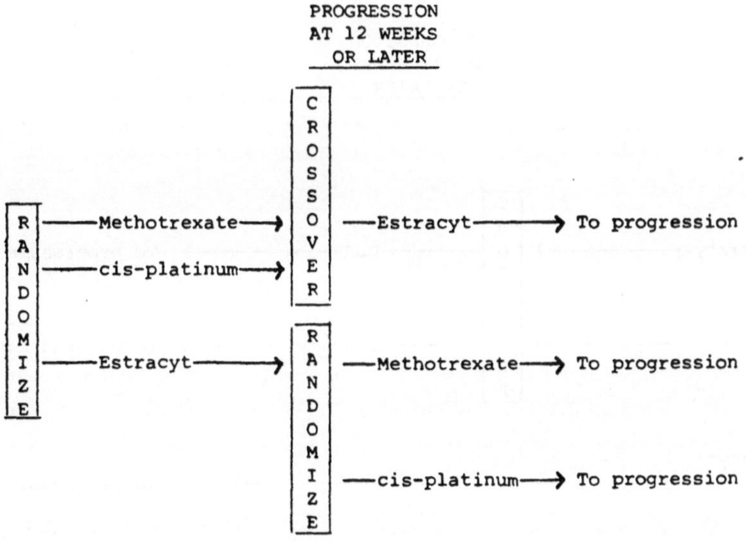

PROGRESSION
AT 12 WEEKS
OR LATER

Fig. 11.   National Prostatic Cancer Project.   Protocol 1100.

A COMPARISON OF ESTRACYT (NSC 89199) VERSUS CIS-DIAMMINEDICHLOROPLATINUM
(DDP) (II NSC 119875) VERSUS ESTRACYT PLUS DDP IN PATIENTS
WITH ADVANCED CARCINOMA OF THE PROSTATE WHO HAVE HAD
EXTENSIVE IRRADIATION TO THE PELVIS OR LUMBOSACRAL AREA

Schema

Estracyt, 600 mg/M^2 p.o. daily in three
divided doses

vs

DDP - prehydrate the patient over 60 minutes prior to DDP with 500 ml of
5% dextrose/½ normal saline (D5/½NS). Place 60 mg/M^2 of DDP in 100 ml D5/½NS
for I.V. infusion over 15 minutes. Follow the DDP with 3 hours of I.V.
infusion with 1000 ml of D5/½NS + 40 meq KCl + 37.5 gm mannitol. Give
Compazine at 10 mg I.M. q 4 hours around the clock on the day of DDP therapy
then q 4 hours PRN. DDP will be given on days 1, 21 and then once every
month. Prevent exposure of DDP to light and do not bring DDP into direct
contact with equipment containing aluminum.

vs

Estracyt plus DDP, administer both agents
as noted above.

PROGRESSION
AT 12 WEEKS
OR LATER

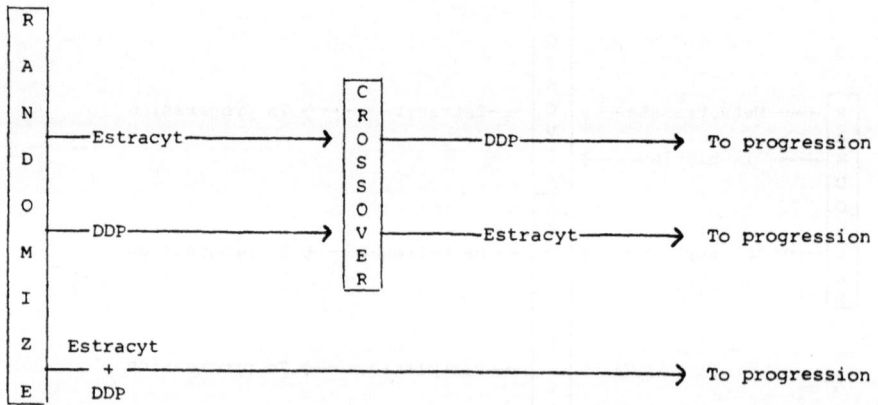

Fig. 12. National Prostatic Cancer Project. Protocol 1200.

A COMPARISON OF DIETHYLSTILBESTROL (DES) OR ORCHIECTOMY
VS CYCLOPHOSPHAMIDE + 5-FLUOROURACIL (5-FU) + DES OR ORCHIECTOMY VS
ESTRACYT ALONE IN NEWLY DIAGNOSED PATIENTS WITH
CLINICAL STAGE D CANCER OF THE PROSTATE WHO HAVE
NOT HAD PRIOR HORMONAL TREATMENT OR CHEMOTHERAPY

Schema

Diethylstilbestrol (DES), 1 mg t.i.d. p.o.
or orchiectomy

vs

Estracyt, 600 mg/M^2 p.o. daily

vs

DES, 1 mg t.i.d. p.o. or orchiectomy
plus
5-fluorouracil (5-FU), 350 mg/M^2 I.V. weekly
plus
Cytoxan, 650 mg/M^2 I.V. q 3 weeks

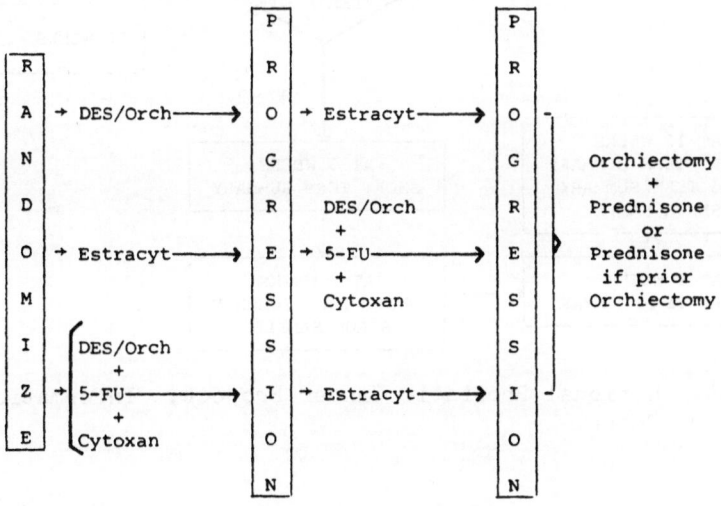

Fig. 13. National Prostatic Cancer Project. Protocol 1300.

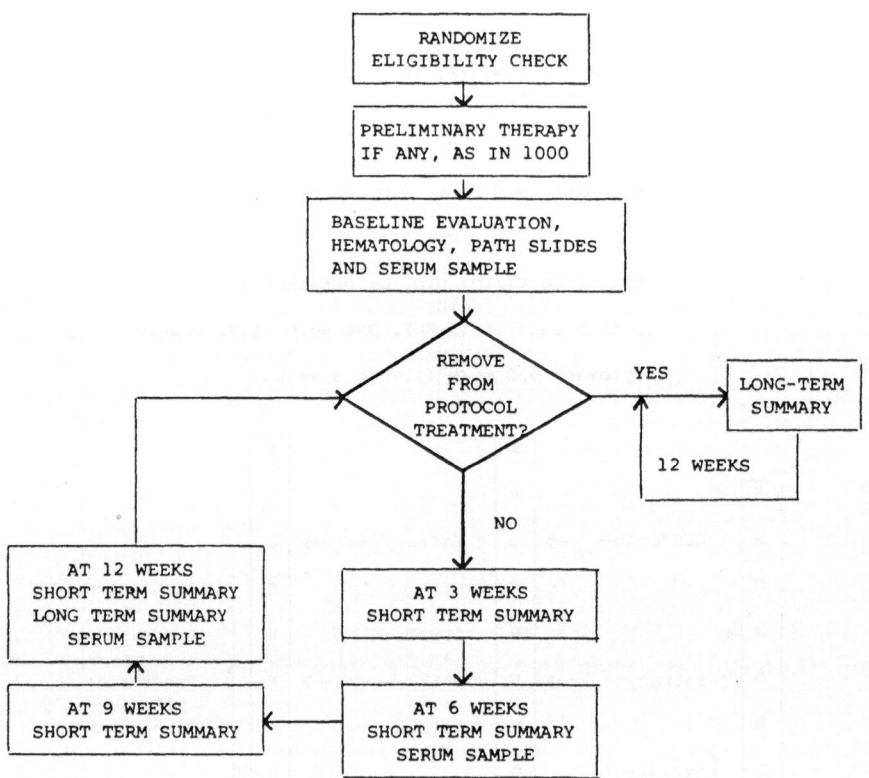

Fig. 14.   National Prostatic Cancer Project.   Information Flow
          Chart.

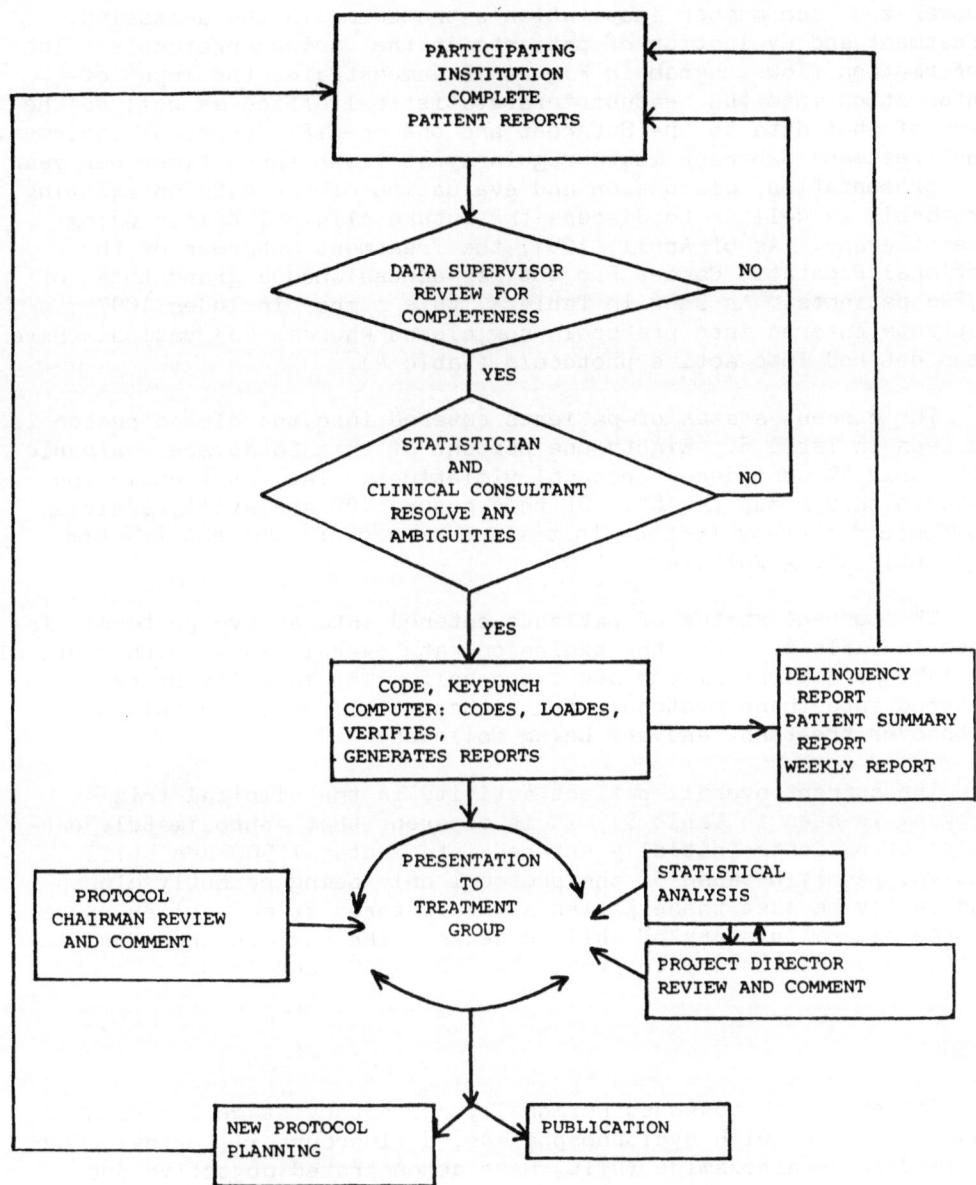

Fig. 15. National Prostatic Cancer Project Treatment Group Information Flow.

METHODS OF PROCEDURE AND PATIENT ACTIVITY

The information flow chart (Figure 14) diagrammatically summarizes each member institution's procedure in the accession, treatment and evaluation of patients in the various protocols. The information flow diagram in Figure 15 demonstrates the input of information into the headquarters statistical office as well as the flow of that data to the Subgroup and the specific protocol chairmen. The Treatment Subgroup meets regularly at least three times per year for presentation, discussion and evaluation of the data on existing protocols as well as to discuss the future clinical trials using chemotherapy. As of April, 1981, the Treatment Subgroup of the National Prostatic Cancer Project has accessioned a grand total of 1,748 patients. As seen in Table 3, this number includes 1097 patients entered into protocols now closed whereas 651 patients have been entered into active protocols (Table 4).

The current status of patients entered into the closed protocols is seen in Table 5. Eighty-one percent of this total are evaluable with only 4% considered protocol violations. The total exclusion rate in this group is 18%. Of this group, 12% are still receiving randomized therapy (either initial or crossover) whereas 22% are currently being followed.

The current status of patients entered into active protocols is seen in Table 6. Here the exclusion rate overall is 9% with protocol violations accounting for about one-half. The majority of patients entered into these protocols are either still receiving initial or crossover treatment and are being followed.

The current overall patient activity in the clinical trials program is seen in Table 7. It is apparent that approximately one-third of patients initially entered into Protocol 500 are still active, partly because of the protocol only being recently closed and partly because these patients were entered at an earlier phase in the natural history of their disease. The same is true for patients accessioned into protocols 900, 1000, and 1300.

RESULTS

Patients with advanced hormonally-refractory stage D prostatic cancer, treated with cyclophosphamide, 5-fluorouracil, methyl-CCNU or imidazole-carboxamide (DTIC) have demonstrated objective and subjective response rates higher than similar patients treated with standard therapy (8). Procarbazine and hydroxyurea were associated with increased toxicity yet response rates were no better than standard therapy. Agents currently under investigations in this category include methotrexate, estramustine phosphate and cis-platinum (Table 8).

Table 3. National Prostatic Cancer Project

Patient Entry for Each Participating Institution to Closed Protocols

Institution	Protocol Number							Total
	100	200	300	400	500	700	800	
M. D. Anderson	41	42	37	27	-	9	30	186
Univ. of Iowa	19	10	38	13	55	11	7	153
Mason Clinic	26	42	49	57	21	15	31	241
Mass. General	20	8	13	6	46	14	8	115
Johns Hopkins	19	23	22	18	15	22	13	132
Univ. Tennessee	-	-	2	10	28	22	8	70
U. C. San Diego	-	-	4	4	49	16	20	93
Tulane Medical	-	-	-	-	28	7	3	38
Wayne State	-	-	-	-	46	9	1	56
Roswell Park	-	-	-	-	6	-	-	6
Baylor College	-	-	-	-	6	-	-	6
Walter Reed	-	-	-	-	1	-	-	1
Total	125	125	165	135	301	125	121	1097

Table 4. National Prostatic Cancer Project

Patient Entry for Each Participating Institution to Current Protocols as of April, 1981

Institution	Protocol Number						Total	Grand Total
	600	900	1000	1100	1200	1300		
M.D. Anderson	-	-	-	-	-	-	-	186
Univ. of Iowa	28	21	7	18	8	8	90	243
Mason Clinic	8	-	5	109	31	2	65	306
Mass. General	8	-	-	-	3	10	21	136
Johns Hopkins	20	-	4	21	17	5	67	198
Univ. Tennessee	51	-	11	27	11	12	112	182
U. C. San Diego	13	2	18	9	7	2	51	144
Tulane Medical	15	28	11	11	1	5	71	109
Wayne State	8	7	15	6	1	9	46	102
Roswell Park	4	6	8	14	6	3	41	47
Baylor College	2	-	-	3	3	9	17	23
Walter Reed	2	3	7	8	9	5	34	35
Rush-Presbyterian	-	2	1	3	-	5	11	11
U. C. Los Angeles	8	1	-	2	8	6	25	25
Total	167	70	87	141	105	81	651	1748

Table 5. National Prostatic Cancer Project

Status as of September 26, 1980 Closed to Patient Entry

| | Protocols | | | | | | | |
	100	200	300	400	500	700	800	Total
Entered	125	125	165	135	301	125	121	1097
Exclusions								
Protocol Violations	3	2	2	5	19	9	8	48
No Treatment (TRT)	4	6	7	6	7	7	5	42
Received <3 Wks TRT	8	12	25	8	24	11	18	106
Insufficient Information For Evaluation	0	0	2	0	14	0	0	16
Evaluable	110	105	116	129	237	98	90	885
Currently on TRT*	0	0	1	0	123	0	3	127
Currently Being Followed	2	2	7	3	200	13	15	242

* May Include Crossover TRT

Table 6. National Prostatic Cancer Project

Total Patients Entered and Status of Current NPCP Protocols as of April, 1981

	Protocol						
	600	900	1000	1100	1200	1300	Total
Entered	167	70	87	141	105	81	651
Exclusions							
Protocol Violations	14	7	1	–	2	–	24
No Treatment (TRT)	1	2	2	9	1	–	15
Received <3 Wks TRT	7	–	–	5	6	–	18
Evaluation Pending	26	9	14	40	31	54	174
Evaluable	119	52	70	87	65	27	420
Currently on TRT*	58	41	62	63	40	74	338
Currently Being Followed	94	70	87	93	71	78	493

* May Include Crossover Treatment

Table 7. National Prostatic Cancer Project

Clinical Trials Program - Patient Activity

May, 1981

Closed Protocols	Patients Active	Total Accessioned
500	113	301
700	0	125
800	3	121

Open Protocols		
600	58	169
900	42	72
1000	61	90
1100	64	148
1200	39	108
1300	99	86

Table 8. Average Response Rates and Major Toxicities of All
Patients Randomized to Date in Each Drug Category
(Endocrine-Refractory Patients - No Significant
Irradiation Therapy).

April, 1981

Agent (No. Patients)	Response Rate Objective/Subjective	Toxicity
Cyclophosphamide (119)	35%/41%	35%
5-Fluorouracil (33)	36%/47%	35%
Methyl-CCNU (27)	30%/41%	56%
DTIC (55)	28%/35%	26%
Standard (36)	19%/22%	14%
Hydroxyurea (28)	15%/19%	46%
Procarbazine (38)	13%/21%	30%
Methotrexate (34)	50%/15%	41%
Cis-platinum (27)	26%/12%	32%

Table 9. Average Response Rates and Major Toxicities of All
Patients Randomized to Date in Each Drug Category
(Endocrine-Refractory Patients with Prior
Significant Irradiation Therapy).

April, 1981

Agent (No. Patients)		Response Rate Objective/Subjective	Toxicity
Streptozotocin	(38)	32%/28%	23%
Estramustine phosphate	(86)	26%/23%	35%
Standard	(21)	19%/19%	22%
Vincristine	(34)	15%/31%	32%
Leo-1031	(62)	13%/35%	17%
Cis-platinum	(22)	23%/ 8%	35%
Cis-platinum plus estramustine phosphate	(20)	45%/22%	46%

In those patients with advanced relapsing stage D prostatic
cancer who have had extensive pelvic irradiation, objective and
subjective response rates have been higher with treatment using
stretozotocin or estramustine phosphate compared to patients receiving standard therapy (8). Prednimustine (Leo-1031), either alone or
in combination with estramustine phosphate, and the agent vincristine
were not as effective as standard therapy. Cis-platinum alone and
combined with estramustine phosphate is currently under study in this
patient population (Table 9).

REFERENCES

1. W.W. Scott, R.P. Gibbons, D.E. Johnson, G.R. Prout, Jr.,
    J.D. Schmidt, J. Saroff, and G.P. Murphy, The continued evaluat-
    ion of the effects of chemotherapy in patients with advanced
    carcinoma of the prostate, J. Urol. 116:211 (1976).
2. G.P. Murphy, R.P. Gibbons, D.E. Johnson, S.A. Loening,
    G.R. Prout, J.D. Schmidt, D.S. Bross, T.M. Chu, J.F. Gaeta,
    J. Saroff, and W.W. Scott, A comparison of estramustine phosphate
    and streptozotocin in patients with advanced prostatic carcinoma
    who have had extensive irradiation, J. Urol 118:288 (1977).

3. J.D. Schmidt, W.W. Scott, R.P. Gibbons, D.E. Johnson, G.R. Prout, Jr., S.A. Loening, M.S. Soloway, T.M. Chu, J.F. Gaeta, N.H. Slack, J. Saroff, and G.P. Murphy, Comparison of procarbazine, imidazole-carboxamide and cyclophosphamide in relapsing patients with advanced carcinoma of the prostate, J. Urol. 121:185 (1979).

4. S.A. Loening, J.B. deKernion, R.P. Gibbons, D.E. Johnson, J.E. Pontes, G.R. Prout, Jr., J.D. Schmidt, W.W. Scott, M.S. Soloway, N.H. Slack, and G.P. Murphy, A comparison of hydroxyurea, methyl-CCNU and cyclophosphamide in patients with advanced carcinoma of the prostate, J. Urol. In Press.

5. G.P. Murphy, R.P. Gibbons, D.E. Johnson, G.R. Prout, J.D. Schmidt, M.S. Soloway, S.A. Loening, T.M Chu, J.F. Gaeta, J. Saroff, Z. Wajsman, N. Slack, and W.W. Scott, The use of estramustine and prednimustine versus prednimustine alone in advanced metastatic prostatic cancer patients who have received prior irradiation, J. Urol, 121:763 (1979).

6. M.S. Soloway, J.B. deKernion, R.P. Gibbons, D.E. Johnson, S. Loening, J.E. Pontes, G.R. Prout, J.D. Schmidt, W.W. Scott, N.H. Slack, and G.P. Murphy, Comparison of Estracyt and vincristine alone or in combination for patients with advanced hormone-refractory, previously irradiated carcinoma of the prostate, J. Urol. In Press.

7. J.D. Schmidt, W.W. Scott, R. Gibbons, D.E. Johnson, G.R. Prout, Jr., S. Loening. M. Soloway, J. deKernion, J.E. Pontes, N.H. Slack, and G.P. Murphy, Chemotherapy programs of the National Prostatic Cancer project, Cancer 45:1937 (1980).

8. R.P. Gibbons and Investigators, National Prostatic Cancer Project Cooperative Clinical Trials: Cooperative clinical trial of single and combined agent protocols: Adjuvant protocols, Urology (Suppl.), 17:48 (1981).

COMBINATION OF CHEMOTHERAPY AND HORMONES IN PROSTATIC CANCER

J. D. Schmidt

University of California Medical Center
San Diego
U.S.A.

ABSTRACT

The National Prostatic Cancer Project in a four-year period has accessioned 301 patients with newly diagnosed Stage D-2 prostatic cancer into a treatment protocol comparing cyclophosphamide (Cytoxan) plus estramustine phosphate (Estracyt) versus Cytoxan plus diethylstilbestrol (DES) versus either DES or bilateral orchiectomy. The three treatment arms appear comparable in terms of entry criteria with the exception of elevated acid phosphatase for one arm which as yet has not influenced the response rates. Thus far, toxicities to the chemotherapy combination treatment arms have not been excessive although more prevalent than in the DES/orchiectomy arm. Major toxicities have been anemia, leukopenia and nausea and vomiting. Preliminary data show that the treatment arm consisting of DES plus Cytoxan is showing a slight but non-significant advantage in delaying progression of the disease compared to the other two treatment arms at the initial 12-week evaluation. Patient follow-up and data collection is still not complete for the assessment of survival and response durations. Approximately one-third of patients entered into the study are still on original or crossover therapy with 75% of patients still in that category. More complete and meaningful data should be available in another 18 months.

INTRODUCTION

In early 1973, the National Prostatic Cancer Project (NPCP) initiated a series of four chemotherapy protocols designed exclusively for those patients with metastatic carcinoma of the prostate (Stage D-2) who had failed to respond or who no longer

responded to endocrine therapy (1). One of the initial and ongoing
objectives of the program was to determine the efficacy and safety
of single agents in the treatment of advanced prostatic carcinoma
resistant to endocrine manipulation, with the hope that this in
turn would lead to effective combination treatment for all stages
of prostatic cancer.

From the results of protocol 100, "A Comparison of
5-Fluorouracil and Cytoxan in Patients with Advanced Carcinoma of the
Prostate," it was determined that Cytoxan (cyclophosphamide) is a
useful chemotherapeutic agent in relapsing Stage D prostatic
carcinoma. From Protocol 200, "A Comparison of Estracyt and
Streptozotocin in Patients with Advanced Prostatic Cancer who have
had Extensive Irradiation," sufficient data was gathered under-
scoring the efficacy of Estracyt (estramustine phosphate) in this
group of patients. Based on these data and pilot studies at
Roswell Park Memorial Institute and elsewhere documenting the
activity as well as relative lack of hematologic toxicity of
Estracyt, the use of both these agents in earlier phases of Stage D
prostatic cancer seemed justified.

Treatment utilizing exogenous estrogens, generally diethylstilbestrol 1 mg. t.i.d., has been accepted for approximately 40
years (2,3). Estrogens can arrest the progress of prostatic cancer
and in many cases reverse the progression of Stage D disease for
variable intervals. Similarly, bilateral orchiectomy has been
widely utilized for patients with advanced prostatic cancer (4).

Based on the above information, the Treatment Subgroup of the
NPCP felt the need to design chemotherapy trials for patients who
had not had prior endocrine therapy and for whom earlier treatments
with combination chemotherapy and endocrine therapy might be of
greater benefit (5,6). This protocol (Protocol 500) was designed
to compare two combinations of agents in a randomized fashion with
either diethylstilbestrol or bilateral orchiectomy. A crossover
design was included to allow a second episode of treatment for
patients removed from initial treatment because of disease
progression and/or toxicity.

SCHEMA AND DOSAGE

Protocol 500 compares the efficacy of Cytoxan + Estracyt versus
Cytotoxan + diethylstilbestrol (DES) versus either DES or bilateral
orchiectomy alone in patients with newly diagnosed Stage D-2
prostatic cancer who have not had prior endocrine therapy.
Cytoxan is administered intravenously at a dose of 1 g/m^2
every three weeks, Estracyt is given at a dose of 600 mg/m^2 orally
every day in three divided doses, and DES is given in the standard
dose fashion 1 mg. t.i.d. orally. Patients randomized to the

endocrine therapy only arm receive either DES or bilateral
orchiectomy based on the option of the investigator and patient
(Appendix 1).

PATIENT SELECTION

     Criteria for eligibility in this study include (a) patients
diagnosed within 30 days of entry with histologically confirmed
prostatic cancer with bone or soft tissue metastases; (b) an
expected survival of at least 90 days; (c) an entry white blood
cell count of 4,000/mm^3 or greater and platelets of 100,000/mm^3 or
greater; (d) freedom from significant infection and satisfactory
recovery from any recent surgery; and (e) fully informed written
consent for the study.

     Ineligibility criteria include (a) history of prior treatment
with either Cytoxan, Estracyt, DES or orchiectomy. (A history of
radiation therapy does not in itself exclude a patient from entry
into this study); (b) presence of another malignancy except non-
melanomatous skin cancer; and (c) patients who, in the opinion of
the investigators, have other significant medical diseases making
the patient a poor risk for possible chemotherapy.

BASELINE LABORATORY STUDIES

     All patients entered into this study have been required to
have the following tests performed within two weeks of initiation
of treatment. These include complete history and physical examination with special attention paid to the prostatic findings,
urinalysis, hemoglobin, leukocyte count, platelet count, differential count, serum creatinine or BUN, serum bilirubin, acid and
alkaline phosphatases, serum glutamic oxaloacetic transaminase
(SGOT), prothrombin time, chest x-ray, either radionuclide bone
scan or skeletal survey, excretory urogram (IVP) and documentation
of the histologic diagnosis by appropriate slide material which in
turn is sent to the NPCP headquarters.

     Following the initiation of treatment, patients receive follow-
up blood studies at three-week intervals and all baseline studies
are performed at 12-week intervals to assess both response to
treatment and toxicities.

EVALUATION OF RESPONSE TO THERAPY

     In this study, patients are evaluated for their response to
treatment according to the National Prostatic Cancer Project
criteria for objective reponses (1). These include complete
objective regression, partial objective regression, objective
stability and objective progression. The criteria for each of
these response categories are included in Appendix 2. In addition,

Table 1: NPCP Chemotherapy Protocol – 500

Status of Patients Entered
As of April 10, 1981

Category	Treatment			
	DES or Orchiectomy	DES + Cytoxan	Estracyt + Cytoxan	Total
Patients on study after 3 or more weeks of treatment	82	75	80	237
Protocol Violations	10	6	3	19
No Treatment	4	1	2	7
Removed before 3 weeks	3	10	11	24
Insufficient data for Evaluation	2	4	8	14
Total	101	96	104	301

the duration of response is tabulated for those patients so designated.

CROSSOVER DESIGN

As indicated in the schema (Appendix 1), the initial treatment may be discontinued either because of objective disease progression or toxicity. Patients initially treated with the combination of Cytoxan and Estracyt may then be crossed over to receive DES. Patients initially treated with the combination of Cytoxan and DES are crossed over to receive Estracyt. Lastly, patients initially treated with either DES or bilateral orchiectomy can then be crossed over to receive the combination of Cytoxan and Estracyt. Following discontinuation of the second treatment because of either progression or toxicity, all patients are followed indefinitely and are treated at the option of the investigators.

CURRENT RESULTS

Protocol 500 was activated on July 1, 1976, and closed to patient entry on August 31, 1980. Since that time, patients with similar eligibility criteria have been entered into a new protocol (Protocol 1300).

A total of 301 patients have been accessioned to Protocol 500 (Table 1). Information of on-study variables is now available for 287 patients, with response and toxicity data available for 237 patients. The exclusion rate has been approximately 17% in each of the three arms. Approximately one-third of all patients are still being treated with either the initial or crossover therapies.

As shown in Figure 1, age distributions are similar in all three treatment arms. All other on-study variables seem to be equal for the three arms with the exception of a greater proportion of patients with increased acid phosphatase activity in the Estracyt plus Cytoxan arm.

At this time 19 patients have been reported as complete objective regressions (Table 2). These include seven patients treated with either DES or bilateral orchiectomy (9%), five patients treated with a combination of DES and Cytoxan (7%) and seven patients treated with a combination of Cytoxan and Estracyt (9%). Partial responses have been reported for 58 patients or 24% of the total. These include 24 patients treated with either DES or bilateral orchiectomy (29%), 20 patients treated with DES plus Cytoxan (27%) and 14 patients receiving Cytoxan and Estracyt (18%). Objective stability has been recorded for 121 patients or 51% of the total. Included are 35 patients in the endocrine therapy arm (43%), 41 patients receiving Cytoxan plus DES (55%) and 45 patients receiving Estracyt plus Cytoxan (56%). Objective

Table 2: NPCP Chemotherapy Protocol – 500

Objective Response According to Treatment, April 1981

Response	Treatment							
	DES or Orchidectomy		DES + Cytoxan		Estracyt + Cytoxan		Total	
	No.	%	No.	%	No.	%	No.	%
Complete	7	9	5	7	7	9	19	8
Partial Regression	24	29	20	27	14	18	58	24
Stable	35	43	41	55	45	56	121	51
Progression	16	20	9	12	14	18	39	16
Total	82		75		80		237	

Table 3: NPCP Chemotherapy Protocol - 500
Response and Evaluation Status of Patients in the DES/Orchiectomy Treatment Arm

Category	DES No.	DES %	Orchiectomy No.	Orchiectomy %	Total
Complete	5	9	2	8	7
Partial	16	29	8	31	24
Stable	26	46	9	35	35
Progression	9	16	7	27	16
Total	56		26		82
Exclusions	11	16	5	15	16
Incomplete	1	1	2	6	3
Total	68	(67)[a]	33	(33)[a]	101

a Percentage of 101 entered to this treatment arm

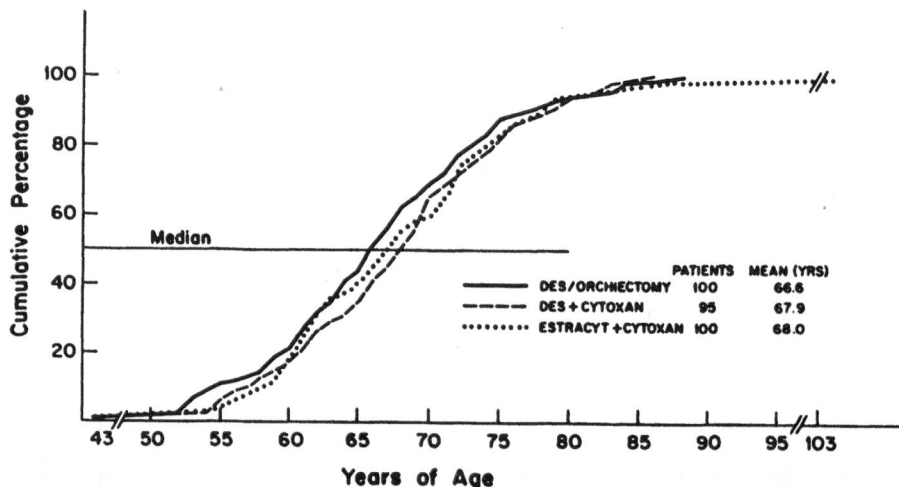

Fig. 1.   Age Distribution According to Treatment

progression on the initial randomized treatment has been reported
for 39 patients or 16% of the total. These include 16 patients on
endocrine therapy (20%), 9 patients on DES plus Cytoxan (12%) and
14 patients on Estracyt plus Cytoxan (18%).

Crossover responses have been reported in 36 of 63 patients
so treated (50% response rate). These include patients who
progressed on their initially randomized therapy as well as patients
who initially responded then progressed and responded to the
crossover treatment. Most of the crossover responses to date have
been in the stable category.

The response rates to either DES or bilateral orchiectomy are
similar to date, namely 84% for DES and 73% for orchiectomy
(Table 3). In a small subset of patients with only soft tissue
metastases, the response rates to date are greater but not
statistically significant compared to the vast majority of patients
with bony metastases alone or the combination of skeletal and soft
tissue metastases. Subjective responses such as improvements in
performance status and pain are relatively the same in all three
treatment arms.

Major toxicities thus far include the tendency to lowering of
hemoglobin in the patients treated with Estracyt and Cytoxan, more
leukopenia in patients treated with the combination of DES and

Table 4: NPCP Chemotherapy Protocol - 500

Reasons for discontinuing randomized treatments for evaluable patients

Reasons	Treatment						
	DES or Orchiectomy		DES + Cytoxan		Estracyt + Cytoxan		Total	
	No.	%	No.	%	No.	%	No.	%
Still on Treatment	45	55	25	33	27	34	97	41
Progression	33	40	22	29	25	31	80	34
Nausea - Vomiting	-		7	9	10	12	17	7
Other Toxicities	4	5	11	15	11	14	26	11
Death	-		6[a]	8	3[b]	4	9	4
Other	-		4	5	4	5	8	3
Total	82		75		80		237	

a Five of the six were still in response at death, one due to auto accident, two to myocardial infarction, and one to congestive heart failure, and one to erythroleukemia.

b One was stable at death from heart failure, one to non cancer causes that were unspecified and one of unknown cause.

Cytoxan, and a very few instances of thrombocytopenia, mostly in patients treated with DES plus Cytoxan.

Nausea and vomiting have been predominant (66% incidence) in the two arms employing Cytoxan but have been infrequent (20%) in the patients receiving only endocrine therapy.

Patients initially treated with either DES or orchiectomy have been crossed over to Cytoxan and Estracyt mainly because of disease progression, with a smaller subset crossed over because of cardio-vascular toxicity of DES (Table 4). On the other hand, both drug toxicity and disease progression have been prominent reasons for discontinuation of treatment in the two arms utilizing Cytoxan.

At this early date, 75% of patients responding to treatment are still responding (Figure 2). Only 24% of patients entered into the study have died (Figure 3). At this time there is no advantage for either DES or orchiectomy regarding survival for patients treated in the endocrine arm (Figure 4). Survival in general has been equal for all three arms of the study with a transient advantage in the second year of treatment for those patients receiving DES plus Cytoxan (Figure 3). Based on the experience to date with patients accessioned, another 18 months of patient follow-up and data collection will be necessary to lead to meaningful results and conclusions.

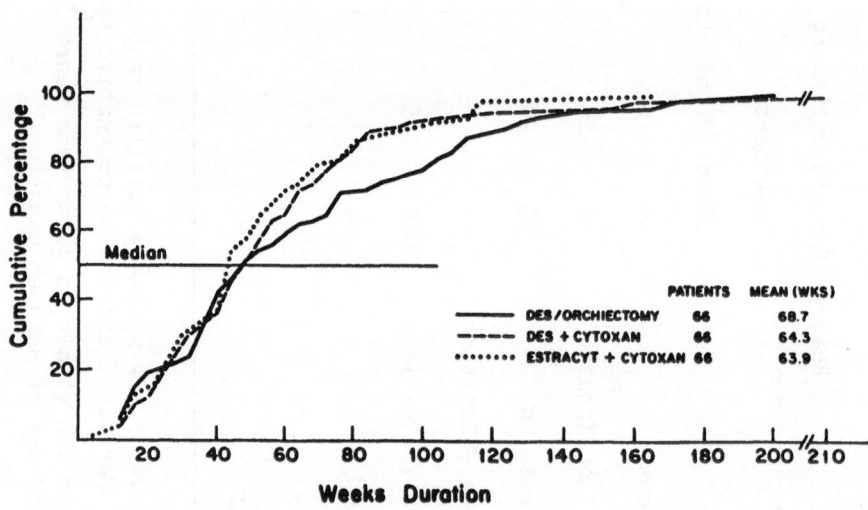

Fig. 2. Distributions of Response Duration for Responders
(Complete, Partial Regression) According to Treatment.

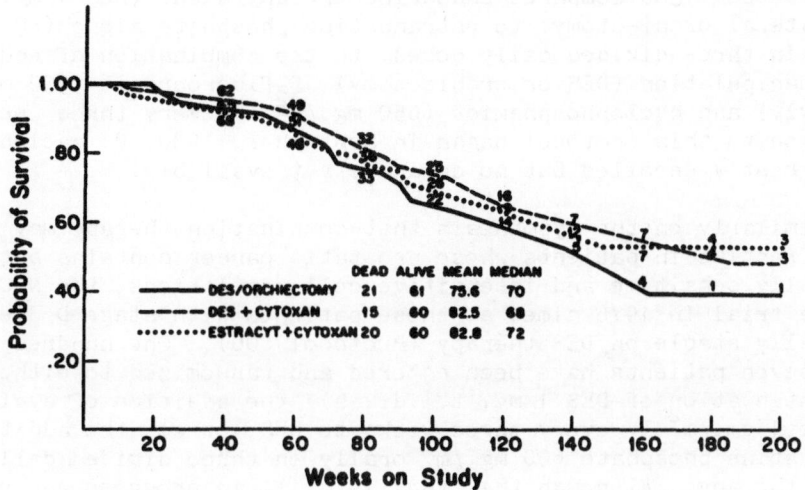

Fig. 3. Probability of Survival for Randomized Treatment Groups
(April 1980).

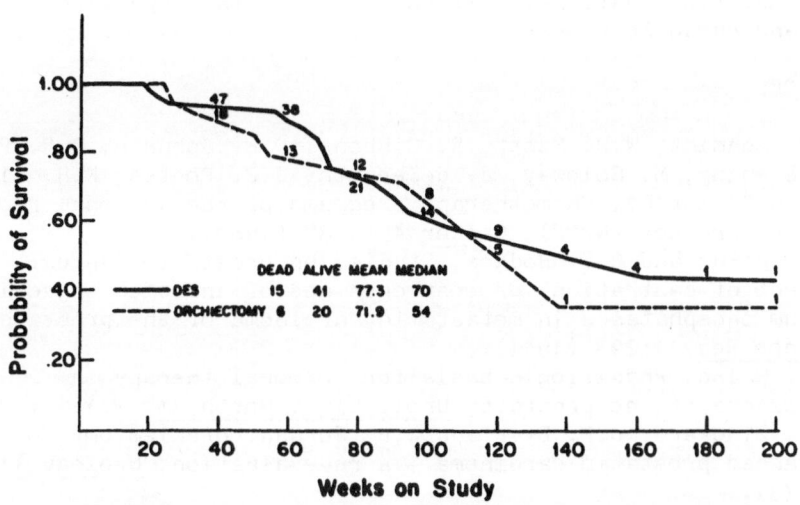

Fig. 4. Probability of Survival for Patients Electing DES or
Orchiectomy in the DES/Orchiectomy Arm.

OTHER CURRENT STUDIES

Protocol 1300 compares endocrine therapy alone (DES 1 mg. t.i.d. or bilateral orchiectomy) to estramustine phosphate alone (60 mg./m^2 orally in three divided daily doses) to the combination of endo-crine manipulation (DES or orchiectomy), 5-fluorouracil (350 mg./m^2 IV weekly) and cyclophosphamide (650 mg./m^2 IV every three weeks). Accession to this protocol began in September, 1980, 81 patients are currently enrolled but no data are yet available.

Similarly on the hypothesis that combination therapy may be more effective in patients whose prostatic cancer contains both hormonally sensitive and insensitive cell populations, the NPCP began a trial in 1976 aimed at those patients with stage D disease clinically stable on DES therapy (Protocol 600). One hundred and sixty seven patients have been entered and randomized to either: a) continuation of DES 1 mg. t.i.d., b) the addition of cyclophos-phamide 1 gm./m^2 IV every three weeks to DES, or c) the addition of estramustine phosphate 600 mg./m^2 orally in three divided daily doses to DES therapy. Although the study is still in progress and results are not complete, preliminary data suggest that the addition of cyclophosphamide to DES reduces the rate of progression compared to DES alone.

This work was supported in part by Public Health Service Grant CA 21428 through the National Prostatic Cancer Project, National Cancer Institute, National Institutes of Health, Department of Health and Human Services.

REFERENCES

1. J.D. Schmidt, W.W. Scott, R. Gibbons, D.E. Johnson, G.R. Prout, S. Loening, M. Soloway, J. deKernion, J.E. Pontes, N.H. Slack and G.P. Murphy, Chemotherapy programs of the National Prostatic Cancer Project (NPCP), Cancer 45:1937 (1980).
2. C. Huggins and C.V. Hodges, Studies on prostatic cancer: Effect of castration, of oestrogen and of androgen injection on serum phosphatases in metastatic carcinoma of the prostate, Cancer Res. 1:293 (1941).
3. P.C. Walsh, Physiologic basis for hormonal therapy in carcinoma of the prostate, Urol. Clin. North Am. 2:125 (1975).
4. C.E. Blackard, D.P. Byar and W.P. Jordan, Orchiectomy for advanced prostatic carcinoma - a re-evaluation, Urology 1:553 (1973).
5. J.D. Schmidt, Chemotherapy of prostatic cancer, Urol. Clin. North Am. 2:185 (1975).
6. J.D. Schmidt, Developments in the endocrine therapy of prostatic cancer, Reviews on Endocrine-Related Cancer 5:13 (1980).

APPENDIX 1

Schema

National Prostatic Cancer Project

Protocol 500

Cytoxan, 1 gm/m^2 I.V. every three weeks
plus
Estracyt, 600 mg/m^2 orally daily in three
divided doses

vs

Cytoxan, 1 gm/m^2 IV every three weeks
plus
Diethylstilbestrol 1 mg t.i.d. orally

vs

Diethylstilbestrol 1 mg t.i.d orally
or
Orchiectomy (Investigator's Option)

APPENDIX 2

Response Criteria

National Prostatic Cancer Project

Protocol 500

OBJECTIVE REGRESSION

All of the following criteria:

Complete

Absence of any clinically detectable soft tissue tumor mass. This may include the primary tumor.

Return of an elevated acid phosphatase to normal level.

The recalcification of all osteolytic lesions if present.

No evidence of progression of osteoblastic lesions, if any are present.

If hepatomegaly is a significant indicator, there must be a complete reduction in liver size, and normalization of all pretreatment abnormalities of liver function.

Partial

A 50% reduction in measurable or palpable soft tissue tumor mass when present.

Return of an elevated acid phosphatase to normal.

The recalcification of some osteolytic lesions if present.

If hepatomegaly is a significant indicator, there must be a reduction in liver size and at least a 30% improvement of all pretreatment abnormalities of liver function.

There must be no increase in any other lesion and no new areas of malignant disease may appear.

No significant deterioration in weight (greater than 10%), symptoms, or performance status (one score level).

OBJECTIVELY STABLE

All of the following criteria:

Insufficient regression of primary indicator lesion to meet criteria above.

Less than 25% increase in any measurable lesion.

No significant deterioration in weight (greater than 10%), symptoms or performance status (one score level).

OBJECTIVE PROGRESSION (or also Relapse after Adequate Therapy)

Any of the following criteria:

Significant deterioration in symptoms related to prostatic cancer, decrease in weight, decrease in performance status, or pain requiring medication.

Development of recurring anemia, secondary to prostatic cancer (not chemotherapy).

Development of ureteral obstruction.

Appearance of new areas of malignant disease.

Increase in any previously measurable lesion (soft tissue and lung, excluding bone) by greater than 50% in two perpendicular diameters.

Increase in osseous metastases as shown by scan.

An increase in acid or alkaline phosphatase alone is not to be considered an indication of progression. These should be used in conjuction with other criteria.

STRATEGY OF TREATMENT IN THE ADVANCED STAGES - ROUND TABLE REPORT

J. P. Blandy[1] and M. Pavone-Macaluso[2]

1. The London Hospital
   London, U.K.

2. The University of Palermo
   Palermo, Italy

Although cancer of the prostate is completely preventable by castration before puberty, prevention at such a price is obviously out of the question. Equally, in later life, it is necessary to weigh up the cost to the patient, in terms of quality of life, of any slight extension of its duration. Denis reminded us that in autumn it is not the length of days but their freedom from distress which should be our primary concern.

Advanced local disease without detectable metastases(T3. MO).

1. The value of lymph node staging

We discussed at length the necessity for lymph node staging. Several proponents took the view that there was no value (to the patient) of knowing the precise N staging, since such knowledge would not alter treatment, and Bagshaw, speaking from his considerable experience, had reached the conclusion that when the acid phosphatase was elevated and the tumour grade was undifferentiated, then nothing was to be gained by node dissection since the nodes were bound to be involved by tumour. After discussion it was felt that perhaps there was a place still remaining for node dissection as a preliminary step in exploration prior to an attempt at a "salvage prostatectomy", if such an operation were to be contemplated.

2. Local radiotherapy for T3 tumours

Most surgeons would agree, it seemed, that radical prostatect-

omy was out of the question for T3 tumours, and Bagshaw was asked
whether he thought these growths were suitable for radiotherapy.
He replied that in his hands they seemed to do reasonably well, and
added that in many of these cases, local extension beyond the
normal limits of his small field of irradiation, or the demonstration
in CAT or lymphangiogram of involvement of pelvic lymph nodes,
could be included in the area to be irradiated by adjustment of the
treatment field.

Since radiotherapy was so dependent upon the bulk of the
tumour, Altwein asked whether we should not try to shrink the bulky
T3 tumours by preliminary estrogens or cyproterone acetate prior to
radiation, particularly in patients whose grossly swollen prostates
were accompanied by outflow obstruction. Bagshaw agreed that this
was useful in practice, and from the discussion that followed, it
seemed clear that the optimum combination of radiotherapy and
hormones was still an area worth studying in clinical trials.

The comparable use of hormones to shrink the "inoperable"
prostate in order to render it suitable for radical perineal
prostatectomy was referred to by Schmidt, and Dr Goodwin reminded
us of the earlier attempts by Dr Winfield Scott to achieve just
this goal, but added that he thought most surgeons had abandoned
this procedure.

3.   Salvage prostatectomy after "failed" radiotherapy

The discussion then turned naturally to the place of "salvage
prostatectomy" after a course of radiotherapy which had been followed
by persistence or return of tumour in the irradiated field. Jacobi's
important finding, that when cancer cells were found in fine-needle
aspiration smears from prostates two years after completion of
radiotherapy, such patients nearly always were found to grow widespread metastases within the next few years, emphasised the real
risk that these "silent" cancer cells posed for the patient. With
this view Andersson agreed, particularly when the cytological
features of these tumours were less than well-differentiated. The
place of salvage prostatectomy remained in question, and again the
question of the price the patient would have to pay in terms of
operative morbidity would need to be submitted to carefully
controlled trials before it could be taken up with any enthusiasm.

Metastatic Disease

1.   Timing for therapy

Nothing raised so much argument among the participants as the
timing of treatment of metastases. Many favoured immediate treatment, arguing classically that those that were smallest should
respond best; others took the view that treatment ought to be

deferred until symptoms occurred. On a show of hands (in the absence of hard evidence) the room was equally divided.

2. Significance of a raised acid phosphatase

Byar's interesting observations that showed such a close relationship between very small elevations of serum acid phosphatase (measured by the old enzymatic method) and the subsequent fate of patients in long term follow up, led to a stimulating discussion as to the role of acid phosphatase, and in particular, to a renewed respect for the traditional enzymatic method. If Byar's observations were confirmed, then one should perhaps regard even a very small elevation of acid phosphatase as a sinister harbinger of occult metastases.

3. Orchidectomy or estrogens?

Having dodged the question of when to start to treat metastases, we turned to the choice of which method of hormone treatment - and in particular, what was the place of orchidectomy? In the VACURG studies it was clear that those assigned to the orchidectomy group in the initial randomisation did less well than those offered estrogen or estrogen plus orchidectomy. Despite a few rather curious claims that orchidectomy was somehow cheaper (for whom?) than estrogen therapy, the consensus of the discussion was that orchidectomy ought to be restricted to those patients who were not reliable pill-takers or for whom the cardiovascular complications of estrogens made them contraindicated.

4. Which estrogen?

None of the alternatives to cheap, simple, old-fashioned DES seemed, from the results of the endless clinical trials that we had listened to, to be any better. Unfortunately, it appeared from the discussion that because DES was so cheap, no manufacturer had much interest in making it, and worse, the risk of stilboestrol being added to cattle food had led to it being banned in certain European countries. Other "natural" estrogens, if pregnant mares' urine can be regarded as natural for mankind, gave equally good, but no better results. There was no advantage in using TACE or cyproterone acetate in the first instance.

5. Chemotherapy

When the claims of the US National Prostatic Studies were critically evaluated, it was pointed out that none of the results justified the use of any chemotherapeutic agent in the first line treatment of metastases. The estrogen-mustard combinations might however have a place, Andersson argued, in the initial treatment of metastases when the tumour grade was especially anaplastic. The

proper place for chemotherapy, at this time, seemed to belong to
the treatment of patients whose tumours had "escaped" from
estrogen therapy. Even here, as emerged very clearly from Schmidt's
reports on the clinical trials, some of these "escapers" were, in
fact, men who had failed to take estrogen therapy as prescribed.
At this stage the discussion came near the brink of the treatment
of "failed estrogen therapy" which was the proper subject of the
next round table, as a result of which this one came to its
natural conclusion.

STRATEGY OF TREATMENT IN PROSTATIC CANCER - A CONTRIBUTION TO THE DISCUSSION

L. Denis

A.Z. Middelheim
Antwerp
Belgium

Appropriate therapy of patients with prostatic cancer with the multitude of existing modalities depends on three important factors - the general condition of the patient, the stage of the cancer and the biological potential of the tumor.

The general condition of the patient should be judged on age, index of vitality, and the presence or absence of associated disease especially cardio-vascular disease; the interest of the patient in sexual activity should also be noted.

The stage of disease should be based on physical findings, laboratory tests, medical imaging techniques and surgical evaluation in some instances. These examinations should result in reliable and reproducible parameters to measure existing or progressive disease.

The biological potential of the tumor should currently be based on a satisfactory tissue specimen and a consultation with the pathologist. A Gleason scale of 9 or 10 seems to be an accurate prognostic factor (1).

Based on this information we should be able to classify patients with prostatic carcinoma as having local or systemic disease. A reasonable effort to collect information on the possible invasion of the regional lymph nodes includes the study of prognostic factors in lymphatic spread, lymphangiography and fine needle biopsy and/or lymphadenectomy (1,2). However, accumulated data would indicate that no local treatment be it radical surgery, interstitial radiotherapy or external beam radiation brings disease control when cancer is present in the local regional nodes (3,4,5).

An international pathology reference system and a referee pathologist are essential to accurate statistical evaluation of any trial concerning prostatic cancer. Another problem of the pathology is that with the exception of the poorly differentiated lesions prostatic <u>micro</u>carcinoma should be eliminated from our clinical data.

True localized cancers can be treated by total or radical prostatectomy, external beam irradiation or interstitial radiotherapy. Total prostatectomy seems the best treatment for the localized nodule (6).

Systemic disease is a problem whose natural history varies according to the different characteristics of the tumor and its host. Hormonal treatment in its diverse forms aims to abolish the physiologic effect of circulating androgenic hormones. Bilateral orchiectomy is indicated in patients with prostatic cancer in relapse where serum testosterone is not reduced to anorchic levels (7). The debate on late or early hormonal treatment is by no means completely resolved (8). Finally, the value of multi-modal hormonal treatment and adjunctive chemotherapeutic treatment can best be determined by future randomized trials and seem to offer the only solution to the dilemma of the management of prostatic cancer.

REFERENCES

1. D.E. Paulson, P.V. Piserchia, and W. Gardner, Predictors of lymphatic spread in prostatic adeno-carcinoma: Uro. Oncology Research Group study, <u>J. Urol</u>. 123:697 (1980).
2. T. Sherwood and E.P.N. O'Donoghue, Lymphograms in prostatic carcinoma: false positive and false-negative assessments in radiology, <u>Brit. J. Rad</u>. 54:15 (1981).
3. G.R. Prout, Jr., J.A. Heaney, P. Griffin, J.J. Daly, and W.U. Shipley, Nodal involvement as prognostic indicator in patients with prostatic carcinoma, <u>J. Urol</u>. 124:226 (1980).
4. W.F. Whitmore, M. Batata, and B. Hilaris, Prostatic irradiation: Iodine-125 implantation, <u>in</u>:"Cancer of the Genito-Urinary Tract," D.E. Johnson and M.L. Samuels, Raven Press, New York, (1979), p.195.
5. D.F. Paulson, Multimodal therapy of prostatic cancer, supplement to <u>Urology</u> 17:53 (1981).
6. P.C. Walsh and H.J. Jewett, Radical surgery for prostatic cancer, <u>Cancer</u> 45:1906 (1980).
7. L. Denis and P. Nowé, Bilateral orchiectomy in patients with progressive advanced prostatic cancer, <u>Acta Urol. Belg</u>. 48:113 (1980).
8. D.S. Coffey and J.T. Isaacs, Prostate tumor biology and cell kinetics theory, supplement to <u>Urology</u> 17:40 (1981).

ON THE METHODOLOGY OF CONTROLLED CLINICAL TRIALS

R. Sylvester

EORTC Data Centre
Brussels
Belgium

INTRODUCTION

A wide and varied literature exists on the appropriate methodology that one should employ in the design and analysis of clinical
trials. As many concepts are somewhat controversial in nature and
not widely accepted or understood by many researchers, this paper
will present a very general overview of the underlying principles
involved in the design and analysis of clinical trials.

THE PROTOCOL

The most important document pertaining to any trial is the
protocol, a self contained description of the rationale, objectives
and logistics of the study. The protocol provides the scientific
basis for the study and describes how the trial is to be carried
out. Staquet, Sylvester and Jasmin (1) have published practical
guidelines for the preparation of cancer clinical trial protocols.
They provide precise suggestions concerning the contents of the
chapter headings found in Table 1 along with a large bibliography
of papers related to the design and analysis of cancer clinical
trials.

PUBLISHING TRIAL RESULTS

One of the main problems encountered in interpreting the
results of a clinical trial is due to the wide variability that
exists in the methods used to assess treatment efficacy and in the
manner in which one publishes trial results. It is often difficult
to place a trial in its proper perspective due to an inconsistent
or incomplete reporting of the patient population under study, the

Table 1: Protocol contents

1. Background and Introduction

2. Objectives of the Trial

3. Selection of Patients

4. Design of the Trial (Including a Schema)

5. Therapeutic Regimens and Toxicity

6. Required Clinical Evaluations, Laboratory Tests and Follow-Up

7. Criteria of Evaluation

8. Registration and Randomization of Patients

9. Forms and Procedures of Collecting Data

10. Statistical Considerations

11. Administrative Responsibilities

12. References

    Appendices: Performance Status Scales

                 TNM or Other Classifications

treatment administered, toxicities observed, or the statistical
methods employed to assess treatment efficacy. In addition there
may be important differences from one trial to another in defining
what constitutes a response to treatment, especially in advanced
disease when there are multiple lesions. Some standardization in the
reporting of treatment results in cancer patients is required if
the results of published trials are to be properly interpreted.

The World Health Organization has attempted such a standardization by publishing the WHO Handbook for Reporting Results of
Cancer Treatment (2). This handbook proposes a minimum data set
which should be reported and provides definitions for terms such as
response, duration of response and duration of survival. In addition
a grading system for the reporting of toxicity is provided. As
the WHO Handbook deals with the reporting of cancer treatment
results in general rather than in the specific setting of a clinical
trial, Kisner and Sylvester (3) have proposed a set of guidelines
based on the WHO Handbook but adapted specifically to cancer clinical
trials. These works should be consulted not only at the time when
the trial is to be analyzed and the results published, but also when
designing new protocols since the definitions proposed in these
papers should be incorporated into the protocol and data forms at
the design stage.

PHASE I, II AND III TRIALS

In cancer research one encounters Phase I, Phase II and
Phase III trials. What is the purpose of each type of trial and
how do they differ?

In its simplest terms a Phase I trial may be thought of as a
toxicity screening trial where after testing in animals, the drug
is administered for the first time in man in order to determine
the maximum tolerated dose. Several patients are treated at each
of a series of increasing dosage levels in order to determine
which level should be tested in a Phase II trial. It should be
emphasized that the assessment of treatment efficacy is not an
endpoint of interest in Phase I trials as we are at this point
only dealing with the initial human clinical pharmacological
evaluation of the drug.

Once a maximum tolerated dose is determined from a Phase I
study, the drug is screened for potential anti-tumour activity in
a Phase II trial in a limited number of patients with advanced
measurable disease. The purpose of a Phase II trial is to see
whether or not the drug has sufficient activity to warrant further
testing in a larger number of patients. A Phase II study is not
an absolute test of the drug's efficacy but rather a screen of the
drug at a given dose in a given group of patients. For example,
a drug may initially be tested in 20 patients and rejected from

further study if no responses are observed.

One problem encountered in Phase II trials is that patients entered in such a trial have usually failed on a number of previous treatments and may be in such poor condition that the chances of their responding to any treatment, even an active one, are very low. Thus a negative result in a Phase II trial does not exclude the possibility that the drug might be active in previously un- treated patients or in patients with less advanced disease.

Once a drug has shown some degree of activity in a Phase II trial at an acceptable level of toxicity, the next step is to introduce the drug into a Phase III trial. The purpose of a Phase III trial is to determine the relative effectiveness of the new treatment by comparing the new drug or perhaps a combination containing the new drug to the classical or best available treat- ment in a large number of patients. The rest of this paper will deal specifically with the design and analysis of Phase III trials.

DESIGNING PHASE III STUDIES

Randomization

When one wishes to compare two or more different treatments in a clinical trial, the treatment groups to be studied should be as similar as possible with respect to all factors, whether known or not, which might affect a patient's response to treatment. Randomization is used as a method of assigning treatment to patients that permits valid statistical comparisons to be drawn without making any special assumptions (4).

Randomization has three primary advantages over using historical controls:

1. An investigator cannot either consciously or subconsciously assign more patients of a certain type to receive a particular treatment. Thus bias is eliminated in the assignment of treatments.

2. The process of randomization tends to balance the distribution of the various prognostic factors, whether known or not. in the various treatment groups. Thus the treatment groups to be compared will tend to be truly comparable.

3. The process of randomization allows one to calculate the so called P-value, the probability of obtaining a difference at least as large as that actually observed in the trial if in fact the treatments are equivalent.

While there are many other advantages to randomization they will not be discussed here. The interested reader is referred to

Byar et al (4) for further details. In any multicenter study
a centralized randomization where participating institutions contact a central office by telephone or telex is to be preferred to
a system of envelopes for the following reasons:

1. A centralized randomization ensures that the randomization is
done correctly. A system of envelopes is to be discouraged as this
method can easily be abused.

2. With a centralized randomization one knows at all times exactly
how many patients have been entered on study and who they are.

3. With a centralized randomization it is possible to request over-
due forms for all patients entered on study.

Stratification

     When one analyzes in a statistical model the effect that
various prognostic factors and treatment may have on a patient's
response to treatment, it is often found that even if there is a
significant treatment effect, several of the prognostic factors
may be more important than the treatment itself. Performance status
for example is an important prognostic factor in determining the
duration of survival in prostatic cancer patients as shown in
figure 1. You will not often find treatment differences of this
magnitude in a clinical trial. It is clear that any imbalance in
the distribution of the performance status in the various treatment groups to be compared will seriously bias the treatment
comparisons unless an adjustment for the performance status is
made. In the case of a retrospective study, data on prognostic
factors such as the performance status are not usually available
for each patient so that no correction for such biases is possible.

     In a randomized prospective trial it is possible to take into
account the effect of various prognostic factors by means of
stratification, either at the time of randomization or at the time
of analysis. Stratification at the time of randomization for the
one or two most important prognostic factors ensures that no
major imbalances in the number of patients receiving each treatment
will occur in these prognostic subgroups.

     While stratification at randomization is beneficial, over-
stratification may actually turn out to provide a worse balance
than if no stratification at all had taken place. After a certain
point, overstratification becomes equivalent to no stratification
at all and may by chance turn out to be worse.

     In determining the number of strata one should estimate the
expected number of patients that will fall into each stratum and
combine those strata which are expected to contain only a few

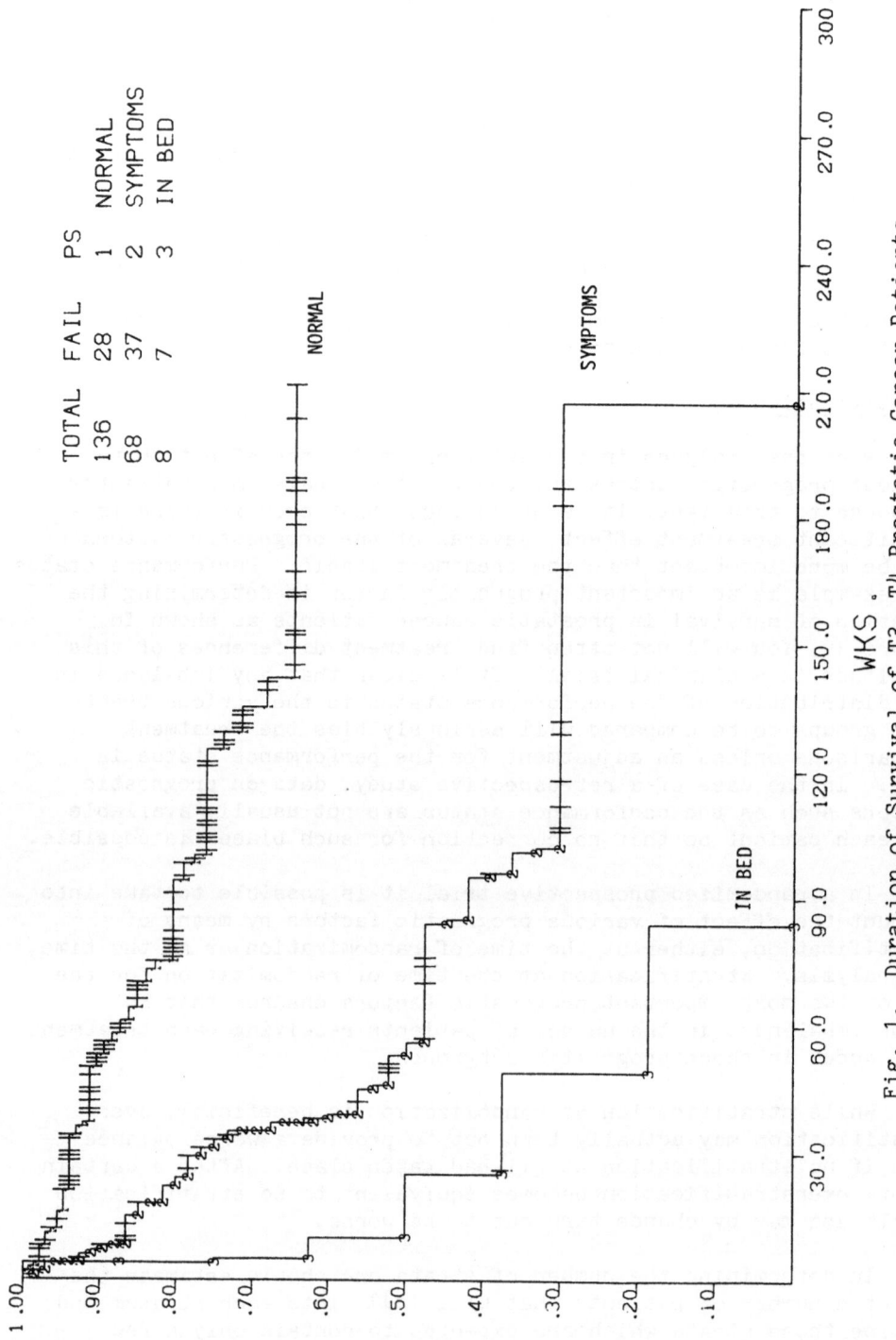

Fig. 1. Duration of Survival of T3, T4 Prostatic Cancer Patients
According to Performance Status (PS).

patients. In a multicenter study I would recommend stratifying by institution and then generally by the one variable thought to be the most important.

Independently of whether or not one has stratified at the time of randomization, it is important to stratify at the time of analysis for those variables which prove to be of prognostic importance (5). In this manner you adjust for the effect that a variable might have on the endpoint of interest. While a moderate imbalance in the distribution of a prognostic factor in the various treatment groups is not a serious problem, stratification at randomization guards against any large imbalances that might arise and for which adjustment procedures may no longer be adequate.

ANALYZING PHASE III STUDIES

Excluding Patients from the Analysis

Perhaps one of the most controversial and misunderstood concepts in the analysis of comparative Phase III trials is the question of excluding non-evaluable patients from the treatment results. When analyzing clinical trial data exclusion of patients for any reason other than ineligibility may no longer permit an unbiased evaluation of the results since the reason for exclusion may be correlated with the treatment group and the endpoints under study.

In the case of an adjuvant study suppose patients are randomized to receive either adjuvant chemotherapy or no adjuvant treatment after removal of the primary tumour. One is tempted to exclude from the statistical analysis those patients who for one reason or another did not receive chemotherapy in accordance with the protocol or who received a reduced number of cycles due to early death or toxicity. On the other hand the same patient, if he had been randomized to the no treatment control group, would have been considered to be fully evaluable and included in the statistical analysis. Excluding patients from the chemotherapy group will result in comparing all the patients of the control group to only a selected subset of the patients randomized to receive chemotherapy, i.e. the chemotherapy patients with the best prognosis. Such a practice will lead to biased results since the two treatment groups will no longer be comparable. In this case it is not surprising that a significant difference may be obtained in favour of adjuvant chemotherapy even if the treatment is of no real benefit. In order to avoid this situation all eligible randomized patients should be included in the statistical analysis. In this manner the balance established by the randomization will be maintained and you are answering the more realistic question: "Is the policy of giving adjuvant chemotherapy whenever possible better than the policy of giving no adjuvant treatment?" It is unrealistic to think that in practice all patients will receive chemotherapy exactly as specified in the protocol. While this example involved a non treated control group, the same principles would apply in the comparison of two or more treatments.

In the analysis of studies of advanced disease the same problem exists. However here it might be stipulated in the protocol that a patient must receive a certain minimal amount of treatment before the patient can be evaluated for tumour response. Even in this case care should be taken to determine whether or not the reason for exclusion is related to the treatment group or the disease in question. If more patients are excluded in one treatment group than in the other, the results may be subject to bias. When publishing trial results it is of utmost importance to account for every patient entered in the trial.

Analysis of Survival Data

A survival curve or a survival distribution is simply a graph or table giving an estimate of the proportion of patients in a specified group who are still alive at different times after randomization or start of treatment. Any technique used in the calculation of survival curves must take into account the possibility that a particular patient's death may not have been observed yet at the time of analysis. For patients who are still alive or lost to follow up at the time of analysis, the only information that is available is the date that the patient was last known to be alive. This is usually referred to as the date of censoring. In constructing a survival curve, the Kaplan-Meier Product Limit method is to be preferred (6).

If we want to compare the effect on survival of two different treatments, it is not sufficient to simply count the number of deaths in each treatment group, but it is also necessary to take into consideration the time of death and for those patients who are still alive, the duration of follow up for each patient.

In testing whether or not there is a significant difference between two or more survival curves, tests which utilize the entire curve should be employed rather than tests which just compare the curves at a specific point or points in time.

Two tests to be preferred are the Log Rank (Mantel-Haenszel) Test and the Gehan Generalized Wilcoxon Test, more fully considered by Peto et al in 1977 (5).

CONCLUSION

A wide number of topics pertaining to the methodology of controlled clinical trials have been discussed in this paper but only in a very general and somewhat superfical manner. Some very basic guidelines have been presented but it is now up to the reader to consult the references provided in order to obtain a fuller understanding of the appropriate techniques to employ in the design and analysis of such trials.

REFERENCES

1. M. Staquet, R. Sylvester and C. Jasmin, Guidelines for the preparation of EORTC cancer clinical trial protocols, Europ. J. Cancer, 16:871 (1980).

2. WHO Handbook for Reporting Results of Cancer Treatment, WHO Offset Publication No. 48, World Health Organization, Geneva (1979).

3. D. L. Kisner and R. J. Sylvester, Guidelines for Reporting Cancer Clinical Trials. Colloque INSERM/Direction de la Pharmacie, Evaluation des Medicaments, INSERM, Paris, Vol 96:477 (1980).

4. D. P. Byar, R. M. Simon, W. T. Friedewald, J. J. Schlesselman, D. L. De Mets, J. H. Ellenberg, M. H. Gail and J. H. Ware, Randomized clinical trials: Prespectives on some recent ideas, New Engl. J. Med. 295:74 (1976).

5. R. Peto, M. C. Pike, P. Armitage, N. E. Breslow, D. R. Cox, S. V. Howard, N. Mantel, K. McPherson, J. Peto and P. G. Smith, Design and analysis of randomized clinical trials requiring prolonged observation of each patient. II. Analysis and examples, Brit. J. Cancer 35:1 (1977).

6. R. Sylvester, D. Machin and M. Staquet, A comparison of the alternative methods of calculating survival curves arising from Clinical Trials. Biomedicine Special Issue, 28:49 (1978).

THE E.O.R.T.C. PHASE II STUDIES IN

ADVANCED PROSTATIC CANCER

G. Stoter, and the E.O.R.T.C. Urological Group

Department of Oncology
Free University Hospital
Amsterdam

The E.O.R.T.C. Urological Group has had many difficulties in the evaluation of the treatment results of their phase II and III trials in prostatic cancer.

In phase II studies, the main problem in the assessment of the response to treatment, is the rarity of measurable metastases in this disease. The majority of the patients present with only evaluable lesions, such as bone metastases, hepatomegaly, ureteric obstruction, lymphangitic spread to the lungs, lymphoedema, and other evaluable features such as elevations of alkaline and acid phosphatase, weight loss, anemia and pain.

The available literature on the efficacy of chemotherapy in prostatic cancer is confusing as a result of poorly defined response criteria that differ from one study to another. For example, Yagoda (1) and Merrin (2) have independently examined the value of cisplatin in advanced prostatic cancer. Yagoda reported 3/25 (12%) partial remissions, whereas Merrin achieved partial remissions in 13/45 (29%).

What criteria did they use? Merrin observed remissions at the following sites: disappearance of lymphoedema of the legs (5 patients), decrease of hepatomegaly (1 patient), recalcification of a lytic bone metastasis or disappearance of a lesion on bone scan (3 patients), disappearance of lung and mediastinal lesions and ureteric obstruction (1 patient), disappearance of malignant effusions (2 patients) and disappearance of supraclavicular lymph nodes (1 patient). With the exception of the supraclavicular lymph nodes, all parameters used are evaluable rather than measurable. Yagoda observed remissions at the following sites: skin and subcutaneous

lesions, lymph nodes, and nodular lung metastases. All these
metastases were measurable. A partial remission denotes a decrease
of 50% or more in the sum of the products of the cross-diameters of
measurable metastases. Obviously the results of Merrin and Yagoda
are not comparable due to the different response criteria. This
example reflects in a nutshell the problems of the interpretation of
the literature on chemotherapy of prostatic cancer.

Several other sets of response criteria are being used. Each
one depends at least partly on evaluable instead of measurable indicator lesions. N.P.C.P.'s parameters (3) may include measurable soft
tissue lesions, but usually the indicator lesions are only evaluable.
E.C.O.G.'s criteria (4) are based on measurable lesions, but if no
measurable lesions are present, a 50% reduction of the serum acid
phosphatase is considered a response. This is suprising since E.C.O.G.
itself (5) has shown that there is no good correlation between the
response in measurable metastases and the reduction in acid phosphatase. The ancillary scoring system (A.S.S.) of Kvols (6) does not
take measurable lesions into consideration at all.

The goal of phase II studies is to measure the anti-tumor
effect of a cytotoxic or a drug combination. The E.O.R.T.C. Urological Group has recognized this and accepts for their phase II
studies only patients with bidimensionally measurable indicator
lesions. These are superficial lymph node metastases, para-aortic and
mediastinal lymph nodes, nodular lung metastases, skin and subcutaneous lesions and demarcated liver metastases. Apparently, CT scanning
and ultrasonography are frequently necessary in the diagnostic work-
up.

A recent analysis of a phase III study of the E.O.R.T.C.
Urological Group has shown a close correlation between the response of
the primary prostatic tumor and survival (7). Therefore, the Group
feels justified in accepting the prostate as an indicator lesion
provided that it can be measured by intrarectal ultrasonography.

In addition to this set of study parameters, E.O.R.T.C. has
adopted the W.H.O. definitions of response for bidimensionally
measurable tumors (8).

Presently, the Group is executing a study to examine the anti-
tumor effect of Vindesine. It is expected that the results of this
study will become available in 1981. The successive study will
examine the value of Mitomycin-C in prostatic cancer.

In conclusion, the use of the strict criteria and study
methods mentioned will lead to the collection of unequivocal data that
meet scientific requirements for clinical research. CT scanning and
ultrasonography should be used more frequently to demonstrate
measurable metastases.

REFERENCES

1. A. Yagoda, R.C. Watson, R.B. Natale, W. Barzell, P. Sogani,
    H. Grabstald, and W.F. Whitmore, A Critical Analysis of Response
    Criteria in Patients with Prostatic Cancer Treated with Cis-
    diammine-dichloro-platinum II, Cancer 44:1553 (1979).
2. C.E. Merrin and S. Beckley, Treatment of Estrogen-resistant Stage
    D Carcinoma of the Prostate with Cis-diammine-dichloro-platinum,
    Urology 13:267 (1979).
3. J.D. Schmidt, D.E. Johnson, W.W. Scott, R.P. Gibbons, G.R. Prout,
    and G.P. Murphy, Chemotherapy of Advanced Prostatic Cancer,
    Urology 12:602 (1976).
4. W.D. DeWijs, M. Bauer, J. Colsky, R.A. Cooper, R. Creech, and
    P.P. Carbone, Comparative Trial of Adriamycin and 5-Fluorouracil
    in Advanced Prostatic Cancer - Progress Report, Cancer Treatment
    Rep. 61:325 (1977).
5. W.D. DeWijs and C.B. Begg, Comparison of Adriamycin and 5-Fluoro-
    uracil in Advanced Prostatic Cancer, Abstract Amer. Soc. Clin.
    Oncol. 19:331 (1978).
6. L.K. Kvols, R.T. Eagan, and R.P. Myers, Evaluation of Melphalan,
    ICRF-159, and Hydroxyurea in Metastatic Prostate Cancer: a
    Preliminary Report, Cancer Treatment Rep. 61:311 (1977).
7. R. Sylvester, E.O.R.T.C. Data Center, Personal Communication,
    (1981).
8. Definitions of Objective Response, in:"W.H.O. Handbook for
    Reporting Results of Cancer Treatment," W.H.O. Offset Publication,
    Geneva, 48:23 (1979).

PRELIMINARY RESULTS OF TWO EORTC RANDOMIZED TRIALS IN PREVIOUSLY

UNTREATED PATIENTS WITH ADVANCED T3 - T4 PROSTATIC CANCER

M. de Pauw[1], S. Suciu[1], R. Sylvester[1], P.H. Smith[2],
M. Pavone-Macaluso[3], and participants in the EORTC Genito-
Urinary Tract Cooperative Group[4].

1. EORTC Data Center, Brussels, Belgium
2. St. James's University Hospital, Leeds, U.K.
3. University of Palermo, Italy
4. Participants listed in Tables 2 and 7

INTRODUCTION

At the end of 1976 and the beginning of 1977 respectively, the
EORTC Genito-Urinary Tract Cancer Cooperative Group started two randomized phase III protocols in previously untreated patients with
advanced T3-4 prostatic cancer (1-3). The first trial, 30762, compared Stilboestrol and Estracyt, while the second, 30761, was a randomized comparison of Stilboestrol, Cyproterone Acetate and Medroxyprogesterone Acetate. Both trials have now been closed to patient
entry and the principal endpoints of the studies analyzed. This
paper will present the interim results which have emerged from these
two studies.

PROTOCOL 30762 (Study Coordinator: P.H. Smith, St. James's University
Hospital, Leeds)

MATERIAL AND METHODS

Protocol 30762 is a randomized phase III study comparing Estracyt
(estramustine phosphate) and Stilboestrol (DES) with respect to the
objective response rate, duration of response, duration of survival,
and the toxicity observed. Estracyt was taken at an initial dose of
280 mg. twice a day for the first eight weeks followed by 140 mg.
twice daily while the dose of DES was 3 x 1 mg/day.

Patients were selected for the study according to the inclusion
and exclusion criteria listed in Table 1 and treated for a minimum of

433

Table 1.   Protocols 30761 and 30762 - Selection Criteria

CRITERIA FOR INCLUSION :

1. NO PREVIOUS TREATMENT FOR PROSTATIC CANCER (except for non-
   radical prostatectomy)

2. HISTOLOGICALLY PROVEN CARCINOMA OF THE PROSTATE

3. CATEGORY T3 : TUMOUR EXTENDING BEYOND THE CAPSULE WITH OR
   WITHOUT INVOLVEMENT OF THE LATERAL SULCI AND/OR SEMINAL
   VESICLES

   CATEGORY T4 : TUMOUR FIXED OR INVADING NEIGHBOURING STRUCTURES

4. ALL N M P AND G CLASSIFICATIONS

CRITERIA FOR EXCLUSION :

1. LIFE EXPECTANCY OF < 90 DAYS

2. CARDIOVASCULAR DISEASE WHICH IN THE OPINION OF THE INVESTIGATOR
   PRECLUDES THE ADMINISTRATION OF DES.

3. EXPECTED DIFFICULTIES OF FOLLOW-UP RELATED TO-PSYCHIATRIC
   DISORDERS, MARKED SENILITY OR TOO LARGE A DISTANCE HOME-
   HOSPITAL

4. PRESENCE OF ANOTHER NEOPLASM EXCEPT NON-MELANOMA SKIN CANCER

eight weeks before being evaluated for tumour response. If a response was observed, treatment was to be continued until progression.
In the case of no change, treatment was to be continued or crossed
over at the investigator's discretion while patients who progressed
were to be crossed over to the other protocol therapy and reevaluated
after eight more weeks. However the number of patients in whom
treatment was actually crossed over after eight weeks was so small
(5/248 patients) that this information was disregarded.

The protocol was started in November 1976 and closed to entry in
June 1980. Patients are still being followed for duration of remission and duration of survival. A total of 336 patients were entered
by 13 institutions. Unfortunately six centers were excluded due to
institutional problems which reduced the total number of patients
under study to 248, 125 and 123 on Estracyt and DES respectively.
Table 2 shows that 90% of the patients were entered by four British
institutions. Patient characteristics at entry on study are presented in Table 3; 51% of the patients were between 71 and 80 years
old and 65% had a normal performance status. A T3 tumour was present
in 71% of the patients while 49% had distant metastases.

Table 2.   Protocol 30762 - Patient Distribution
by Treatment and by Institution

INSTITUTION	ESTRACYT	DES	TOTAL
C. BOUFFIOUX, LIEGE	7	8	15
B. LARDENNOIS, REIMS	6	4	10
PH. SMITH, LEEDS	27	25	52
M. ROBINSON, CASTLEFORD	39	36	75
B. RICHARDS, J.R.G.BASTABLE, YORK	36	39	75
R.W. GLASHAN, HUDDERSFIELD	10	11	21
T O T A L	125	123	248

RESULTS

As of April 1981 a total of 45 and 57 patients were still being
treated with Estracyt and DES respectively as indicated in Table 4.
The remaining 146 patients went off study mainly due to progression
(43%), excessive toxicity (16%) and non cancer related deaths (15%).

Side effects

Side effects can be broken down into three principal categories:
painful gynecomastia, gastro-intestinal and cardiovascular. Overall
there was no significant difference between the two treatments with
respect to the number of patients who developed painful gynecomastia.
Gastro-intestinal side effects were however reported more frequently
by the patients treated with Estracyt than those treated with DES:
26% against 11% respectively. In addition they were more severe on
Estracyt which had to be stopped in 8% of the patients(against none
taking DES) due to severe abdominal and epigastric pain, gastro-
intestinal distress, diarrhea and nausea and vomiting.

The incidence of cardiovascular side effects during treatment
was 32%, namely 28% on Estracyt and 36% on DES (Table 5). Out of the
13 cardiovascular deaths which occurred during treatment, three were
reported on Estracyt against 10 on DES. If we look separately at the
patients according to whether or not they had a history of cardiovascular disease at entry on study, no difference has been observed
between the treatments in the incidence of cardiovascular side effects
for those patients without previous cardiovascular history. However,
the percentage of patients with a previous history of cardiovascular
disease who developed cardiovascular complications during treatment
is higher on DES (52%) than on Estracyt (26%). This difference is
not statistically significant (p= .10) but nevertheless suggests that
those patients with a previous history at entry on study tend to

Table 3. Characteristics at entry on study

	PROTOCOL 30761	PROTOCOL 30762
	PERCENTAGES	
METASTASES		
YES	52	49
NO	44	50
UNKNOWN	4	1
PAIN		
YES	24	32
NO	76	68
HISTOLOGY		
G1	23	23
G2	48	41
G3	24	34
GX	5	2
T CLASSIFICATION		
T0-2	1	2
T3	79	71
T4	20	27
SIZE OF PROSTATIC TUMOUR		
$1 - 9$ cm^2	46	28
$10 - 19$ cm^2	26	27
$20 - 29$ cm^2	19	31
> 30 cm^2	9	14
PERFORMANCE STATUS		
NORMAL ACTIVITY (1)	40	65
SYMPTOMS BUT AMBULATORY (2)	50	31
IN BED < 50% OF TIME (3)	10	4
AGE		
40 - 60	7	10
61 - 70	34	31
71 - 80	49	51
80 +	10	8
CHRONIC DISEASES		
YES	62	53
NO	38	47
CARDIOVASCULAR DISEASES		
YES	32	25
NO	68	75

Table 4. Protocol 30762 - Reasons for going off study
(stopping treatment)

REASON OFF-TREATMENT	ESTRACYT	STILBOESTROL	TOTAL
STILL ON TREATMENT	45	57	102
PROGRESSION (Including deaths due to prostatic cancer)	39	24	63
EXCESSIVE TOXICITY	15	9	24
DEATH (Not due to cancer)	8	14	22
INELIGIBILITY	8	9	17
TREATMENT AND/OR EXAMINATIONS REFUSED	4	4	8
LOST TO FOLLOW UP	-	2	2
PROTOCOL VIOLATION	-	2	2
OTHER	6	2	8
T O T A L	125	123	248

Table 5. Protocol 30762 - Cardiovascular side effects

TREATMENT	NO HISTORY OF CARDIOVASC. DISEASE		HISTORY OF CARDIOVASC.DISEASE		TOTAL		TOTAL
	SIDE EFFECTS		SIDE EFFECTS		SIDE EFFECTS		
	NO	YES	NO	YES	NO	YES	
ESTRACYT	57	23(29%)	20	7(26%)	77	+ 30(28%)	107
STILBOESTROL	56	26(32%)	12	13(52%)	69	++ 38(36%)	107
T O T A L	113	49(30%)	32	19(37%)	146	68(32%)	214

+   3 cardiovascular deaths
++ 10 cardiovascular deaths

develop more cardiovascular side effects when treated with DES than with Estracyt.

Of the cardiovascular side effects reported during treatment with Estracyt or DES, 52% consisted of fluid retention (heart failure, hypertension, oedema, dyspnoea and cramps), 25% of venous thromboembolism (deep venous thromboembolism, pulmonary embolism, cerebrovascular accidents and thrombophlebitis) and 21% of ischemic heart disease (infarctions, ventricular ectopic beats, S T segment and R.B.B.B.). No significanct difference in the type of cardiovascular complications was noted between the two treatments.

Tumour Response

The response of the prostatic tumour and the response of the bone metastases were analyzed separately. The response of the prostatic tumour is based on rectal palpation findings after a minimum of two months of treatment and is defined as complete remission (CR)- absence of any clinically detectable prostatic tumour mass; partial remission (PR)- 50% decrease of the product of the two maximum perpendicular diameters; no change (NC)- a change of less than 50%- and progression (PROGR)- a 50% increase of the product of the two maximum perpendicular diameters. All patients with follow up data at two months or for whom progression is known to have occurred prior to two months were taken into consideration.

The overall response rate (CR + PR) of the prostatic tumour is 42% (36% on Estracyt and 48% on DES Table 6) with no significant difference between the two treatments (P =0.13).

Table 6.   Protocol 30762 - Overall best
           response of the prostatic tumour

TREATMENT	CR	PR	NC	PROGR.	TOTAL	% CR + PR
ESTRACYT	6	27	48	11	92	36
STILBOESTROL	2	44	44	6	96	48
TOTAL	8	71	92	17	188	42

P = .13

ADJUSTED FOR PERFORMANCE STATUS P = .18
ADJUSTED FOR G GRADE   P = .17

Analyses of the potential factors related to the response of the prostatic tumour revealed that the size of the prostatic tumour, the performance status and the G grade are the most important prognostic factors. After adjustment for performance status and G grade, the P values are P =0.18 and P =0.17 respectively. Adjustment for tumour size gives P =0.05 in favour of DES although this does not take into account the imbalance of either the performance status or the G grade in the two treatment groups.

The response of the bone metastases is based on the results of an extramural review of all scans and/or X-rays. So far only 69 patients have been evaluated. The overall response rate is 30% (30% for Estracyt and 31% for DES). Adjustment for the performance status, the most important prognostic factor for the response of the bone metastases also reveals no difference (P =0.91) between the two treatments.

Since the presence or absence of pain was related to the patient's metastatic status, the percentage of patients with relief of pain at two months was also analyzed. Among the 65 patients who complained of pain at entry on study, 33 on Estracyt and 32 on DES, relief of pain at two months was observed in 61% of the patients treated with Estracyt and in 69% of the patients treated with DES.

Survival

Out of the 214 eligible patients for whom follow up has been received, 74 patients (35%) have died as of April 1981.

Figure 1 presents the duration of survival by treatment group taking into consideration all causes of death. Forty-three patients have died in the Estracyt group as opposed to 31 patients on DES. While there appears to be a difference between Estracyt and DES in favour of DES, adjustment for the most important diagnostic factor for survival - performance status, shows in fact that there is no significant difference between the two treatments (P =0.57, Logrank Test). If now one considers only those deaths due to malignant disease, the difference between Estracyt and DES is likewise non significant after adjustment for the performance status with P =0.39. This example shows very clearly how incorrect conclusions might be drawn even in a randomized trial if one does not adjust at the time of the analysis for those factors which are of prognostic importance.

If one considers now only those deaths due to cardiovascular disease, six in the Estracyt group and 11 in the DES group, there is no significant difference between the two treatments (P =0.28, Logrank Test) with respect to the duration of survival. An adjustment for the patient's age, the most important prognostic factor related to cardiovascular deaths, likewise did not reveal a significant difference between the two treatments (P =0.18, Logrank Test).

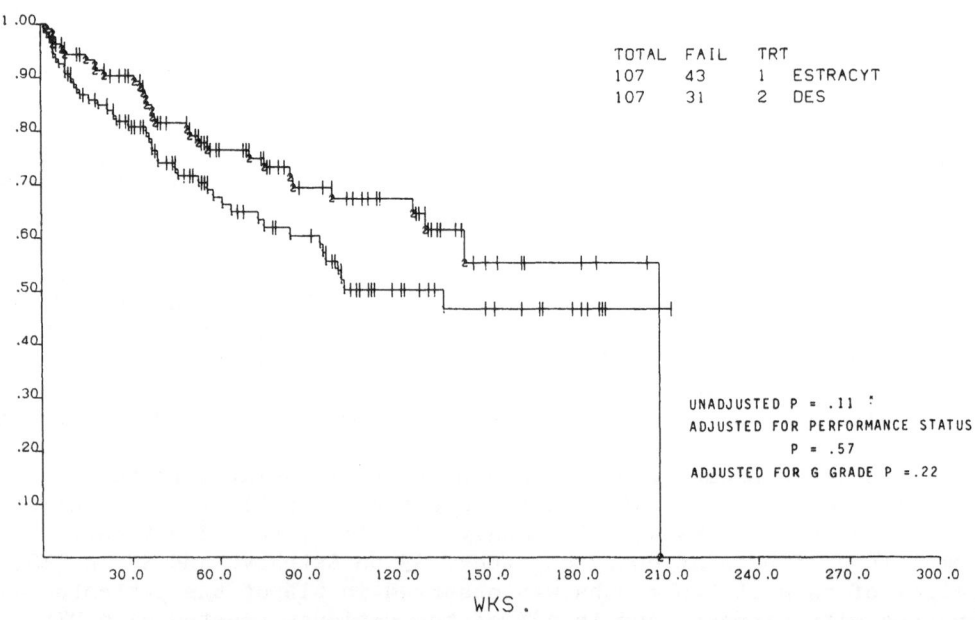

Fig. 1.   Protocol 30762 - Duration of survival by treatment
           considering all causes of death.

CONCLUSIONS

        Gastro-intestinal side effects were reported more frequently and
were more severe in degree in the patients treated with Estracyt.
On the other hand this trial suggests that patients with a previous
cardiovascular history tend to develop more cardiovascular complications when treated with DES than with Estracyt.

        So far comparisons of the response rates of the prostatic tumour
and the bone metastases as well as the duration of survival have not
shown any statistically significant difference between Estracyt and
DES once one adjusts for the performance status.

PROTOCOL 30761 (Study Coordinator: M. Pavone-Macaluso, University
of Palermo)

MATERIAL AND METHODS

        Protocol 30761 is a randomized phase III study comparing Cypro-
terone Acetate (CPA) 250 mg/d·, Medroxyprogesterone Acetate (MPA)
500 mg. I.M. 3 x weekly for the first eight weeks followed by 100 mg.
orally twice a day and Stilboestrol (DES) 3 x 1 mg/d.   The purpose
of this trial, the patient selection criteria (Table 1) as well as
the design are identical to protocol 30762 with the exception that
there was no possibility of crossing over patients to another proto-

col arm.   This protocol was started in February 1977 and was closed
to patient entry in April 1981 at the time of this analysis.

A total of 314 patients were randomized by 29 institutions from
eight countries. However four institutions representing 19 patients
have thus far been excluded due to institutional problems, reducing
the total number of patients under study to 295. The participating
investigators with the number of patients entered are listed in
Table 7. Almost half of the patients or 49% were entered by 10
Italian institutions.

Table 7.   Protocol 30761 - Participating Institutions

INSTITUTIONS	TOTAL NUMBER OF PATIENTS RANDOMIZED
ITALY	
G. VIGGIANO, MESTRE	34
ZOLFANELLI, BARASOLO, VERCELLI	24
S. LEONE, GENEVA (S.M.NUOVA)	22
M. PAVONE, PALERMO	17
C. BONDAVALLI, MANTOVA	11
F. GASTALDI, GENOVA (OSP. CELESIA)	10
F. MERLO, BIELLA	8
M. PORENA, TERAMO	8
L. MARCO, TORINO	6
V. NADALINI, GENOVA (SAN MARTINO)	6
THE NETHERLANDS	
H. DE VOOGT, LEIDEN	31
J. ALEXIEVA-FIGUSCH, ROTTERDAM	21
FRANCE	
B. LARDENNOIS, REIMS	32
P. FARGEOT, DIJON	6
ENGLAND	
B. RICHARDS, YORK	11
M. ROBINSON, CASTLEFORD	9
D. NEWLING, HULL	7
Ph. SMITH, LEEDS	1
SPAIN	
M. PINEIRO, MADRID	12
L.R. ESTEVE, MADRID (CRUZ ROJA)	3
A.E. BARRILERO, MADRID (RAMON Y CAJAL)	2
BELGIUM	
C. SCHULMAN, BRUSSELS	4
C. BOUFFIOUX, LIEGE	3
PORTUGAL	
F.CALAIS DA SILVA, LISBON	5
AUSTRIA	
R. KOHLE, SALZBURG	2
T O T A L	295

Table 3 presents the distribution of patient characteristics at entry on study. Half of the patients entered the study with symptoms but were ambulatory (performance status 2), 49% were between 71 and 80 years old, 52% had metastatic disease, and 79% of the patients had a T3 tumour.

RESULTS

As of April 1981 a total of 42, 34 and 37 patients are still being treated with CPA, MPA and DES respectively. The remaining 182 patients went off study mainly because of progression (46%) or because they were lost to follow up (16%) (Table 8). Nineteen patients were ineligible and should not have been entered in the protocol while six patients were taken off treatment due to toxicity, three on MPA (pulmonary embolism, retinal atrophy, acute aortic insufficiency), two on DES (hepatic toxicity and phlebitis, thrombophlebitis) and one on CPA (Meniere's syndrome).

Table 8.   Protocol 30761 - Reasons for going off study
(stopping treatment)

REASON OFF TREATMENT	CPA	MPA	DES	TOTAL
STILL ON TREATMENT	42	34	37	113
PROGRESSION (Including deaths due to prostatic cancer)	26	35	24	85
LOST TO FOLLOW UP	16	8	6	30
INELIGIBILITY	4	9	6	19
TREATMENT REFUSED	6	5	3	14
DEATH (Not due to cancer)	4	2	4	10
EXCESSIVE TOXICITY	1	3	2	6
PROTOCOL VIOLATION	1	1	1	3
OTHER	3	4	8	15
T O T A L	103	101	91	295

Side Effects

Painful gynecomastia was more frequent on DES than on the other two arms being reported by 40% of the patients treated with DES against only 6% of the patients treated with CPA or MPA.

On the other hand gastro-intestinal side effects were almost negligible and did not require the treatment to be permanently stopped in any patients. Only 2% of the patients taking DES or CPA reported any gastro-intestinal side effects as opposed to 8% of the patients on MPA.

The total incidence of cardiovascular side effects reported in this study was 25%, namely 14, 23 and 38% on CPA, MPA and DES respectively (Table 9). The difference between CPA and DES is significant at P = 0.01 and indicates that patients treated with DES have a significantly higher chance of developing cardiovascular side effects than patients treated with CPA. If we now look separately at those patients without a history of cardiovascular disease at entry on study, the frequency of cardiovascular side effects reported during treatment in 8 ,26 and 32% for CPA, MPA and DES respectively and again the difference between CPA and DES is significant (P =0.02). In the patients with a history of cardiovascular disease, no statistically significant difference was observed between the treatments although the data again suggest that DES patients tend to develop more cardiovascular side effects than the patients treated with MPA or CPA.

Table 9.   Protocol 30761 - Cardiovascular side effects

TREATMENT	NO HISTORY OF CARDIOVASC. DISEASE		HISTORY OF CARDIOVASC. DISEASE		TOTAL		TOTAL
	SIDE EFFECTS		SIDE EFFECTS		SIDE EFFECTS		
	NO	YES	NO	YES	NO	YES	
CPA	37	3(8%)	12	5(29%)	49	+ 8(14%)	57
MPA	28	10(26%)	21	5(19%)	49	++ 15(23%)	64
DES	25	12(32%)	11	10(48%)	36	+++ 22(38%)	58
T O T A L	90	25(22%)	44	20(31%)	134	45(25%)	179

+   4 cardiovascular deaths
++   1 cardiovascular death
+++   2 cardiovascular deaths

Of the cardiovascular side effects reported during treatment, 42% involved fluid retention: heart failure, hypertension, oedema and dyspnoea while ischemic heart disease (infarctions, R.B.B.B., ventricular ectopic beats) and venous thromboembolism (thrombophlebitis, deep venous thromboembolism, cerebrovascular accidents, pulmonary embolism) were each reported by 28% of the patients who developed cardiovascular side effects. Four cardiovascular deaths were reported on CPA as opposed to one on MPA and two on DES.

Tumour Response

Since this protocol was closed to patient entry only recently, a separate analysis of the response of the prostatic tumour and the bone metastases has not yet been carried out. Therefore, the criteria of response in this protocol are different compared to the criteria of protocol 30762, first because no distinction between local and distant disease is made and second because any increase in size of a lesion is sufficient to consider that lesion as progressive as opposed to a 50% increase in protocol 30762. The criteria of response adopted in this study are presented in Table 10. One hundred and sixty-five patients with follow up data at two months or for whom progression is known to have occurred prior to two months are included in the treatment comparison. The overall response rate (CR + PR) is 32%, namely 33, 18 and 44% on CPA, MPA and DES respectively (Table 11). The difference between MPA and DES is significant at P =0.005 in favour of DES. None of the other treatment differences are statistically significant at this time. However we would like to emphasize again that extramural review of scans and/or X-rays is planned for determing the response of the bone metastases while the response of the prostatic tumour will be reassessed according to the criteria of protocol 30762. Consequently, the response rates given in Table 11 must be considered as very preliminary. The amount of follow up data is not sufficient yet to enable a meaningful comparison of the three treatments with respect to the duration of survival.

CONCLUSIONS

Since this protocol was closed to patient entry only recently, a considerable amount of patient follow up data must still be received and the current results must be considered as being more preliminary than those reported in protocol 30762.

Painful gynecomastia was reported more frequently by the patients treated with DES while gastro-intestinal side effects were almost negligible. Patients treated with DES tended to develop more cardiovascular side effects than those patients treated with MPA or CPA, independently of whether or not a patient had a previous history of cardiovascular disease.

Table 10. Protocol 30761 – Criteria of overall response
(local + distant)

COMPLETE REMISSION

1. Absence of any clinically detectable soft tissue tumour mass
2. Recalcification of all osteolytic lesions if present
3. No evidence of progression of osteoblastic lesions if any are present

PARTIAL REMISSION

1. A significant decrease in size in at least 50 % of all soft tissue lesions
   - measurable lesions : decrease of 50 % of the product of the 2 largest tumour diameters
   - non-measurable lesions : reduction of at least three-fourths of the estimated volume
2. Recalcification of some osteolytic lesions if present

- No increase in any other lesion and no new areas of malignant disease may appear
- No significant deterioration in weight (> 10 %), symptoms or performance status (one score level)
- Return of an elevated acid phosphatase to normal
- If hepatomegaly is a significant indicator, there must be a reduction in liver size and at least a 30 % improvement of all pretreatment abnormal liver function tests.

NO CHANGE

- No new lesions appear and no lesion increases in size
- No significant deterioration in weight, symptoms or performance status

PROGRESSION

- Any lesion increases in size or any new lesion appears, regardless of what the response of the other lesions may have been
- Significant deterioration in symptoms, decrease in weight or decrease in performance status
- An increase in acid or alkaline phosphatase alone is not to be considered as an indication of progression.

Table 11. Protocol 30761 – Overall response rates
(local + distant)

TREATMENT	CR	PR	NC	PROGR.	TOTAL	% CR + PR
CPA	2	15	14	21	52	33
MPA	-	10	23	23	56	18
DES	7	18	18	14	57	44
TOTAL	9	43	55	58	165	32

OVERALL RESPONSE RATE : MPA VS DES, $P = .005$
CPA VS DES, $P = .32$
CPA VS MPA, $P = .12$

The overall response rates (CR + PR) of both the prostatic tumour and the bone metastases indicate that DES is significantly superior to MPA (P =0.005) while no other statistically significant differences have been observed.

REFERENCES

1. M. Pavone-Macaluso, F. Lund, J.H. Mulder, P.H. Smith, M. de Pauw, R. Sylvester, and EORTC Urological Group, EORTC Protocols in Prostatic Cancer, An Interim Report, Scand. J. Urol. Nephrol. Suppl. 55: 163 (1980).

2. P.H. Smith, A. Akdas, M.K. Mason, B. Richards, M. Robinson, M. de Pauw, and R. Sylvester, Hormone therapy in prostatic cancer, Acta. Urol. Belg. 48: 282 (1980).

3. M. de Pauw, C. Bouffioux, J. Casselman, C. Schulman, B. Vergison, and L. Denis, The European Organisation for Research on Treatment of Cancer. Genito-Urinary Tract Cancer Cooperative Group, Acta. Urol. Belg. 48: 285 (1980).

This investigation was supported by Grant No. 5R10 - CA11488 - 12, awarded by the National Cancer Institute, DHEW.

Editorial Note - P.H.S.

Although not directly comparable, these two trials have many features in common. They represent an attempt to compare the effectiveness of agents which are potential alternatives to conventional oestrogen therapy and which are all significantly more expensive. Also, patients entered into the studies show similar characteristics in relation to age, T, G, and M categories, prostatic size, and the incidence of pain. However, those entered to the study comparing Estracyt and Stilboestrol had a somewhat higher performance status - 65% vs 40% having a normal status.

The evaluation of the results of therapy is very difficult in patients with prostatic cancer since objective remission of the commonest metastatic lesions - those in bone - is slow and difficult to measure with accuracy.

These very preliminary results have however shown that a dose of DES of 1 mg tds carries a distinct cardiovascular risk, especially in those with a previous history of cardiovascular disease. This showed clearly in each study. However, it seems likely that patients receiving DES will prove to show the highest incidence of objective remission, a point which can be determined only at subsequent analysis where other critical factors, including time to progression and survival will be assessed.

The best treatment for metastatic prostatic cancer is still by no means clear and further studies of low dose Stilboestrol (1 mg daily), other agents, orchiectomy and chemotherapy, alone or in combination, will be required to clarify the situation.

THE VALUE OF THE ANCILLARY FACTOR SCORING SYSTEM

S. Suciu,[1] M.R.G. Robinson,[2] and participants in the
EORTC Genito-Urinary Tract Cancer Cooperative Group
Protocol 30762*

1. EORTC Data Center
    Brussels
    Belgium

2. Pontefract General Infirmary
    Pontefract, U.K.

INTRODUCTION

An accurate objective assessment of the response to treatment
in patients with advanced prostatic cancer is not an easy task. The
problems associated with the evaluation of treatment response have
been considered by Eagan, Hahn and Myers (1) and Kvols, Eagan and
Myers (2) who developed a scoring system which they used in an
attempt to assess a patient's response to treatment. An overall
ancillary score was calculated based on changes in the value of six
different ancillary factors. This score was then used to assess a
patient's response to treatment.

In order to determine the validity and suitability of this
system for assessing response to treatment and for comparing two or
more different treatments, the EORTC Genito-Urinary Tract Cancer
Cooperative Group applied this scoring system to one of its ongoing
trials. The purpose of this paper is to present the results of
this investigation and discuss how such an index might be improved.

THE ANCILLARY FACTOR SCORING SYSTEM

The objective measurement of tumour response in prostatic
cancer patients is difficult at best due to problems in accurately
measuring the primary lesion and due to difficulties in interpreting
successive bone scans. It is thus natural to attempt to assess a
patient's response to treatment in terms of those aspects of the

disease which can be accurately and objectively measured and which are correlated with the objective tumour response.

Eagan, Hahn and Myers (1) and Kvols, Eagan and Myers (2) proposed a scoring system to be used in assessing response to treatment for patients with advanced metastatic disease. As shown in Table 1 this system is based on information provided by six ancillary factors: pain, performance status, weight, hemoglobin and the total alkaline and acid phosphatase levels. Scores are computed for each factor based on the change in the factor relative to its initial value. For a given factor, a score of zero at follow up represents a normal value for the factor and a score of one represents an improvement without returning to normal. No change in an abnormal factor is scored as a two while worsening of the factor is coded as a four. A total ancillary score is then calculated by summing the scores for each individual factor. A low total ancillary score suggests that the patient has improved during the course of the study while a high score indicates an overall worsening of the patient's condition. Kvols et al (2) found that among the seven patients who were considered to have responded using conventional evaluation criteria, all seven had total ancillary scores of less than ten.

The EORTC Genito-Urinary Tract Cancer Cooperative Group has applied a slightly modified version of this scoring system (Table 2) to data from its trial comparing Stilboestrol and Estracyt in previously untreated T3, T4 prostatic cancer patients (3). The score for weight had to be modified since only a patient's initial weight was available at entry on study and not his normal weight. In addition alkaline and acid phosphatase were considered separately and a change of 50% rather than 25% was required for the change to be considered significant.

CORRELATION OF THE ANCILLARY FACTOR SCORES WITH CLINICAL RESPONSE

Local Response

In order to determine whether or not a correlation exists between the ancillary scores and the response of the primary tumour as measured by rectal palpation, scores for each factor were calculated at the time of the local response. The guidelines of the World Health Organization (4) were used to assess a patient's response to treatment, except that an increase of 50% in the cross product of the two largest perpendicular diameters was required in order to demonstrate a progression. The following response categories were determined based on changes in the size of the prostatic lesion:

1. Complete response (CR): complete disappearance of the local tumour
2. Partial response (PR): decrease of at least 50% in the cross product of the two largest perpendicular diameters

Table 1. Ancillary scoring system (all changes
relative to starting value) (2)

Ancillary factors	Scores and Changes			
	0	1	2	4
Pain	None	Improved	Stable	Worse
Performance status (ECOG)	Asymptomatic	Improved	Stable	Worse
Weight (%)	Normal	Increased >5	Stable (≤ 5)	Decreased >5
Hemoglobin (g/100ml)	Normal*	Increased >1	Stable (≤ 1)	Decreased >1
Total alkaline and acid phosphatase levels (%)	Normal	Decreased >25	Stable (≤25)	Increased >25

An overall score of ≤ 9 considered a response; overall score of 10-14
considered stable; and an overall score ≥15 considered progression.

*13g/100ml

Table 2. Ancillary factor scoring system studies
by the EORTC GU Group

Ancillary Factors	Scores and Changes			
	0	1	2	4
Pain	None	Improved	Stable	Worse
Performance status	Asymptomatic	Improved	Stable	Worse
Weight	Stable or increase	–	–	Decrease ≥5%
Hemoglobin	Normal[+]	Increase ≥10%	Stable	Decrease ≥10%
Alkaline phosphatase	Normal*	Decrease ≥50%	Stable	Increase ≥50%
Acid phosphatase	Normal*	Decrease ≥50%	Stable	Increase ≥50%

[+]13g/100ml Equivalent, *Hospital limits

3. No change (NC): less than 50% increase or decrease in the
    cross product of the two largest perpendicular diameters
4. Progression (PROG): increase of at least 50% in the cross
    product of the two largest perpendicular diameters.

Patients were initially evaluated at two months and then again at
six months and every six months thereafter as long as the patient
remained on-study. If the response of the local lesion was CR, PR
or PROG, then the ancillary scores for each factor were calculated
at the moment of the response. If a patient's response to treatment
was NC, then the ancillary scores were calculated at six months, or
at two months if no data at six months were available.

   One hundred and eighty-seven patients receiving Estracyt or DES
and for whom the required data are available are included in this
analysis. The complete and partial responders were grouped together
for analysis purposes. Table 3 presents the local response and the
corresponding total ancillary factor score calculated at the time of
the response. Patients are divided into three categories according
to the value of the total score: 0-3, 4-7 and ≥8. While this division into three groups is somewhat arbitrary, it was chosen for
statistical reasons which will not be detailed here. While there is
a significant correlation between a patient's response to treatment
and his total score (P = .0003), a closer investigation of this table
reveals that the total score is not very informative and cannot be
used to accurately assess a patient's response to treatment. First
it should be noted that 53% of the patients fall in the NC category
with only a slight variation as the score increases. For patients
with a total score of ≥8, approximately the same percentage responded as those who progressed. Thus no discrimination between
responders and failures is possible in this group of patients. While
in each of the categories 0-3 and 4-7 patients are more likely to
respond than to progress, no discrimination between responders and
patients with no change is possible. Thus from a practical point of
view, knowledge of the total ancillary factor score does not allow
one to accurately determine a patient's response to treatment.

   An examination of the individual ancillary factor scores for
each factor included in the total score reveals that only the ancillary score for the performance status is highly correlated (P =
.0006) with the response of the local tumour. However once again
one cannot accurately determine the response of the local lesion
based on the knowledge of the ancillary factor score for performance
status. From these analyses it is evident that knowledge of the
total ancillary factor score or of any of its components cannot be
used to assess a patient's response to treatment.

Table 3. Local response by total ancillary factor score

Score \ Response	CR – PR	NC	PROG	TOTAL
0 – 3	34 (48%)	32 (45%)	5 (7%)	71
4 – 7	27 (41%)	36 (55%)	3 (5%)	66
$\geq$ 8	9 (18%)	31 (62%)	10 (20%)	50
Total	70 (37%)	99 (53%)	18 (10%)	187

Test for correlation
Kendall's TAU = .23   P = .0003

Distant Response

As in the case of the local lesion, ancillary scores were calculated at the time of the response of the distant lesions for the 87 patients with bone metastases. An extramural review committee evaluated the scans and X-rays of 66 of the patients in order to determine their response to treatment. For the remaining 21 patients a review was not available and the evaluation of the local investigator was used. As there was only a small number of patients with a complete response of their distant lesions, complete and partial responders were grouped together for analysis purposes.

The distribution of the distant response to treatment according to the total ancillary factor score is presented in Table 4. Once again there is a significant correlation (P < .0001) between a patient's response and his total score; however the score's usefulness in assessing response remains limited. Fifty-seven percent of the patients were classified as NC with little variation according to the score.

Although only three patients with a total score of 0-3 progressed and only one patient with a score of $\geq$ 8 responded to treatment, Table 4 reveals that in patients with a score of 0-3, no discrimination is possible between CR-PR and NC. In addition there is a similar percentage of responders and failures in the group with a score of 4-7 and in the group $\geq$ 8 no discrimination between NC and PROG can be made. As before the usefulness of the total score remains limited. When analyzing each ancillary factor separately, it was found that there was a significant correlation between the response to treatment of the bone lesions and the ancillary scores for performance status (P = .0001), weight (P = .0004), alkaline phosphatase (P = .004) and

Table 4. Distant response (bone lesions) by
total ancillary factor score

Response Score	CR - PR	NC	PROG	TOTAL
0 - 3	15 (41%)	19 (51%)	3 (8%)	37
4 - 7	5 (18%)	19 (68%)	4 (14%)	28
$\geq$ 8	1 (5%)	12 (55%)	9 (41%)	22
Total	21 (24%)	50 (57%)	16 (18%)	87

Test for correlation
Kendall's TAU = .38   P = < .0001

pain (P = .005). These correlations are deceptive however as one
cannot accurately determine a patient's response to treatment based
on the scores for any of these variables.

ASSESSMENT OF THE ANCILLARY FACTOR SCORING SYSTEM

Although there is a significant correlation between the total
ancillary factor score and a patient's response to treatment, the
ancillary factor scoring system as developed by Kvols and Eagan is
not recommended for use in clinical trials as an alternative method
for assessing a patient's response to treatment for the following
reasons:

1.   This scoring system does not adequately take into consideration
a patient's initial disease status. It makes no distinction between
a patient who initially has an abnormal value for a factor which
returns to normal at the time of response and a patient who initially
has a normal value for the factor and which remains at a normal level
during the course of the trial. Thus two patients with the same
score might have had quite different amounts of tumour growth or
shrinkage. In addition one patient may achieve a lower score than
another patient simply because he was in better overall condition
at the start of the study.

2.   Secondly, this scoring system assumes that the six factors
which comprise it are all of equal importance with respect to assessing a patient's response to treatment. It was found that only the
score for the performance status was correlated with the response of
the local lesion while for the distant metastases, four of the
factors were found to be of importance. Yet all six factors are

given equal weight in computing the total score. In addition one
might expect several of the factors to be correlated with each other
so that information provided by some of the individual scores may be
redundant. There is no justification for assigning equal weights to
the six ancillary factors.

Since this scoring system does not adequately take into consideration a patient's disease characteristics at entry on study and
since it has no statistical basis, it should not be used to assess
a patient's response to treatment or to compare the relative efficacy
of two or more different treatments.

DEVELOPING AN ANCILLARY FACTOR SCORING SYSTEM

In constructing an index to aid an investigator in assessing a
patient's response to treatment, it is logical to restrict oneself
to those factors which are of prognostic importance with respect to
the endpoint under study. The prognostic importance of the baseline
values of the following variables has been studied using Cox's proportional hazards regression model and linear logistic regression:

1.   T category
2.   M category
3.   G category
4.   Age
5.   Performance status (E.C.O.G. scale)
6.   Chronic diseases
7.   Weight
8.   Pain
9.   Hemoglobin
10.   Alkaline phosphatase
11.   Acid phosphatase
12.   Size of the primary lesion

Taking into account the correlation between these variables,
Table 5 presents in the order of their relative importance those
variables which are of prognostic importance with respect to the
duration of survival and the response to treatment of the local and
distant lesions. It is seen from this table that the most important
ancillary factor for both survival and response to treatment is the
patient's performance status at entry on study. Thus any scoring
system would most likely give the greatest weight to changes in this
variable. Although the size of the local lesion is positively correlated with the response rate, the significance of this variable
remains unclear as only a very small change which may be due to
measurement error is required for a response or progression in very
small lesions.

Based on these observations one should correlate the response
to treatment with changes in a patient's performance status,

Table 5. Prognostic factors in prostatic cancer

Duration of survival		Response	
All causes of death	Death due to malignant disease	Local lesion	Distant metastases
1. Performance status	1. Performance status	1. Size of local lesion	1. Performance status
2. Presence or absence of chronic diseases	2. G category	2. Performance status	2. Acid phosphatase
3. G category	3. Presence or absence of pain	3. G category	

G category, pain and acid phosphatase levels and construct an index using these variables or a subset of them. The practical problem of how to construct such an index or how to measure changes in the factors retained are important problems which will not be discussed here.

DISCUSSION

It may be questioned whether or not one should attempt to assess a patient's response to treatment by taking various ancillary factors into account or whether one should rely only on objective tumour measurements, however accurate or inaccurate they may be. Despite the fact that measurement of the primary lesion by rectal palpation is criticized as being subject to considerable measurement error, we have found a significant correlation between the response of the local tumour as measured by rectal palpation and the patient's over-all duration of survival. Thus it is important to assess the response of the primary tumour even if only by rectal palpation. However newer techniques such as ultrasonography should permit a more accurate and objective evaluation of the prostate than is possible by palpation.

The EORTC Genito-Urinary Group has set up a central review of all patient's scans and X-rays in order to assess the response of the bone metastases. While the conclusions concerning the problems in interpreting successive scans and X-rays and their reliability are still pending, it is felt that the review has provided an important standardization in the assessment of the distant lesions.

No ancillary factor scoring system can at this time replace the classical techniques of tumour evaluation since no satisfactory scoring system currently exists. However the information provided by changes in factors such as a patient's performance status and degree of pain should not be neglected when assessing a patient's overall well being and quality of life as these factors provide supplementary information concerning a patient's progress under treatment.

REFERENCES

1.   R.T. Eagan, R.G. Hahn, and R.P. Myers, Adriamycin versus 5-Fluorouracil and Cyclophosphamide in the Treatment of Metastatic Cancer, Cancer Treat. Rep. 60: 115 (1976).
2.   L.K. Kvols, R.T. Eagan, and R.P. Myers, Evaluation of Melphalan, ICRF-159, and Hydroxyurea in Metastatic Prostate Cancer: A Preliminary Report, Cancer Treat. Rep. 61: 311 (1977).
3.   M. Pavone-Macaluso, F. Lund, J.H. Mulder, P.H. Smith, M. De Pauw, R. Sylvester, and EORTC Urological Group, EORTC Protocols in Prostatic Cancer: An Interim Report, Scand. J. Urol. Nephrol. Suppl. 55: 163 (1980).
4.   WHO Handbook for Reporting Results of Cancer Treatment, WHO Offset Publication No. 48, World Health Organization, Geneva, (1979).

*Participants in the EORTC Genito-Urinary Tract
 Cancer Cooperative Group Protocol 30762 -

York District Hospital - B. Richards and J. Bastable
Castleford, Normanton and District Hospital - M. Robinson
St. James's University Hospital - P.H. Smith
Huddersfield Royal Infirmary - R. Glashan
Hopital de Baviere - C. Bouffioux
C.H.U. de Reims - B. Lardennois

This investigation was supported by Grant No. 5R10-CA11488-12, awarded by the National Cancer Institute, DHEW.

THE CORRELATION BETWEEN GRADING AND CLINICAL RESPONSE

R. Sylvester

EORTC Data Center
Brussels
Belgium

INTRODUCTION

The prognostic importance of the histological grading of prostatic cancer has received considerable attention during the past decade. Classification systems such as those developed by Gleason (1), Mostofi (2) and Gaeta et al (3) have shown a direct correlation between a patient's histological pattern and his prognosis, especially with respect to duration of survival.

The EORTC Genito-Urinary Tract Cooperative Group has adopted the histological grading system published by the International Union Against Cancer (UICC) in the TNM Classification of Malignant Tumours (4). A G grade is determined based on the worst degree of tumour differentiation which can be identified:

GO : No evidence of anaplasia

Gl : High degree of differentiation

G2 : Medium degree of differentiation

G3 : Low degree of differentiation or undifferentiated

GX : Grade cannot be determined

The usefulness of this classification scheme as an indicator of a patient's prognosis was studied in a randomized trial comparing Estracyt to Stilboestrol in previously untreated prostatic cancer patients with advanced T3 or T4 disease (5). The purpose of this paper is to present some interim results of the prognostic importance of this grading system.

459

Table 1.   Correlation Between Grading and Biopsy Procedure

	NEEDLE	TUR	TUR + NEEDLE	TOTAL
G1	15 (33%)	21 (23%)	8 (13%)	44 (22%)
G2	12 (27%)	49 (53%)	25 (40%)	86 (43%)
G3	18 (40%)	23 (25%)	29 (47%)	70 (35%)
TOTAL	45	93	62	200

Test for Correlation Between Grading and Biopsy Procedure

Kendall's TAU B = .13   P = .02

DISTRIBUTION OF G GRADE AT ENTRY ON STUDY

Out of the 248 patients entered in this study, data concerning the initial G grade are available for 220 patients.   Table 1 presents the distribution of the G grade by biopsy procedure in the 200 G1, G2 or G3 patients for whom the grading at entry on study was determined by needle biopsy, TUR or TUR plus needle biopsy.   As can be seen from the table, 22% of the patients were G1, 43% were G2, and 35% were G3.   This table shows however that the G grade is correlated with the biopsy procedure and appears to depend on the amount of material available for the biopsy.   Patients with a TUR plus needle biopsy have a worse average G grade than patients with either a TUR or needle biopsy alone (P = .01).   In addition it is seen that the percentage of G1 patients decreases as the amount of material for the biopsy procedure increases, going from 33% for needle biopsy alone to only 13% for TUR plus needle biopsy.

The above analysis is however subject to bias as the choice of biopsy procedure may depend on the patient's clinical characteristics. The correlation between the biopsy procedure and the G grade might be due to the correlation of the G grade with the T classification, the M classification and a patient's performance status or perhaps with other variables not taken into account.   However further analyses revealed that after adjustment for the T classification, the M classification, the performance status and the presence or absence of pain and urinary symptoms that the correlation between the biopsy procedure and the G grade persists and that the G grade thus appears to be influenced by the biopsy procedure employed.   This analysis suggests that with either TUR or needle biopsy alone, a significant proportion of the patients may be understaged, thus leading to an incorrect prognosis for the patient.

Table 2.   Correlation Between Grading and Response of the
           Local Prostatic Tumour.

	CR	PR	NC	PROG	TOTAL
G1	2	22	23	1	48
G2	5	29	33	7	74
G3	1	16	34	8	59
TOTAL	8	67	90	16	181

Test for Correlation

Kendall's TAU C = 0.165 $P < 0.01$

THE PROGNOSTIC IMPORTANCE OF THE G GRADE

     The importance of the G grade in determining a patient's resp-
onse to treatment was studied by first considering the G grade
separately and then by considering its relative importance when other
clinical variables were accounted for.   Table 2 presents the correlation between the grading and the response of the primary lesion.
The response criteria are based on those of the World Health Organisation (6).   A 50% response rate was observed among G1 patients,
46% for G2 patients and 29% for G3 patients.   A test for an overall
correlation between the response to treatment and the G grade, taking
the ordering of both variables into account, is significant at $P < .01$.
If one considers the correlation between the grading and the response
of the primary separately for each type of biopsy procedure, it was
found that a significant correlation exists only for those patients
who had both a TUR and a needle biopsy at entry on study.   The misclassifications which may result when patients are biopsied by TUR
or needle alone tend to conceal the true importance of the G grade
as a prognostic factor in these patients.   This analysis thus shows
that the G grade is an important prognostic factor with respect to
the response of the prostatic tumour.

     The distribution of the response of the bone metastases according
to the grading of the primary tumour is shown in Table 3.   As can be
seen from this table the correlation between these two variables is
not statistically significant;   however it is based on a relatively
small number of patients and no adjustment for type of biopsy procedure has been made.   Thus while the grading of the primary tumour
appears to be of no direct prognostic importance with respect to
whether or not the bone metastases respond to treatment, further follow up is required before a definite analysis can be carried out.

Table 3.   Correlation Between Grading and Response of the
           Distant Metastases

	CR	PR	NC	PROG	TOTAL
G1	2	2	11	1	16
G2	1	10	8	6	25
G3	1	4	14	6	25
TOTAL	4	16	33	13	66

Test for Correlation

Kendall's TAU C = 0.128   P = 0.12

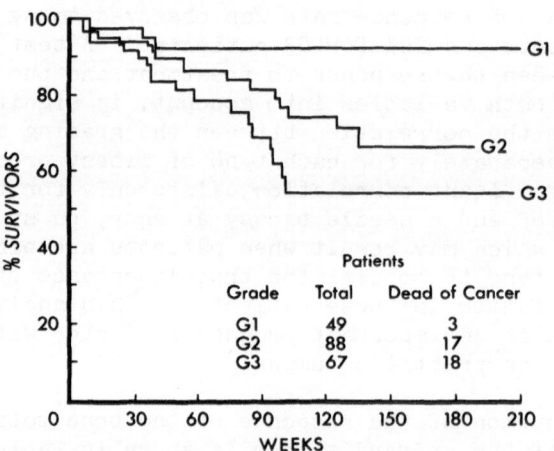

Grade	Total	Dead of Cancer
G1	49	3
G2	88	17
G3	67	18

Fig 1.   EORTC Protocol 30762.   Duration of survival of T3, T4.
Prostatic cancer patients according to G grade and deaths
from prostatic cancer (April 1981).

Figure 1 presents the duration of survival by G grade where now we are considering only those deaths due to malignant disease. As seen from this figure the duration of survival is directly related to the G grade (P <.01, Logrank Trend Test) with the relative death rate for G2 and G3 patients being respectively twice and three times that for G1 patients. Similar results are obtained if we consider all causes of death, rather than just those due to malignant disease. When we consider the correlation between the grading and the duration of survival for each biopsy technique separately, the difference between the curves is significant at the 5% level after adjustment for the performance status only for those patients with a TUR and needle biopsy. Considerably less of a separation between the curves is noted for patients with a TUR or needle biopsy alone.

These results show that despite possible inaccuracies in assessing the G grade, which means that a certain percentage of patients will inevitably be understaged, the G grade is an important prognostic factor when considered by itself with respect to the response rate of the prostatic tumour and a patient's duration of survival. The importance of the grading would be even more dramatic if all patients were correctly staged without error since such misclassifications only mask to some degree the true prognostic importance of this variable.

No analysis would be complete however without considering the importance of the histological grading relative to other clinical variables which may influence a patient's prognosis. Any effect attributed to the grading may in practice be due to its correlation with other more important variables.

When considering the correlation between the grading and other clinical variables, it was found that the G grade was correlated with a patient's performance status (P <.01), the T classification (P <.01) the level of acid phosphatase (P = .02) and to a lesser extent, the M classification (P = .06) and the patient's degree of pain (P = .08). No correlation was detected between the G grade and the patient's age, weight, associated chronic diseases, the size of the primary lesion or the level of alkaline phosphatase. A lower degree of differentiation was associated with a worse performance status, a higher T classification, a higher level of acid phosphatase, a greater probability that distant metastases are present and a higher degree of pain.

Since the G grade is correlated with several variables of prognostic importance, it is essential to determine the relative importance of the G grade with respect to these variables. One must verify whether or not the G grade retains its importance as a prognostic factor once these variables are taken into account.

Linear logistic regression was used to determine the relative importance of the G grade with respect to the response of the local and distant lesions while Cox's proportional hazards regression model

Table 4. Prognostic Factors in Prostatic Cancer

Duration of Survival		Response	
All Causes Of Death	Death Due To Malignant Disease	Local Lesion	Distant Metastases
1. Performance Status	1. Performance Status	1. Size of Local Lesion	1. Performance Status
2. Presence or Absence of Chronic Diseases	2. G Grade	2. Performance Status	2. Acid Phosphatase
3. G Grade	3. Presence or Absence of Pain	3. G Grade	

was used for the same purpose with regard to the duration of survival.
Table 4 presents the results of this analysis. For each endpoint,
response rate or duration of survival, this table presents those variables which are of prognostic significance in the order of their relative importance. Thus if one considers death due to malignant disease, the performance status is the most important variable. However
once one adjusts for the performance status, the G grade becomes the
next most significant prognostic factor. Despite the correlation of
the G grade with a patient's performance status, the additional information provided by the G grade over and above that given by the
performance status improves one's ability to predict a patient's overall duration of survival.

This table shows that in spite of the correlation of the G grade
with other prognostic factors, the G grade remains of prognostic
importance with respect to the response rate of the primary tumor
and a patient's duration of survival. Thus the significance of the
G grade is not simply due to its correlation with other variables
but it is an important prognostic factor in its own right even once
these other factors have been considered. Thus assessment of the
G grade plays a vital role in the patient's evaluation. Despite
the inaccuracies inherent in its determination, the G grade is shown
here to be more important than either the T or M classification in
predicting a patient's local response or duration of survival.

The EORTC attempted in this protocol to correlate the local
tumour response with the change in the G grade at eight weeks. However since there was no standardization of the successive biopsies,

it is not surprising that no significant correlation was detected. While a needle biopsy was routinely performed at eight weeks, only 22% of the patients had their G Grade at entry on study determined by a needle biopsy alone. For this reason no conclusions can be drawn concerning the usefulness of a follow-up biopsy in assessing a patient's response to treatment.

DISCUSSION

Due to its prognostic importance, it is mandatory that the G grade be accurately assessed in all patients with prostatic cancer. This requires a standardization of biopsy techniques and a central review of all slides. Only in this manner can a patient's prognosis adequately reflect the importance of the histological grading and the appropriate treatment be chosen. Without this knowledge we may be under staging and under treating our patients and neglecting what is one of the most useful indicators of a patient's overall prognosis.

Editorial Comment (C.B. and P.H.S.)

This paper clearly emphasizes the importance of the G grade in the prognosis of prostate cancer. We were however surprised to find no correlation between grade and type of biopsy or amount of tumour thereby made available. This might be due to: a) Selection of patients - those who have a TUR having a more advanced local tumour, or b) Alteration of the tissue sample by electroresection leading to the appearance of a more undifferentiated tumour.

REFERENCES

1.   D.F. Gleason, Classification of Prostatic Carcinomas, Cancer Chemo. Rep. 50:125 (1966).
2.   F.K. Mostofi, Prostatic Carcinoma: Significance of Histopathological Findings, in "Cancer of the Genito-Urinary Tract, D.E. Johnson and M.L. Samuels (eds), Raven Press, New York, (1979) p. 189.
3.   J.F. Gaeta, J.E. Asirwatham, G. Miller and G.P. Murphy, Histologic Grading of Primary Prostatic Cancer: A New Approach to an Old Problem, J. Urol. 123:689 (1980).
4.   T.N.M. Classification of Malignant Tumours, M.H. Harmer (ed), International Union Against Cancer, 3rd Edition, Geneva (1978).
5.   M. Pavone-Macaluso, F. Lund, J.H. Mulder, P.H. Smith, M. De Pauw, R. Sylvester and the E.O.R.T.C. Urological Group, E.O.R.T.C. Protocols in Prostatic Cancer: An Interim Report, Scand J. Urol. Nephrol. 55:163 (1980).
6.   WHO Handbook for Reporting Results of Cancer Treatment, WHO Offset Publication No. 48, World Health Organisation, Geneva. (1979).

ACKNOWLEDGMENTS

This investigated was supported by grant number 5R10-CA11488-12, awarded by the National Cancer Insitute, D.H.E.W.

CRITERIA FOR EVALUATING RESPONSE TO TREATMENT IN PROSTATIC CANCER

J.D. Schmidt and J.J. Pollen

University of California Medical Center
San Diego
U.S.A.

ABSTRACT

Better delineation of criteria for both objective and subjective responses to treatment of prostatic cancer will aid in evaluating new cytotoxic agents as well as combinations of endocrine manipulation and chemotherapy. The inclusion of the radionuclide bone scan in such criteria will help in the evaluation of the many patients with skeletal involvement only.

The need for criteria of response to treatment of prostatic cancer has arisen only in the past few years. Between the early 1940's and the early 1970's when endocrine manipulation (bilateral orchiectomy and/or exogenous estrogens) was the only treatment available for advanced prostatic cancer, only a rare patient could be identified as becoming tumor-free. When endocrine therapy was started, generally in patients suffering from some clinical disability, e.g., bone pain or urinary tract obstruction, a beneficial response of uncertain duration could be predicted in about 75% of men. Clinical responses were most often subjective in nature including alleviation of pain, improvement in voiding, weight gain and a feeling of well-being.

Another significant problem with which many cooperative groups and individual investigators have been grappling recently, is the difficulty in making objective assessments of a patient with advanced prostatic cancer (1). The primary tumor, if not removed by total prostatectomy, is notoriously difficult to measure. Notwithstanding recent attempts utilizing ultrasonography or computerized tomography, the margin of error in such measurements is great. Soft tissue lesions (enlarged lymph nodes, pulmonary

467

nodules and other masses) are infrequently seen even in advanced prostatic cancer; thus few patients in this category are available for treatment and assessment of their responses.

The use of the serum acid and alkaline phosphatase activities for assessment of response to therapy has had its pitfalls. Perhaps 20 to 25% of patients with Stage D prostatic cancer will never demonstrate an elevated serum acid phosphatase by any method. Changes in elevated serum acid phosphatase activity, whether increases or decreases, have been interpreted by varying individual criteria, e.g., serum acid phosphatase activity decreasing to normal and for various durations or simply a decrease in activity to a level greater than 50% of the pretreatment value.

The alkaline phosphatase activity is also unreliable since the source of this enzyme may be other than bone. Important to note is the classical paradoxical increase of an already elevated serum alkaline activity in response to hormonal therapy; here the increased activity represents a "healing reaction" of normal bone. Yet in the same patient, at a later date, an increased alkaline phosphatase activity may represent increasing osseous metastatic disease.

Until the advent of reproducible high-quality technetium bone scanning, the common osteoblastic metastases of prostatic cancer were followed as unreliable indicators of disease activity vis a vis response to treatment. Osteoblastic metastases often increase dramatically in patients who otherwise are "doing well" (2), and only a rare patient demonstrates complete disappearance of such metastases. The less common osteolytic metastases need to be observed for recalcification, a somewhat subjective interpretation.

In the United States, the National Prostatic Cancer Project (NPCP) has focused on these problems by setting down criteria in various categories of objective response: complete response (CR), partial response (PR), stable disease (S) and progression (P). These criteria have slowly evolved and continue to be modified (3). In addition, criteria for subjective responses have been formulated. The current NPCP criteria for objective and subjective responses are presented in Table 1-5. Recently the NPCP has demonstrated that survival is similar for patients considered stable and in partial regression compared to those in progression according to the response criteria as listed (4).

To further the input of radionuclide bone-scanning in evaluating treatment responses, the NPCP in 1980 held a workshop to study this aspect of diagnosis (5). Criteria of response utilizing the bone scanner are listed in Table 6. Employing these criteria solely, we recently evaluated 41 patients with stage D prostatic cancer receiving various treatment including chemotherapy and/or hormones and compared their responses to survival. The Figure identifies the

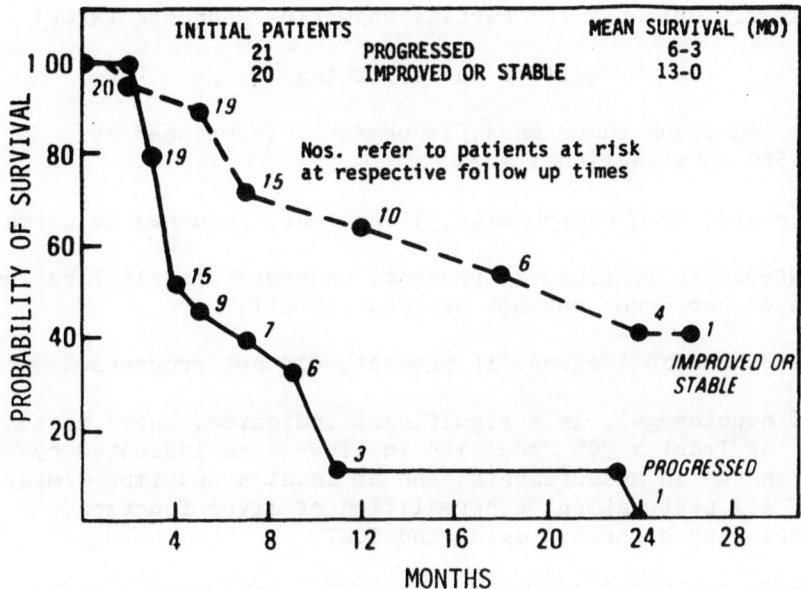

Fig. 1. Survival of 41 patients with stage D prostatic
cancer evaluated according to response on radionuclide
bone scan.

Table 1. Criteria for Complete Objective Regression (NPCP)

(All of the following must be present)

1. Tumour masses, if present, totally disappeared and no new
   lesions appeared. The primary tumor is included.

2. Elevated acid phosphatase, if present, returned to normal.

3. Osteolytic lesions, if present, recalcified.

4. Osteoblastic lesions, if present, disappeared.

5. If hepatomegaly is a significant indicator there must be
   a complete return in liver size to normal, i.e., no
   distention below both costal margins at the mid-clavicular
   lines and from the tip of the xiphoid process during quiet
   respiration without liver movement, and normalization
   of all pretreatment abnormalities of liver function
   including bilirubin mg/dl and SGOT.

6. No significant cancer related deterioration in weight
   ($>$10%), symptoms, or performance status.

Table 2. Criteria for Partial Objective Response (NPCP)

(All of the following)

1. At least one tumor mass, if present, is reduced by
    $>$ 50% in x-sectional area.

2. Elevated acid phosphatase, if present, returned to normal.

3. Osteolytic lesions, if present, underwent recalcification
    in one or more, but not necessarily all.

4. Osteoblastic lesions, if present, did not progress.

5. If hepatomegaly is a significant indicator, there must
    be at least a 30% reduction in liver size indicated by
    a change in measurements, and at least a 30% improvement
    of all pretreatment abnormalities of liver function,
    including bilirubin mg/dl and SGOT.

6. There may be no increase in any other lesion and no new
    areas of malignant disease may appear.

7. No significant cancer deterioration in weight ($>$ 10%),
    symptoms, or performance status.

Table 3. Criteria for Objective Stable Disease (NPCP)

(All of the following)

1. No new lesions occurred and no measurable lesions
    increased more than 25% in x-sectional area.

2. Elevated acid phosphatase, if present, decreased.

3. Osteolytic lesions, if present, did not appear to
    worsen.

4. Osteoblastic lesions, if present, remained stable.

5. Hepatomegaly, if present, did not appear to worsen by
    more than a 30% increase in the measurements, and
    hepatic abnormalities did not worsen including
    bilirubin mg/dl and SGOT.

5. No significant cancer related deterioration in weight
    ($>$ 10%), symptoms, or performance status.

Table 4. Criteria for Objective Progression (NPCP)

(Any of the following)

1. Significant cancer related deterioration in weight (>10%), symptoms or performance status.

2. Appearance of new areas of malignant disease.

3. Increase in any previously measurable lesions by greater than 25% in x-sectional area.

4. Increase in osseous metastases as shown by scan.

Note: An increase in acid or alkaline phosphatase alone is not to be considered an indication of progression. These should be used in conjunction with other criteria.

Table 5. Criteria for Subjective Response (NPCP)

(At least 2 of the 3 criteria must be present)

1. Weight gain of 3% in any 4 week period without evidence of edema.

2. Correction of anemia (hemoglobin > 10.5 grams%).

3. Relief of pain on a scale 1-4, with 4 being maximum relief.

Table 6. Objective Response Criteria Utilizing Bone-Scanning

Complete Response (CR):		No evidence of metastases
Partial Response (PR):		(a) Reduction in intensity of uptake
	or	(b) Reduction in extent of uptake
	or	(c) Disappearance of some metastases
	and	(d) No new lesions
Stable (S):		No significant change in uptake pattern
Progression (P):		(a) Increase in intensity of uptake
	or	(b) Increase in extent of uptake
	or	(c) Appearance of new lesions

strikingly improved survival of patients considered as objectively improved or stable via bone scan criteria compared to those patients considered in progression. Clearly this is a preliminary observation and will need to be clarified and confirmed by other investigators. Problems to be worked out include standardization of scanning techniques and equipment, differences in radiopharmaceuticals, time intervals between scanning procedures and reproducible means of quantitation of bone scan changes.

This work was supported in part by Public Health Service Grant CA 21438 through the National Prostatic Cancer Project, National Cancer Institute, National Institutes of Health, Department of Health and Human Services.

REFERENCES

1. J.D. Schmidt, D.E. Johnson, W.W. Scott, R.P. Gibbons, G.R. Prout, Jr., and G.P. Murphy, Chemotherapy of advanced prostatic cancer, evaluation of response parameters, Urology 7:602 (1976).
2. J.J. Pollen, and W.J. Schlaer, Osteoblastic response to successful treatment of metastatic cancer of the prostate, Amer. J. Roentgenol. 132:927 (1979).
3. J.D. Schmidt, W.W. Scott, R. Gibbons, D.E. Johnson, G.R. Prout, Jr., S. Loening, M. Soloway, J. deKernion, J.E. Pontes, N.H. Slack and G.P. Murphy, Chemotherapy programmes of the National Prostatic Cancer Project (NPCP), Cancer 45:1937 (1980).
4. N.H. Slack, A. Mittelman, M.F. Brady, G.P. Murphy, and Investigators in the National Prostatic Cancer Project: The importance of the stable category for chemotherapy treated patients with advanced and relapsing prostate cancer, Cancer 46:2393 (1980).
5. N.H. Slack, J.P. Karr, T.M. Chu, G.P. Murphy, and Investigators in the National Prostatic Cancer Project: An assessment of bone scans for monitoring osseous metastases in patients being treated for prostate carcinoma, The Prostate 1:259 (1980).

Editorial Note (P.H.S.) This paper and that by the same author on combinations of chemotherapy and hormones in prostatic cancer illustrates some of the work of the National Prostatic Cancer Project. It is clear that the NPCP is as concerned as the EORTC about the problems of evaluation of response in prostatic cancer.

The concept of stable disease as an objective response is attractive but even though it is clear that patients showing stable disease survive longer than those who continue to progress, it is

by no means certain that this finding can yet be attributed to the
treatment given.

The criteria of response as listed in the two articles vary
slightly and presumably patients with recurring anaemia or who
develop ureteral obstruction will no longer be regarded as
progressing. This is likely to increase the number of patients
with "stable disease" but may reduce any difference in survival
between the two groups. It is unlikely that cytotoxic or other
therapy will be of real value unless the patients show large numbers
of complete or partial objective responses and it may be preferable
to limit the term "objective response" to these two categories.

CANCER OF THE KIDNEY

AETIOLOGY OF KIDNEY TUMOURS

M. Pavone-Macaluso, G.B. Ingargiola and M. Lamartina

Institute of Urology
University of Palermo
Italy

Surveys of possible aetiological factors were made by one of us in 1963 and in 1967 (1,2), reviewing 441 articles hoping to find some clues to the causes of tumours of the kidney.

It is apparent that, from the aetiological standpoint, renal cell carcinoma must be kept separate from nephroblastoma, transitional cell carcinoma, sarcoma and other types of renal neoplasia, although in rare instances the same cause was experimentally found to be responsible for the occurrence of renal tumours of different histotypes. For instance, benzpyrene was found to produce renal cell carcinoma, kidney sarcoma or squamous cell carcinoma of the renal pelvis, depending on the experimental animal or on the route of administration.

Apart from this, and other exceptions, it was apparent that adenoma and adenocarcinoma (renal cell carcinoma) were often caused by the same factors, whereas Wilms' tumours and the other neoplasias were related to different aetiological factors.

1. Nephroblastoma Nephroblastoma is not infrequently congenital and bilateral. It can be associated with various congenital malformations especially hemihypertrophy and aniridia. It has been suggested that the presence of aberrant embryonal germ cells or the abnormal growth of multipotent cells during foetal life, might be responsible for their formation. Heredity may represent a predisposing factor, whereas geographical and environmental conditions, including chemical carcinogens and hormones, do not appear to play a significant role in their aetiology. It is extremely difficult to produce Wilms' tumour experimentally, although a virus-induced nephroblastoma could be obtained in the fowl by the myeloblastosis

avian tumour virus (3).

2. <u>Squamous Cell Carcinoma</u> has been described in patients as a
late complication of retrograde pyelography with a radioactive
compound, thorotrast. Squamous cell carcinoma has also been produced experimentally by the intrarenal administration of chemical
carcinogens. Renal stones, infection and other factors producing
"chronic irritation" are likely to play a role in the development of
both squamous cell carcinoma and mucus-secreting adenocarcinoma of
the renal pelvis.

3. <u>Transitional Cell Carcinoma</u> of the renal pelvis can be produced
by the same carcinogens, either exogenous or endogenous, that are
held responsible for the induction of bladder tumours. Papillary
tumours of the renal pelvis have been produced experimentally using
2-naphthylamine and have been detected in workers exposed to
industrial carcinogens. Urothelial carcinoma of the renal pelvis
has often been found in association with two types of chronic
interstitial nephritis, namely Balkan nephropathy, and nephritis
due to prolonged use of phenacetin-containing analgesics.

4. <u>Renal Adenoma and Adenocarcinoma</u> A more detailed discussion will
be devoted to the spontaneous occurrence of renal adenocarcinoma in
animals, as well as to the various aetiological factors that have
been investigated in different animal species. Adenoma and adenocarcinoma will be considered together, as we believe that there is
no clear distinction between the two conditions and that the
traditional differentiation based only on the size of the tumours is
arbitrary. In addition, both adenoma and carcinoma can be produced
by the same carcinogen in various animal models and serial transplantation of renal adenoma may give rise to a frankly malignant
carcinoma. In the following lines only the term "adenocarcinoma"
will be employed. It includes adenoma and is considered synonymous
with "renal cell carcinoma."

A. <u>Spontaneous Renal Tumours in Animals</u>

Spontaneous renal tumours are relatively rare, both in wild and
domestic animals. Among the latter ones, poultry, horses and swine
are affected most frequently. Although mixed tumours, similar to
Wilms' nephroblastoma and renal urotheliomas have been occasionally
found, only adenocarcinoma will be considered here. The incidence
of renal adenocarcinoma in rats ranges between 0.0004 to 0.2% in
various strains. Genetic as well as hormonal factors seem to play
a role in a strain of Wistar rats in which 24% of males and 51% of
females were affected (4). Similarly in mice the overall incidence
is 0.02% (5), but a given strain was found to be affected in about
one half of the animals (6). Spontaneous adenocarcinoma has been
found in 0.5% of hamsters (7). The occurrence of renal adenocarcinoma in frogs will be discussed as an example of viral aetiology.

B. Association of Renal Tumours with Other Pathological Conditions

Horseshoe kidney and other congenital malformations are
occasionally associated not only with nephroblastoma but also with
renal cell carcinoma. According to Patoir (8), who collected 30
such cases in the medical literature up to 1959, the incidence of
renal tumours of horseshoe kidneys is higher than in the average
population. Unilateral or bilateral renal cancer has also been
observed in association with polycystic disease of the kidneys (9,
10), multilocular cystic disease (11), diabetes mellitus (12) and
a variety of other diseases (2). It has also been suggested that
adenomas are more likely to arise in atrophic kidneys with focal
tubular hyerplasia than in normal organs. It is difficult to be
certain that such associations are due to a cause-effect relationship, rather than merely being coincidental. There are however
two conditions in which renal tumours, often bilateral, are
significantly more frequent than in the non-affected population:
a) renal hamartomas in Bourneville's tuberous sclerosis and b)
renal adenocarcinomas in von Hippel-Lindau's haemangioblastoma. For
an extensive bibliography concerning these pathological associations,
see refs. 1 and 2.

C. Possible Aetiological Factors for Renal Adenocarcinoma

Such factors include race, heredity, viruses, alterations in
the host's immunological reactivity (renal transplantation),
irradiation, hormones, endogenous and exogenous carcinogens,
smoking habits, beverages, food and other environmental factors.
A detailed discussion of these factors is beyond the scope of the
present article. For detailed information and bibliography the
reader is referred not only to our previous reviews (1,2) but also
to more recent papers on closely related topics (13,14). Only
brief comments and recent references will be given here.

C1. Race, epidemiology and other environmental factors
Epidemiological studies, with regard to renal cancer, are relatively
scarce (15). It does not seem, however, that racial factors play
a major role. In the United States no significant difference in
the frequency of renal tumours was observed among Caucasian, Negro
and Mexican ethnic groups, although the incidence in the Japanese
population has been reported to be slightly higher. As far as
geographic distribution is concerned, only minor fluctuations have
been described. Comparison of mortality rates from renal malignancies
in selected countries permitted a distinction between three different groups (16). a) countries showing low rates (Ireland, Italy,
Japan, Spain, Venzuela) b) countries showing high rates (Denmark,
Norway, Scotland, New Zealand) c) countries with an intermediate
incidence (Belgium, Holland, France, England, Wales, Australia,
the U.S.A.). It can be inferred that the highest frequency of
carcinoma of the kidney is found in the industralized countries of

western Europe, especially in the northern areas (Scandinavia and
Scotland) and, to a lesser degree, in the U.S.A.

Urbanization and high social class appear to be associated
with a comparatively high incidence of renal cancer. This does not
appear to be related to animal protein but rather to fat intake. A
positive correlation with obesity has been suggested. No correlation
with coffee consumption has been found. The role of smoking is
still controversial, although some reports show a greater incidence
of renal tumours not only in cigarette but especially in cigar and
pipe smokers. This may depend, at least in part, on the fact that
tobacco smoking leads to increased absorption and inhalation of
"renal carcinogens", such as methylnitrosamine and cadmium, as well
as to enhanced urinary excretion of 3-hydroxyanthranilic acid and
other abnormal tryptophan metabolites. Occupational hazards should
also be considered and workers involved with coke ovens appear to
be especially at risk (17).

C2 <u>Heredity</u> This is not usually considered of primary importance
in this context, although genetic factors have been shown to play
a definite role, not only in rats and mice, but also in Rhesus
monkeys. In the latter species, a family has been described in
which four animals were affected by renal adenocarcinoma (18).

In humans there are also several observations of renal adenocarcinoma in members of the same family. Brinton in 1960 (19)
described a family in which at least four persons died from kidney
carcinoma in two different generations. Ten people in three
generations were found to be affected in a more recent report (20).
The role of genetic factors is stressed by the higher incidence in
subjects with blood group A, as well as by the reports of cases of
hereditary renal cell carcinoma associated with chromosome trans-
locations (21) and with colour blindness (22). Reddy (23), in
addition to his own observation of <u>bilateral</u> renal cell carcinoma
in a father and his two sons, reported 114 cases of familiar renal
cancer that he had been able to find in the English literature up
to 1981. The problem of heredity in renal cancer should be
investigated with greater attention in the future, especially in
cases of bilateral tumours.

C3 <u>Irradiation</u> Whole body irradiation induced renal adenocarcinoma
in 30% of intact mice and in 53% of animals with single kidneys (24).
Fast neutrons lead to similar results. A case of renal adenocarcinoma following retrograde pyelography with thorotrast, a
colloidal suspension of radioactive throrium dioxide, has also been
described (25), in addition to the more numerous cases of squamous
cell carcinoma, which can be ascribed to the same aetiological
factor. Radioactive compounds, such as Polonium-210 and Strontium
90, have also been incriminated in renal carcinogenesis.

C4 <u>Viruses</u> The viral aetiology of a spontaneous renal carcinoma (Lucké's tumour) occurring in the North American leopard frog (Rana pipiens) has been demonstrated beyond doubt. The lesions are well differentiated adenocarcinomas which, under favourable conditions, metastasize in 80% of cases. When adult frogs are kept in the laboratory for eight months, the incidence may be as high as 25%, whereas the field incidence is between 3 and 9%. An updated review was presented in 1980 by Beckley (26). Already in 1938, Lucké (27) had demonstrated that this tumour is strictly species-specific. If its cells or their extracts are injected into green frogs (Rana clamitans), bull frogs (Rana catesbiana), or even into a different sub-species of Rana pipiens, none of the frogs of foreign species develop renal cancer. The aetiological agent has been identified as a herpes simplex virus (28). Interestingly enough, in a recent investigation by Cocchiara, Tarro et al (29) herpes simplex virus (HSV) specific antigens were identified in a human adenocarcinoma of the kidney. As the presence of HSV tumour- associated antigens has been described in a variety of human tumours, it remains uncertain whether or not this really represents the demonstration of their viral aetiology. Renal tumours can also be produced by the polyoma virus, the simian virus (SV 40) and by the adenovirus-7 in hamsters and in other rodents. They are usually different from adenocarcinoma, a sarcomatous pattern being the most frequent histotype.

C5 <u>Hormones</u> It has been known for many years that renal adenomas and adenocarcinomas can be provoked by prolonged administration of both natural and synthetic oestrogens in the male golden Syrian hamster. A recent report suggests that renal tumours can also be consistently induced in the European hamster (30). It appears that the male hamster is the only animal species in which renal tumours are caused by oestrogens. If administration of hormones is stopped even after long periods of time, regression of the tumours will take place. These tumours are similar to adenocarcinoma of the human kidney, including the high lipid content of the tumour cells. They are often multiple and bilateral. Their growth is initially expansive and eventually becomes infiltrative. True metastases are rare. If the oestrogenic treatment is extended for at least 250 days, kidney tumours develop in about 97% of treated males. No tumours appear in organs other than the kidneys. Oestrogen-induced renal adenocarcinoma may develop, not only in intact male hamsters, but also in castrated males. In females, oestrogens can induce renal tumours only before the onset, or after the cessation, of sexual activity.

The tumours can be serially transplanted into other male hamsters provided the recipient animals are also treated with oestrogens. Such hormone-dependence, however, can be lost after several passages in animals, so that, after many transfers, takes can be obtained even if the recipient animals are not given oestrogens.

This animal model lends itself to attempts at treatment with a variety of hormone manipulations. Thus, it has been shown that deoxycorticosterone inhibits the growth of renal carcinoma in oestrogen-treated male hamsters (31). By transplantation of an oestrogen-independent tumour into animals treated with various hormones or submitted to endocrine ablation procedures (32), it has appeared that a) cortisone produces marked tumour inhibition, b) a progestational agent, if used without the concurrent administration of cortisone has comparatively little effect upon the tumour growth rate, c) adrenalectomy produces growth reduction, d) orchidectomy is followed by inhibition of tumour development and by prevention of further growth in established transplants, e) the effect of orchidectomy can be abolished by the administration of testosterone or oestrogens, f) bromocryptine inhibits primary renal tumours induced by DES. The above-mentioned experiments have been followed by many attempts to treat human renal adeonocarcinoma with hormones. Medroxyprogesterone acetate, testosterone and cortisone or related steroids have been used for this purpose. Human renal adenocarcinoma has long been considered to be responsive to hormonal treatment and even to be a hormone-dependent tumour. This view was recently supported by the finding of hormone receptors in normal kidney tissue and in renal cancer (33). This has however been challenged in the last few years, due to conflicting clinical and experimental results (34). This topic will form the object of a more thorough discussion elsewhere in this book.

There seems to be little doubt that human renal adenocarcinomas are under some sort of hormonal influence. There is a significant sex ratio, the tumour being more frequent in males than in females. In the series of Pignalosa and Fernandez (35) 69.9% of renal tumours were found in males. This difference tends to increase after menopause, reaching a male to female ratio of 4:1. The dependence of "hypernephromas" on endocrine disturbances has often been postulated. It was claimed, for instance, that renal adenocarcinoma is more frequent in patients with hypercorticism or other hormonal imbalance states than in the average population. It has also been hypothesized that spontaneous regression of renal tumours may be under the influence of endocrine changes (36). The relationship between hormones and renal cancer remains a controversial issue. Oestrogen-induced renal carcinoma in the male hamster is an important experimental model but this animal is unique in showing this particular behaviour. The gap still remains to be filled between laboratory animals and human beings and, in our view, it is doubtful whether conclusions drawn from investigations performed in the hamster can be safely applied to renal tumours in man.

C6 <u>Chemicals</u> Endogenous carcinogens may be involved not only in the production of urothelial tumours but also in that of renal parenchymal cancer. A case of an adenocarcinoma associated with increased urinary excretion of Tryptophan metabolites was described

in 1963 (37) but, to our knowledge, this finding has not been
confirmed in subsequent years. This remains, however, a very
interesting avenue for future research. A larger number of observations has been obtained with regard to exogenous chemical
carcinogens. A table with a long list of substances having been
tested for renal carcinogenic activity was presented in our review
of 1967 (2). Further data from the current literature were reviewed
by Sufrin in 1980 (14).

It has been shown that several exogenous chemical carcinogens
are able to produce renal tumours in various laboratory animals.
There are also some interesting clinical observations that this may
also be true in the human being. Among the substances that are
carcinogenic for the kidney, nitroso-compounds, aromatic amines,
hydrazines, alkylating agents, anticancer chemotherapeutic agents,
metals and natural compounds deserve special attention. A few
miscellaneous agents will also be considered.

a. N-nitroso compounds

Nitrosamines are currently employed in rubber vulcanization and
textile fibre industries.

Dimethylnitrosamine (DNM) has for many years been known to be a
potent oncogenic agent. The chronic administration of DMN to the
rat gives rise to degenerative changes and to neoplasms in the liver
and lungs. In acute experiments with high doses of DMN, the liver
undergoes marked regression without secondary tumour formation.
Instead, renal adenoma or adenocarcinoma appear in about one half of
the surviving animals. Even a single dose of DMN will produce renal
tumours in 63% of female rats, in spite of the fact that DMN is
rapidly excreted and metabolized. In other animal species, DMN
feeding induces renal adenocarcinoma in 72% of Swiss mice, but is
ineffective in European hamsters. The renal tumours induced by DMN
and related compounds are of two main histological types, i) a
differentiated neoplasm, resembling clear cell carcinoma and ii) an
anaplastic infiltrating tumour.

Diethylnitrosamine, if given by a single intravenous bolus to
Sprague-Dawley rats induces bilateral and multifocal renal tumours
in 30% of males and 80% of females. Tumours tend to be present in
other organs too. The same compound is also effective in inducing
renal adenocarcinoma in either sex in the golden Syrian hamster.

Nitrosomethylurea gives rise to anaplastic or sarcomatous renal
tumours if administered to adult rats, whereas adenocarcinoma can
be obtained in 25% of Wistar rats treated at birth or within the
first days of life. Similar results were obtained in mice.

Nitrosethylurea Following treatment with this compound rats develop nephroblastoma, but mice develop adenocarcinoma. This is another interesting confirmation that the same oncogenic agent can produce various tumour histotypes if employed under different experimental conditions and in different animal species.

b. Aromatic amines

4 fluoro-4-aminodiphenyl This amine induces renal adenocarcinoma in 80% of treated male Wistar rats. They are often bilateral and multi-focal and are usually associated with tumours of other organs. Similar tumours that can be serially transplanted are induced in rats by a closely related compound, N-(4-fluoro-4-biphenyl) acetamide.

2-Acetylaminofluorene This compound is a well known carcinogen which is responsible for the induction of transitional cell carcinoma from the urothelium of bladder and renal pelvis. It can also induce renal adenocarcinoma in 10% of treated rats.

c. Hydrazines

Renal adenocarcinomas were obtained in 80% of Sprague-Dawley rats treated with formic acid-nitrofuryl-thiazolyl hydrazide (FNT). The other hydrazines tested so far appear to be less effective.

d. Alkylating agents

An alkylating agent, the flame retardant tris (2,3-dibromo-propyl) phosphate (TBP), if given in high doses, is capable of inducing renal adenocarcinoma in 39% of rats and in 21% of mice. As recently pointed out by Reznick et al (38) the use of flame re-tardants has greatly increased in recent years, following the intro-duction of U.S. federal regulations concerned with fabric flammability, particularly those requiring treatment of all children's sleepwear. In addition, TBP is used in carpets, plastics, house furnishings and in building materials. The oncogenic effects of TBP in rodents occur not only after oral administration, but also if it is painted on the skin of experimental animals. This has created great concern in the United States for fear that a carcinogenic substance might enter the bodies of children by being absorbed through the skin or by being ingested by children sucking their clothing. TPB was therefore banned from commerce starting April 1977. Interestingly enough, large quantities of children's pyjamas treated with flame retardants, are now being exported from the U.S.A. to Europe. This fact has even led to an official investigation in March 1981 by a member of the European Parliament. Flame retardants are certainly toxic. They cause testicular atrophy and chronic interstitial nephritis in rabbits. If traces of TPB (1 p.p.m.) are added to the water containing goldfish, all the fish die within five days. There is however no proof until now that TBP and related compounds are responsible for the induction of renal cancer in man.

e. Anticancer agents

Streptozotocin, administered by a single intravenous dose, induces diabetes mellitus immediately and causes delayed renal adenocarcinoma in 50% of treated male Holzinan rats. Only 7% of Wistar rats are affected, suggesting an important strain difference.

Daunorubicin an anthracycline anti-tumour antibiotic closely related to doxorubicin (adriamycin), if administered to Sprague-Dawley rats, has been reported to produce chronic glomerulonephritis in nearly all animals, as well as renal adenocarcinoma in 21% of treated rats (39).

f. Metals

Lead In 1962 Kilham et al (40) reported that a high prevalence of renal tumours had been observed in wild rats living in a suburban industrial area, in the vicinity of burning refuse dumps containing substantial amounts of lead. The lead content of various tissues was abnormally high and typical lead inclusions were discovered in the renal tubular cells of these animals. Furthermore, it was demonstrated that prolonged administration of lead acetate or phosphate results in the development of kidney adenocarcinomas in the rat. Hyperplastic and cystic lesions occur after short periods of treatment. Such tumours can be obtained only in rats and mice, probably because of their tolerance of high doses which would be lethal to other animals.

Attempts to ascertain if chronic lead intoxication is a factor in the development of renal tumours in man have yielded negative results so far. Despite marked reduction of saturnism in the typographic industry, chronic lead poisoning is still possible. Work involving soldering, painting, battery changing and insecticide spraying are particularly hazardous from this standpoint. Heavy air pollution in most cities, especially since lead tetraethyl is used as an additive to petrol, is a factor to be kept in mind. This may be a possible explanation for the higher incidence of renal cancer in urban than in rural areas. However, follow up studies of workers exposed to lead vapour inhalation have failed to demonstrate any greater incidence of renal tumours among those workers than in the general population.

Cadmium A relatively high incidence of renal cancer has been described in workers exposed to cadmium poisoning (15). This metal is also being suggested as a possible oncogenic factor for prostatic adenocarcinoma. It is of interest that the incidence of both cancers is especially high in Sweden where chronic cadmium poisoning represents a very severe problem. Exposure to this substance may occur in the manufacture of almost all industrial products from cameras to aircraft brakes, from semi-artificial agricultural

fertilizers to dyes and washing machines. It has been reported that
Sweden actually uses from 80 to 100 tons of cadmium yearly and that
the manufacturing process often gives rise to highly toxic clouds.
It has also been calculated that its concentration in the ground rises
yearly by a factor of 0.5%. It has more than doubled within the
last 40 years. A similar trend has also been observed in other
countries. This should lead to a more careful search for a correlation between exposure to cadmium and renal oncogenesis so that
timely preventive measures can be taken, if this correlation can be
confirmed.

g. Natural products

Cycas Circinalis is a palm-like plant which is used as a source of
starch among the Chamorro, the indigenous population of Guam,
Mariana Islands. There is evidence to indicate that the seed of
this plant can induce a high yield of kidney and liver tumours when
incorporated in the diet of rats. The renal tumours correspond
even ultrastructurally to human adenocarcinomas (41). The responsible
substance is a glycoside named cycasin. Its hydrolysis liberates
the active aglycone, methyl-azoxy-methanol (MAM). Intraperitoneal
MAM induces renal adenocarcinoma or, less frequently, a renal
sarcoma in 78% of rats. The tumours are bilateral in 57% of cases.
The incidence of MAM on cycosin-induced tumours is much lower in
mice and hamsters.*

Aflatoxin produced by the fungus Aspergillus flavus which not
rarely contaminates peanut meal has also been shown to be able to
produce renal adenocarcinoma in rats.

h. Miscellaneous compounds

A list of substances experimentally found to be capable of
inducing renal cancer would not be complete without ochratoxin A,
safiole, niridazole, urethane and elaiomycin. The potent and
almost ubiquitous polycyclic aromatic hydrocarbon carcinogens,
benzpyrene, 20-methylcholanthrene and dibenzanthracene are rather
ineffective as renal oncogens since less than 1% of treated animals
develop kidney adenocarcinomas.

Finally a recent WHO report, quoted in the Bulletin of the
Italian Ministry of Health (41) suggests that chloroform is also a
relatively potent agent responsible for experimental induction

------

* There is not yet any clear-cut evidence that the population of
  Guam presents a strikingly high incidence of renal cancer.
  However the frequently held view that normal, unadulterated
  foodstuff is always free from carcinogenic hazards is no
  longer tenable.

of renal adenocarcinoma in rats and mice. In the rat, renal cancer
was obtained in 8% and 24% of animals treated with daily doses of
90 and 180 mg/kg respectively. Higher doses induced liver carcinoma.
In the mouse renal adenocarcinoma developed in 10-25% of males
treated with 60 mg/kg/day. Chloroform has therefore been considered
as a potential carcinogenic agent in man and the U.I.C.C. has
suggested that all pharmaceutical products containing chloroform
should be withdrawn from free commercial distribution. This
recommendation has been put in practice in Canada, the U.S.A.,
Japan, Norway, Poland, Sweden and Switzerland. The European
Community has however not restricted the use of tooth paste containing 4% chloroform, postponing final decisions until January 1981.
In the United Kingdom a maximum chloroform concentration of 0.5% is
still allowed in pharmaceutical products pending more definitive
information about its actual carcinogenic risk in man. Again, as
noted with regard to flame retardants, no controls or restrictions
are requested in European countries belonging to the Common Market
with regard to products imported from abroad.

Conclusions

    In conclusion, a few interesting animal models have emerged
from the study of spontaneous and experimental animal tumours. They
are appealing, in spite of the obvious reservations and limits, for
the investigation of potential forms of treatment (43). They have
however given us relatively little insight into the unsolved
problem of aetiology of renal cancer in man. Important information
on the early events in renal carcinogenesis has resulted. It is
of interest that damage to the tubular cells appears to be the
first recognizable event and that the appearance of cystic lesions
often precedes that of adenoma and adenocarcinoma in a few experimental renal tumours. Species or strain specificity and sex also
appear to play a significant role. It is likely that in man
heredity, coexistence of other diseases, smoking and, in rare
instances, irradiation represent possible aetiological factors.
It also appears that hormonal, chemical and other environmental
factors can play a role. The importance of herpes virus in renal
adenocarcinoma needs to be elucidated. Many suspects are at hand,
but a major villain still remains to be identified. It is hoped
that further research will be continued, so that data obtained
from experimental work can lead to a better understanding of
aetiology and hopefully to clues for prevention of human renal
cancer.

REFERENCES

1. M. Pavone-Macaluso, L'étiologie et la pathogénie des tumeurs
    du rein. Les tumeurs expérimentales, Gazette Médicale de
    France 70:1143 (1963).

2. M. Pavone-Macaluso, Etiology of kidney tumors, in:
    "Renal Neoplasia", J.S. King, ed., Little, Brown and Co.,
    Boston (1967) p 247.

3. H. Ishiguro, D. Beard, J.R. Sommer, U. Heine, G. de Thé and
    J.W. Beard, Multiplicity of cell response to the BAI strain A
    (myleloblastosis) avian tumor virus. I: Nephroblastoma (Wilms'
    tumor) gross and microscopic pathology, J. Nat. Cancer Inst.
    29:1 (1962).

4. R. Eker, Familial renal adenoma in Wistar rats, Acta Path.
    Microbiol. Scand. 34:554 (1954).

5. H.A. Horn and H.L. Stewart, A review of some spontaneous tumors
    in non-inbred mice, J. Nat. Cancer Inst. 13:591 (1952).

6. A. Claude, Adénocarcinome rénal endémique chez une souche de
    souris, Rev. Franc. Etudes Clin. Biol. 3:261 (1958).

7. J.A. Fortner, A.G. Mahy and R.S. Cotron, Transplantable tumors
    of the Syrian golden hamster. Part II: Tumors of the hema-
    topoietic tissues, genito-urinary organs, mammary glands and
    sarcomas, Cancer Res. 21:199 (1961).

8. G. Patoir, Les tumeurs du rein en fer à cheval, J. Urol. Méd.
    Chir. 65:799 (1959).

9. A. Tallarigo, Su un raro caso di associazione tra rene poli-
    cistico e tumore ipernefroma, Riv. Anat. Patol. Oncol. 3:510
    (1950).

10. A. Puigvert, Polykystose rénale et cancer bilatéral, J. Urol.
    Méd. Chir. 64:30 (1958).

11. J.B. Beckwith, Multilocular renal cysts and cystic renal tumors,
    Amer. J Roentgenol. 136:435 (1981).

12. R. Churalla, Fenomeni endocrini nell' ipernefroma del rene,
    Urologia 20:9 (1953).

13. A.F. Kantor, Current concepts of epidemiology and etiology of
    primary renal cell carcinoma, J. Urol. 117:415 (1972).

14. G. Sufrin, Spontaneous, hormonal and chemically induced animal
    models of renal adenocarcinoma, in: "Renal Adenocarcinoma"
    G. Sufrin and S.A. Beckley, eds., U.I.C.C., Geneva (1980) p 2.

15. F. Berrino, Epidemiologia e patogenese dei tumori maligni del
    rene: Presented at the 22nd course of the Istituto Nazionale
    Tumori, Milano, 1981 (to be published).

16. R.A.M. Case, Mortality from cancer of the kidney in England
    and Wales with data from other countries for comparison in:
    "Tumours of the Kidney and Ureter", E. Riches, ed.,
    Livingstone, Edinburgh, (1964) p 1.

17. Redmond, J. Occ. Med. 9:277 (1965) quoted by Berrino (15).

18. H.L. Ratcliffe, Familial occurence of renal carcinoma in Rhesus
    Monkey (macaca mulatta), Amer. J. Pathol.16:619 (1940).

19. L.F. Brinton, Hypernephroma: familiar occurrence in one family,
    J. Amer. Med. Assoc. 173:889 (1960).

20. S.M. Goldman, Renal cell carcinoma diagnosed in three gener-
    ations of a single family, South Med. J. 72:1457 (1979).

21. A.J. Cohen, F.B. Li, S. Berg, D.J. Marchetto, S. Tsai,
    S.C. Jacobs and R.S. Brown, Hereditary renal cell carcinoma
    associated with a chromosome translocation, New Engl. J. Med.
    301:592 (1979).

22. J.P. Griffin, G.V. Hughes and W.B. Peeling, A survey of the
    familial incidence of adenocarcinoma of the kidney, Brit. J.
    Urol. 39:63 (1967).

23. E.R. Reddy, Bilateral renal cell carcinoma, Unusual occurrence
    in three members of one family, Brit. J. Radiol. 54:8 (1981).

24. V.J. Rosen and L.J. Cole, Accelerated induction of kidney
    neoplasms in mice after X-radiation and unilateral nephrectomy,
    J. Nat. Cancer Inst. 28:1031 (1962).

25. W. Freidrich, Hypernephroides Carcinom nach Thorotrastanwendung
    und eosinophiles Adenom der Hypophyse, Krebsforsch 63:456 (1960).

26. S. Beckley, Viral models of renal adenocarcinoma, in: "Renal
    Adenocarcinoma", G. Sufrin and S.A. Beckley, eds., U.I.C.C.
    Geneva (1980) p 28.

27. B. Lucké, Carcinoma in the leopard frog. Its probable
    causation by a virus, J. Exp. Med. 68:457 (1938).

28. A. Granoff, Herpes virus and the Lucké tumor, Cancer Res.
    33:1431 (1973).

29. R. Cocchiara, G. Tarro, G. Flaminio, M. Di Gioia, R. Smeraglia
    and D. Geraci, Purification of herpes simplex virus tumor
    associated antigen from human kidney carcinoma, Cancer 46:1594
    (1980).

30. H. Reznick-Schuller, Carcinogenic effect of diethylstilbestrol
    in male Syrian golden hamsters and European hamsters, J. Nat.
    Cancer Inst. 62:1083 (1979).

31. M.C. Rivière, I. Chouroulinkov and M. Guerin, Action inhibante
    de la désoxycorticosterone sur la production de tumeurs rénales
    chez le hamster mâle traité par un oestrogen, C.R. Soc. Biol.
    154:1415 (1960).

32. H.J.G. Bloom, C.E. Dukes and B.C.V. Mitchley, Hormone-dependent
    tumours of the kidney: I. The oestrogen-induced renal tumour
    of the Syrian hamster. Hormone treatment and possible relation-
    ship to carcinoma of the kidney in man, Brit. J. Cancer 17:611
    (1963).

33. G. Concolino, A. Marocchi, C. Conti, R. Tenaglia, F. di
    Silverio and U. Bracci, Human renal carcinoma as a hormone-
    dependent tumour, Cancer Res. 38:4340 (1978).

34. F. di Fronzo, Estrogen receptors in renal carcinoma, Eur.
    Urol. 6:307 (1980).

35. M. Pignalosa and M. Fernandez, "Tumori del Rene", L. Capelli,
    Bologna (1938) p 37.

36. O. Bantley and G.T. Hultquist, Spontaneous regression of hyper-
    nephromas, Acta Pathol. Microbiol. Scand. 27:448 (1950).

37. W.K. Kerr, M. Barkin, J.A.D. Todd and Z. Menczyk, Hypernephroma
    associated with elevated levels of bladder carcinogens in the
    urine: case report, Brit. J. Urol. 35:263 (1963).

38. G. Reznick, J.M. Ward, J.F. Hardisty and R. Russfield, Renal carcinogenic and nephrotoxic effects of the flame retardant Tris (2,2 -dibromopropyl) phosphate in F344 rats and (C57BL/ (6N x C3H/HeN) F₁ mice, J. Nat. Cancer Inst. 63:205 (1979).

39. S.S. Sternberg, F.S. Philips and A.P. Cronic, Renal tumors and other lesions in rats following a single intravenous injection of daunomycin, Cancer Res. 32:1029 (1972).

40. L. Kilham, R.J. Low, S.F. Conti and F.D. Dallenbach, Intra-nuclear inclusions and neoplasms in the kidneys of wild rats, J. Nat. Cancer Inst. 29:863 (1962).

41. W. Gusek, Die Ultrastruktur Cycasin induzienter Nierenadenome, Virchows Arch. Abt. A. Pathol. 365:221 (1975).

42. D. Poggiolini, ed., Cloroformio - Bollettino d'informazione sui farmaci, Ministero della Sanita 4 (11):5 (1980).

43. R. de Vere White, A spontaneously arising renal cancer in the rat. A model for drug sensitivity studies, in: "Cancer of the Prostate and Kidney," P.H. Smith and M. Pavone-Macaluso, eds., Plenum Press, London and New York (1982).

RENAL CANCER: IN VITRO MODELS AND ANIMAL TUMORS

F. H. Schröder, M. G. Weissglas and K. H. Kurth

Erasmus University
Rotterdam
The Netherlands

Model systems for human tumors are necessary tools of basic and clinically related research that can not be carried out in humans. It is desirable that these models reflect the properties of the human tumor as closely as possible. Before assuming that results obtained with a tumor model are relevant to the management of patients, a model system has to be characterized, and the similarity of the model with the human situation has to be firmly established. In the case of human renal carcinoma (RC) research with tumor models could be oriented in the directions indicated in this diagram:

Renal Carcinoma

Tumor Models

Characterization ——————————— Therapeutic Studies

Basic Research

Prior to considering treatment studies, characterization is an obligatory step. There should be correlation with the basic research that can be conducted with established models.

ANIMAL MODELS

Review of the literature reveals a large number of available animal tumor models and surprisingly little work that has been done with relation to human RC.

Spontaneous tumors occur in rats, mice and in the Syrian golden hamster (1,2,3,4). Kidney tumors with great morphological similarity to RC can be induced in Syrian golden hamsters by prolonged estrogen treatment (5). This tumor has been shown also to depend on progesterone, androgens and glucocorticoids in a complex manner (6).

Virally induced tumors occur in the frog rana pipiens (7) and have also been described in hamsters, mice, rats and chicken.

Chemically induced kidney tumors have frequently been found in chemical carcinogenesis studies in various animals. They usually occur together with other malignant tumors which determine the prognosis of the laboratory animals. The renal tumors are a by-product found at autopsy. Two rat tumor lines induced by mono- and diaminobiphenyl compounds (MK1 and MK3) have been well characterized and have proved to be useful for chemotherapy studies (8,9). This subject has recently been reviewed by Sufrin (10).

Human tumor transplants in animals. Heterotransplantation of human RC tissue has occasionally been possible. Katsuoka described five transplantable lines in 'nude' mice. He attempted transplantation of 24 different tumors, a success rate of about 20% (11). The tumor line NC 65 has, together with a more recent line, been isolated in our own laboratory (12). The results obtained with the NC 65 line which has also resulted in two cell culture lines will be described in greater detail. Recently Day et al. (13) mentioned the use of two new RC lines in nude mice on which chemotherapy experiments were performed. The transplantation of the RC cell lines CAKI 1 and 1072 F into the cheek-pouch of the hamster, an immunologically privileged site, has been accomplished and used for the study of cholesterol metabolism by Clayman (14).

Selected Results

Animal tumors. The Syrian golden hamster RC has been subject to a large number of publications which were recently reviewed by Sufrin (10). This tumor, which has great morphological similarity to human RC can be induced in male hamsters by the application of natural or synthetic estrogens in 9-12 months. The same techniques fail to induce RC in intact female animals. However, if the females are pre-treated by androgens immediately after birth, if the estrogen treatment is initiated in pre-puberal animals or after castration, RC will also develop in females exposed to estrogen. The agent that protects intact female animals from getting the tumor has been identified as being progesterone. Simultaneous application of progesterone with estrogen in intact males or castrated females prevents tumor induction. Also testosterone, deoxycorticosterone, bromoergocryptine 20-methylcholanthrene and nafoxidine prevent tumor induction if concurrently administered with an estrogenic hormone. Cortisone enhances tumor induction, prolactin has no effect. The induced RC

requires estrogen for its maintenance. The tumors spread and infiltrate locally, rarely metastasize but eventually kill the animals.

Estrogen induced hamster RC shows strong morphological and biochemical similarities with human RC. The possibility of progesterone
dependence of human RC has been deduced from this model. Unfortunately, the initial enthusiasm for gestagenic treatment of RC has been
shown to be unjustified. Only an occasional patient responds to this
treatment and it must be concluded that endocrinologically the
similarities between estrogen induced hamster RC and human RC are
limited. Review of the literature has not revealed any application of
chemotherapy to this model system.

A large volume of work has been carried out to characterize the
two chemically induced rat RC lines MK1 and MK3 biochemically,
morphologically and genetically. Furthermore biochemical parameters
such as enzymes of glucose, pyrimidine and purine metabolism have
been studied in these slow growing, well differentiated adenocarcinomas and have been compared to the same parameters in normal human
and rat kidney and to human RC.

The pertinent findings have been recently reviewed by Weber (9).
The studies show convincing similarities between the MK1 and MK3
transplantable lines and human RC. The findings obtained led Weber
and his research group to the conclusion that "the reprogramming of
gene expression manifested in the enzymatic imbalance in human RC in
a large extent was similar to that observed in the chemically induced
rat kidney carcinomas". The strongest linkage between renal neoplasia
and enzymatic changes was found for the increased activities of
pyruvate kinase, uracil phosphoribosyl transferase, IMP dehydrogenase
and AMP deaminase. A number of enzyme ratios were found to be
increased and some enzymes of glucose metabolism were decreased in
activity.   The strategy of this research lies in identifying
"Key enzyme systems" which are essential for DNA replication and
which can not be replaced by salvage pathways. Such systems can then
be used as targets for chemotherapy which can be specifically
designed. This highly sophisticated approach could make clinical
research for chemotherapy more efficient and cut down on the need for
clinical experimentation if it proves successful.

In 1973 Murphy and Hrushesky (15) described a tumor line which
was derived from a spontaneous, transplantable RC of a BALB/c Cr
mouse. The tumor metastasizes and grows fastest when transplanted
under the renal capsule. Presence of the tumor leads to an increase
of the hematocrit by secretion of "erythrocyte stimulating factor".
The tumor is fast growing and kills all animals. Its growth is
enhanced by exogenous testosterone and DES but it is unaffected by
gestagens. This model has recently been used by Sufrin in chemotherapy studies and serves presently as a model for immunotherapy in
the hands of Pontes (16). CCNU, BCNU and adriamycin were active

agents; cytosine arabinoside, bleomycin and cyclophosphamide showed little activity.

Soloway and Myers (17) studied the effect of hormones in another mouse tumor line (BALB/c/cf/cd) named MKT-Cd1. They found suppression of growth by estrogen and testosterone.

White and Oson (18) characterized and used for chemotherapy experiments a spontaneous RC tumor line growing in Wistar Lewis rats. The tumor resembles human RC morphologically, it metastasizes and kills the animals. Preliminary chemotherapy studies were carried out.

Human RC in "Nude mice". In a recent review of this subject (19) only 11 human RC lines were found in the literature. It seems that with the techniques used at this time a take rate of 20% in human RC is the maximum that can be expected. Only one of these lines has been characterized to some extent and it will therefore serve as an example.

The transplantable tumor line NC65 was initiated in 1976 from a moderately differentiated RC and from a hilar lymph node metastasis (20). The tumor has also given origin to two permanent cell culture lines which bear the same name. The animal tumor will readily grow in culture but culture lines cannot be transplanted successfully back into the mice. Morphologically the tumor can easily be recognized as RC. It consists of clear and granular cells growing in trabecular fashion. The speed of growth and the morphological appearance have remained remarkably stable over the years. The doubling time varies between four and six days. The tumor has been characterized biochemically and genetically (21,22). It was proven by chromosone analysis that the tumor derives its stroma from the mouse. The model shows very strong similarity with human RC and is presently used for chemotherapy studies.

CELL-CULTURE

A large number of normal animal kidney cell lines are available and have been recently reviewed (19). Also, at least 10 cell lines have been isolated from human RC and have at least been partially characterized (19). Very little has been done to establish their possible usefulness as models for RC. Some of these lines are transplantable into 'nude' mice.

Organ cultures and short term cell cultures of RC can be established with a good chance of success; however very little work has been done in this field. Atkins (23) has shown in organ cultures that human RC tissue remains functionally active and produces prostaglandin E_2 leading to bone resorption in co-cultivated mouse calvaria.

RC cells may be clonogenic in soft agar (24). Also micro-transplantation under the renal capsule is applicable to trans-plantable lines and perhaps to fresh tissue (25). These techniques may prove to be useful for therapy studies; preliminary results will be reviewed.

Proper attempts to characterize these models have been carried out only in very few instances. Many potential markers are available in human RC and need to be exploited. The development of new markers is one of the important aspects of this research.

Selected Results

At least 12 cell lines have been isolated from human RC. Few attempts to characterize cell lines have been made. As already mentioned, a cell line also resulted from the tumor which gave origin to the transplantable line NC 65.

This cell line was initiated from tissue of the primary tumor; attempts to grow cells from hilar metastases were unsuccessful. Within the cell population marked morphological differences were seen and in the 25th passage cloning was undertaken which resulted in one line consisting of round cells called NC 65 R and another consisting of spindle cells called NC 65 SP. Another line, NC 65 V, could be initiated from the nude mouse line which was originally grown from the hilar metastases. This line consisted only of granular cells and the cell culture line NC 65 V only of round cells. All three lines were characterized genetically. They were shown to possess a human karyotype, at least three common marker chromosomes being identified. These studies suggest that the NC 65 R and V cells may be identical with granular cells and that the NC 65 SP cells are derived from the clear cells of the tumor. Confirmation by re-transplantation has not yet been obtainable.

Long term cell lines are ideal models for the study of in vitro killing conditions by cytostatic drugs. Lines have been used to set up such studies which can then be used for freshly grown cells from individual tumors.

Short term cultures from human RC can be established with a good chance of success. Such cultures have been shown to carry on the abnormal pattern of lipid metabolism which is typical for human RC (26). Short term culture has been widely used in immunological studies (19). Some renal carcinomas have been shown to be clonogenic in soft agar (24) and this property is now widely exploited for in vitro chemotherapy studies.

CLINICAL APPLICATIONS

As mentioned above animal and in vitro models have been successfully used to identify endocrine properties of RC. Marker substances such as prostaglandins, parathormone and other peptide hormones have been identified. Human cell lines and transplantable tumors should be especially suitable material for the search for marker substances. Such research is presently conducted in some laboratories at a low scale and should be encouraged.

The endocrine and immunological properties of human RC are still unclear. Well documented evidence suggests that such properties can be used at least in some instances for controlling growth in patients with metastatic disease. Animal and culture models should be suitable to investigate this important field in a more conclusive way with the goal of identifying tumor and host factors which can be manipulated for controlling growth in patients.

Chemotherapy testing has become a vast field of research. Some laboratories feel that the suitability of available techniques should be further documented, whilst others have immediately applied experimental results to patient management to try to correlate these results retrospectively to patient response. In the U.S. soft agar cloning assays have already become commercially available.

Four testing systems are presently used experimentally:

1. Soft agar clonogenic assay (23,26).
2. ^{3}H uridine incorporation assay (27).
3. Measurement of subcutaneous nude mouse transplants.
4. Microtransplantation under the renal capsule of nude mice (24).

Space does not permit a detailed review of the reported results. In summarizing the available information it can be stated that up to now no effective single agent has been identified. Sarosdy et al. (28) feel that individual tumors will require individual treatment and that RC is less sensitive to commonly used drugs than other solid tumors. This observation made with the soft agar assay is confirmed by Day et al. (13). Extensive drug resistance has also been reported by Lieber (29).

Belitsky et al (30) linked Adriamycin to an antirenal carcinoma antibody and were able to target the drug into the renal carcinoma of BALB/c mice. They were able to inhibit tumor growth more effectively than by using the non-conjugated drug. This technique could be a major break-through if it proves to be applicable to human RC.

REFERENCES

1. G.W. McCoy, A Preilimary Report on Tumors Found in Wild Rats,
    J. Med. Res. 21:285 (1909).
2. R. Eker, Familial Renal Adenocarcinoma in Wistar Rats, Acta
    Pathol.Microbiol.Scand. 34:554 (1954).
3. H.Z. Ratcliffe, Spontaneous Tumors in Two Colonies of Rats of
    the Wiston Institute of Anatomy and Biology, Am.J. Pathol. 16:
    237 (1940).
4. J.G. Fortner, A.G. Mahy, and R.S. Cotron, Transplantable Tumors
    of the Syrian Golden Hamster, Part II: Tumors of the Hemato-
    poietic Tissues, Genitourinary Organs, Mammary Glands and
    Sarcomas. CS 199, Cancer Res. 21:199 (1961).
5. V.S. Matthews, H. Kirkman, and R.L. Bacon, Kidney Damage in the
    Golden Hamster Following Chronic Administration of Diethyl-
    stilbestrol and sesame oil, Proc. Soc. Exp. Biol. Med. 66:195
    (1947).
6. E.S. Horning, Observations on Hormone-Dependent Renal Tumours
    in the Golden Hamster, Brit. J. Cancer 10:678 (1956).
7. B. Lucké, A Neoplastic Disease of the Kidney of the Frog Rana
    Pipiens, Amer. J. Cancer 20:352 (1934).
8. H.P. Morris, B.C. Wagner, and D.R. Meranze, Transplantable
    Adenocarcinomas of the Rat Kidney Possessing Different Growth
    Rates, Cancer Res. 30:1362 (1970).
9. G. Weber, Enzymatic Programs of Human Renal Adenocarcinoma,
    in:"Renal Adenocarcinoma," G. Sufrin and S.E. Beckley, eds.,
    UICC technical Report Series, Geneva (1980), p.44.
10. G. Sufrin, Spontaneous, Hormonal and Chemically Induced
    Animal Models of Renal Adenocarcinoma, in:"Renal Adenocarcinoma,"
    G. Sufrin and S.A. Beckley, eds., UICC Technical Report Series,
    Geneva Vol. 49:2 (1980).
11. Y. Katsuoka, S. Baba, M. Hata, and H. Zaki, Transplantation of
    Human Renal Cell Carcinoma to the Nude Mice: As an Intermediate
    of in vivo and in vitro Studies, J. Urol. 115:373 (1976).
12. W. Höhn and F.H. Schröder, Renal Cell Carcinoma. Two New Cell
    Lines and a Serially Transplantable Nude Mouse Tumor (NC 65),
    Invest. Urol. 16:106 (1978).
13. J.W. Day and D.F. Paulson, In vivo Confirmation of in vitro
    Chemotherapy Testing. Abstract, American Urological
    Association, No. 134 (1980).
14. R.V. Clayman, M. Dempsey, and R. Gonzalez, Cholesterol
    Accumulation in Renal Cell Carcinoma: A clinical Assessment.
    Abstract, American Urological Association, No. 137 (1980).
15. G.P. Murphy and W.J. Hrushesky, A Murine Renal Cell Carcinoma,
    J. Natl. Cancer Inst. 50:1013 (1973).
16. J.E. Pontes, M Goldrosen, and G.P. Murphy, Immunological
    Response to Tumor Ischemia in a Murine Renal Cell Carcinoma,
    Abstracts, American Urological Association, No. 420 (1981).
17. M.S. Soloway and G.H. Myers, The Effect of Hormonal Therapy on
    a Transplantable Renal Cortical Adenocarcinoma in Syngeneic

Mice, J. Urol. 109:356 (1973).

18. R.V. White and C.A. Olsson, Renal Adenocarcinoma in the Rat, Invest. Urol. 17:405 (1980).

19. F.H. Schröder and K. Oishi, Renal Adenocarcinoma-Immuno-Deficient Systems, in:"Renal Adenocarcinoma," G. Sufrin and S.A. Beckley, eds., UICC Technical Report Series, Geneva Vol. 49:114 (1980)

20. G. Popelier, R. Geers, G. Verdonck, F.H. Schröder, and W. Höhn, The Biochemical Profile of the Tissue of a Human Renal Cell Xenograft on the Nude Mouse (NC 65) Compared to the Profile of Human Renal Cortex (RCX) and Renal Cell Carcinoma (RCC), Urol. Res. 8:233, No. 4 (1980)

21. A Hagemeyer, W Höhn, and E.M.E. Smit, Cytogenetic Analysis of Human Renal Cell Carcinoma Cell Lines of Common Origin. (NC 65)., Cancer Res. 39:4462 (1979).

22. D. Atkins, K.J. Ibbotson, K. Hillier, N.H. Hunt, J.C. Hammonds, and T.J. Martin, Secretion of Prostaglandins as Bone-resorbing Agents by Renal Cortical Carcinoma in Culture, Brit.J. Cancer 36:601 (1977).

23. M.M. Lieber and J.S. Kovach, Drug Sensitivity Testing in vitro with a Soft Agar Stem Cell Colony Assay. Abstracts, American Urological Association, No. 133 (1980).

24. H.E. Bogden, A Rapid Screening Method for Testing Chemothera-peutic agents against Human Tumor Xenografts, in:"Symposium on the use of Athymic "Nude" Mice in Cancer Research," D.H. Houckens and A.A. Ojevera, eds., New York (1978).

25. R. Gonzalez and M.E. Dempsey, Sterol Synthesis in Cultured Human Renal Cell Cancer, J. Urol. 117:708 (1977).

26. A.W. Hamburger and S.E. Salmon, Primary Bio Assay of Human Tumor Stem Cells, Science 197:461 (1977).

27. S. Shrivastav and D.F. Paulson, In Vitro Chemotherapy Testing of Transitional Cell Carcinoma, Invest. Urol. 17:395 (1978).

28. M.F. Sarosdy, D.L. Lamm, H.M. Radwin and D.D. von Hoff, In vitro Clonal Assay and Chemosensitivity Testing of Human Urologic Malignancies. Abstract, American Urological Association, No.418 (1981).

29. M.M. Lieber and J.S. Kovach, Soft Agar Clonogenic Assay for Primary Human Renal Carcinoma: In vitro Chemotherapeutic Drug Sensitivity Testing. Abstract, Americal Urological Association, No. 531 (1981).

30. P. Belitsky, T. Ghose, K. Vaughan, H. Nolido, and T. van Zoost, Inhibition of a Mouse Renal Carcinoma with Adriamycin Linked Anti-renal Carcinoma Antibody. Abstracts, American Urological Association, No. 421 (1981).

THE EVALUATION OF CHEMOTHERAPY IN A MURINE RENAL ADENOCARCINOMA

R. deVere White,[1] C.A. Olsson,[1] R. Babyian[2]

1. College of Physician & Surgeons
   New York, U.S.A.

2. Boston University Medical Center
   Boston, Massachusetts, U.S.A.

A spontaneously arising renal adenocarcinoma in a male Wistar-Lewis rat has been used over the past three years as a testing system for various chemotherapeutic agents, used alone or in combination. We have also utilized this model in an effort to evaluate the ability of cytoreductive surgery to render chemotherapy more effective. Finally, we have looked at the sensitivity of this tumor to hyperthermia delivered alone or in combination with cyclophosphamide.

DEVELOPMENT OF TUMOR MODEL

We have previously described in detail the method by which a nodule and metastatic model were produced (1) and will only outline them here in brief.

Nodule Model

0.06 to 0.08 grams of the spontaneously arising renal adenocarcinoma is taken from a single donor and placed subcutaneously in the flank of a syngeneic rat anesthetized with ether. The incision is closed with a single clip. Three weeks later 90% of animals will have palpable tumors.

Metastatic Model

Male Wistar-Lewis rats, anesthetized with ether, underwent splenectomy after which 0.06 to 0.08 grams of tumor, taken from a single donor animal, was placed intra-peritoneally. The peritoneum and skin were closed with clips and treatment began five weeks later at which time 90% of animals had metastatic intraperitoneal tumor growing.

SINGLE AGENT STUDIES

Nodule Model

In order to test the effectiveness of single agents against this tumor system, the tumor was implanted in the flank of the rat and allowed to grow for a week. The animals were then treated with intraperitoneal (IP) injections of various agents on weeks one, two and three. On week four the animals were sacrificed, the tumor removed and the wet tumor weight recorded. The effectiveness of the chemotherapy was measured by the reduction in the number of animals bearing tumor at this time compared with their own controls and in the reduction of the tumor weight as compared to its own controls. The results can be divided into the agents that were or were not effective in the dosages and time sequence utilized. Ineffective agents included 5-fluorouracil, cis-platinum, bleomycin, hydroxyurea, streptozotocin, neocarzinostatin, chlorzotocin, carminomycin and methyl-GAG. Maytansine did not reduce the number of tumors present, but did significantly reduce the weight of the tumor present in comparison to its own control. The agents which appeared effective either by reducing tumor weight or by reducing the amount of tumor surviving at the time of sacrifice were cytoxan, adriamycin, vinblastine and vindesine. By far the most effective agents, both reaching statistical significance, were cytoxan and vindesine.

Metastatic Model

The obvious limitations of a nodule model is that it does not metastasise and therefore does not in any way reproduce the situation in humans. For this reason, a metastatic model was utilized to further evaluate the efficacy of the agents which had proven effectiveness in the nodule model, these agents being used either alone or in combination. In the drug regimens utilized, the tumor was allowed to grow for five weeks post implantation and then treated for three weeks with intraperitoneal injections. The animals were sacrificed the following week, which in most cases was the ninth week following implantation. The effectiveness of the single agent or combination therapy was judged by assessing the number of animals that had tumor in comparison to their own control or by the wet weight of the tumor present. This was gauged by the removal of all visible tumor, obtaining a wet weight and comparing this to the wet weight of the removed tumor in that animal's own control. Agents employed were: cytoxan alone, vindesine alone, cytoxan and cis-platinum, cytoxan and vinblastine, cytoxan and adriamycin, and cytoxan, adriamycin and vinblastine. The problem with all the combinations was that 80 - 100% of the animals had persistent tumor present at the time of sacrifice and those combinations which produced any marked decrease in tumor weight had an unacceptably high animal mortality.

Following this vindesine, cytoxan and vindesine, cytoxan, vindesine and cis-platinum were tried in various combinations. By far the most effective combination tested was vindesine 0.5 mg/kg on weeks five and seven, with cis-platinum 5 mg/kg and cytoxan 40 mg/kg on week six and eight, the animals being sacrificed on week nine. Of the forty rats so treated, 51% had no evidence of tumor at the time of sacrifice and in those in whom tumor was present, the weight ranged from 6.5 to 15 grams as compared to the control in which the weight of tumor ranged between 36 and 143 grams. The average reduction in tumor weight compared to its own control was 90% - the reduction in the incidence of tumor and in the tumor weight reaching significance.

The extrapolation of any results from animals to human is always fraught with danger and in renal cancer the ideal animal tumor model system should (a) arise spontaneously, (b) be histologically a pure adenocarcinoma, (c) have a predictable growth rate, (d) have the capacity to metastasize, (e) be hormonally independent and (f) respond to chemotherapeutic agents as does the disease in humans. This present model does have some of these characteristics. It arose spontaneously, is histologically a pure adenocarcinoma, and has a predictable growth rate. It does not metastasize from the flank but produces a metastatic disease model if placed intraperitoneally. The tumor was tested for its hormonal responsiveness and was found initially to be hormonally independent. Interestingly, in later generations its growth in females appears retarded although the tumor histologically has not changed. Regarding the tumor's response to chemotherapeutic agents, it has, like its human counterpart, remained resistent to most chemotherapeutic agents - cytoxan being the only exception. This tumor certainly appears more sensitive to this alkylating agent than its human counterpart.

THE EFFECT OF CYTOREDUCTIVE SURGERY ON
THE TUMOR'S RESPONSE TO CHEMOTHERAPY

In order to see if debulking would improve the effectiveness of vindesine (VDR), 22 male Wistar-Lewis rats were innoculated with tumor to produce both a flank and a metastatic tumor model. Seven weeks later the rats were divided into three groups, six designated as controls, eight receiving vindesine 0.5 mg/kg IP at week seven and week nine, and eight having cytoreductive surgery. In this last group the flank tumor was removed prior to a similar dose of vindesine IP at week seven and nine. At week ten all animals were sacrificed, the tumor removed and the wet weight recorded in grams. Values representing mean and standard error are shown in Table 1. The reduction in flank, IP and total tumor weight between the control and VDR animals was in cases significant ($p < 0.05$, < 0.25 and < 0.001

Table 1. Tumor Weight at 10 Weeks

	Flank Tumor Wt.	IP Tumor Wt.	Total Tumor Wt.
Control	44.83 ± 7.84	46.5 ± 12.45	91.33 ± 10.15
VDR	23.95 ± 6.52	14.21 ± 5.2	35.16 ± 5.87
VDR & Debulking		39.64 ± 8.67	39.64 ± 8.67

respectively). In contrast, in the debulked group, the IP tumor
weight was similar to that of controls and significantly larger than
the IP tumor weight in the VDR group, ($p < 0.025$). The IP tumor
weight in the debulked group was the same as the total weight (flank
+ IP tumor) in the vindesine group. Therefore in this, albeit small,
study debulking did not appear to statistically increase the effectiveness of the chemotherapeutic agent, in this case vindesine, against
the remaining intraperitoneal tumor. Certainly from this experiment
it could be suggested that surgery and/or anesthesia had nullified
the effectiveness of vindesine against IP tumor growth. Further
studies have been done and in none of these have we found that debulking in any way improved the effectiveness of vindesine.

SUSCEPTIBILITY OF TUMOR TO HYPERTHERMIA

These experiments were carried out on the flank nodule. The
tumor was allowed to grow to a diameter of $1\frac{1}{2}$ to 3 cm and was then
subjected to localized hyperthermia to a temperature of 43° for
twenty minutes at weekly intervals. The hyperthermia was delivered
via a focus ultrasound machine which was constructed by a Professor
Lele at the Massachusetts Institute of Technology. The heat was
confined strictly to the tumor nodule (2). Tumor size was measured
weekly by three perpendicular diameters with Vernier calipers. Tumor
sensitivity was assessed by differences in the tumor size between
the treated and control animals. In the ten animals treated, there
was a 41% reduction in tumor volume after one week; 43.3% reduction
after two weeks and 71.3% reduction after three weeks of hyperthermia.
The control animals uniformly showed progressive increase in their
tumor size.

The experiment was then repeated, but on this occasion with
four groups of animals, one group treated with hyperthermia, one
group treated with cyclophosphamide, one group treated with hyperthermia and cyclophosphamide and a control group. Though these
studies are still in a pilot stage, the combination of hyperthermia
40° for twenty minutes and cyclophosphamide (20 mg/kg IP weekly)
showed a greater decrease in tumor size than when the hyperthermia

or chemotherapy were used alone. Cytoxan alone produced a 40% decrease in tumor size as compared to the controls, hyperthermia alone a 47% reduction and cytoxan and hyperthermia 85% reduction.

REFERENCES

1. R. deVere White and C.A. Olsson, Renal adenocarcinoma in the Rat, Invest. Urol. 17: 204 (1980).
2. P.P. Lele, Induction of deep, local hyperthermia by ultrasound and electromagnetic fields, Radiat. Environ. Biophys. 17: 204 (1980).

Editorial Note (M.P.)

Dr. deVere White and his colleagues deserve to be congratulated on this very careful study. There is certainly a great need for studies of this type, in the hope of finding a reliable animal model for therapeutic research on renal cancer.

Unfortunately, as the authors rightly point out, there is a large gap to be filled between in vitro or animal studies and the clinical situation in man and attempts to extrapolate results from animals to humans are fraught with danger. This murine tumor is responsive to both cyclophosphamide and vindesine. Unfortunately, there is no evidence that this is also true for human renal cancer. Probably cyclophosphamide has not been sufficiently evaluated in man, but the few available results in small series do not indicate a significant activity. Vindesine is currently being evaluated by the EORTC Urological Group. It is too early to reach any conclusions but the preliminary results do not appear to be encouraging apart from an occasional response. The neurotoxicity is not negligible. The correspondence between response in this animal model and that obtained in humans seems to be imperfect.

EPIDEMIOLOGY OF RENAL TUMORS

C.R. Bouffioux

University of Liège
Liège
Belgium

INTRODUCTION

Many different tumors may arise within the kidney. Although the commonest are tumors of epithelial origin including adenoma (benign) and adenocarcinoma (also called hypernephroma or Grawitz' tumor) together with tumors of the renal pelvis (transitional cell, squamous or undifferentiated) one must not forget nephroblastoma, also called Wilms' tumor, and its variants. Less commonly benign and malignant mesenchymal tumors may be found. The benign include leiomyoma, leiomyolipoma, angiomyolipoma, hemangioma, juxta-glomerular tumor, lymphangioma, fibroma and the malignant, leiomyosarcoma, rhabdomyosarcoma, liposarcoma, angiosarcoma, fibroxanthosarcoma, oesteogenic sarcoma and hemoblastoses.

EPIDEMIOLOGY

A.   Benign mesenchymal tumors are rare. Most are detected incident-ally at autopsy and usually being too small to produce clinical symptoms during life. In some cases, they give hematuria or hyper-tension; they are more frequent in women than in men.

Malignant mesenchymal tumors are also rare. The leiomyosarcoma is that most frequently formed but less than 100 cases have been reported in the literature and with the exception of well-known association of angiomyolipomas with Bourneville's tuberous sclerosis, no data are available on the epidemiology of these tumors (1).

B.   Nephroblastoma or Wilms' tumor is usually discovered during infancy or childhood. It is a malignant embryonic tumor originating from metanephrogenic blastema. Although it represents 6% of all

503

malignant neoplasms in children below the age of 15 years, it is a rare tumor and its incidence is approximately one case per 150,000 children per year.   The incidence is the same in boys and in girls.

Ten per cent are discovered during the first year of life;   50% before the third year and 80% before the fifth year.   A few cases have been reported in adults (approximately 3%).   Nearly 5% of the cases are initially bilateral.

The constancy of incidence in every nation and race indicates that the tumor is not dependent on any kind of carcinogenic influence but that it results from a stable endogenous process.   Its association with various malformations or other tumors and familial incidence indicate the importance of genetic factors in the occurence of this type of tumor.

C.   Tumors of the renal pelvis are about three times less frequent than adenocarcinomas of the kidney.   They are histologically identical to tumors of the ureter or of the bladder and their epidemiologic and etiologic factors are also the same (2).   They have been extensively discussed.

D.   <u>Adenocarcinoma of the kidney</u>

Erroneously called "hypernephroma" as it was formerly considered to be derived from vestiges of ectopic adrenal tissue, renal cancer is now recognized to be derived from the epithelial cells of the proximal convoluted tubules.

In many epidemiological reports, renal cell carcinoma is grouped together with pelvic tumors, nephroblastoma and the more rare forms under the general definition of renal cancer, which makes a correct evaluation of the incidence of the disease rather difficult.

In the United States (3,4), cancer of the kidney is slightly more common among white males - the age standardized incidence rate being 8.6/100,000 as compared with 7.6/100,000 in the black male.

The incidence of white and black males is twice as high as in white and black females (4 and 3.8/100,000 respectively).

Table 1 gives the age-specific and age-standardized incidence rates (per 100,000 person-years) of renal cancer in the United States (4).

Figure 1 clearly shows that the incidence of cancer of the kidney in the United States (1969-71) is related to age in both sexes and races.   Extremely rare before 40 years, it reaches a plateau at about 75-80 years;   the incidence is then about 50 cases per 100,000 person-years in white males.

Table 1. Age-specific and age-standardized incidence
(per 100,000 person-years) of renal cancer
in the United States of America.

AGE	MALE		FEMALE	
	WHITE	BLACK	WHITE	BLACK
15	0.9	1.1	1.1	1.0
15-29	0.2	0.7	0.2	0.7
30-39	1.6	0.9	1.0	1.2
40-49	7.2	8.6	3.2	3.0
50-59	16.7	17.2	8.5	9.4
60-69	33.6	25.3	14.0	12.5
70-79	46.0	40.7	19.7	14.3
80-84	52.5	26.7	24.4	27.7
85+	53.5	17.3	22.3	5.5
All ages*	8.6	7.6	4.0	3.8

* Standardized to the 1970 U.S. standard population

In blacks, the incidence falls after this age but it is probable
that this decrease is due to failure of diagnosis in many and to the
fact that fewer black males survive beyond this age.

In Belgium, 451 cases of renal carcinoma were reported in 1975
but only 59 cases of pelvic (and ureteral) cancer (5). The incidence rate for renal cancer is 6.1/100,000 in males and 4.4/100,000
in females. If we exclude the tumours of the renal pelvis and
ureter, the incidence rate is 5.6/100,000 in men and 4/100,000 in
women. When compared with those in the United States the rates are
slightly higher for women and lower for men. The distribution of
the cases in the different regions (mainly industrial and urban or
rural) does not show any significant differences suggesting that
industrial carcinogens play no obvious role in the development of
renal cancer.

Table 2 illustrates the age-standardized incidence rate (cases
per 100,000 person-years) in several countries (6).

The incidence rates are higher in North America and South
America. The difference is similar to, but much less marked than
that seen in similar geographical areas in prostatic cancer. The
sex ratio varies from 1.3 to 2.4, but in every country, the incidence is higher among men.

Table 2.   Age-standardized incidence of renal cell cancer
by country (cases/100,000 person-years).

COUNTRY	MALE	FEMALE	SEX RATIO
DENMARK	7.2	5.1	1.4
USA (ALAMEDA COUNTY, CALIFORNIA)			
White	7.1	3.6	2.0
Black	6.0	2.5	2.4
FINLAND	6.3	3.9	1.6
BELGIUM	6.1	4.4	1.4
ENGLAND AND WALES	4.4	2.0	2.2
YUGOSLAVIA	3.5	1.8	1.9
ISRAEL			
Jews born in Israel	3.7	2.8	1.4
Jews born in Europe	7.2	4.3	1.7
JAPAN	1.5	1.2	1.3
HAWAII (Japanese)	4.0	1.5	2.6

The difference observed between people of different origins but
living in the same country (e.g. Jews in Israel) or people of the
same origin but living in different countries (e.g. Japanese in Japan
and in Hawaii), suggest that genetic and environmental factors probably play a part in the occurence of this disease.

Finally, time trends of incidence and mortality rates show a
doubling among men from the mid-1930's to the mid-1950's.   Thereafter, there has been little change, and it is very probable that

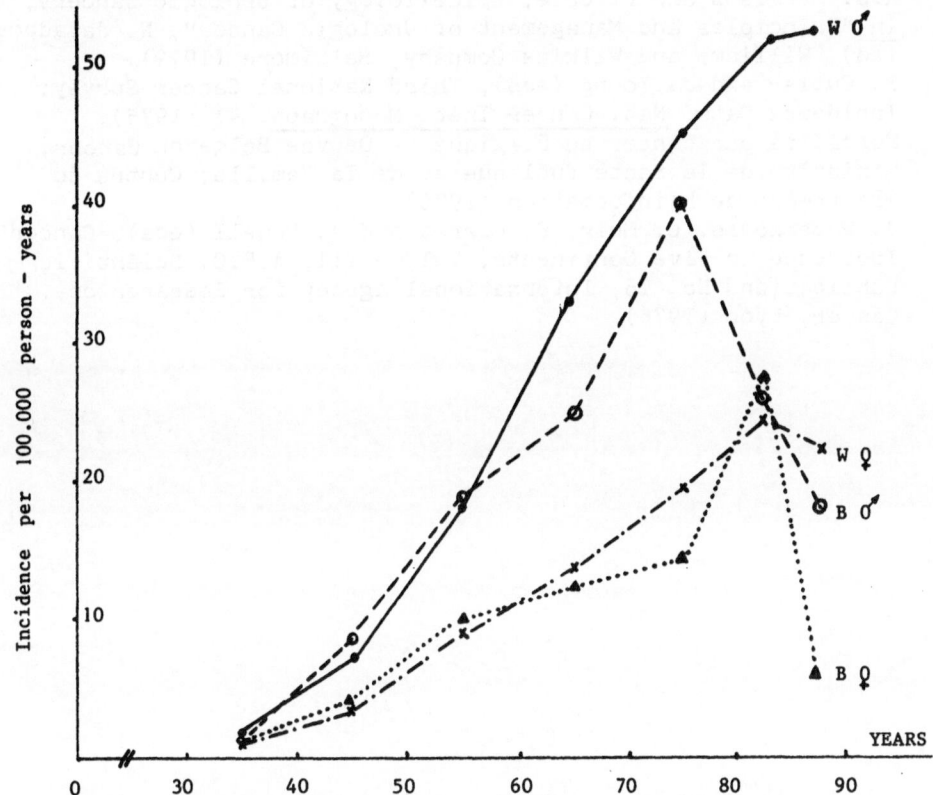

Fig. 1.   Incidence of cancer of the kidney in the United
           States of America (1969-71) by age, sex and race.
           (B = black;   W = white).

this increase is fictitious and related to improvements in the
diagnostic methods.

REFERENCES

1.   L. Leder, H. Richter and C. Stambolis, Pathology of Renal and
      Adrenal Neoplasm, in "Renal and Adrenal Tumors", E. Löhr (ed),
      Springer-Verlag, Berlin (1979).
2.   L. Wahlqvist, Chemical Carcinogens - A Review and Personal
      Observations with Special Reference to the Role of Tobacco and
      Phenacetin in the Production of Urothelial Tumours, in "Bladder
      Tumors and Other Topics in Urological Oncology", M. Pavone-
      Macaluso, P.H. Smith and F. Edsmyr (eds), Plenum Press, New
      York (1980).

3.   A.S. Morrison and P. Cole, Epidemiology of Urologic Cancers,
     in "Principles and Management of Urologic Cancer", N. Javadpour
     (ed), Williams and Wilkins Company, Baltimore (1979).
4.   S. Cutler and J. Young (eds), Third National Cancer Survey:
     Incidence Data, Nat. Cancer Inst. Monograph. 41 (1975).
5.   Morbidité par cancer en Belgique. Oeuvre Belge du Cancer,
     Ministère de la Santé Publique et de la Famille, Centre du
     Traitement de L'information (1975).
6.   J. Waterhouse, C. Muir, P. Correa and J. Powell (eds), Cancer
     Incidence in Five Continents, Volume III, A.R.C. Scientific
     Publications No. 15, International Agency for Research on
     Cancer, Lyon (1976).

UNRECOGNIZED RENAL CELL CARCINOMA

S. Hellsten, T. Berge, L. Wehlin

Malmö General Hospital
Malmö
Sweden

In a series of 16,294 autopsies, 350 cases of renal cell carcinoma were found. Of these tumours 235, i.e. two-thirds, were unrecognized during the patients' lifetime. Metastatic spread was revealed in 56 patients with unrecognized renal cell carcinoma (24%) and was the main cause of death in 49 patients (21%).

The number of metastasizing tumours increased significantly with the size of the primary tumour. Local aggressiveness of the primary tumour was also more common in large tumours but was much more closely correlated to metastatic spread than to size. Invasion of the renal vein by tumour was significantly more common in metastasizing tumours than in non-metastasizing lesions.

The present study confirms that an analysis of local aggressiveness of the primary renal tumour is of prognostic value and might be useful in defining the group of patients who may benefit from adjuvant treatment such as radiation therapy, chemotherapy and immunotherapy.

Editorial Note (P.H.S.)

If further autopsy studies in other parts of the world prove that renal cell cancer is three times as common as the clinical incidence suggests, one can justifiably argue both for non treatment in the elderly patient, as suggested by Denis at this meeting (especially if the diagnosis is made by chance in a patient free from symptoms) and also for an effective screening programme as suggested by Blandy in this volume, since the tumour is the cause of death in 21% of the affected patients.

THE USE OF ELECTRON-MICROSCOPY IN THE CONTROVERSY OF RENAL ADENOMA VERSUS CARCINOMA

M. Tannenbaum and S. Tannenbaum

Columbia-Presbyterian Medical Center
New York
N.Y., U.S.A.

The debate as to whether or not renal adenomas are benign or malignant tumors is of great academic and epidemiological importance. Within Bennington and Beckwith's Tumor Fascicle on Kidney, Renal Pelvis, and Ureter (1), it is stated (and these authors concur) that the so-called renal adenomas are more frequent than renal adenocarcinomas. They believe, as we do, that renal adenoma is a small carcinoma and that whatever the etiological agents, it is through this evolutionary stage that renal adenocarcinomas develop. Unfortunately, in terms of time sequence, the surgical pathologists see these tumors as slow-growing. One may expect that with increased longevity in our growing geriatric age group, the incidence of clinically apparent renal adenocarcinomas will increase and the earlier diagnosis of these small cortical glandular tumors will become more important. Bennington and Beckwith (1) have gathered an impressive array of facts that demonstrate very clearly the similarity between the so-called renal adenomas and the renal adenocarcinomas, including the following:-

1.   Both renal adenomas and adenocarcinomas arise from cells of the proximal convoluted tubule. This has been demonstrated both immunologically and ultrastructurally by several groups of workers (2,3).
2.   There are no light histology, histochemistry, or electron microscopic features that distinguish an adenoma from a clear cut similar cell type carcinoma of the kidney either in the human or in experimental animals.
3.   Adenomas occur more frequently in a kidney containing a renal adenocarcinoma (4).
4.   Adenoma and adenocarcinoma occur in the same age group and Bennington and Beckwith state that they are rarely found before the age of 30. They also show a marked predisposition for the human male (2-4:1).

5.   Both renal adenomas and adenocarcinomas occur with the same increased frequency among tobacco users. Bennington and Laubscher (5)
have done extensive epidemiological research concerning this issue.
6.   There is a direct relationship between tumor size and frequency
of metastases considering all the renal cortical glandular tumors (6).

      Bennington and Kradjian (7) also present convincing evidence that
there are no correlative/morphological criteria that can distinguish
renal adenomas from the small cortical glandular tumors that manifest
their aggressiveness by perforating their capsule. They have shown
that a small renal adenoma (< 1.5 cm) demonstrates perforation of the
tumor capsule at several points. This is one of the important criteria for the diagnosis of cancer, i.e. the ability to break out of
tissue architecture. They believe that the so-called adenoma is
actually a small renal adenocarcinoma which, in many instances, has
not yet metastasized. They also point out that the small renal cortical glandular tumors that are < 3.0 cm in greatest diameter are
almost invariably an incidental finding at autopsy so that their
classification is of no clinical consequence to the patient. However,
when such a tumor is found at surgery, the diagnostic terminology
becomes more important. If one gives a diagnosis of renal adenoma,
it signifies a benign tumor, but it occasionally metastasises. On
the other hand, a diagnosis of renal adenocarcinoma unlikely to
metastasise, portends lifelong overtones of cancer for the patient
and his family. When they are found in surgery, these authors, like
Bennington and Beckwith (2) feel that it is best to diagnose such
small cortical glandular neoplasms of the kidney as renal adenocarcinomas. It is imperative for all concerned that the tumor diameter size also be reported to make the urologisit or the oncologist
aware that their patient's tumor may not have reached the minimal
invasive size. Bennington and Beckwith (1) point out that enough
sections should be taken to determine whether this "renal adenoma"
is truly invasive into the surrounding parenchyma or through its
tumor capsule. Such tumors offer an excellent prognosis and a comment
may also be reported in the diagnosis but with the stipulation that
tumors of this size may occasionally metastasize. Unfortunately,
one cannot predict histologically which will behave in this way but
the mention of the possibility that metastases might occur allows
the urologist to plan careful follow up for the patient.

      Briefly, we would like to discuss the ultrastructural pathology
of human renal tumors. For several years, there have been extensive
review articles and original research on the ultrastructural pathology
of renal neoplasms (8). The clear and granular cell tumors are the
predominant cell types in most renal carcinomas. They are found
either in the tubular or papillary form. We, like several other
investigators, feel that renal carcinomas do arise from the renal
tubular epithelium and prefer the term "renal cell carcinoma" to be
appended to the surgical pathology reports. Many observations of
light histology patterns support the renal tubular epithelial origin

of renal cell carcinomas. These patterns may mimic normal tubular
structures or they may exhibit transitions from normal tubules to
those arranged in a papillary or cord-like fashion. There is even
further support for this concept of origin. Electron microscopic
studies demonstrate many similarities between renal carcinoma cells
and the normal epithelial cells of the proximal convoluted tubule (8).

Before discussing the ultrastructural pathology of the granular
cell tumors that are found both in renal cell carcinomas and in adenomas, a brief resumé of the ultrastructure of the normal renal tubules seems warranted. The appearance of the different parts of the
tubules in man does not differ significantly from that found in
animals. The main distinguishing features of the proximal convoluted
tubules of the kidney are:-

1.   The presence of a brush-border containing many tightly packed
microvilli which contain filaments.
2.   Invaginations of the apical plasmic membrane provided with membrane coatings.
3.   The occurrence of vesicles or vacuoles with a characteristic
structure in the apical cytoplasm.
4.   An abundance of mitochondria.
5.   Deep invagination of the basal plasma membrane creating slender
cytoplasmic compartments.

Cells of the distal tubules do not demonstrate any of these
apical cytoplasmic specialties. However, they contain abundant mitochondria and show deep basal plasma membrane invaginations. In the
other parts of the tubular system, the cells are less specialized and
show a similar structure of the plasma membrane as well as of the
cytoplasm.

When the granular cell tumors of either the adenoma or carcinoma
are examined, they are found to contain mitochondria. Occasional
granules interposed between these organelles and interpreted as glycogen are also seen in the clear cell carcinomas. These granules are
PAS-positive. In the cytoplasm of many of these tumor cells, there
is marked infolding of the nuclear membrane with deep invaginations
of the cytoplasm into these structures. The cytoplasm of many of
these tumors contains intracytoplasmic well differentiated, brush-
border like structures similar to those previously mentioned. In
several instances where serial sectioning of the same block is performed, these intracytoplasmic brush-border lumens do not communicate
with the exterior of the cell. At this institution, this attempt at
brush-border formation seems to be more prevalent within the granular
cell tumors than in the clear cell carcinomas of the kidney. These
cells, i.e. the granular cells found both within the granular cell
adenomas and granular cell carcinomas of the kidney are identical in
morphology. We and Bennington (personal communication) have likened
these granular cells to those of the proximal convoluted tubules of
the normal kidney because of the similarities that would be found:-

1.   Microvilli and brush-border elements.
2.   Membrane associated vesicles which might be involved in pino-
     cytosis.
3.   Membrane coatings.
4.   Basal infoldings of the plasma membrane.
5.   Intercellular junctions and most important of all
6.   Abundant mitochondria.

     As now seems to be the prevalent feeling, there is a continuum
between adenomas of the granular cell type and carcinomas of the
kidney. As a result, more definitive epidemiological and ultrastructural analyses can be done in terms of time sequence studies of
various agents that might be considered important in renal cell carcinomas.

REFERENCES

1.   J.L. Bennington and J.C. Beckwith, "Atlas of Tumor Pathology:
     Tumors of the Kidney, Renal Pelvis, and Ureter," Armed Forces
     Institute of Pathology, Washington, D.C. (1975).
2.   E.R. Fisher and B. Horvat, Comparative ultrastructural study of
     so-called renal adenoma and carcinoma, J. Urol. 108: 382 (1972).
3.   A.C. Wallace and R.C. Nairn, Renal tubular antigens in kidney
     tumors, Cancer 29: 977 (1972).
4.   D.S. Cristol, J.R. McDonald, and J.L. Emmett, Renal adenomas in
     hypernephromatous kidneys: A study of their incidence, nature
     and relationship, J. Urol. 55: 18 (1946).
5.   J.L. Bennington and F.A. Laubscher, Epidemiologic studies on
     carcinoma of the kidney. I. Association of renal adenocarcinoma
     with smoking, Cancer. 21: 1069 (1968).
6.   E.T. Bell, "Renal Disease," Lea & Febiger, Philadelphia (1950).
7.   J.L. Bennington and R.M. Kradjian, "Renal Carcinoma,"
     W.B. Saunders Co., Philadelphia (1967).
8.   M. Tannenbaum, Ultrastructural pathology of human renal cell
     tumors, Pathol. Annual 6: 249 (1971).

RENAL ONCOCYTOMA

R.J. Macchia

Downstate Medical School
Brooklyn
New York, U.S.A.

An oncocytoma is a neoplasm composed <u>entirely</u> of oncocytes. Oncocytes are cells rich in mitochrondria but sparse in other organelles. Oncocytoma has been described in many organs. Interest in oncocytoma of the kidney was recently revived by Klein and Valensi (1). They proposed that renal oncocytoma be considered a proximal tubule adenoma with oncocytic features. The importance of renal oncocytoma is as follows.

These tumors are solid and frequently large, i.e., > 5 cm. Klein and Valensi proposed that they are essentially benign tumors. Their differentiation from renal carcinoma is then of more than academic interest. If oncocytoma is presently being confused with carcinoma, needless nephrectomies are being performed. Finally, are survival statistics for various modes of therapy being favourably influenced by the unwitting inclusion of oncocytoma?

We may pose several questions concerning oncocytoma. Is this a sufficiently well described entity to allow for consistent diagnosis by an informed pathologist? What percentage of clinically detected solid renal masses represents oncocytoma? Can the diagnosis be established with confidence without surgery? Klein and Valensi propose that their data suggest a recent increase in the incidence of this disease. Is this correct? Klein and Valenis also propose that the clinical history, specifically the lack of hematuria, might be a useful diagnostic clue. Is this correct? Under what circumstances, if any, can the diagnosis of oncocytoma be established by frozen section? Finally, is this invariably a benign disease?

The following abbreviated case report may illustrate the

challenge and opportunity presented by this disease. The full case
report is awaiting publication (2). The patient was a 42 year old
white married nulliparous previously healthy female. She complained of colicky left flank pain and was admitted to a local
hospital with the presumptive diagnosis of a left ureteral calculus.
The admitting physical examination and laboratory data were within
normal limits except for microhematuria. An excretory urogram
revealed a large middle pole mass of the left kidney and a smaller
upper pole mass of the right kidney. Sonography revealed both
masses to be solid. An aortogram and bilateral selective renal
arteriograms were performed. An evaluation for metastases was
negative. The patient was referred to us with a diagnosis of
bilateral renal cell carcinoma.

Our evaluation of the patient failed to reveal any evidence of
von Hippel-Lindau disease or tuberous sclerosis. Ultrasonograph-
ically controlled "skinny" needle aspiration cytology of the masses
was negative for malignant cells from the right and technically
unsatisfactory from the left kidney.

Since in our opinion the most likely diagnosis was malignancy
with, however, the remote possibility of an unusual benign tumor we
chose to approach the problem by performing a radical nephrectomy
of the kidney with the greatest tumor burden, i.e., the left. We
modified the procedure, however, by leaving the vessels intact until
we had mobilized the entire specimen. We then secured the vessels,
removed the specimen and immediately perfused the kidney via the
renal artery with cold Collin's solution. The mass was shelled out
with a combination of blunt and sharp dissection. The entire mass
which weighed almost 400 grams and was 10.5 cm in diameter was
given to our pathologist (Dr A Nicastri). Frozen section was
interpreted as a benign tumor. The kidney was reconstructed and
then autotransplanted into the left iliac fossa by our transplant
surgeon, Dr Khalid Butt. The regional lymph nodes looked and felt
normal and this together with the frozen section report of benign
disease prompted us not to perform a lymphadenectomy. The patient
was discharged on the eleventh post-operative day. The final
pathological diagnosis was oncocytoma.

The patient was re-admitted 35 days after her initial discharge.
We performed a simple enucleation of the right kidney mass and a
second previously undetected mass. Again the frozen and permanent
section diagnosis was oncocytoma.

We believe this is the first report of bilateral renal
oncocytoma. Forty eight months have now elapsed since her surgery
and the patient has no evidence of malignant disease.

An attempt will now be made to answer the questions posed in
the initial part of this article. Based on a review of the

literature, I am of the opinion that a well informed competent
pathologist can be expected to reliably establish the diagnosis
especially when the entire tumor is available for study. Reports
in the literature have suggested that the percentage of clinically
detected solid renal masses which subsequently prove to be oncocytoma ranges between 5-15%. It is our opinion that no publication
has documented a reliable method of establishing the diagnosis
prior to surgery. Publications subsequent to that of Klein and
Valensi (1) have failed to confirm their suggestion that the
incidence of this tumor may be increasing. Klein and Valensi also
suggested that these tumors might have a characteristic clinical
history. Most significantly they suggested a lack of hematuria.
This case report, however, and many other reports in the literature
document that the clinical history does not differ significantly
from that of renal cancer. A frozen section based on a small
volume of tissue as obtained from, for example, a needle biopsy,
is unlikely to be of value because needle biopsy is highly selective. The current definition of an oncocytoma requires that the
tumor be entirely composed of oncocytes. If, as in this case, the
entire tumor can be examined closely by the pathologist and frozen
sections taken, then frozen sections may be reliable.

Until the recent report from the Mayo Clinic by Lieber et al
(3) no oncocytoma had been reported to have produced metastases.
They reported 90 cases divided in two groups - 62 cases with what
they categorise as Grade I oncocytoma and 28 cases with Grade 2
disease. No case in the Grade I group developed metastases, but
six of the Grade 2 group did. Their report suggests that a
spectrum of clinical behaviour exists for these tumors.
Confirmation of the malignant potential of Grade 2 oncocytomas as
noted by the Mayo Clinic group is currently lacking.

The use of radical nephrectomy and autotransplantation in the
management of renal masses of uncertain nature has been previously
discussed (4) and is of considerable value in certain cases.

REFERENCES

1. M. J. Klein and J. Valensi, Proximal tubular adenomas of
    kidney with so-called oncocytic features, Cancer 38:906 (1976).
2. R. J. Macchia, K. M. H. Butt, A. D. Nicastri and C. Chen,
    Bilateral renal oncocytoma, J. Urol. (submitted for publication).
3. M. M. Lieber, K. M. Tomera and G. M. Farrow, Renal oncocytoma,
    J. Urol. 125:481 (1981).
4. G. P. Kearney, E. M. Mahoney and J. Dmochowski, Radical
    nephrectomy, bench surgery and autotransplantation in the
    potentially malignant mass, J. Urol. 116:375 (1976).

CIRCULATION TIME AND RENAL BLOOD FLOW IN KIDNEY CARCINOMA

G. Lingårdh and S.O. Hietala

Regionsjukhuset, Örebro and
University of Umeå
Sweden

Renal carcinomas are often highly vascular tumours. From angiographic as well as from direct pathologic examinations it is well known that some tumours show arteriovenous shunts (1,2). A rapid opacification of the renal vein is sometimes seen indicating shunt flow. However, as a rather large amount of contrast medium is needed to visualize the renal vein, the incidence of arteriovenous shunts might be much more common than is shown by angiography. Information on renal blood flow and arteriovenous shunts is of basic interest in conjunction with the development of future alternative therapeutic methods in inoperable cases of renal carcinoma. Thus, dose calculations for direct arterial infusion of chemotherapeutic agents or embolization with microseeds loaded with cytostatic or radioactive material might be dependent on the knowledge of tumour blood flow.

MATERIAL AND METHODS

Renal circulation was studied in 15 patients with renal carcinoma by a dye-dilution technique at the time of angiography. No premedication was given. Both the renal artery and the renal vein were catheterized and a bolus injection of indocyanine green was given into the artery while blood was continuously sucked from the renal vein through a spectrophotometer. The resulting concentration curves facilitate the calculation of renal blood flow, appearance time of dye in renal vein and disclose, by curve irregularities, shunt flow which in many cases can be calculated and separated from total renal blood flow too (3,4). The vasularity of the tumours and the size of the kidneys were determined from the angiograms.

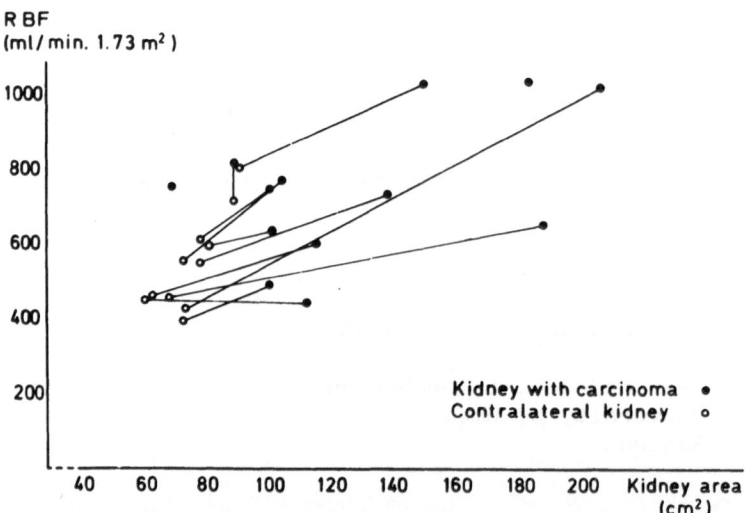

Fig 1.   Renal blood flow (RBF) in tumour kidneys compared to contra-
         lateral kidneys and plotted against the size of the organs
         as measured from the angiograms.   In all but one case the
         tumour kidney had the highest blood flow.

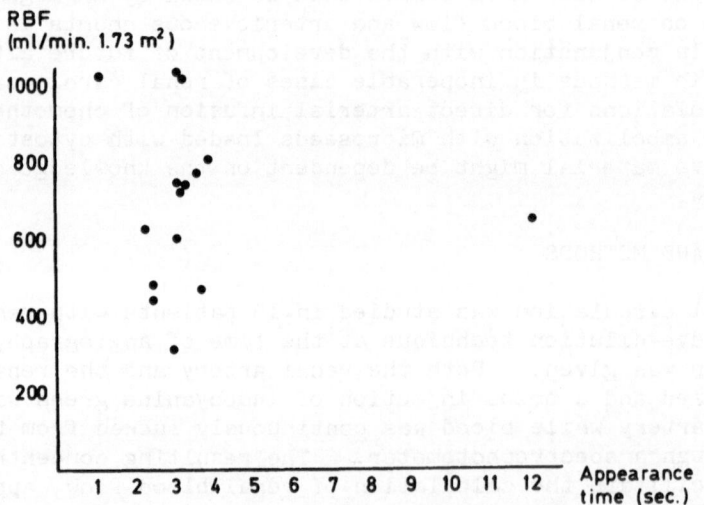

Fig 2.   RBF in tumour kidneys plotted against appearance time of dye
         in the renal vein.   No correlation was seen between RBF and
         appearance time, which was extremely short only in one case
         and was prolonged in one case in spite of a rather high RBF.

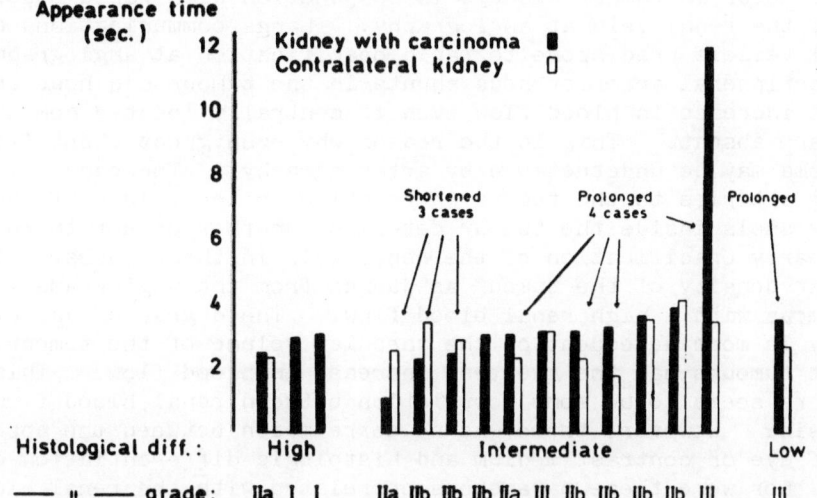

Fig 3.   Appearance time of dye in tumour kidney compared to the
         contralateral one.   Three cases had a shorter appearance
         time on the tumour side and five had a prolongation, while
         it was approximately the same in the others.   (In three
         patients the contralateral kidney could not be studied for
         technical reasons.)

RESULTS

     The total renal blood flow was as a rule increased on the tumour
side.   Large tumours had the greatest blood flow.   In three cases
the blood flow was more than 1000 ml. per minute (fig 1).   One of
these tumour kidneys had a rapid appearance of dye in the renal vein
but no correlation was seen between appearance time of dye and increase in renal blood flow (fig 2).   In all but one kidney obvious
curve irregularities showed the occurence of abnormal shunt flow.
Compared to the appearance time of the contralateral kidney the tumour
kidney had a shorter time in three cases and a longer in five.   In
the other cases the differences were small (fig 3).   There was no
correlation between the appearance time of dye or contrast medium
and histologic differentiation or grade;   nor were these parameters
correlated to the renal blood flow.

CONCLUSION

     Angiography gives mainly morphologic information on renal car-
cinomas and tumour vessels and is only able to reveal a few cases of
arteriovenous shunting.   All renal carcinomas, except for those
totally necrotic, can be shown to have pathological arteriovenous
tumour shunts.   Massive increase in total renal blood flow may or

may not occur in tumour kidneys in conjunction with rapid opacification of the renal vein at angiography.   Large communications between
central vessels predispose to rapid opacification at angiography.
Large peripheral arteriovenous shunts in the tumour can however give
a great increase in blood flow even if centrally located communications are absent.   This is the reason why even great shunt flow in
carcinoma may be undetectable by arteriography.   The capacity of the
feeding arteries to the tumour in relation to the volume of the sinus-
oidal vessels inside the tumour determine whether or not there will
be an early opacification of the renal vein in these cases.   A high
vascular density of the tumour as judged from the angiograms is not
synonymous with a high renal blood flow.   The degree of vascular
density is more dependent on the vascular volume of the tumour.   The
largest tumours had the greatest increase in blood flow.   This is
why there seems to be some correlation between renal blood flow and
prognosis.   However, there was no correlation between the appearance
time of dye or contrast medium and histologic differentiation or
grade;   nor were these parameters correlated with the renal blood
flow.

REFERENCES

1.   E. Boijsen and J. Folin, Angiography in the Diagnosis of Renal
      Carcinoma, Radiologe 1:173 (1961).
2.   M.E. Siegel, F.A. Giargiana and H.M. Wagner Jr., Verification
      and Quantification of Anatomic Arteriovenous Shunting in a Hyper-
      nephroma, J. Urol. 112:16 (1974).
3.   G. Lingårdh, B. Lindqvist and B. Lundström, Renal Arteriovenous
      Fistula Following Puncture Biopsy.   A Hemodynamic and Functional
      Study in Four Cases, Scand. J. Urol. Nephrol. 5:181 (1971).
4.   G. Lingårdh and B. Lundström, Renal Blood Flow in Man Studied
      with a Dye-Dilution Method, Scand. J. Urol. Nephrol. 6:54 (1972).

HISTOCHEMICAL DETECTION OF STEROID BINDING SITES IN HUMAN RENAL TISSUE AND RENAL CELL CARCINOMA: A PRELIMINARY REPORT OF WORK IN PROGRESS

R.J. Macchia,[1] L.P. Pertschuk,[1] G.J. Wise,[2] and P. Shapiro[1]

1. The State University of New York
   Downstate Medical Center
   Brooklyn, New York, U.S.A.

2. The Maimonides Medical Center
   Brooklyn, New York, U.S.A.

The degree of interest in the hormonal milieu as a factor influencing the natural history of renal cell carcinoma is, perhaps, out of proportion to what is warranted by the cumulative experience. Controversy regarding this topic might best be relegated to the medical equivalent of Shakespeare's "Much Ado About Nothing". As a minor offshoot of our binding site studies involving prostatic cancer (described in another section of this book: see 'Histochemical determination of androgen binding in prostatic adenocarcinoma: clinical correlation') we succumbed to this apparently irresistable phenomenon. The following is a preliminary report on work in progress.

Using the histochemical technique, eighteen non-cancerous kidneys were analyzed for estrogen, progesterone and testosterone binding sites. This work has been previously published (1). Binding of all three hormones was detected in eight of eighteen specimens, 5/18 exhibited various combinations of binding and 5/18 were negative. The predominant site of binding was the epithelial cells within the glomerular capillary loops. Binding was also frequently seen in Bowman's capsule. Almost half of the positive specimens showed additional binding in the epithelial cells of the proximal and/or distal convoluted tubules. The results of competitive and non-specific binding studies have been published (1).

Thirty-six specimens of either primary site or metastatic renal cell carcinoma were assayed histochemically but only for estrogen binding. The results, previously unpublished, were as follows: 2/36 necrotic - not assayable; 9/36 negative;

4/36 - low level binding (circa 10% of cells positive); 4/36 - 25%
of cells positive; 3/36 - 50% of cells positive; 14/36 - 75% of cells
positive. Most cells that were positive exhibited predominantly
nuclear binding. Assuming that no nuclear estrogen receptor assay
is usually performed with biochemical methods, only 4/36 specimens
exhibited significant enough numbers of positive cells to have
potentially detectable cytoplasmic binding by the usual biochemical
methods.

Preliminary clinical correlation was available in fifteen of
these thirty-six cases. In twelve cases the specimens were of the
primary site, i.e. kidney, and in three of metastatic deposits. Of
the group of twelve primary cases, eight were men and four were women.
The average age was sixty-four years. Table 1 shows the level of
estrogen binding as a function of stage of disease. Table 2 relates
the subcellular location of estrogen binding to binding intensity.
Table 3 studies the same relationship but for the specimens of
metastatic disease.

Our work is still at too preliminary a stage to draw any meaningful conclusions. The potential role played by steroid hormones
in the kidney has been discussed (1).

Table 1. Level of Estrogen Binding Relative to Disease Stage

	Low	Moderate	High	Total
Localized to Kidney	-	-	6	6
Beyond Kidney	-	2	4	6
Total	-	2	10	12

Table 2. Renal Cell Carcinoma - Binding Site Study
(Primary Tumours)

Binding	Nuclear	Cytoplasm	Mixed	Total
Low <10%	-	-	-	-
Moderate 10-49%	1	-	1	2
High > 50%	8	-	2	10
Total	9	-	3	12

Table 3. Renal Cell Carcinoma - Binding Site Study
(Metastatic Lesions)

Binding		Nuclear	Cytoplasm	Mixed	Total
Low	< 10%	-	-	-	-
Moderate	10-49%	1	-	-	1
High	> 50%	-	1	1	2
Totals		1	1	1	3

REFERENCES

1. L.P. Pertschuk, E.E. Carvounis, E.H. Tobin, and E. Gaetjens,
Renal glomerular steroid hormone binding. Detection by fluorescent microscopy. J. Steroid Biochem. 13: 1115 (1980).

Editorial Note (M.P.)

Although the authors state that their results are still preliminary, their 36 cases of renal cancer, that have been assayed for
estrogen receptors by histochemical technique, lend themselves to
some considerations.

It is hard to establish any correlation between this and the
conventional biochemical techniques as the latter, as indicated by
the authors, are unable to identify the presence of nuclear receptors,
but merely reflect the presence of receptors in the cytoplasm. In
the present series, fluorescence in the cytoplasm was found, along
with nuclear fluorescence, only in three out of 36 patients. This
would appear to confirm the findings of those workers who were unable to detect biochemically significant amounts of estrogen receptors in the cytosol of renal adenocarcinoma in humans.

The clinical significance of the relatively high number of cases
showing nuclear binding sites by histochemical techniques needs to
be clarified if the findings are confirmed by further study. It is
also of interest that estrogen receptors in the normal kidney seem
to be located more in the glomerular tuft and in Bowman's capsule
than in the convoluted tubules from which renal adenocarcinomas
originate. This work does not help to unveil the mystery of the role
of hormones in the natural history and in the treatment of renal cell
cancer.

HORMONE THERAPY AND RECEPTOR STUDIES IN HUMAN RENAL CELL CARCINOMA

G. Pizzocaro and the Lombardy Study Group*

Istituto Nazionale Tumori
Milan
Italy

INTRODUCTION

There is very clear experimental evidence of the hormone-dependence of renal cancer in the male hamster (1-5) but little evidence of the effectiveness of hormone therapy in humans. Opinions are controversial and Hrushesky & Murphy (6) pointed out that the cumulative reported response rate to either progesterone or androgen therapy in advanced renal cell carcinoma was 17% in the literature up to 1971 and less than 2% afterwards. In recent years, antiestrogens have been tried and the response rate reported in the largest published series (7) is 4% objective remission and 28% subjective improvement. Different criteria of evaluation may be responsible for the widely differing results reported in the older literature.

In recent years steroid receptors have been widely studied in renal cancer and normal kidney parenchyma. With the exception of Concolino et al (8,9), who faithfully trust in the hormone-dependence of human renal cancer, high affinity binding sites to estrogens (ER) and to progesterone (PR) are found at a very low concentration in a small proportion of kidney tumor cytosols (10,11). In particular, estrogen treatment does not induce PR synthesis in human renal cancer (12) and both ER and PR binding is higher in the normal kidney than in the tumor (13). Recently a significant concentration of binding sites to androgens (AR) and glucocorticoids (GR) has been demonstrated in both the tumor and in normal tissue (13-17), while renal cancer appears not to contain binding sites to mineral corticoids (MR) (17).

PERSONAL EXPERIENCE

In a preliminary investigation of the hormone-dependence of human renal cell carcinoma, we studied the ER content in both the

527

tumor mass and the surrounding healthy parenchyma of 31 kidneys consecutively removed at the Istituto Tumori for cancer (18). ER were non negative in 12/31 neoplastic tissue cytosols (38%) and in 13/26 normal tissue samples (50%). Of these patients, 10 also had metastatic disease and were given high dose Medroxyprogesterone Acetate (MPA) as post operative treatment (19). Stabilization of the disease was achieved in two of five patients whose tumors were not ER negative. These preliminary results persuaded us to undertake a prospective cooperative study in Lombardy starting in July 1979; this is sponsored by the Consiglio Nazionale delle Ricerche (CNR), Rome.

The design of the study is outlined in Fig. 1. Every patient with renal cancer amenable to surgery undergoes a radical transperitoneal nephrectomy. No pre-operative embolization is allowed. Tissue samples are immediately taken from the tumor mass and the surrounding healthy parenchyma and stored at $- 70^{\circ}C$. Receptor studies are carried out in the laboratory of the Istituto Tumori. ER, PR and AR are currently studied by the dextran-coated charcoal (DCC) technique as previously described (18). A further purification of the cytosol by precipitation with $(NH4)_2SO_4$ 35-50% was introduced in order to remove the steroid binding plasma proteins, as the kidney is a very vascular organ.

Up to March 31st 1981, 79 patients have entered this study (Table 1). Randomization of the 62 category MO patients is quite satisfactory (Table 2). ER and PR have been studied in 59 samples of neoplastic tissue and in 32 normal parenchyma. AR were studied in a smaller number of tissue samples (Table 3). ER and PR were detectable in 10% of renal cancer studied and in 40% of healthy tissues. AR were present in nearly the same proportions of healthy and neoplastic tissues studied and the concentration in the neoplastic tissue was twice that which was found in the normal parenchyma.

To date, relapses have occurred in 4 of the 46 evaluable category MO patients (8%). All relapses occurred in patients with locally extensive disease, 3 of whom had been randomized to receive MPA postoperatively (Table 4). However, as far as the receptor content in the tumor tissue is concerned (Table 5), relapses occurred only in ER- PR- and AR- patients and no response to hormone therapy could be expected in receptor negative cases. Twelve category M1 patients have been evaluated (Table 6). No objective response was observed, but four patients (33%) had stabilization of the disease for four to more than eight months. No correlation between clinical response and tumor receptor studies could be found. These results are very preliminary, and a larger number of cases must be studied to obtain significant information.

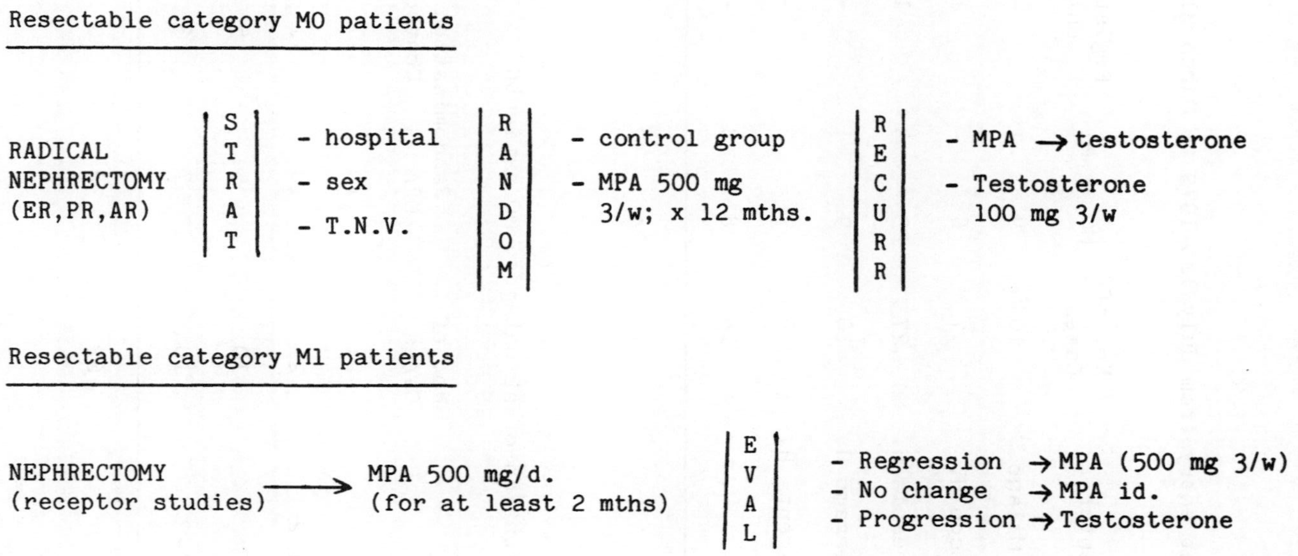

Resectable category MO patients

RADICAL NEPHRECTOMY (ER,PR,AR)

STRAT
S - hospital
T - sex
R - T.N.V.
A
T

RANDOM
R - control group
A - MPA 500 mg
N   3/w; x 12 mths.
D
O
M

RECURR
R - MPA → testosterone
E - Testosterone
C   100 mg 3/w
U
R
R

Resectable category M1 patients

NEPHRECTOMY (receptor studies) ──→ MPA 500 mg/d. (for at least 2 mths)

EVAL
E
V
A
L

- Regression → MPA (500 mg 3/w)
- No change → MPA id.
- Progression → Testosterone

Fig. 1. Prospective Cooperative Study to Evaluate the Hormone-Dependence of Human Renal Cell Carcinoma (Lombardy Group 1979, sponsored by CNR, Rome)

Table 1. Patient entry from July 1st 1979 to March 31st 1981

Participating Center	No. of Cases	M0	M1	Registered only
Univ. Urol. School, Milano	10	9	1	-
Dept. of Urology, Lecco H.	7	6	-	1
Dept. of Urology, Brescia H.	27	23	3	1
Dept. of Urology, Bergamo H.	10	9	1	-
Dept. of Urology, Magenta H.	9	7	2	-
I.N.T. Milano	16	8	8	-
Total	79	62	15	2

Table 2. Distribution of 62 category M0 patients

	Stratification	No. of Cases	Randomisation MPA	Control
M	T1-2, N0, V0	21	10	11
	T3-4, N1-2, V1-2	21	10	11
F	T1-2, N0, V0	10	5	5
	T3-4, N1-2, V1-2	10	7	3
	Total	62	32	30

Table 3. ER, PR & AR Concentration and Binding Affinity in the Normal and Neoplastic Renal Tissue Samples Studied

Receptors	Tissue	Cases Studied	Positive cases No.	Positive cases (%)	F mol/mg prot.	Ka 10^{-9} M^{-1}
E.R.	Normal	32	13	(40)	2.75 ± 0.40	5.11 ± 0.95
	Neoplastic	59	6	(10)	4.34 ± 1.10	5.12 ± 1.02
P.R.	Normal	32	14	(43)	4.37 ± 0.77	3.41 ± 0.59
	Neoplastic	59	6	(10)	3.04 ± 0.92	1.03 ± 0.36
A.R.	Normal	20	6	(30)	5.33 ± 0.96	2.86 ± 1.24
	Neoplastic	47	11	(23)	9.21 ± 1.69	1.65 ± 0.19

Table 4. Recurrences in 46 evaluable category MO patients
according to the extent of the disease

Treatment/Extent		No. of Cases	Relapses	
			No.	(%)
MPA	T1-2, N0, V0	13	-	-
	T3-4, N1-2, V1-2	12	3	(25)
Control	T1-2, N0, V0	10	-	-
	T3-4, N1-2, V1-2	11	1	(9)
	Total	46	4	(8)

Table 5. Relapses in 46 evaluable category MO patients
and receptor studies in their neoplastic tissue

Receptor studies in the neoplastic tissue	No. of Cases	MAP		Control	
		No.	Relapses	No.	Relapses
ER- PR- AR-	26	13	3	13	1
ER- PR- ARx*	7	5	-	2	-
ER- PR- AR+	5	4	-	1	-
ER- PR+ AR-	1	1	-	-	-
ER- PR+ ARx*	1	-	-	1	-
ER- PR+ AR+	1	-	-	1	-
ER+ PR- AR-	2	1	-	1	-
ER+ PR- AR+	2	-	-	2	-
ER+ PR+ AR+	1	1	-	-	-
Total	46	25	3 (12%)	21	1 (5%)

* ARx : AR not studied

Table 6.   Receptor studies in neoplastic tissue and the results
of high dose MPA treatment in 12 category M1 patients

Pt.	Sex	Receptors			Distant metastases	Response to MPA	Duration (months)	Survival (months)
		E	P	A				
1	M	−	−	−	adrenal (removed)	no change	8 +	8 +
2	M	−	−	−	paratesticular (removed)	"	5 +	5 +
3	M	+	+	+	bone	progression	−	3
4	M	−	−	−	bone and lung	"	−	6
5	M	+	−	+	lung	"	−	4
6	M	−	−	−	lung	"	−	15 + *
7	F	−	+	x	bone	no change	7	11
8	F	−	−	x	lung	"	4	6 +
9	F	−	−	−	lung	progression	−	11 + *
10	F	−	−	x	lung	"	−	13 + *
11	F	−	−	−	lung	"	−	3
12	F	−	−	−	bone	"	−	10

* 3 patients achieved stabilization by subsequent androgen therapy.

CONCLUSIONS

There is some evidence that a weak hormone dependence may exist
in human renal cell carcinoma. Further studies are needed to investigate the mechanism of action of steroid hormones in this tumor,
with particular reference to the possibility of inducing PR synthesis
by tamoxifen administration (20) and to the significance of the high
GR content in renal cancer.

* The Lombardy Study Group includes -

Dr. G. Di Fronzo[1], Dr. E. Ronchi[1], Dr. L. Piva[2], Dr. E. Lasio[3],

Dr. U. Maggioni[3], Dr. A. Giongo[4], Dr. E. Mastroberandino[4],

Dr. V. Maffeis[5], Dr. C. Guzzetti[5], Dr. U. Fontanella[6],

Dr. A. Zanollo[6], Dr. E. Dormia[7], Dr. S. Minervini[7].

1. Dept. of Experimental Oncology C, Istituto Naz. Tumori, Milano
2. Section of Urologic Oncology, Istituto Nazionale Tumori, Milano
3. Dept. of Urology, University School of Medicine, Milano
4. Dept. of Urology, General Hospital, Brescia
5. Dept. of Urology, General Hospital, Bergamo
6. Dept. of Urology, General Hospital, Magenta
7. Dept. of Urology, General Hospital, Lecco

REFERENCES

1. H.J.G. Bloom, G.E. Dukes, and B.C.V. Mitchley, Hormone-
    dependent tumours of the kidney, Br. J. Cancer 17: 611 (1963).
2. H. Kirkman, Estrogen induced tumours of the kidney in the
    Syrian hamster, Nat. Cancer Inst. Monogr. 1: 1 (1959).
3. J.J. Li, D.J. Talley, S.A. Li, and C.A. Villee, Receptor charac-
    teristic of specific estrogen binding in the renal adenocarcin-
    oma of the golden hamster, Cancer Res. 36: 1127 (1976).
4. J.J. Li, T.L. Curthbertson, and S.A. Li, Specific androgen bin-
    ding in the kidney and estrogen-dependent renal carcinoma of
    the Syrian hamster, Endrocrinology 101: 1006 (1977).
5. S.A. Li and J.J. Li, Estrogen-induced progesterone receptor in
    the Syrian hamster kidney. I. Modulation by antiestrogens and
    androgens, Endocrinology 103: 2119 (1978).
6. W.J. Hrushesky and G.P. Murphy, Current status of the therapy
    of advanced renal carcinoma, J. Surg. Oncol. 9: 277 (1977).
7. M. Al-Sarraf, The clinical trial of Tamoxifen in patients with
    advanced renal cell cancer in South West Oncology Group Study,
    Proc. Am. Assoc. Cancer Res. 20: 378 (1979).
8. G. Concolino, A. Marocchi, C. Conti, R. Tenaglia, F. Di Silverio,
    and U. Bracci, Human renal cell carcinoma as a hormone-dependent
    tumor, Cancer Res. 38: 4340 (1978).
9. G. Concolino, F. Di Silverio, A. Marocchi, and U. Bracci, Renal
    cancer steroid receptors: Biochemical basis for endocrine
    therapy, Eur. Urol. 5: 90 (1979).
10. H. Bojar, R. Dreyfürst, K. Balzer, W. Staib, and J.C. Wittliff,
    Oestrogen-binding components in human renal cell carcinoma,
    J. Clin. Chem. Clin. Biochem. 14: 521 (1976).
11. H. Bojar, K. Maar, and W. Staib, The endocrine background of
    human renal cell carcinoma - I - Binding of the highly potent
    progestin R 5020 by tumor cytosol, Urol. Int. 34: 302 (1979).

12.   H. Bojar, K. Maar, and W. Staib, The endocrine background of
      human renal cell carcinoma. II. Attempt to induce the R 5020
      binding components by oestrogens, Urol. Int. 34: 311 (1979).

13.   G.P. Hemstreet, J.L. Wittliff, A.M. Sariff, M.C. Hall,
      L.J. McRae, and J.R. Durant, Comparison of steroid receptor
      levels in renal cell carcinoma and autologous normal kidney,
      Int. J. Cancer 26: 769 (1980).

14.   H. Bojar, K. Maar, and W. Staib, The endocrine background of
      human renal cell carcinoma. IV. Glucocorticoid receptors as
      possible mediators of progesterone action, Urol. Int. 34: 330
      (1979).

15.   H. Bojar, K. Maar, and W. Staib, The endocrine background of
      human renal cell carcinoma. V. Binding of the highly potent
      androgen methyltrienolone (R1881) by tumour cytosol, Urol. Int.
      35: 154 (1980).

16.   L. Chen, F.R. Weiss, S. Chaichik, and I. Keydar, Steroid
      receptors in human renal carcinoma, Isr. J. Med. Sci. 16:
      756 (1980).

17.   M.E. Rapertin-Oblin, C. Roth-Mayer, M. Claire, A. Michaud,
      E. Baviera, J.M. Brisset, and P. Corvol, Are mineral corticoid
      receptors present in human renal adenocarcinoma? Clin. Sci.
      57: 421 (1979).

18.   G. Di Fronzo, E. Ronchi, F. Bertuzzi, P. Vezzoni, and
      G. Pizzocaro, Estrogen receptors in renal carcinoma, Eur. Urol.
      6: 307 (1980).

19.   G. Pizzocaro, M. Valente, I. Cataldo, P. Vezzoni, and
      G. Di Fronzo, Estrogen receptors and MPA treatment in met-
      astatic renal carcinoma. A preliminary report. Tumori 66:
      739 (1980).

20.   M. Namer, C. Lalanne, and E.E. Baulieu, Increase of proges-
      terone receptor by tamoxifen as a hormonal challenge test
      in breast cancer, Cancer Res. 40: 1750 (1980).

(This paper is supported by grant no. 80.01620.96, CNR, Rome.)

DIAGNOSTIC INVESTIGATIONS IN RENAL CANCER. ADVANCES IN DIAGNOSIS INCLUDING RADIOLOGY, LYMPHOGRAPHY, PERCUTANEOUS PUNCTURE ULTRA-SONOGRAPHY AND COMPUTED TOMOGRAPHY

L. Denis and L. Mortelmans

Academic Hospital
Free University of Brussels
A.Z. Middelheim Antwerp, Belgium

INTRODUCTION

The classical clinical triad of flank mass, pain and hematuria is seen in a small minority of patients. More than half the diagnosed renal masses, including tumors, are incidental findings during a urological investigation carried out for some other purpose or the result of a stubborn search for the aetiology of the origin of a variety of paraneoplastic symptoms or signs. In this respect renal cancer earns the nickname of the internist's tumor.

HISTORY AND PHYSICAL EXAMINATION

Hematuria is the initial symptom in about half the patients and is total in nature. Flank pain, usually dull or of a colicky nature when clots are passed, is another symptom leading to the diagnosis of renal cancer. Extra-renal signs, such as low grade fever, increased sedimentation rate, an expression of metastatic disease or one of the many para-neoplastic syndromes point in a slow but constant percentage of patients to the diagnosis (1). Physical examination allows the detection of a mass in a minority of patients. Edema of the lower extremities and weight loss are signs of advanced disease. As a rule we accept that a renal cyst of benign nature, a common disease in elderly people, should be considered as an incidental event and extreme caution is advised before attributing any of the aforementioned symptoms to this benign condition. Cukier et al (2) reviewed 184 cases of renal cancer and found hematuria (50%), flank pain (10%) and alteration of the physical status (10%) as the initial symptoms. In a retro-spective study of 50 cases of renal cancer (from 1975-1980) and

50 cases of renal cysts (from 1977-1980) we found as the initial
symptom of the 50 patients with renal cancer: 28 with hematuria
(56%), pain of a dull nature in eight (16%), renal colic in another
eight (16%) and an altered physical condition in three (6%). Only
three of the 50 cases with renal cancer were referred with the
diagnosis of flank mass and only two of the 50 cases with renal cyst
presented symptoms that were attributable to the cyst. The
sedimentation rate was elevated in all but three patients with renal
cancer. A list of manifestations described in patients with renal
cancer is presented in Table 1.

MEDICAL IMAGING STUDIES

Intravenous Urography and Nephrotomography

These studies are essential to an evaluation of the basic
problem and their quality usually determines the chain of events
leading to final diagnosis. To repeat an improperly executed
intravenous urography (IVU) is good clinical practice. Irregularity
of the excreting system by tumor invasion points to the diagnosis of
transitional cell cancer. The real adenocarcinoma is revealed by
the euphemistically called "space occupying lesion" with distortion
of the collecting system and an enlarged displaced or non functioning kidney. In general one can state that regular, smooth and well
defined masses are usually benign whilst irregularity, calcifications,
amputations and variation in deformity are suggestive of neoformations. A typical renal cyst as an incidental finding can be
demonstrated as a radiolucent mass, sharply defined against the
normal parenchyma. In elderly persons we do not hesitate to accept
this as a final diagnosis and avoid further investigations.
Additional confirmation can be obtained in this examination by abdominal compression and mobility of the affected kidney (3). Normal
variants which may mimic calyceal distortion such as exaggerated

Table 1: Clinical Manifestations in Renal Cancer

G.U.	Systemic Toxicity	Endocrine
Hematuria	Anemia	Erythrocytosis
Pain	Weight Loss	Hypercalcemia
Mass	Neuromyopathy	Hypertension
Varicocele	Fever	Ectopic HCG Production
AV Shunting	Amyloidosis Hepatic Dysfunction Increased Sedimentation Rate	

renal lobes or renal sinus fat deposit in the aged are typical and
should be recognised. A renal scan may solve the problem in an
individual case. Retrograde pyelography provides sharp definition
by filling the collecting system but there is really no need for
this investigation except for the collection of biopsy material
in cases supected of having urothelial tumors. The variability of
the collecting system and the variations in vascularity and excretion
pattern appeal to the lyricism of the radiologist or to the logic of
the computer (4) but the IVU is only the first step in a diagnostic
pathway (Fig. 1) and a well educated guess with a lack of accuracy
in a small but constant percentage of patients with renal masses.
The prime example to illustrate the fallacy of tumor diagnosis on
IVU only has been demonstrated by a review of 19 misdiagnosed cases
in the National Wilms Tumor Study (5). An expert panel despite
knowledge of the intent of the review, could not correct all the
errors.

Ultrasonography and Computed Tomography

Ultrasonography (US) and Computed Tomography (CT) brought a
new kind of diagnostic imaging, the cross-sectional display of
organs and body. The physical basis of both techniques and the
clinical priniples, limitations and applications in urological
practice have been described elsewhere (6-8).

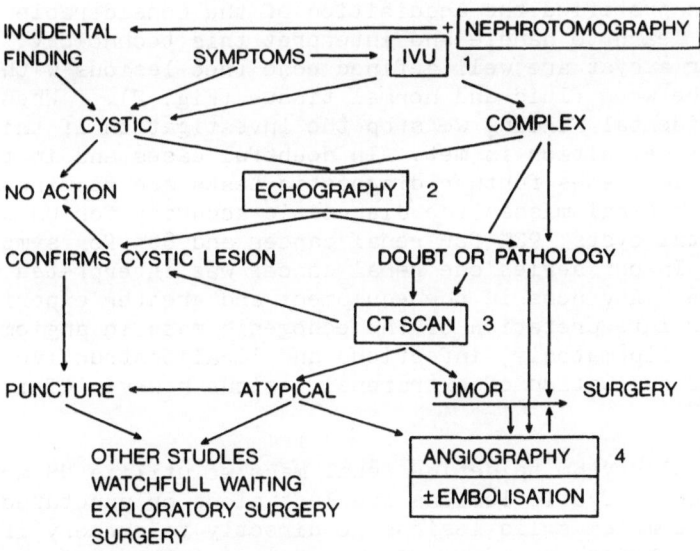

Fig. 1. Diagnostic Algorythm of Renal Mass

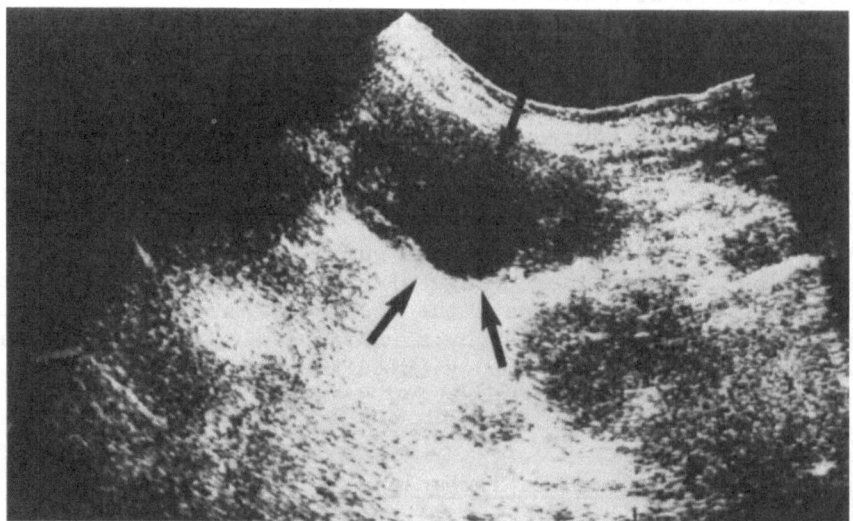

Fig. 2. Renal Cyst. Criteria on Ultrasonography include echo free
         lesions, sharp interfaces and enhanced transmission of
         sound through cystic space.

     US became a natural second choice in the evaluation of renal
masses because of its unusual accuracy in defining cystic
structures, the commonest finding in renal masses. The complete
absence of side effects, the low cost and the possibility of serial
examinations justified the acquisition of the considerable skill
required to learn to handle and interpret this technology. The US
criteria for a cyst are well defined echo free lesions with sharp
interfaces between fluid and normal tissue (Fig. 2). When dealing
with an incidental finding we stop the investigation if this simple
and clearcut definition is met. In doubtful cases and in those
with echogenic masses further diagnostic tests are required. In a
series of 266 renal masses the diagnostic accuracy for US was 100%
for incidental cysts, 92% for renal cancer and 80% for symptomatic
cysts (9). In our series one renal cancer was interpreted as a
cyst in 1976. Advances in the equipment and greater experience
allow better interpretation of the echogenic mass in angiomyolipoma
(10), pelvic lipomatosis, infections and local obstructive uropathy
(7). In the evaluation of extrarenal lesions however CT is superior
to US (11,12).

     In our algorythm to define renal mass we utilize US as a
revolving door. Cystic lesions are left alone or punctured.
Doubtful or complex solid lesions go directly to surgery if renal
cancer looks obvious or go to CT or preoperative arteriography for
further evaluation.

Compared to US the CT is more costly and requires the use of radiation and contrast media. However this technique is easier in operation and image interpretation and less limited by bowel arte-facts and not at all by bone, fat or gas. In addition it is acknowledged that CT allows easy visualization of complete body slices with information on the suspected lesion and its adjacent structures. Staging of renal cancer and serial follow-up with ac-curate patient positioning seems to be superior by CT evaluation (13,14). Though we usually refer our doubtful or solid images on US to CT it is established that CT allows for accurate diagnosis of renal cysts. Here the mass lesion is well rounded with a uniform density close to that of water. This density does not increase after the administration of contrast material unlike that of the adjacent parenchyma. The cyst walls are not detectable outside the kidney structure. False negatives do occur when the cyst diameter is smaller than the slice thickness. The presence of a dense rim is suggestive of tumor especially when it is thick and irregular. Again a solid neoplastic mass is determined by its irregular form. Here the decreased area of density lies between the cyst pattern and normal parenchyma.(Fig. 3). Variation in these density readings usually indicate necrosis or hemorrhage.

It should be noted that small areas of calcification are easily detected on CT. The demonstration of extrarenal extension is opti-mal with CT including venous invasion, lymph node involvement and

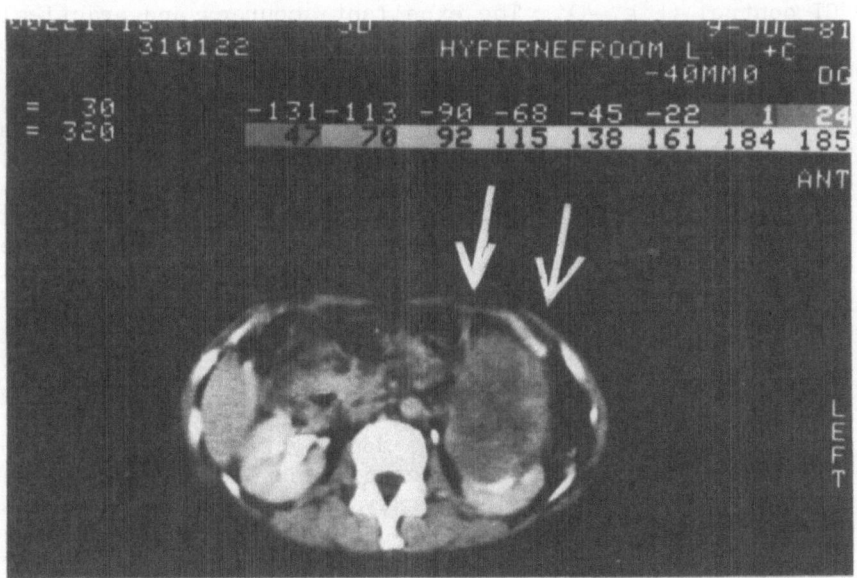

Fig. 3.   Renal tumor is suggested by the irregular form and inter-
          mediate density on CT scan.

liver metastases. It is true that all these features are detectable
by US subject to the skill and patience of the operator. We think
however that US is more useful in detecting the presence of fluid
collections such as abscesses, hematoma and urinoma around the
kidney. In clinical practice CT proves invaluable since radiation
treatment planning can be performed on the newest CT scanners (15).
A tissue specificity with the exception of the typical angiomyolipomas is not possible and the etiology of extensive retroperitoneal
tumors may be attributed to lymphoma, kidney, pancreas, retroperitoneal tissue, adrenals and metastatic disease. This lack of tissue
specificity leaves us with the problems of indeterminate renal
masses especially inflammatory disease that may mimic the characteristics of renal cancer on US or CT. It is at this point that the
clinical evaluation of the individual patient requires further
investigation or treatment by puncture and / or angiography.

Cyst Puncture and Aspiration Test Complex (CPATC)

Puncture of renal lesions is primarily reserved for the confirmation of cystic lesions by the aspiration of clear fluid without
positive histochemical and cytologic examination. A cyst fluid
culture is usually requested as a precaution. The histochemical
analysis determines fat, protein, amylase and lactic dehydrogenese
content. Cytologic examination establishes the presence of malignant or inflammatory cells (16). Contrast medium is instilled
until the cyst is completely filled to reproduce the renal mass.
The procedure is extremely simple and can be done under fluoroscopic,
US or CT control (Fig. 4). The excellent accuracy and practical
lack of complications leads automatically to a fine needle puncture
in complicated cysts of an inflammatory or hemorrhagic nature. If
the needle is in the lesion and no fluid is aspirated (a dry tap)
a solid lesion is present. Aspiration biopsies by a thin needle
technique are attempted in inflammatory lesions and hematomas (16).
The hazard of puncturing a renal cancer is small indeed and only
one case of needle tract seeding has been reported (17). We try to
avoid the puncture of an obvious cancer but fine needle puncture
aiming for cytological material is sometimes preferred to angiography in the elderly patient. False negative results occur but
false positive results have not yet been seen. Negative cytological
results after fine needle biopsy allow a wait and see attitude which
we prefer to explorative surgery, a type of surgery which is costly
to the patient and of poor diagnostic contribution. Cyst aspiration
is without therapeutic benefit since most cysts recur after simple
aspiration which is only to be expected. Therefore large cysts
causing renal parenchymal atrophy or cysts in a perapelvic position
should be excised.

Lymphangiography

The evaluation of suspected lymph nodes is based on lymph-

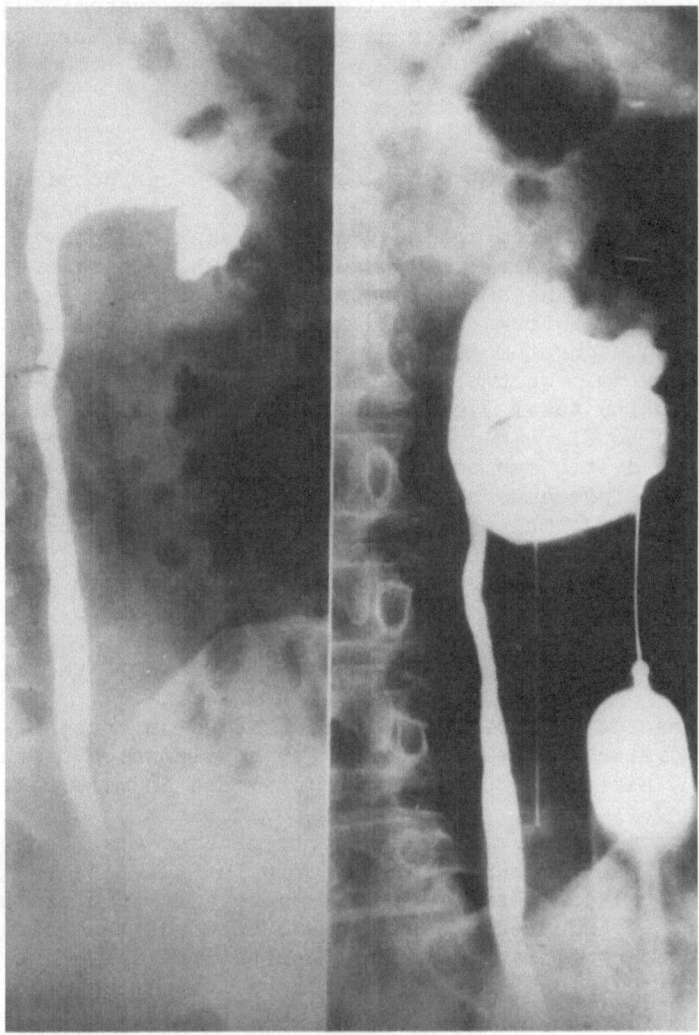

Fig. 4. Cyst puncture includes cytology, culture and chemical
        analysis of the fluid and radiological investigations.

angiography, CT scan, occasionally US and as an extremely rare
event on physical examination. The problem of course with CT and
US is the minimal mass required for discovery. The interest in
lymphangiography is waning due to the number of false positive and
false negative results and few centers perform this examination in
patients with renal cancer (18). Many centers carry out a more or
less extended lymphadenectomy after removal of the renal tumor. The
therapeutic value of lymphadenectomy is not however clearly established (19). We continue to practice limited regional lymphadenectomy since we feel that the presence of tumor indicates dissemin-

ated disease which should be treated in a more systemic way. This kind of staging procedure adds no morbidity to the surgery and provides reliable data for final staging and treatment.

DISCUSSION

Ultrasonography and CT were instituted in our hospital in 1975 and 1976 respectively. They share cross-sectional images, non invasive characteristics and many similar applications in clinical organ imaging. Together, they changed the whole diagnostic pathway to the solution of the space occupying lesions in the kidney. Accurate clinical information and a perfectly performed intravenous urography with nephrotomography constitutes the first and basic step in this algorythm. We prefer US as our next step in the investigation due to its total lack of side effects and its relative low cost compared to CT. The diagnostic accuracy is near 100% for the uncomplicated cystic lesion, a prevalent renal mass in elderly people. In the presence of symptoms, in case of doubt or in solid lesions CT brings complementary and sometimes invaluable information.

CT is superior in the demonstration of extrarenal growth, the relation and assessment of other retroperitoneal structures and the confirmation of the cystic, solid or mixed state of the mass.

The enhanced possibility of percutaneous puncture of all and especially cystic structures allows for confirmation of the diagnosis. This technique should be utilized in more cases with contradictory findings. In a recent round table on diagnostic problems in renal tumors it became evident that most centers experienced special problems where US, CT or both failed to suggest the correct diagnosis or worse were misleading. Typical examples were presented (2). Enhanced experience and improved technology will diminish these problems. However a constant reassessment with clinical controls is necessary for proper evaluation. Newer and refined technology has changed our possibilities for proper evaluation six times in the last five years for US and three times for CT. At this moment we utilize the Aloka SSD 60 C and the Philips Sonodiagnost B 7000 for US evaluation of the kidney and, for CT, the ACTA Scan 200 F.S. The participation of many centers is required to evaluate future trends in cross-sectional imaging to define the exact clinical applications to give the greatest advantage to the individual patient and the least expenditure to an increasingly cost conscious society.

REFERENCES

1. R. Ghozlan, Syndromes Paranéoplastiques et Cancer du Rein in "Tumeurs du Rein," L. Boccon-Gibod and A. Steg, eds, Expansion Scientifique Française, Paris (1979) p 111.

2. J. Cukier, B. Pascal and P.H. Mangin, La semiologie revelatrice
    du cancer du rein chez l'adulte, Acta Urol. Belg.: In press.

3. A. Steg, Diagnostic d'une tumeur du rein de l'adulte en 1979,
    in: "Tumeurs du Rein," L. Boccon-Gibod and A. Steg, eds.,
    Scientifique Française, Paris (1979) p 7.

4. L.R. Bigongiari, D.F. Preston, L. Cook, S.L. Dwyer, S. Fritz,
    D.G. Fryback and J.R. Thornbury, Uncertainty / information as
    measures of various urographic parameters: An information theory
    model of diagnosis of renal masses, Invest. Radiol. 16:77 (1981).

5. R.M. Ehrlich, S.D. Bloomberg, M.T. Gyepes, S.B. Levitt, S. Kogan,
    M. Hanna and W.E. Goodwin, Wilms tumor, misdiagnosed preoperat-
    ively: A review of 19 national Wilms tumor study I cases, J. Urol.
    122:790 (1979).

6. L. Appel, J. Broos, G. Declercq and L. Denis, Evaluation of upper
    urinary tract by CT scan and ultrasonography, Comp. Tom. in press.

7. H. Watanabe, J.H. Holmes, H.H. Holm and B.B. Goldberg,
    "Diagnostic Ultrasound in Urology and Nephrology," Igaku-Shon,
    Tokyo (1981).

8. M.I. Resnick, Advances in imaging techniques, Urol. Clin. North
    America, 6:305 (1979).

9. F. Richard, C. Chatelain, A. Jardin, J.P. Grellet, Ph. Curet
    and R. Küss, Résultats comparatifs de l'echotomographie, de la
    tomodensitométrie et de l'artériographie dans l'exploration des
    masses rénales, in: "Séminaires d'Uro-Néphrologie," R. Küss and
    M. Legrain, eds., Masson, Paris (1981) p 1.

10. W.R. Pitts Jr., E. Kazam, G. Gray and E.D. Vaughan Jr., Ultra-
    sonography, computerized transaxial tomography and pathology of
    angiomyolipoma of the kidney: Solution to a diagnostic dilemma,
    J. Urol. 184:907 (1980).

11. W. Jaschke, G. van Kaick and H. Palmtag, Vergleich der Wertigkeit
    von Echographie und Computertomographie bei der Diagnostik
    raumfordernder Prozess der Nieren, Fortschr. Röntgenstr. 132:
    145 (1980).

12. E. Levine, N.F. Maklad, S.J. Rosenthal, K.R. Lee and J. Weigel,
    Comparison of computed tomography and ultrasound in abdominal
    staging of renal cancer, Urology 16:317 (1980).

13. W.D. Fuchs, Radiologic diagnosis of renal mass lesions: A
    rational approach, in "Renal and Adrenal Tumors," E. Löhr, ed.,
    Springer-Verlag, Berlin, Heidelberg, New York (1979).

14. M. Haertel, P. Probst, M. Bishop, E. Zingg and W.A. Fuchs,
    Renal Computerotomographie, Deutsche Med. Wochenschr. 16:54
    (1981).

15. L. Love, C.J. Reynes, R. Churchill and M. Rogelio, Third
    generation CT scanning in renal disease, Radiol. Clin. North
    America 17:77 (1980).

16. E.K. Lang, Röntgenologic approach to the diagnosis and manage-
    ment of cystic lesions of the kidney: Cyst exploration
    mandatory?, Urol. Clin. North America 7:677 (1980).

17. W.H. Bush, L.L. Burnett and R.P. Gibbons, Needle tract seeding
    of renal cell carcinoma, Am. J. Röntgenol. 129:725 (1977).

18. J. Auvert, Second Congress of the European Association of
     Urology: Lymphadenectomy in urological cancer, European Urology
     4:149 (1978).
19. J.B. deKernion, Lymphadenectomy for renal cell carcinoma:
     Therapeutic implications, Urol. Clin. North America 7:697 (1981).
20. C. Bouffioux, P. Godechard, J. Jadot and L. Pender, Reflexions
     sur les problèmes diagnostiques des tumeurs rénales. Intérêt
     et insufficances de l'echotomographie et de la tomographie axiale
     computerisée, Acta Urol. Belg.: In press.

ARTERIOGRAPHY, VENOGRAPHY AND RADIO-ISOTOPES IN THE DIAGNOSIS OF CANCER OF THE KIDNEY

C. Bollack[1], J. Wenger[2] and J.C. Grob[3]

1. Department of Urology
2. Department of Radiology
3. Centre Paul Strauss

Strasbourg
France

ARTERIOGRAPHY

In 1981, renal angiography is no longer necessary in order to make a diagnosis and to institute appropriate treatment for renal cancer. However it remains of great value in the diagnosis of extension of the tumour and for the knowledge of the arterial and venous disposition which the surgeon will encounter. From a technical point of view, this information is important.

TECHNIQUE

As with all invasive tests, arteriography involves certain risks. However in the hands of experienced operators, these are minimal. Our arteriographic team has done over 7,000 diverse angiographies and has experienced approximately one complication per 1,000 cases.

After puncturing the femoral artery according to the classical Seldinger technique, the aorta is catheterized after which:

(a) <u>Aortography</u> (Fig 1) allows one to visualize the entire abdominal arterial vessels to isolate the tumour, its pedicle or pedicles and to show an extension, particularly to the mesenteric territory, the adrenals, the contralateral kidney or the liver. It also allows the discovery of other vascular lesions.

(b) <u>Selective opacification of the renal arteries</u> (Fig 2a) should always be carried out, injecting a large quantity of

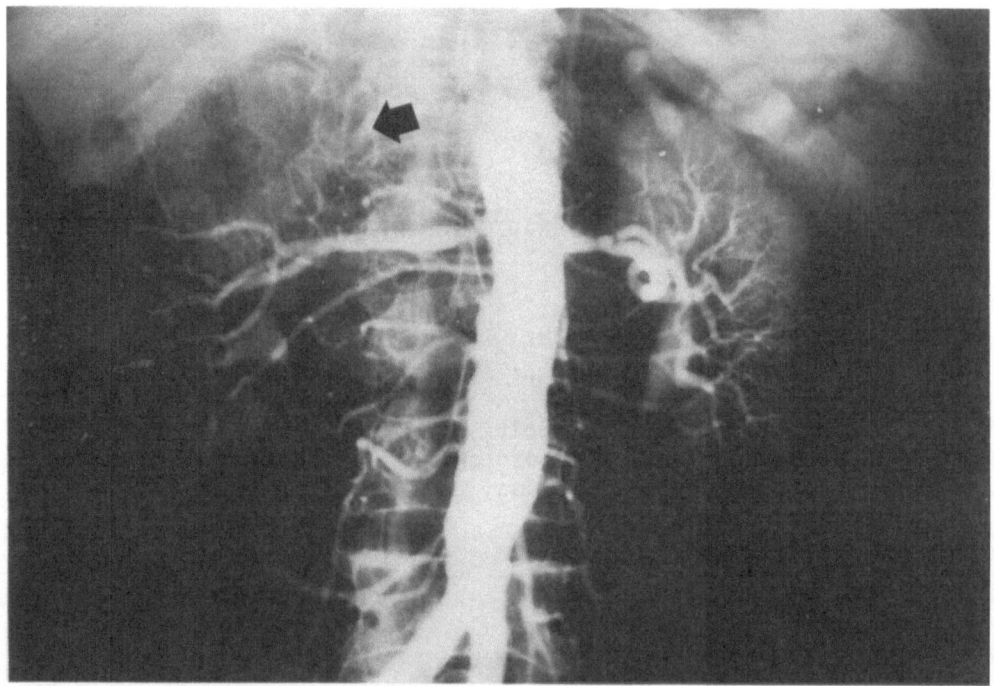

Fig. 1.   Translumbar aortography - shows two right renal arteries
          with stenoses of the main right renal artery and of the
          left renal artery in a patient with a tumour of the upper
          pole of the right kidney (arrow).

contrast medium in order to obtain a venous return that can be
analyzed (Fig 2b).

     It also allows the utilisation of drugs to modify arterial
function, if, after standard posterior, anterior and lateral views,
the diagnosis remains uncertain. Selective exploration of the
celiac trunk is desirable in order to search for a neighbouring
extension of the primary tumour or of metastases (especially hepatic
lesions).

RESULTS

     If a diagnosis appears evident after angiography, the X-rays
should be analyzed methodically starting with the trunk of the
renal artery to the trunk of renal vein: vessels penetrating the
tumour and their extension, tumorography, the peritumoural venous
circulation and the large venous axes.

     Angiographically, there are two different forms of renal

cancer, the hypervascular tumour, where all the signs of malignancy
are formed and appear evident from the test injection on, and
the hypovascular cancer in which there are discrete anomalies
which only a methodical search can discover.

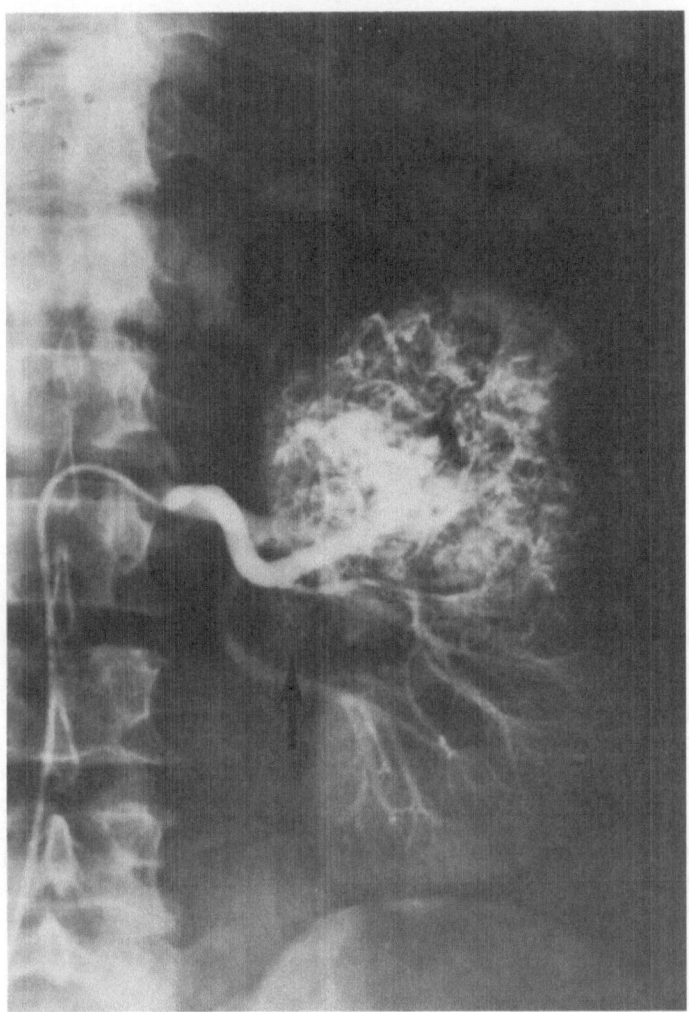

Fig. 2a. Left selective renal arteriogram - large hypervascular
          tumour at the upper pole of the left kidney with some
          new blood vessel formation in the renal hilum (arrow).

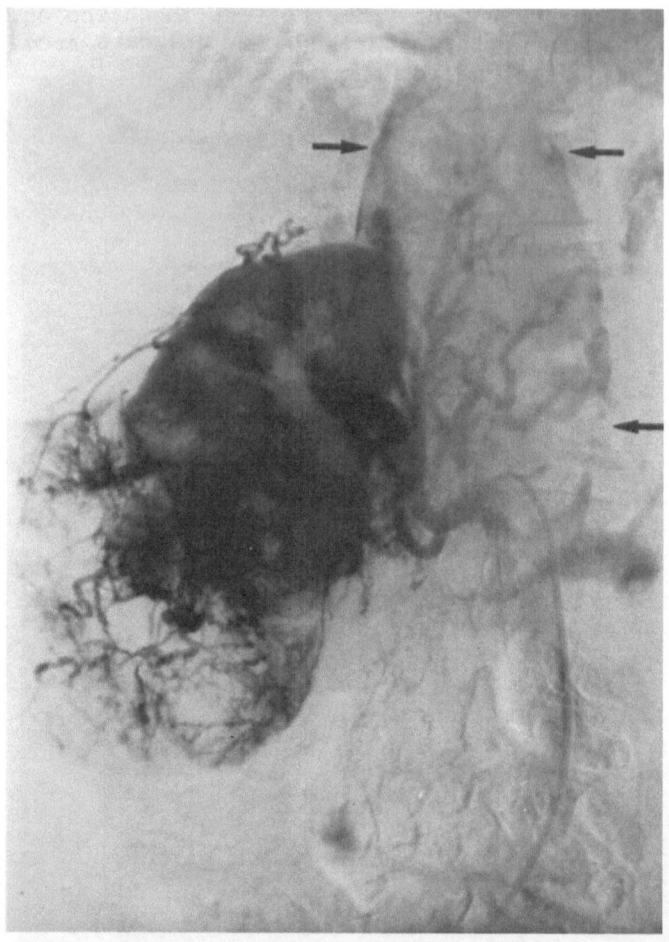

Fig. 2b. Right selective renal arteriogram - large tumour of the
          lower pole of the right kidney with obvious extension in
          the inferior vena cava. The neoplastic growth extending
          into the vena cava is partially vascularised by branches
          of the right renal artery. This permits the identification
          of the position of the inferior vena cava which is dis-
          placed medially. Only a slight amount of contrast medium
          is visible in the left renal vein.

     (a) The Hypervascular Syndrome This combines all (or almost
all) signs of renal cell carcinoma:

- augmentation of the size of the renal artery and its bifurcations
- displacement of the peritumoural arteries (less than in the case
  of a cyst)

- amputation of arteries or arterial branches
- neovascularization or anarchic distribution, the vessels being irregular in their direction, their caliber, and their divisions and sometimes forming sanguinous lakes
- very obvious tumorography, most often heterogenous with vascular zones corresponding to necrosis, sometimes well delimited and separated from non invaded renal parenchyma
- an abundant peritumoral venous circulation arising because of an obstruction of normal venous drainage: neoplastic outgrowth extending more or less towards the vena cava, which can be confirmed by the analysis of venous return during selective arteriography.

The diagnosis of adenocarcinoma of the kidney creates few problems of differential diagnosis in hypervascularized tumours. A hamartoma (angio-myolipoma) can have a similar angiographic appearance and biopsy alone will confirm the diagnosis if tomo-densitometry is not conclusive.

(b) Hypovascular Cancer The diagnosis is more difficult and in doubtful cases necessitates special radiological manoeuvres, often the injection of vasoconstrictors into the renal artery or its branches (angiotensin, norepinephrine). In these patients:

- vascular spreading seems to be incomplete and some branches appear to penetrate the tumour
- neovascularization is seen mainly by arterial amputation and irregularities of the vascular pathway
- tumorography is absent but the parenchymal space occupying lesion "is regular". This aspect is different than that of a cyst.
- venous invasion is less frequent than in hypervascularized tumours.

The diagnosis of malignancy is more difficult to establish in these cases and will also be more difficult to relate to a specific pathological lesion. One can discuss various diagnoses including clear cell carcinomas with necroses, undifferentiated adeno-carcinoma or basophilic cell tumour, renal metastasis of various tumours (gastro-intestinal, ENT, pulmonary) or of a hemolymphopathy, a mesenchymal tumour and of course cancer of the excretory pathway. Usually, however, these transitional cell lesions are recognized before arteriography is undertaken. If arteriography is carried out, it can show neovascularization which does not appear unless functional vascular modifiers are injected. Arteriography is of secondary importance in the diagnosis of excreto-urinary cancer, but it can help in resolving problems of non secreting kidneys.

Nephroblastoma is rare in adults and is usually seen in an extensive hypovascular lesion. The arteries are irregular and are spread out by the tumour formation. Neighbouring extension is

frequent, as well as metastasis to the contralateral kidney.
However, these properties do not always confirm the diagnosis of
nephroblastoma in adults.

CONCLUSION

Arteriography is no longer an indispensable test to establish
the diagnosis of cancer of the kidney. This diagnosis can easily
be made using non invasive methods such as intravenous urography
and echography and eventually confirmed by CT scan which will show
up extracapsular extension.

The value of arteriography is no longer to confirm a diagnosis
but to add further information to a diagnosis already known or
uncertain. Angiography allows one to appreciate with precision
the size of the tumour in the frontal plane and its extension to
other viscera. It also maps out the arterial and venous area that
the operator will encounter during surgery.

PHLEBOGRAPHY

It is helpful to know the venous network in order to know the
extent of spread of the renal cancer, to specify a prognosis, and,
to establish a rational operative approach.

Usually, the nephrogram phase of renal arteriography gives a
good visualisation of the venous bed. If the renal vein or veins
are not well seen after arteriography or if an important collateral
venous circulation is discovered, cavography (Fig 3a) or eventually
venography (Fig 3b) are indicated.

For certain difficult diagnoses, selective phlebography of the
trunk of the renal veins is indicated, especially for hypovascular
tumours, for example, even if the venous bed can be seen during
arteriography.

TECHNIQUE

In order to avoid dislodging a neoplastic thrombus, angiography
of the inferior vena cava always precedes selective opacification
of the renal vein but may be carried out by canulation via the
superior vena cava and right auricle (Fig 4).

(a) The Inferior Vena Cava Cavography is usually performed
after puncture of a femoral vein. The permeability of the iliac
axis is verified by a test injection of the contrast medium. A
catheter is placed in the inferior vena cava after having verified
the permeability of this large venous trunk while the patient is
performing a Valsalva manoeuvre: afterwards, the renal vein is
selectively catheterized.

(b) The Renal Vein The technique of pre-operative arterial
embolisation has the same effect on phlebography as does intra-
arterial injection of angiotensin. As a result of the absence of
arterial flow, venous reflux from the inferior vena cava into the
renal vein is established. Therefore one can obtain good visualisation of the venous pedicle and its tributaries. Opacification
of the intra-renal venous network is obtained using pharmaco-
angiography (intra-arterial injection of angiotensin) or by using a
catheter with a balloon which occludes the trunk of the renal vein.

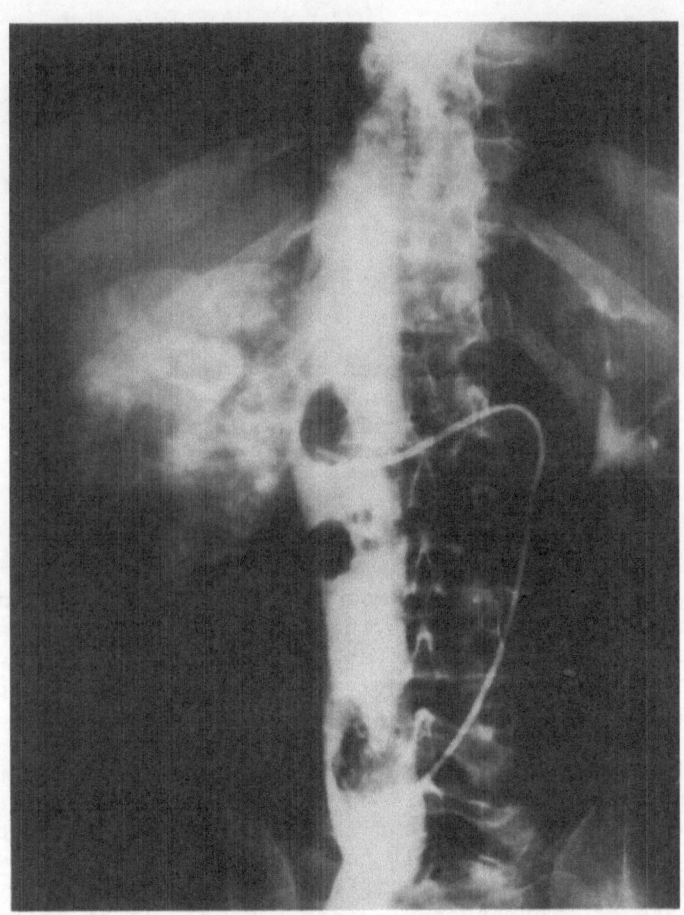

Fig. 3a.   Inferior vena cavography after puncture of the right
           femoral vein. Multiple filling defects in the vena cava
           arising from a right renal tumour. This example under-
           lines the importance of cavography before selective
           renal vein catheterisation.

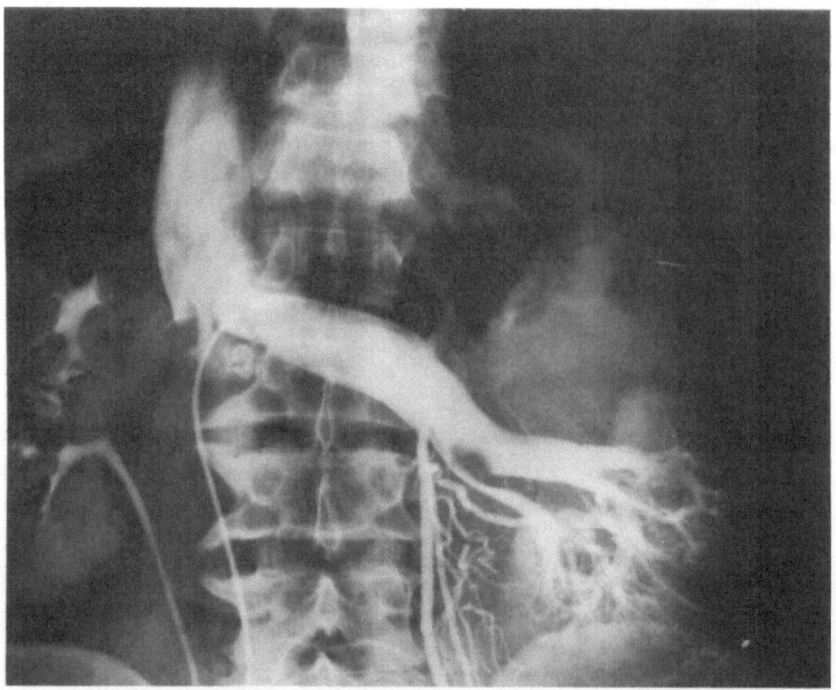

Fig. 3b.   Selective catheterisation of the left renal vein - shows
           a filling defect in a branch of the renal vein, correspond-
           ing to the region of hilar vascularity shown in the
           arteriogram in figure 2a.

RESULTS

    Invasion of the vena cava presents as a constant well defined
sometimes polycyclic space occupying lesion. A differential
diagnosis, but easy enough to establish with lateral view cavography,
is the compression of this venous axis by metastatic adenopathies
with give the false impression of space occupying lesions.

    Within the renal veins, the radiological signs of a tumour includes
irregular narrowings, interruptions of the venous axes, lateral
imprinting of the venous wall and sometimes images of different
density which are very difficult to diagnose. Certain renal vein
space occupying lesions can be difficult to understand and correspond
to the drainage of a hypervascularized tumour. It is important to
compare arteriography and selective phlebography: an accelerated
flow of venous drainage usually corresponds to hypervascularisation
at the level of the renal parenchyma, due to actual intra-tumoral
arterio-venous communications. This observation sometimes allows
one to confirm an otherwise uncertain diagnosis of cancer of the
kidney.

CONCLUSION

Plebography is no more essential than arteriography as an aid for the surgeon who is about to carry out an ablation for cancer of the kidney. However, phlebography is useful in that it allows one to appreciate the vascular extension of a cancer and to establish a rational operative approach.

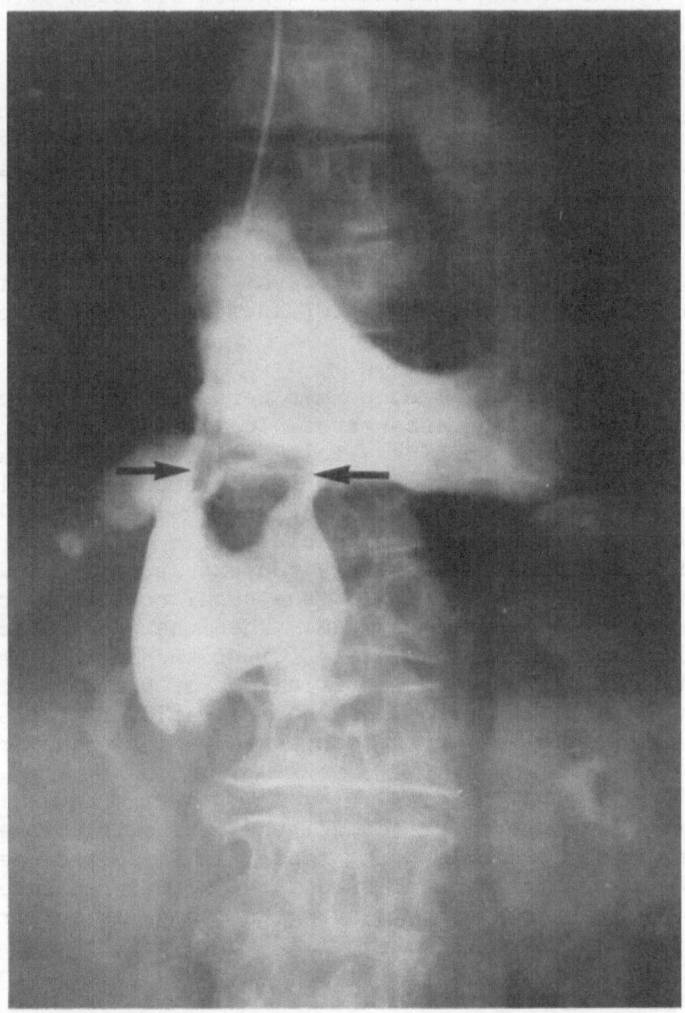

Fig. 4. Opacification of the inferior vena after catheterisation
via the superior vena cava and right auricle. The
extension into the inferior vena cava extended up to the
right auricle and is revealed by the contrast.

RADIO-ISOTOPES

Diagnosis of the Primary Tumour

Renal investigation with radiopharmaceuticals provides a reliable, easy and non invasive method for appreciating renal morphology and estimating renal function. Because of revolutionary developments in echographic techniques (specially real time scanning) and in computed X-ray tomography, the renal scan has lost some of its interest for demonstrating anatomical defects although it may be helpful as the first approach. It is however increasingly used for the determination of divided renal function.

Static renal imaging technique. Until the early 1970's, the agent used to demonstrate the renal parenchyma was usually an organic mercury compound: Neohydrin labelled with Hg 203 soon replaced by Hg 197 labelled organomercurials. The molecules are filtered through the glomeruli and tightly bound in the tubules. They show relatively slow excretion - approximately 1% per 24 hours, so that long lasting images could be obtained. However their use was limited by the unfavorable dosimetry of Hg 203 and the suboptimal energy of Hg 197.

As a result the mercurial compounds were replaced by Tc 99 m labelled renal agents, iron ascorbate - Tc 99 m, Gluconate or glucoheptonate Tc 99 m, and DTPA - Tc 99 m (diethylene triamine pentaacetic acid) which is almost completely excreted by glomerular filtration and is used as a standard of glomerular filtration rate. DMSA - Tc 99 m (dimercapto succinic acid), like chlormerodrin, shows high cortical and low medullary concentration and low urinary excretion, allowing visualisation of the renal cortex without interference by the collecting system. When the preparation is injected intravenously, approximately 50% of the administered dose is localized in the kidneys. Quantification of the uptake of DMSA into each kidney is determined and the ratio of counts in each kidney calculated so that we can estimate individual renal function.

Results. When the kidneys are normal, the uptake is homogeneous - sometimes we can see the collecting system as an area of reduced activity. When there is a renal tumor, the normal renal cells concentrate the scanning agent, leaving the tumor as an irregular area of decreased activity. Yet an image of a parenchymal defect is not specific for such a defect may also be an abscess, hematoma or a renal cyst (Figs. 5 and 6).

Diagnosis of Metastases

Pulmonary and bone metastases are quite common in renal cancers. Bone scanning is a necessary technique to ascertain the spread

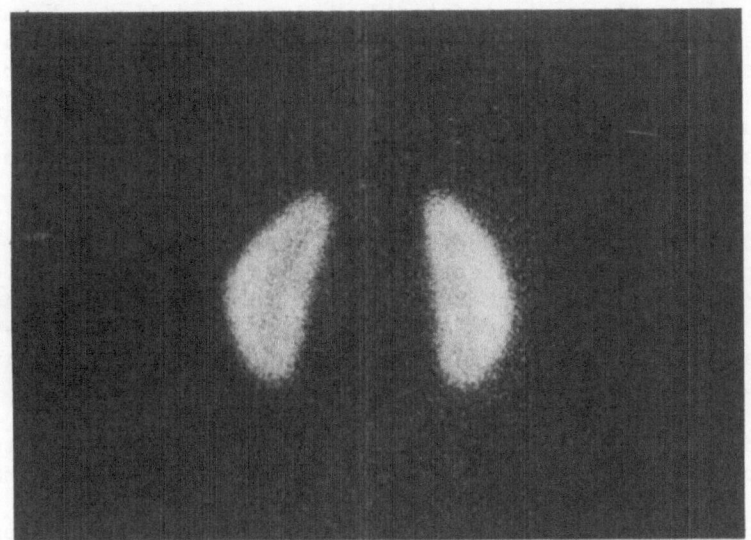

Fig. 5. Normal D.M.S.A. renal scan.

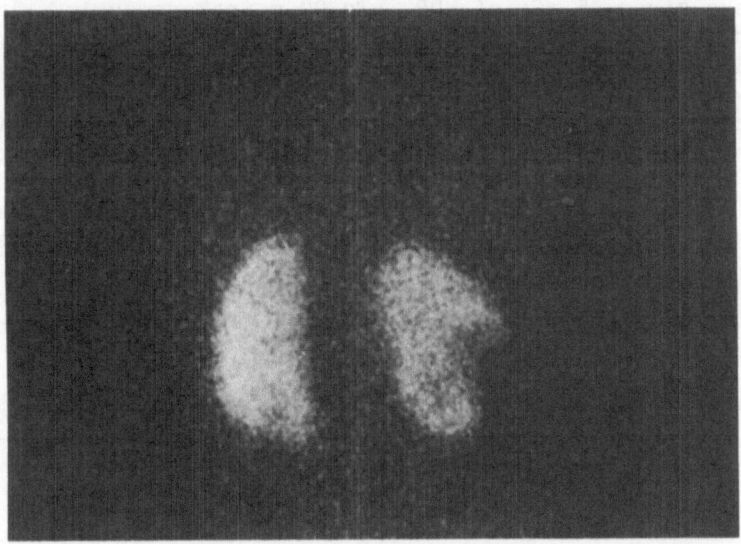

Fig. 6. D.M.S.A. renal scan showing filling defect of the infero-
lateral part of the right kidney.

of bone-seeking cancers. A bone scan proves or excludes the
diagnosis of bone metastases during the initial check-up, detects
new localisations during follow-up and allows one to evaluate the
efficiency of the treatment.

Technique. Bone tissue is constantly being remodelled. Normally
there is an equilibrium between bone crystal and blood so that the
calcium concentration in the skeleton is constant. The tumor takes
the place of the calcium in bone structure, disturbing this
equilibrium. The bone reacts by trying to lay down mineral
substances all around the lesions. The calcium balance may be
either deficient or in excess.

        For bone destruction to be demonstrable by X-rays, the
proportion of calcium in metastatic bone must be different from
that in normal tissue by about 30%. Thus the lesions are discovered
late. By using bone-seeking radio-isotopes, areas of osteolytic
activity are visualized as well as areas of osteoblastic activity.
These "hot spots" are seen early.

        The ideal isotope would be calcium 47 or calcium 45 but the
physical properties are not suitable. Ca 45 has too long a half-
life (165 days) and Ca 47 has too high γ energy (1,3 Mev).
Strontium (Sr 85 or Sr 87 m) follows calcium accurately in bone
metabolism but is not commonly used.

        The discovery of compounds of phosphate labelled with Tc 99 m
allows the widespread use of bone scans. Polyphosphate, pyro-
phosphate and mainly methyldiphosphonate (MPD) are used. The
patients are given 15 mCi of MDP - Tc 99 m intravenously. Imaging
is carried out two or three hours after injection.

        A view of the skeleton is obtained with a camera equiped with
a whole body system after which local views are recorded on film.
Besides the anatomical study, the computer gives a pathological
bone - to - normal bone ratio and a lesion - to - total activity
ratio.   This quantification allows us to follow the development
of metastases and to appreciate the efficiency of the treatment.

Results. Metastases are shown by "hot spots." These areas of
increased radioactivity are seen from three to nine months sooner
than X-ray abnormalities. For each patient the ratios are
calculated every three months. Three groups of patients are found:
those whose pathological bone - to - normal bone ratio decreases,
those whose ratio stays unchanged and those whose ratio increases.
In this last group the treatment is not effective.

SUMMARY

        Quantified bone scanning, with the computation of activity

ratios between pathological bone area and normal bone area, can be done every three months, and leads to an appreciation of the development or regression of bone metastases under treatment.

IS ARTERIOGRAPHY ANY LONGER NECESSARY IN THE ASSESSMENT OF RENAL CANCER?

S. Khoury, F. Richard and R. Küss

Hôpital de la Pitié
Paris
France

The process of diagnosis of renal tumors is usually triggered by the finding of a space occupying lesion at IVP.   In the past the definitive diagnosis of the lesions depended most of the time on surgical exploration or needle aspiration.

Later the introduction of arteriography represented a major step forward in the diagnostic field of renal tumors.   In the last few years, however, the development of ultrasonography and computerized tomography (CT scan) have dramatically changed the diagnostic approach to kidney tumors and rendered arteriography unnecessary in the majority of cases.

The diagnostic approach in kidney tumors must assure:

1.   highest confidence level

2.   least invasive diagnostic studies

3.   minimal risk to patient

4.   lowest price in time and money.

On every one of these criteria the association of ultrasonography and CT scan can score better than arteriography as we shall try to demonstrate.

In space occupying lesions of the kidney ultrasonography is a good screening study to differentiate between cysts and solid tumors. The confidence level is excellent in <u>asymptomatic</u> masses (the risk of finding a cancer is those cases is about 5%).   Under such

561

conditions an unequivocal ultrasonic diagnosis of a cyst may be
accepted as definitive.   In our experience of 220 cases there was
virtually no risk of missing a solid tumor.

If ultrasonography suggests a solid tumor and in patients with
symptomatic lesions the confidence level of ultrasonography is no
longer acceptable.   These lesions should be explored further.
Should such exploration be by arteriography, by CT scan or both?
That is the question - or more precisely that was the question, for
now we have the answer.   CT scan is the best routine exploration
for kidney tumors, arteriography being reserved as an additional
study in a few particular cases since -

(i)   CT scan can diagnose renal masses more accurately than
arteriography.

At La Pitié Hospital in Paris 137 kidney tumors were explored
by CT scan and 116 by arteriography (most of them had both investigations).   Diagnosis was ultimately confirmed by surgical exploration
and/or a two year follow up in cases not treated surgically.

This study showed that CT scan gave the exact diagnosis in 95%
of cases and arteriography in only 79% of cases (Table 1).   Details
of the seven patients with erroneous or uncertain diagnosis on CT
scan is given in Table 2.   Details of the 21 patients with an
erroneous or uncertain diagnosis at arteriography is given in Table 3.

Table 1. Diagnosis of Renal Tumors.

	CT Scan	Arteriography
No. of cases	137	116
Diagnosis accurate	130 (95%)	92 (79%)
Diagnosis erroneous or uncertain	7 (5%)	24 (21%)

Table 2. Patients in Whom Diagnosis by CT Scan
          Was Uncertain or Erroneous (7 Cases).

Diagnosis uncertain	5
Failure to differentiate benign and malignant tumors	2
False negative diagnosis of cancer	0

Table 3. Patients in Whom Diagnosis by Arteriography
Was Uncertain or Erroneous (24 cases).

Diagnosis at Arteriography		Diagnosis at Operation	
Cysts	4	Cancers	2
		Bertin *	1
		Normal	1
Cancers	4	Cysts	2
		Angiomyolipoma	1
		Normal	1
Normal	3	Transitional Cell Tumor	2
		Cancer	1
Benign Solid Tumor	1	Cancer	1

12 Lesions of Uncertain Diagnosis

* Hypertrophy of Bertin's column.

(ii) CT scan can assess abdominal disease extension in renal cancer much better than arteriography.   CT scan can study most of the parameters usually considered in the assessment of disease extension while arteriography can only explore the possibility of renal vein invasion or thrombosis (Table 4).

Table 4. Assessment of Possibility of Extension
of Disease in Malignant Renal Tumors.

	CT Scan	Arteriography
Perinephric fat	+	
Renal vein	+	+ (10/18)
Vena cava	+	
Lymph nodes	+	
Extension to adjacent organs	+	
Abdominal wall	+	
Liver metastases	+	

In our experience CT scan gave a correct appreciation of disease extension in the abdomen as confirmed at operation in 85% of
cases of renal cell carcinoma.   Arteriography gave data only on
renal vein involvement and even in this situation the information
was less accurate than that given by CT scan.   In our series arteriography diagnosed renal vein extension in 10 of the 18 surgically
documented cases showing renal vein involvement.   Without CT scan,
cavography must be used together with arteriography to achieve a
good level of confidence as far as renal venous involvement is
concerned.

(iii) CT scan is a non-invasive study and is more comfortable
and much safer than arteriography.   Despite the excellent safety
record of arteriography, complications do occur in 1-2% of cases
reported in the world literature.   In our 116 cases we had two
complications (1.8%), one of septicaemia and one of arterial thrombosis at the injection site that necessitated surgery.

(iv) CT scan is also much cheaper than arteriography (Table 5).
Furthermore, CT scan, by eliminating the need for hospitalization and
reducing the rate of complications, leads to even lower costs in both
money and time.

CONCLUSION

It is for these reasons that, at La Pitié Hospital in Paris,
CT scan is the technique used routinely in the diagnosis of renal
cancer, arteriography being reserved as an additional procedure for
the doubtful case (Fig. 1).   We must point out that arteriography
is undertaken only in 5% of cases for diagnostic purposes.   In a
further 10-15% of cases it is done mainly for therapeutic reasons
(Table 6).

Table 5.   Costs of Ultrasound, CT Scan and
           Renal Arteriography (French Francs).

Ultrasound	CT Scan	Arteriography
200 FF	600 FF	2500 FF + 2 days in Hospital

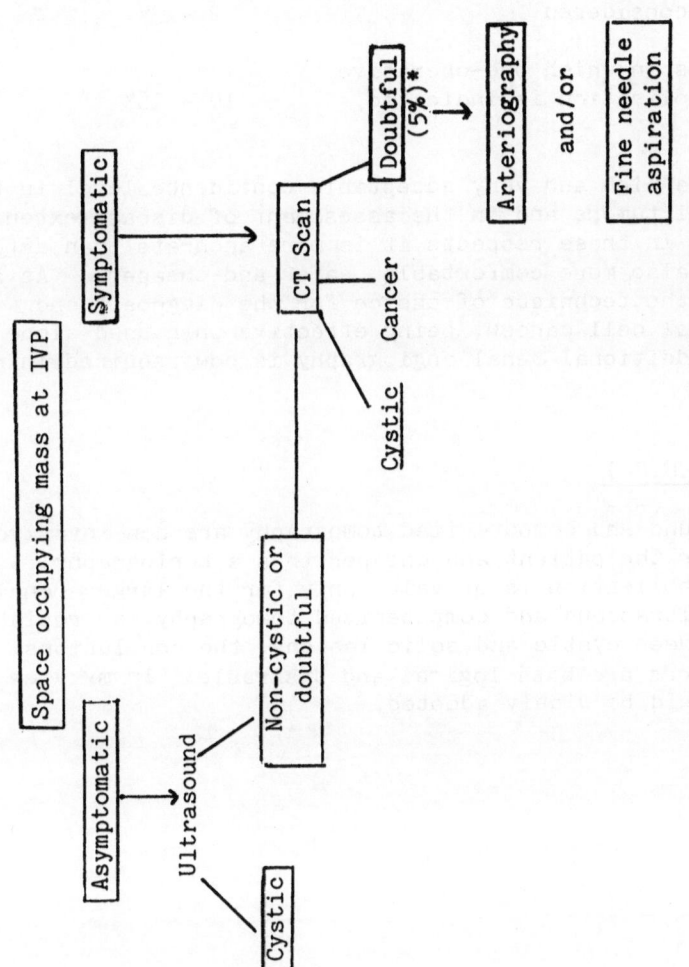

Fig. 1. A Systematic Diagnostic Approach to the Assessment of Renal Mass Lesions.

Table 6.   Indications for Arteriography

1.   Cases unconfirmed by CT Scan   5%

2.   Cases where conservative surgery
        is considered   2 - 3%

3.   Tumors in which pre-operative
        embolisation is indicated   10 - 15%

CT scan has a high and very acceptable confidence level in the diagnosis of renal tumors and in the assessment of disease extension in the abdomen.   In these respects it is more accurate than arteriography.   It is also more comfortable, safer and cheaper.   As a result is is now the technique of choice for the diagnosis and assessment of renal cell cancer, being effective when used alone in 95% of cases.   Additional renal angiography is now required in only 5% of patients.

Editorial Note (P.H.S.)

Both ultrasound and computerized tomography are non-invasive, less demanding for the patient and cheaper than arteriography. Accepting that embolization is of value only for the larger renal tumors and that ultrasound and computerized tomography can reliably differentiate between cystic and solid lesions, the conclusions drawn by the authors are both logical and desirable.   In my view this approach should be widely adopted.

ASPIRATION BIOPSY AND CYTOLOGY OF RENAL CANCER

L. Andersson, T. von Schreeb and S. Franzén

Karolinska sjukhuset
Stockholm
Sweden

INTRODUCTION

In cases of renal carcinoma, preoperative cytologic verification
of the diagnosis and assessment of the malignancy grade by aspiration
biopsy is part of our diagnostic routine. Though echotomography and
computerized tomography have reduced the need of diagnostic verification, there still remain a number of patients with a small tumour
where needle puncture is useful to distinguish between a cyst and
a tumour, sometimes a cystic tumour, and to distinguish adenocarcinoma from renal pelvic cancer. In addition aspiration biopsy
is an easy and reliable method for preoperative malignancy grading.

METHOD

In principle the technique is the same as in aspiration biopsy
of the prostate, introduced by Franzén, Giertz and Zajicek (1).

The puncture is done under television-monitored fluoroscopy and
the kidney located by intravenous urography. In recent years ultrasound scanning has been used more often than fluoroscopy. With the
patient in the prone position and local anaesthesia in the skin a
trocar with a diameter of 1.5 mm is introduced from behind. When
the tip of the trocar lies against the kidney the mandril is removed
and a long thin needle introduced. The needle is attached to a
syringe. Cellular material is aspirated from various parts of the
tumour. The smears are either air-dried and stained by the May-
Grunwald-Giemsa method or fixed in an ether-alcohol mixture and
stained by Papanicolau's technique.

To evaluate the conformity between aspiration biopsy and histo-
pathologic grading von Schreeb, Franzén and Ljungquist (2) performed
puncture of the removed kidney within five minutes of dividing the
blood vessels in 47 patients. In some cases pre-operative
percutaneous puncture was also carried out. The smears were similar
whether the puncture was done percutaneously or on the operative
specimen.

The malignancy grading was determined by a cytologist and the
histo-pathological evaluation by a separate person, a pathologist.
If the smears contained cells of varying degrees of differentiation
the most dedifferentiated cells were taken as indicating the malignancy grade. In the histo-pathological evaluation the highest
malignancy grade also determined the classification.

Table 1 shows a comparison between cytologic and histologic
malignancy grading in the 47 cases. In 36 cases there was agreement
between the cytologic and the histologic evaluation, and in 11 cases
there was a disparity, usually of one grade, but in one case of two
grades. Sometimes tumours with no marked cellular dedifferentiation
but with infiltrative growth are considered highly malignant. This
may be one explanation of the disparity in some cases. Another
explanation is the individual variation of judgement and there is
no escape from the fact that a subjective judgement is part of both
the cytologic and histo-pathologic evaluation.

Like cancer of the prostate, renal carcinoma often has different
cell patterns in different areas. The risk of having a non-
representative aspiration biopsy is however minimized by taking
material from different parts of the tumour.

Table 1.   Correlation Between Cytological and
Histological Grading in 47 Patients

Cytologic Grade	Histologic Grade		
	High	Moderate	Poor
High	4	3	1
Moderate	-	13	6
Poor	-	1	19

Table 2.   Relation between survival, degree of differentiation,
           size of tumour, and macroscopic and microscopic
           delimitation in 172 cases of renal cell cancer
           (from Arner, Blanck and von Schreeb, 1965).

	5 year survival
Histological Differentiation	
Well differentiated	82%
Moderately differentiated	50%
Poorly differentiated	15%
Size (Diameter)	
< 7 cm	69%
7 - 15 cm	40%
>15 cm	29%
Macroscopic delimitation	
Clear demarcation line	62%
No clear demarcation	39%
Microscopic delimitation	
Delimited tumours	61%
Unclear delimitation	31%

In a series of 187 cases of renal carcinoma, subjected to
nephrectomy, Arner, Blanck and von Schreeb (3)   studied the
correlation between survival and various morphologic parameters such
as the degree of cellular differentiation, tumour size and macroscopic
and microscopic delimitation of the tumour, in the 172 patients
surviving more than one month after operation. All these factors are
correlated with survival (Table 2). In the patients with poorly
differentiated carcinoma there was a higher than expected incidence
of large and poorly demarcated tumours.

Another question that has to be answered is whether puncture of the tumour implies risk of seeding tumour cells and producing metastases. In a previous series of renal cancer patients, puncture of the tumour and injection of contrast medium was performed. The needle used for injection had a larger calibre than the needle used for aspiration biopsy. Von Schreeb, Arner, Skovsted and Wikstad (4) compared the 5-year survival of 77 patients without obvious metastases and subjected to renal puncture with the survival of 73 control patients who had no puncture. When tumour size and degree of malignancy were taken into account there was no significant difference in 5-year survival between the two groups. Thus there is no reason to believe that aspiration biopsy involves risk of tumour spread.

Apart from verification of diagnosis and malignancy grading aspiration biopsy may sometimes be helpful to indicate the site of origin of a secondary tumour with a characteristic cell pattern.

SUMMARY

Fine needle aspiration biopsy was found to be a useful method of preoperative cytologic verification of the diagnosis and malignancy grading in patients with kidney tumours. The puncture is done with the aid either of ultrasound scanning or of television-monitored fluoroscopy. The relevance of cytologic grading was investigated by performing aspiration biopsy of tumours immediately after nephrectomy in 47 patients with renal cell carcinoma. In 36 cases there was conformity between the cytologic and the histo-pathologic grading. In the remaining 11 cases there was a disparity of one grade or, in one case, of two grades. There was no evidence of serious complications or tumour spread following the aspiration biopsy.

REFERENCES

1. S. Franzén, G. Giertz, and J. Zajicek, Cytological diagnosis of prostatic tumours by transrectal aspiration biopsy: A preliminary report, Brit. J. Urol. 32:193 (1960)
2. T. von Schreeb, S. Franzén, and A. Ljungquist, Renal adenocarcinoma. Evaluation of malignancy on a cytologic basis: a comparative cytologic and histologic study, Scand. J. Urol. Nephrol. 1:270 (1976).
3. O. Arner, C. Blanck, and T. von Schreeb, Renal adenocarcinoma. Morphology - grading of malignancy - prognosis. A study of 197 cases, Acta. Chir. Scand. suppl. 346:25 (1965).
4. T. von Schreeb, O. Arner, G Skovsted, and N. Wikstad, Renal adenocarcinoma. Is there a risk of spreading tumour cells in diagnostic puncture? Scand. J. Urol. Nephrol. 1:270 (1976).

DYNAMIC COMPUTED TOMOGRAPHY IN RENAL TUMORS

F. Calais da Silva,[1] and L. Aires de Sousa[2]

Civil Hospitals of Lisbon[1]
New University of Lisbon[2]
Portugal

Dynamic Computed Tomography is a method that allows the study of the circulation in both kidneys. We use a General Electric 8800 scanner with an experimental dynamic system. After injecting 50 cc of Uromiron 380 rapidly, we begin the cuts 10 seconds later. The CT scan allows us to obtain six cuts, each one in a scan time of 4.8 seconds and an interscan time of 1.2 seconds.

It is possible to obtain an incrementation scan by moving the patient in an axial direction and to obtain a succession of cuts at one centimetre intervals, or by doing the six cuts at the same anatomic level one can register a density histogram within 35 seconds.

We have applied this technique to 10 patients with renal tumors. It is possible to obtain images of the tumor's vascularization and to define a vascular pattern in the tomographic cuts. It is equally possible to characterize zones of necrosis, a technique which will be useful to control the evaluation of the embolization of tumors.

With the concentration values of contrast in an axial plan, we can construct a density histogram, to study the velocity of the intratumoral circulation, and compare zones with different circulatory velocities. This technique opens a new field in the study of tumor circulation and allows comparison with the anatomo-pathological findings. We are now trying to characterize the curves and relate them to the various types of tumors and their evolution but as yet we have insufficient data.

LIPID ANALYSIS IN CYSTIC RENAL LESIONS

H. Kleist[1], O. Jonsson[1], S. Lundstam[2], J. Nauclér[1],
A.E. Nilson[1] and S. Pettersson[1]

Sahlgrenska sjukhuset (1) and Östra sjukhuset (2)
University of Göteborg
Göteborg,   Sweden

Cystic lesions of the kidney are detected with steadily increasing frequency. Although most are benign, cause the patient no trouble and have significance only in the differential diagnosis of renal carcinoma, it must be accepted that about four per cent of renal carcinomas are cystic. Cystic renal tumours may not be possible to differentiate from benign cysts with modern radiological methods such as ultrasonography and computed tomography. The percutaneous puncture of the cystic lesion will therefore remain as an important technique in the differentiation of a benign cyst from a cystic renal tumour.

Histochemical examination of the lipid content of the cystic fluid was suggested as a possible way of differentiating malignant cystic tumours from simple benign cysts. To obtain a quantitative determination of the lipid content in renal cystic lesions 18 cystic renal tumours and 42 benign cysts were examined biochemically with regard to the total lipid and cholesterol content and the presence of atypical or malignant cells (1).

The total lipid and the cholesterol content was low in the benign cysts (0.30 $\pm$ 0.07 and 0.18 $\pm$ 0.07 mmol/1, respectively) and high in the cystic tumours (13.2 $\pm$ 3.3 and 8.5 $\pm$ 2.4 mmol/1, respectively). No cystic tumour had a total lipid value of <1.6 mmol/1 whilst 29 of 30 benign cysts had a value of <0.8 mmol/1. The cholesterol contents of cystic tumours were always >1.1 μmol/1 and those of benign cysts, with one exception, <0.7 μmol/1. Cytological examination of the fluid showed atypical cells in only two out of 11 cystic tumours.

It is concluded that analysis of the lipid content may increase

the accuracy in the differential diagnosis between renal cysts and
cystic renal tumours. A low lipid value speaks strongly for a
benign cyst. A high lipid value is likely to represent a malignant
lesion, though a false positive lipid test may be obtained in
inflammatory or hemorrhagic cysts. In this study the reliability of
the cholesterol and total lipid estimation was equal and it therefore
seems sufficient to analyze the cholesterol content of the aspirated
cyst fluid, a technique which is available in most clinical chemical
laboratories.

REFERENCE

1. H. Kleist, O. Jonsson, S. Lundstam, J. Nauclér, A.E. Nilson, and
    S. Pettersson, Quantitative lipid analysis in the differential
    diagnosis of cystic renal lesions, Brit. J. Urol (1981).

CANCER OF THE KIDNEY: STAGING

G.D. Chisholm, J.R. Hindmarsh, D.C. Grieve

Western General Hospital.
Edinburgh
Scotland

Staging methods for carcinoma of the kidney continue to be debated due mainly to the difficulty in characterising any deep seated tumour and especially one that is located in the retro-peritoneum. The main staging system, widely used in Europe and N. America, was popularised by Robson et al (1). Four stages are described:-

Stage 1: Tumour within the capsule of the kidney
Stage 2: Tumour has invaded the perinephric fat but is confined within Gerota's fascia
Stage 3: Tumour involvement of regional nodes and/or renal vein and cava
Stage 4: Tumour involves adjacent organs or there are distant metastases

This staging system is based mainly on the pathological findings but it also relies to some extent on the description by the surgeon and the extent of the operative procedure in obtaining lymph nodes from at least the para-aortic region. But the final arbiter is the pathologist who can define precisely the extent of the renal capsular involvement and spread of tumour into the renal vein.

An alternative classification for this tumour was introduced by the UICC using the TNM categories.

The current TNM pretreatment clinical classification is as follows:-

TO   no evidence of primary tumour.
T1   evidence of a small tumour without enlargement of the

kidney. There is limited calyceal distortion or deformity
and circumscribed vascular deformities surrounded by renal
parenchyma.

T2   evidence of a large tumour with deformity and/or enlargement
     of the kidney or calyceal or pelvic involvement. The con-
     tinuity of the cortex is preserved on arteriography.

T3   evidence of spread into perinephric fat, peripelvic fat or
     hilar renal vessels.

T4   evidence of extension into neighbouring organs or abdominal
     wall.

TX   the minimum requirements to assess the primary tumour cannot
     be met.

T CATEGORY

By definition, a T category is a <u>clinical</u> pre-operative assessment of a tumour but from the beginning it was evident that this
would be difficult to apply. Urologists recognise the almost impossible task of assessing the size of a kidney clinically and even a
kidney mass cannot be judged reliably by palpation; thus any attempt
to obtain a T category by this method alone would be doomed. With
the increasing use of arteriography and selective renal angiography
it was decided to include this investigation in the minimum requirements for a T category when this tumour site was first classified by
the UICC in 1973.

Few studies have looked at the usefulness of angiography in
determining a T category, probably because in practice most urologists prefer to wait for the pathologist's report before giving a
post surgical histopathological classification.

In 1977 Das et al (2) reported a study which examined the
accuracy of renal angiography. Thirty-six patients underwent
selective renal angiography prior to nephrectomy for a renal carcinoma. The radiological T category was then compared with the pathological findings in the specimen.

The results showed that there was agreement of T and P category
in 21/36 (58%); there was false pre-operative overstaging in 8/36
(22%) i.e. T ⋗ P; there was a false pre-operative understaging in
6/36 (16%) i.e. T ⋖ P; in one patient the tumour was not diagnosed
on the angiogram. There was therefore a substantial error when
angiography was used to obtain an improved reliability of the T
category.

Because selective angiography is now recognised to be so inaccurate, other imaging techniques have been suggested to improve the
value of a T category. In recent years ultrasound has become a most
important method for the investigation of renal masses but its

special value lies in the distinction of solid from cystic masses. Ultrasound can give useful information about other abnormalities in the retroperitoneum but cannot give the precision to the extent of tumour spread that is required for staging (3).

Computed tomography (CT) is increasingly used to determine the extent of renal tumours (4,5) and a recent report by Khoury (6) indicates an extremely high degree of reliability in staging renal tumours using CT alone.

In a comparative study of the use of CT and ultrasound for staging renal carcinoma Levine et al (7) showed that CT was capable of detecting tumour invasion of perinephric fat and adjacent muscles which could not (usually) be shown by ultrasound. Both CT and ultrasound demonstrated venous and retroperitoneal tumour extension but CT was more reliable because bowel gas often obscured the retroperitoneum for ultrasound scanning. These authors concluded that while ultrasound was helpful in determining the extent of a tumour, CT was the better method for staging purposes.

N CATEGORY

The minimum requirements for N category comprise clinical examination, urography and lymphography (8). Unfortunately, the reliability of these methods is seriously in doubt as indeed are most pedal lymphograms when it comes to providing a reliable measure of lymph node metastases.

In an early study by Hulter et al (9) the lymphographic findings correlated poorly with histologically proved metastases and false positive as well as false negative lymphographic signs occurred frequently. In this study of 22 patients, a retroperitoneal lymph node dissection provided information not only on the correlation with lymphography but also on the site of positive lymph nodes in relation to the renal tumour; the authors demonstrated that if lymph nodes are to be removed as part of a radical nephrectomy, then the dissection should include not only the lumbar nodes bilaterally but also the nodes along the common iliac vessels at least on the homolateral side.

More recent studies of lymph nodes (10) have shown the inaccuracy of pedal lymphography in renal carcinoma and emphasised that the information gained from lymphography has little effect on the treatment. Even the role of lymphadenectomy in renal carcinoma is debatable (11); the procedure provides staging information but whether or not it influences results is uncertain. Survival rates with and without lymphadenectomy suggest that lymphadenectomy enhances survival but the data suffers from being retrospective and not randomised. Thus, the use of node dissection for staging as the possible benefit in treatment has yet to gain general acceptance.

M CATEGORY

The minimum requirements for M category now comprise clinical examination, radiography and, in the more advanced primary tumours or when clinical suspicion warrants, radiographic or radioisotopic studies are recommended. Metastases from renal carcinoma arise most frequently in the lungs followed by the lymph nodes, bones and adrenals. Thus, radiological,and radioisotopic bone studies,are still the main methods for diagnosing and monitoring metastases.

There is at present no tumour "marker" that can be used in this tumour. A variety of abnormalities have been described in association with renal tumours (12) but either they are non specific or the incidence of the abnormality is too infrequent to be of clinical use (13,14).

CONCLUSIONS

The importance of staging tumours is not in doubt but it is evident that attempts to apply the TNM principles have added little to the reliability of staging renal tumours. Recent reports now show that CT provides the best information for a T category but it would make no sense to include this as a minimum requirement as CT is not yet widely available in the Western world and the accuracy of staging described, requires up-to-date CT equipment. However the TNM classification does allow for the inclusion of a C-Factor which refers to the level of certainty. It reflects the information at a point in time and according to the diagnostic methods employed. Degrees of C may be applied to the T, N and M categories and in this way those centres in which special diagnostic methods are available can identify the precision of their categorisation.

Both N and M categories are seen to be very weak in their diagnostic accuracy and reliability. It is hoped that in future years, it might be possible to incorporate some aspect of the paraneoplastic syndromes into diagnosis and monitoring of the tumour, or preferably, a specific tumour marker may be identified.

Meanwhile, the clinician must continue to use the best investigative techniques available to him in order to characterise the extent of the tumour prior to nephrectomy and then to use the evidence provided by the pathologist to place the tumour in the correct stage or pT category.

REFERENCES

1.   C.J. Robson, B.M. Churchill, and W. Anderson, The results of radical nephrectomy for renal cell carcinoma, J. Urol. 101: 297 (1969).

2.   G. Das, G.D. Chisholm, and T. Sherwood, Can angiography stage
     renal carcinoma? Brit. J. Urol. 49: 611 (1977).
3.   N.F. Maklad, V.P. Chuang, B.O. Doust, K.J. Cho, and J.E. Curran,
     Ultrasonic characterization of solid renal lesions: echographic
     angiographic and pathologic correlation, Radiology 123:
     733 (1977).
4.   E. Levine, N.F. Maklad, S.J. Rosenthal, K.R. Lee, and J. Weighel,
     Comparison of computed tomography and ultrasound in abdominal
     staging of renal cancer, Urology 16: 317 (1980).
5.   L. Love, C.J. Reynes, R. Churchill, and R. Moncada, Third gener-
     ation CT scanning in renal disease, Radiol. Clin. N. Am. 17:
     77 (1979).
6.   S. Khoury, F. Richard, and R. Küss, Is arteriography necessary
     any longer in the assessment of renal cancer? in: "Cancer of
     the Prostate and Kidney," P.H. Smith and M. Pavone-Macaluso,
     eds., Plenum Publishing Company, London and New York (1982).
7.   E. Levine, K.R. Lee and J. Weighel, Pre-operative determination
     of abdominal extent of renal cell carcinoma by computed tomog-
     raphy, Radiology 132: 395 (1979).
8.   UICC, TNM Classification of Malignant Tumours, 3rd edition,
     Geneva, UICC (1978).
9.   L. Hulten, M. Rosencrantz, T. Seeman, L. Wahlquist, and
     C. Ahren, Occurrence and localisation of lymph node metastases
     in renal carcinoma, Scand. J. Urol. Nephrol. 3: 129 (1969).
10. M.D. Cosgrove and C.K. Metzger, Lymphangiography in genito-
     urinary cancer, J. Urol. 113: 93 (1975).
11. P.C. Peters and G.L. Brown, The role of lymphadenectomy in the
     management of renal cell carcinoma, Urol. Clin. N. Am. 7: 705
     (1980).
12. G.D. Chisholm, Clinical and biochemical markers in renal carci-
     noma, in: "Renal Adenocarcinoma," UICC Report No. 10,
     G. Sufrin and S.A. Beckley, eds., UICC, Geneva (1980), p. 182.
13. G.D. Chisholm, J.R. Hindmarsh, and T.B. Hargreave, The effect
     of embolisation/nephrectomy for renal carcinoma on the para-
     neoplastic syndromes, in "Cancer of the Prostate and Kidney,"
     P.H. Smith and M. Pavone-Macaluso, eds., Plenum Publishing
     Company, London and New York (1982).
14. M.R.G. Robinson, D. Daponte, and C. Chandrasekaran, Carcinoma
     of the kidney: biological markers, in: "Cancer of the Prostate
     and Kidney," P.H. Smith and M. Pavone-Macaluso, eds., Plenum
     Publishing Company, London and New York (1982).

HISTOPATHOLOGY AND NUCLEAR GRADING IN RENAL CELL NEOPLASMS

M. Tannenbaum and S. Tannenbaum

Columbia-Presbyterian Medical Center
New York
U.S.A.

INTRODUCTION

In most series of renal adenocarcinomas the overall ten year
survival rate is between 18 and 27% (1). Considering that nephrectomy is frequently performed under adverse circumstances and in
spite of metastasis at the time of surgery, the overall survival is
still very high as compared to many other cancers with a similar
clinical stage. This supports the belief that these tumors are
usually slow growing. The poor prognosis is usually not solely attributable to aggressiveness but rather to the large sizes that these
tumors can attain, the frequency of metastases being responsible for
the presenting symptomatology, and the extensive delay before the
patient seeks medical aid (2).

The most important gross features that these kidney tumors
exhibit and which can be related to prognosis have been incorporated
into a very comprehensive and relatively accurate staging system (3).
These features relate primarily to the importance of renal vein and
perinephric fat invasion. The most comprehensive staging system is
that of Robson and associates (4). In their experience, perinephric
fat invasion is less important than renal vein involvement; this is
reflected in their staging system. We should consider their system
in its entirety because it can be related to histological grading.
We would like first to consider several features in relation to the
gross specimen which should be described in the surgical pathology
report because, in many instances, it does relate very closely to
the prognosis.

SURGICAL PATHOLOGY GROSS SPECIMEN FEATURES

Number and Location of Tumors

The differences in number are not great and, at this time, the location of the tumors at either the upper or lower pole does not appear to alter prognosis. The presence of calcification is of very little prognostic significance (5).

Size

There are numerous reports demonstrating that the larger the renal tumor, the worse is the prognosis (6,7). However, the greater the size of the tumor, the greater is the likelihood that there will be vascular invasion, associated local extension and metastases to other parts of the body (8).

Local Extension

If the tumor is well circumscribed and expecially of low grade, then the patient's prognosis is very good. However extension beyond the renal capsule adversely effects patient survival. Kaufman has reported a 56% ten year survival in the absence of perirenal invasion as against 14% with invasion (1). The clinical outcome has an even more ominous prognosis when the tumor, either grossly or microscopically, is seen to infiltrate the surrounding renal parenchyma.

Renal Vein Invasion

Patients with renal vein involvement have a significantly worse prognosis than those whose tumors are confined to the kidney (8). Renal vein invasion however seems to be less important than perirenal invasion (1,5,6), contrary to the views of Robson et al (4).

Regional Lymph Node Metastasis

When the regional lymph nodes are involved, we can expect the same prognosis as that seen in the presence of renal vein invasion (4).

HISTOLOGICAL GRADING AND MICROSCOPIC FEATURES
OF RENAL CARCINOMAS

It is generally agreed that compared to most other carcinomas, renal carcinomas are usually well differentiated with relatively little pleomorphism of their nuclei (2). The cells will usually demonstrate an occasional mitosis. Riches (9) graded 110 renal adenocarcinomas histologically and found that 45% were well differentiated, 36% were of intermediary differentiation and only 18%

were poorly differentiated or pleomorphic. There are many variegated patterns and sometimes histological features can be found. As a consequence, some authors (9,10) have tried to classify these neo- plasms on the basis of cell type and light histology configurations. Many classifications have arisen and are based upon the presence of cystic, solid, tubular, as well as papillary patterns. None has shown an improved statistical correlation with survival. In addition a predominance of clear or granular cell types does not seem to have any prognostic significance (11). Bennington and Beckwith (2) in their extensive monograph on tumors of the kidney, renal pelvis and ureter, have also expressed the opinion that neither the presence of clear or granular cells nor the patterns of organization, i.e. cystic, tubular or papillary, has any prognostic significance. They are also of the opinion that histological grading can be used to assess prognosis but that it has no greater accuracy than staging. In their opinion and that of these authors, it usually requires exten- sive sampling of every tumor and considerable experience for the histological grade to be reliably assessed. Mostofi (12) has also extensively reviewed the subject of histological grading and he states that "grading is both difficult and of very little value" and as a result, he classifies renal adenocarcinomas as either well differentiated or not well differentiated.

     In general, it appears that in the majority of kidney carcinomas which are not Robson stage 1, it is more important to assess prognosis on the basis of further staging, i.e. tumor size, extent of local invasion, vascular involvement and metastases. Many authors (13,14) are of the opinion that it requires less experience, is less time consuming and correlates better with survival than does histological grade. However, with the combined approach of careful physical workups, IVP and urinary cytology, it is possible to detect many more kidney tumors at an early stage. Consequently, there can be an increase in the detection of stage 1 kidney tumors, as has been seen at our institution in the last few years when compared to thirty years ago. It is hoped that quicker and more careful fixation of the surgical specimens will assist computer-based systems in analyzing the multiple variants found both in the gross specimen and in the histological and cytological features of the tumor (15). It is anticipated that there will be a greater degree of accuracy in estimating prognosis if one can numerically assign exact values rather than subjective values for grading renal tumors.

NUCLEAR GRADING AND STAGE IN PROGNOSIS

     Three different groups of workers have attempted to correlate the various stages of kidney carcinomas with nuclear grade and size and to associate this with prognosis (16-18). Fuhrman and Limas (16) have reported recently that morphological parameters are of prog- nostic significance in renal cell carcinomas. Their study evaluated 76 cases of renal cell carcinoma. They classified their tumors in regard to size, cellular arrangement and type (solid, papillary, tubular; clear versus dark) and nuclear grades from 1 - 4. The grade 1 tumors had small nuclei roughly the size of red blood cells with no nucleoli. Grade 2 tumors were twice the size of red blood cells and had very prominent nucleoli. Grade 3 were much larger and had very dark staining nucleoli. Grade 4 were spindle-shaped cells. In their hands, nuclear grading was superior to all other parameters in predicting the development of metastases following radical nephrectomy. When patients with stage 1 tumors were considered (43 cases), none of the grade 1 tumors (9 cases) developed metastases whereas 60% of the grades 2 - 4 did. It was also noted that there was a significant difference in the subsequent metastatic rates for stage 1 tumors when grade 1, as distinct from grade 2, neoplasms were compared (0% metastases for grade 1 and 50% metastases in grade 2).

Fuhrman and Limas also noted that there was an apparent relationship between cell type and prognosis but as a function of nuclear grade and not an independent variable. As an example - in clear cell carcinomas of the kidney, 68% were other than grade 1 and 44% developed metastases. Of the exclusively dark cell tumors, 92% were greater than grade 1 and 81% of them were metastatic. They also noted that their tumors were, in all instances, greater than 3 cm in size with 77% being over 5 cm and 36% being over 8 cm. There was a positive correlation between the size and stage of the tumor at the time of diagnosis but the size of the stage 1 tumors did not correlate with the subsequent development of metastases. Of the parameters which they studied, grade alone was significant in predicting the outcome of stage 1 renal cell carcinomas.

Gilchrist et al (17) retrospectively studied nuclear size as a prognostic discriminator in 44 renal cell carcinomas of Robson stage 1, 2 or 3. They wanted to determine if easily reproducible histological parameters could more finely discriminate for survival than pathological staging. Nuclear grading by relative size was examined at 10 - 20 magnifications. Similar nuclei were essentially equal in size but dissimilar nuclei were greater than twice the length or width of neighboring nuclei. Regions within one field of tumor necrosis were not studied. The designation of nuclear sizing in their study was based on the deviation in nuclear sizes after examination of every available histological section within the primary carcinomas. Correlation of nuclear size with numerous clinical features in their study was unrewarding. Their dissimilar nuclear sizes could not predict any possibility of distant metastases. In another study by Leiber et al (18), 90 cases of exclusively well differentiated eosinophilic granular renal cell carcinomas were studied. They excluded the higher grade tumors, i.e. grades 3 and 4. The clinical, laboratory, pathological and survival features of these patients were analyzed. Their tumors were identified mainly according to cytological features in terms of grading. Grade 1 oncocytic neoplasms or granular cell tumors were composed of closely similar cells

possessing round smooth nuclei and abundant eosinophilic cytoplasm.
The grade 2 tumors had larger, more irregular nuclei and there was
more variation among cells in size and configuration. The grade 3
neoplasms represented a further extension of the morphological depar-
ture from normal and featured very variable cells often with bizarre
nuclear forms. Mitotic figures were abundant in this grade of tumor.
The authors noted that 62 patients had grade 1 tumor and 28 patients
had grade 2 tumors. None of the patients with grade 1 tumors developed metastases. However, 4 of the patients with grade 2 tumors died
of metastatic disease. Survival curves showed no differences between
patients with these renal tumors and age- and sex-matched controls.

SUMMARY

    At the present time, not only is careful processing of the
surgical specimens necessary for determining whether there is any
renal parenchyma or fat invasion but the diagnosis should also be
expressed in terms of grade, especially where the tumor is well
encapsulated and a Robson stage 1. The burden of evidence at the
present time seems to indicate that the higher the grade of the
tumor, especially the stage 1 tumor, the greater is the possibility
that these types of tumors will have a worse prognosis in the
distant future.

    With the advent and use of more definitive morphological instru-
mentation and analysis, differences in nuclear size and/or surface
area can be computerized. The future use of this approach appears
very hopeful. The prognosis of the various stages of the tumor as
they correlate with nuclear grade and histological stage, provided
there is adequate tissue sectioning, can be assessed more critically
and in a more objective statistical fashion.

REFERENCES

1. J.J. Kaufman, Reasons for nephrectomy. Palliative and curative,
    J.A.M.A. 204: 607 (1968).
2. J.L. Bennington and J.C. Beckwith, Atlas of Tumor Pathology:
    Tumors of the Kidney, Renal Pelvis, and Ureter, Armed Forces
    Institute of Pathology, Washington, D.C. (1975).
3. J.M. Holland, Cancer of the kidney - Natural history and
    staging, Cancer 32: 1030 (1973).
4. C.J. Robson, B.M. Churchill, and W. Anderson, The results of
    radical nephrectomy for renal cell carcinoma, J. Urol. 101:
    297 (1969).
5. I.H. Griffiths, "Monographs on Neoplastic Disease at Various
    Sites, Vol. V, Tumours of the Kidney and Ureter,", Williams &
    Wilkins Co., Baltimore (1964).
6. O. Arner, C. Blanck, and T. von Schreeb, Renal adenocarcinoma;
    morphology-grading of malignancy-prognosis, Acta Chir. Scand.
    (Suppl.) 346: 1 (1975).

7.   S. Kay, Renal carcinoma. A 10-year study, Am. J. Clin. Pathol.
     50: 428 (1968).
8.   E.T. Bell, "Renal Disease," Lea & Febiger, Philadelphia (1950).
9.   E.W. Riches, "Monographs on Neoplastic Disease at Various Sites,
     Vol. V, Tumours of the Kidney and Ureter," Williams & Wilkins
     Co., Baltimore (1964).
10. M.M. Melicow and A.C. Uson, Nonurologic symptoms in patients
     with renal cancer, J.A.M.A. 172: 146 (1960).
11. L.E. Bottiger, C. Blanc, and T. von Schreeb, Renal carcinoma.
     An attempt to correlate symptoms and findings with the histo-
     pathologic picture, Acta Med. Scand. 180: 329 (1966).
12. F.K. Mostofi,"Pathology and Spread of Renal Cell Carcinoma,"
     Little Brown & Co. Inc., Boston (1967).
13. R.H. Flocks and M.C. Kadesky, Malignant neoplasms of the kidney:
     an analysis of 353 patients followed five years or more,
     J. Urol. 79: 196 (1958).
14. S.D. Petkovic, An anatomical classification of renal tumors in
     the adult as a basis for prognosis, J. Urol. 81: 618 (1959).
15. H.R. Newman and M.L. Schulman, Renal cortical tumors: a 40-year
     study, Urol. Survey 19: 2 (1969).
16. S.A. Fuhrman and C. Limas, Prognostic significance of morpho-
     logic parameters in renal cell carcinoma, Lab. Invest. 44:
     22A (Abs.) (1981).
17. K.W. Gilchrist, T.F. Hogan, and J. Harberg, Simplified assess-
     ment as a prognostic discriminant in renal cell carcinoma,
     Lab. Invest. 44: 22A (Abs.) (1981).
18. M.M. Lieber, K.M. Tomera, and G.M. Farrow, Renal oncocytoma,
     J. Urol. 125: 481 (1981).

PROGNOSTIC RELEVANCE OF CYTOLOGIC GRADING IN METASTATIC RENAL CELL CARCINOMA

H. Rauschmeier, F. Hofstädter and G. Jakse

University of Innsbruck
Innsbruck
AUSTRIA

INTRODUCTION

In 1932 Hand and Broders stressed the importance in renal cell carcinoma (RCC) of tumor grading in predicting the course of the disease (1) and since then many authors have agreed with that point of view. This observation has induced a previous retrospective study at our department, which included 121 patients who had been treated by radical nephrectomy for RCC (2). At the time of diagnosis 52 patients had metastases. Of these 42 were operated on. In this study we have investigated the survival of these 42 patients in accordance with the histologic tumor grade. The Erlangen histological grading system, proposed by Hermanek and coworkers in 1976 (3), is based on the criteria shown in Table 1. Comparing these different histologic grades with regard to prognosis (fig. 1), we find that the one-year survival rate is significantly worse in G3 tumors than in G2. The difference between G1 and G2 tumors is not statistically significant, possibly due to the small number of patients with G1 lesions.

Thus, if the grade of tumor differentiation could be assessed pre-operatively, a high malignancy grade in metastatic RCC would be of great influence on further therapeutic procedures.

For pre-operative diagnostic assessment of the tumor grade, cytologic specimens obtained by percutaneous fine needle biopsy seems to be the most satisfactory (4), though the reliability of cytologic methods in relation to the histologic evaluation should first be examined. We have attempted to compare the cytological and histological findings in this study.

Table 1. The Erlangen System of Histologic Grading
          of Malignancy in Renal Cell Carcinoma.

Grade 1:   Solid tumors consisting of clear
           and intermediate cells, adenomas
           of doubtful malignancy.

Grade 3:   Tumors of glandular or glandular-
           papillary pattern, tumors showing
           exclusively granular cells or
           sarcoma-like areas.

Grade 2:   All other malignant parenchymal
           tumors.

MATERIAL AND METHODS

    One hundred and five aspiration biopsies were carried out on the
surgical specimens of 21 patients, who had had operations for renal
tumors, using the technique of Franzén and coworkers (5).

    The smear was stained according to the May-Grünwald-Giemsa tech-
nique and classified as proposed by Papanicolaou.   Tumors were classified into two groups of low and high malignancy.   The smear was
then decolourised and stained with Feulgen-reagent.   Thereafter DNA
single cell cytophotometry was performed on a Reichert-Densitometer$^{(R)}$
with connected Hewlett-Packard-computer$^{(R)}$.

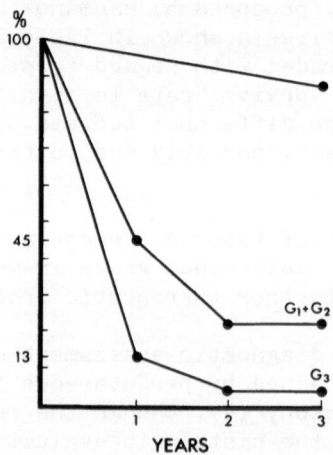

Fig. 1. Survival Rate by Grade in 42 Patients with Metastatic Renal
         Cell Carcinoma (Difference at one year, G2 versus G3,
         p = 0.05).

The classification of the histological specimens was made according to the Erlangen system as mentioned above (Table 1), but based on the non-significant difference in survival rates (fig. 1) grade 1 and 2 tumors were grouped together for correlation with the two classes of cytologic malignancy.

RESULTS

Twenty-one tumor specimens were evaluated. Tumor cells were found in 92 of 105 (87.6%) preparations. Cells of renal cell carcinoma were always identified without doubt.

In cytologic assessment there were 14 tumors of low and seven of high malignancy. On histologic grading, we found 13 grade 1 or 2 and eight grade 3 tumors. If we correlated these two examinations for each tumor, we found corresponding results in 12 tumors with grade 1 or 2 lesions and six in grade 3 tumors (fig. 2) to give a positive correlation rate of 85.7%.

In an attempt to obtain objective results DNA-cytophotometry was performed on cytological specimens. Table 2 shows postulated DNA-distribution for each malignancy grade, according to our previous work (6).

Grade 1 tumor cells (fig. 3) should have a DNA-distribution pattern like normal cells, e.g. leucocytes, in the histogram. The main DNA-content lies about the 2c-value and a tumor stemline cannot be identified. Therefore, SQ, the stemline quotient (which is the value of the tumor DNA-stemline divided by normal DNA-stemline) is about 1.0. The number of tetraploid tumor cells is not significant; therefore, the diploid deviation quotient (DDQ) is also about 1.0. (The DDQ is the average DNA-content per cell divided by normal DNA-value).

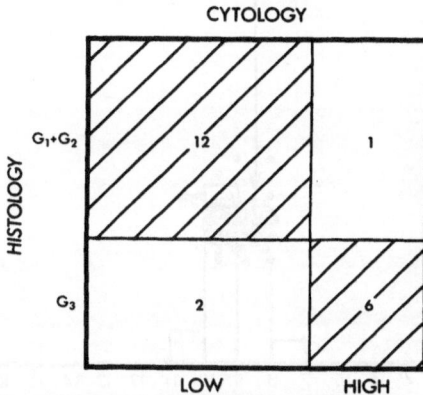

Fig. 2. Correlation Between Malignancy Grading, Obtained by Histologic Versus Cytologic Assessment in 21 Patients. A Positive Correlation was Found in 85.7% of Cases.

Table 2.   Postulated DNA-Distribution Pattern
According to Malignancy Grade in RCC

Grade 1 :   2c - (4c)   SQ = 1.0 $\pm$ 0.2   DDQ = 1.0 $\pm$ 0.2

Grade 2 :   2c - 4c   SQ = 1.0 $\pm$ 0.2   DDQ $\geqq$ 1.2

Grade 3 : .3c....6c..   SQ > 1.2   DDQ > 1.2

Grade 2 tumors (fig. 4) must also show a unimodal DNA-distribution with a SQ about 1.0, but as an expression of their higher proliferation rate, they should have a clearly distinguishable peak at
the 4c-value (DDQ is higher than 1.0).

Finally, grade 3 carcinoma cells (fig. 5) are postulated to have
a bimodal distribution pattern with an own tumor stemline, e.g. at
the 3c-value (SQ higher than 1.2) and another peak for instance at
the 6c-value (DDQ also higher than 1.2).

The two tumors of the study (fig. 2), which gave false negative
results on cytological examination were checked by measurements of
DNA-content.   There we saw DNA-distribution patterns identical with
those found in G3 tumors.   This means that the high malignancy of
these RCC was missed by standard cytology but was identified by cytophotometry.   By combining cytophotometry with cytology, the correla-

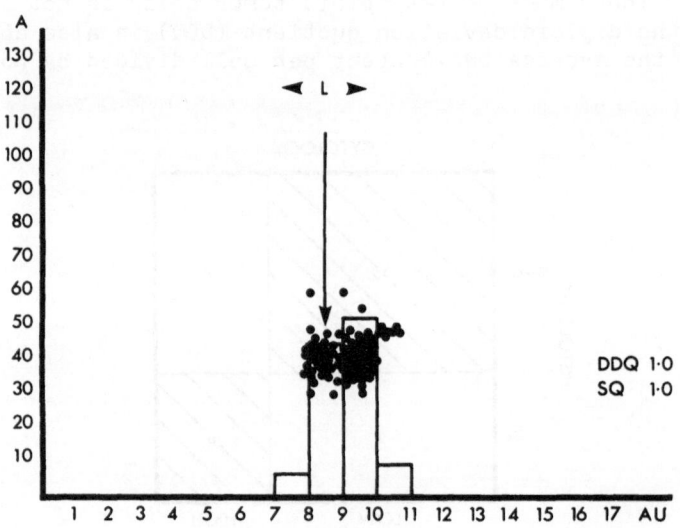

Fig. 3.   DNA Cytophotometry in a Patient with a G1 Renal Cell
Carcinoma.

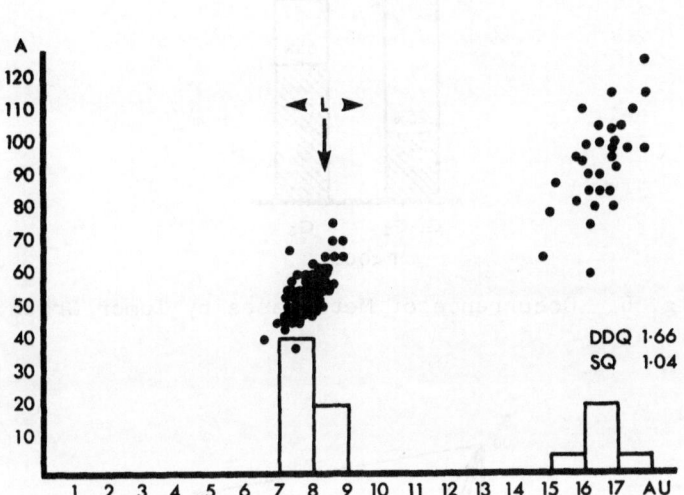

Fig. 4.   DNA Cytophotometry in a Patient with a G2 Renal Cell
          Carcinoma.

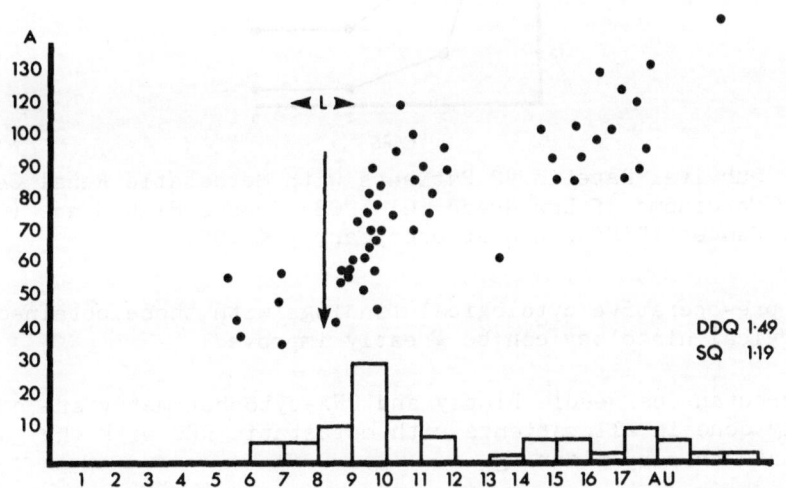

Fig. 5.   DNA Cytophotometry in a Patient with a G3 Renal Cell
          Carcinoma.

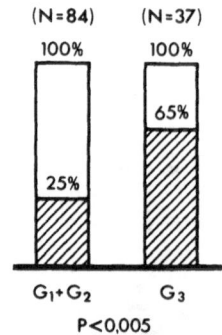

Fig. 6.   Occurrence of Metastases by Tumor Grade.

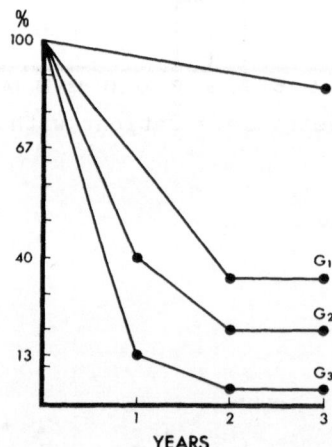

Fig. 7.   Survival Rate in 42 Patients with Metastatic Renal Cell
          Carcinoma of Low Grade (Gl + G2) Versus High Grade (G3)
          Cancer (Difference at one year, p <0.05).

tion of pre-operative cytological findings with those obtained by
post-surgical histology can be greatly improved.

    Percutaneous needle biopsy and DNA-cytophotometry are now
routinely done in all patients with metastatic RCC with the goal of
an adequate therapy planning.

    In our clinical follow up study mentioned above we have also
found a significantly higher tendency to formation of metastases in
patients with highly malignant tumors (fig. 6).   Considering this
and the significantly lower one-year survival rate (fig. 7) in
patients with metastatic G3 tumors compared to metastatic Gl and G2

tumors the importance of a reliable method for evaluation of tumor grading prior to any invasive therapeutic procedure is obvious. Possibly those patients with extremely poor prognosis (G3 tumors) should be excluded from surgical therapy except in cases of uncontrollable bleeding or pain.

CONCLUSIONS

In conclusion there are four points to be stressed:

1. tumor grade is an important factor for survival time.

2. percutaneous needle biopsy should be performed in RCC to assess tumor grade pre-operatively.

3. DNA-cytophotometry can improve cytological results, and

4. patients with poorly differentiated metastatic tumors should perhaps not be submitted to radical nephrectomy.

REFERENCES

1. J.R. Hand and A.C. Broders, Carcinoma of the Kidney: Degree of Malignancy in Relation to Factors Bearing on Prognosis, J. Urol. 28:199 (1932).
2. W. Pauer, G. Mikuz and G. Jakse, Ist Die Nephrektomie Beim Metastasierenden Nierenzellkarzinom sinnvoll? Akt. Urol. in press (1981).
3. P. Hermanek, A. Sigel and S. Chlepas, Histological Grading of Renal Cell Carcinoma, Eur. Urol. 2:189 (1976).
4. V.T. Schreeb, O. Arner, G. Skovsted and N. Wikstad, Renal Adenocarcinoma: Is There a Risk of Spreading Tumor Cells in Diagnostic Puncture? Scand. J. Urol. Nephrol. 1:270 (1967).
5. S. Franzén, G. Giertz and J. Zajicek, Cytological Diagnosis of Prostatic Tumors by Transrectal Aspiration Biopsy: A Preliminary Report, Brit. J. Urol. 32:193 (1960).
6. F. Hofstädter and P. Ehlich, DNS-Feulgenzytophotometrie bei Nierenparenchymkarzinomen Verschiedenen Malignitätsgrades, Verh. Dtsch. Ges. Path. 62:375 (1978).

PROGNOSTIC FACTORS IN RENAL CANCER

B. van der Werf-Messing, R.O. van der Heul,
R. Ch. Ledeboer

Rotterdam Radiotherapy Institute
Rotterdam
Holland

In 1965, Rotterdam urologists and the Rotterdam Radiotherapy Institute started a prospective clinical trial in order to investigate the value of preoperative irradiation in renal cell cancer, to assess the value of the TNM classification of the International Union against Cancer, and to identify prognostic tumor and host factors. In a previous report, preliminary results have been reported (1).

Operable patients - without any evidence of metastasis - were randomized into either simple nephrectomy or preoperative irradiation immediately followed by simple nephrectomy. As a routine no lymph node evaluation was done. Preoperative irradiation consisted of 3000 - 4000 rad in 3 - 4 weeks depending on the side of the affected kidney; on the right side, the liver had to be considered. The irradiation field covered the kidney, the homolateral lymph nodes, and after 1970 also the contralateral lymph nodes.

The decision of "operability" was based on the results of physical examination, routine laboratory tests, routine X-ray investigations including chest X-ray, skeletal survey, intravenous pyelography, and in the majority of cases arteriography.

Routine histology of the operative specimen was done according to rules accepted by all Rotterdam pathologists; in 1977 review took place of all histological slides by one pathologist and of all intravenous pyelographies and arteriographies by one radiodiagnostician.

All patients have been seen at regular intervals for follow up examination. No patient was lost to follow up.

MATERIAL AND METHODS

A total of 206 patients were admitted to the trial. Table 1 lists the most important analyzed tumor and host factors. Thirty-two patients had to be excluded from further analysis for the following reasons: 15 appeared to have metastases prior to operation; five turned out to have a transitional cancer of the renal pelvis; 12 tumors appeared to be either a cyst, hemangioma, or fibroma. These patients were distributed equally over the two treatment modalities. Of the 174 remaining trial patients, 89 received preoperative irradiation while 85 underwent immediately simple nephrectomy.

There were 99 males and 75 females; both sexes had an average age of 59 years.

Table 1. Analyzed Tumor and Host Factors

Admitted to trial	206	P Categories	
Analyzed cases	174	P1	61
		P2	38
Males	99	P3	67
		P4	7
Females	75	Px	1
Preoperative X	89	Renal vein involvement	
No preoperative X	85	V−	105
		V+	64
T Categories		Not known	5
T1	14	Cell type	
T2	47		
T3	66	Granular	17
T4	39	Clear	123
Tx	8	Mixed	22
		Not known	12
ESR		Degree of differentiation	
<30	89		
≥30	83	High	21
Not known	2	Medium	81
		Low	60
		Not known	12

Based on intravenous pyelography and arteriography, the T categories of the primary were defined according to the rules of the International Union against Cancer (2); 14 belonged to the T1 category, i.e. small tumor without enlargement of the kidney; 47 were classified at T2, i.e. large tumor but cortex not broken; 66 were classified as T3, i.e. perinephric or hilar extension; 39 belonged to the T4 category, i.e. extension into neighboring organs. In eight patients no arteriography was done (Tx).

In 89 patients the sedimentation rate was less than 30 after 1 hour (ESR $<$ 30); in 83 patients it was 30 or more after 1 hour (ESR $\geq$ 30). In two patients the ESR was not known.

The P categories of the UICC correspond to the T categories. Their assessment was based on the examination of the nephrectomy specimen.

In 105 patients no renal vein involvement was found in the nephrectomy specimen, whereas in 64 cases renal vein involvement could be demonstrated. In five instances this information was not available.

The distribution of the degree of differentiation and the distribution of the cellular type of the growths are also presented in Table 1.

A detailed statistical analysis was performed in order to assess the prognostic significance of each factor and in order to elucidate the interrelationship between the various analyzed factors.

RESULTS

The actuarial uncorrected survival rate according to Berkson and Gage (3) for all cases is about 50% after 5 years and about 45% after 10 years. Relapse-free survival is continuously 5 - 10% less. The expected survival of the same age group is about 40% higher (Fig. 1).

Preoperative irradiation had no bearing on survival.

The T categories had no bearing on prognosis except for T4 patients who had a poor prognosis (Fig. 2).

Prognosis of females was significantly better than prognosis of males (Fig. 3).

Patients with ESR $<$30 fared significantly better than those with ESR $\geq$30 (Fig. 4).

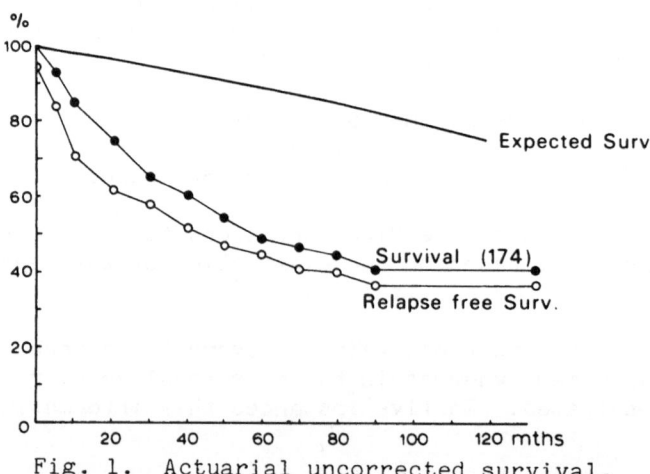

Fig. 1.   Actuarial uncorrected survival.

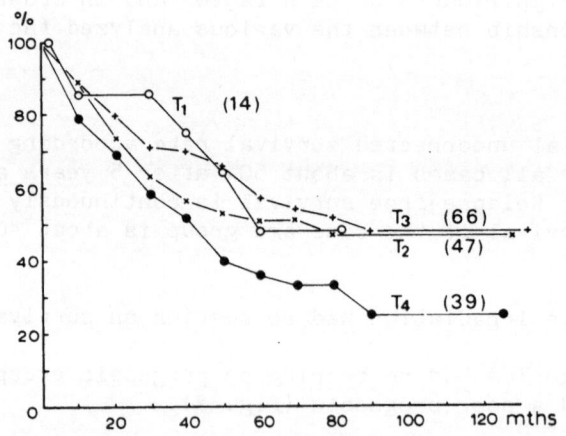

Fig. 2.   Actuarial uncorrected survival by T category.

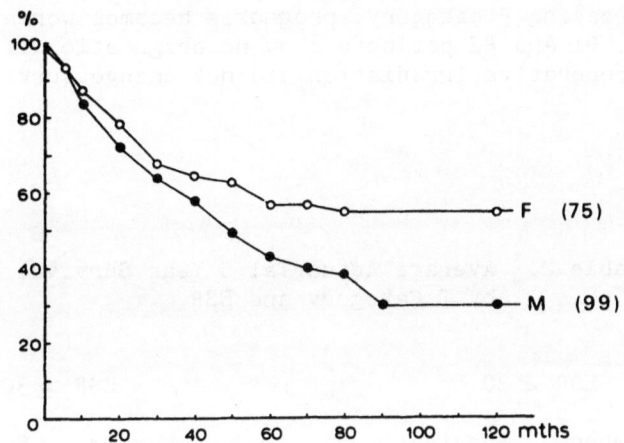

Fig. 3.   Actuarial uncorrected survival by sex.

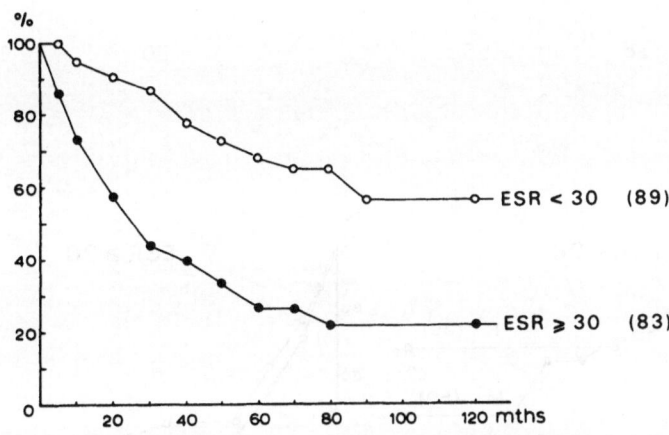

Fig. 4.   Actuarial uncorrected survival by ESR.

There was no correlation between sex and T category or ESR and
T category. In each T category, those with ESR < 30 had a better
prognosis (Table 2). In case of ESR < 30 and especially in case of
ESR ≥ 30, females fared better than males (Fig. 5).

With increasing P category, prognosis becomes worse; however,
after 3 years, P1 and P2 patients show no prognostic difference
(Fig. 6). Preoperative irradiation did not change survival in each
P category.

Table 2. Average Actuarial 5 Year Survival
by T Category and ESR

	ESR < 30			ESR ≥ 30	
	Number Treated	Survival (%)		Number Treated	Survival (%)
T1	11	59		3	0
T2	27	63		20	30
T3	30	85		35	30
T4	18	55		20	10

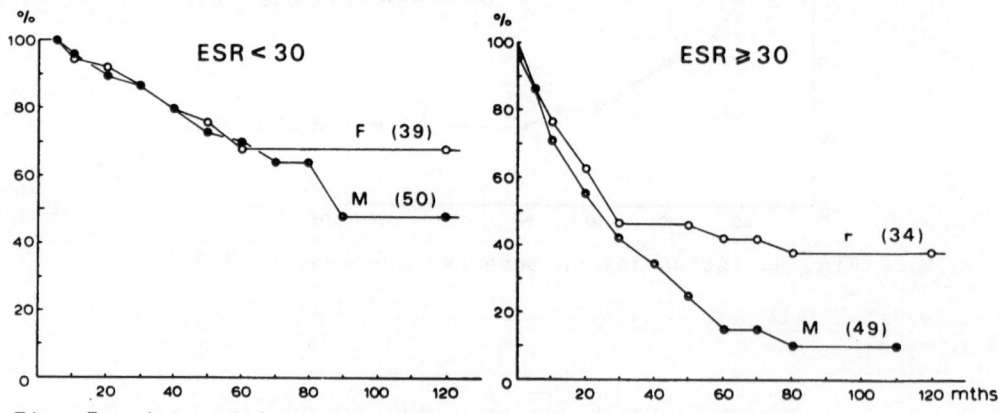

Fig. 5. Actuarial uncorrected survival by ESR and sex.

There was no correlation at all between P and T category: in about 60% of the cases P was smaller than T, in 20% P was larger than T, and only in about 20% P was the same as T (Fig. 7). This finding applied equally to the group with and without preoperative irradiation, indicating that probably preoperative irradiation did not influence visibly the extent of the growth.

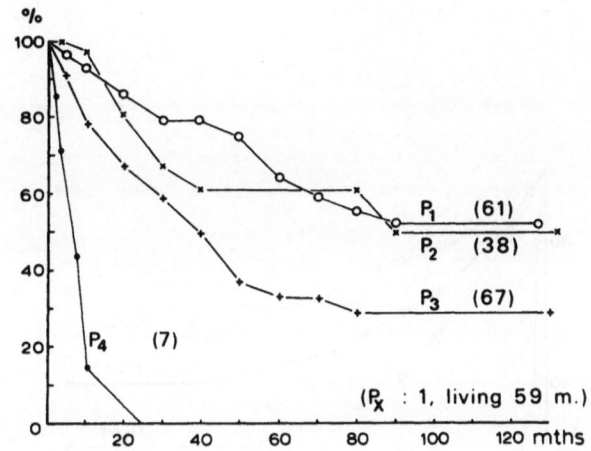

Fig. 6.   Actuarial uncorrected survival by P category.

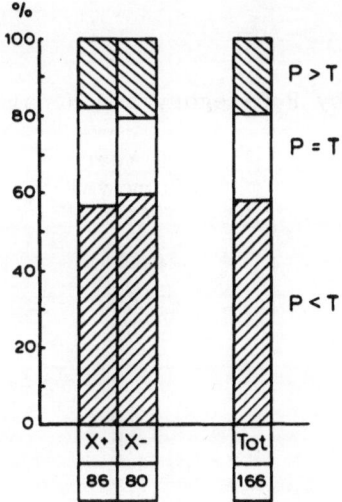

Fig. 7.   Correlation of T and P categories (according to Preoperative Radiotherapy (X)).

Renal vein involvement significantly reduced the chance of cure: with renal vein involvement only 20% of the patients were alive after 10 years, whereas in case of no renal vein involvement about 55% were alive (Fig. 8).   In the subgroups according to renal vein involvement, the P categories had no prognostic influence.   As with increasing P category, there was an increasing incidence of renal vein involvement; apparently the influence of P categories on prognosis is derived from renal vein involvement (Table 3).   Preoperative irradiation had no bearing on the prognostic influence of renal vein involvement.

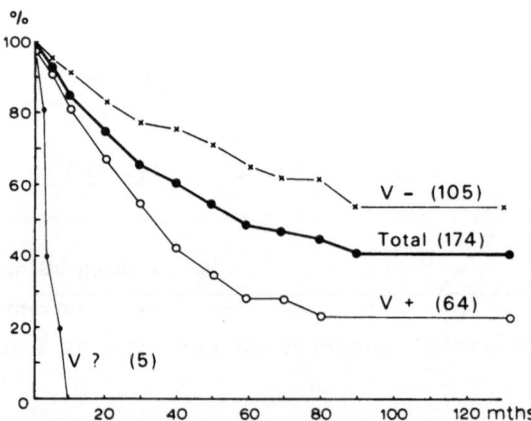

Fig. 8.   Actuarial uncorrected survival by renal vein involvement.

Table 3.   Prognosis by P Category and Renal Vein Involvement

	Number	5 Year Survival (%)	10 Year Survival (%)
P1			
V–	53	65	55
V+	8	40	30
P2			
V–	23	70	55
V+	15	45	40
P3			
V–	28	50	50
V+	39	20	15

Table 4 demonstrates prognosis according to sex, renal vein involvement, and ESR. Only in case of low ESR and no renal vein involvement do females and males have the same prognosis. In all other instances females fare better than males; in each sex, prognosis in case of no vein involvement and ESR$\geq$30 is comparable with prognosis in case of vein involvement and ESR $<$ 30. Prognosis is worst in case of vein involvement and high ESR.

The cellular type, i.e. granular or clear cell carcinoma, had no bearing on prognosis.

The histological degree of differentiation influenced prognosis: with decreasing degree of differentiation survival also decreased. The degree of differentiation had no correlation with either renal vein involvement or sex; the frequency of cases with low degree of differentiation was significantly higher in case of ESR $\geq$ 30 than in case of ESR $<$ 30. In each degree of differentiation the sedimentation rate determined prognosis. Analyzing the effect of degree of differentiation reveals that in each ESR group prognosis is identical for growths of high and of medium degree of differentiation, whereas a low degree of differentiation slightly worsens prognosis in both groups (Table 5).

In the P3 category, 36 patients had received preoperative irradiation. Four of them showed cancer in the plane of resection (11%), whereas of 31 P3 patients without preoperative irradiation 11 showed cancer in the plane of resection (35%). In spite of this apparent benefit from preoperative irradiation, due to small numbers it is not expressed in a better survival of the P3 category after preoperative irradiation.

Table 4. Average Actuarial 5 Year Survival by
Renal Vein Involvement, ESR, and Sex

	ESR $<$ 30		ESR $\geq$ 30	
	Number Treated	Survival (%)	Number Treated	Survival (%)
No renal vein involvement				
Males	38	90	22	20
Females	24	80	19	50
Renal vein involvement				
Males	12	18	26	10
Females	14	60	12	40

Table 5.   Prognosis by Degree of Differentiation and ESR

Degree of Differentiation	Number	5 Year Survival (%)	5 Year Survival (%)
High	21	65	55
Medium	81	55	45
Low	60	40	38
ESR < 30			
High	17	75	63
Medium	44	75	60
Low	24	60	44
ESR ≥ 30			
High	3	35	0
Medium	37	35	25
Low	36	26	25

There was no significant impact on prognosis either by the dose of irradiation (3000 or 4000 rad) or by the size of irradiation field (regional nodes included or excluded).

Apart from inoperable patients, where death is usually due to local growth with or without metastases, death usually is caused by distant metastases without local recurrence. In 38 instances pulmonary metastases were diagnosed during follow up: 23 showed progression; in seven cases there was dubious progression; and in eight cases (31%) there was spontaneous, complete, or partial regression. After pulmonary metastases, the next frequent site for metastasis were the vertebral bodies from cervical 4 to lumbar 2.

Table 6 presents the distribution of pulmonary and vertebral-body metastases according to renal vein involvement, sedimentation rate, and sex.

DISCUSSION

Of the preoperatively assessable tumor and host factors, only sex and sedimentation rate appeared to have a bearing on prognosis: women fared better than men, and patients with a sedimentation rate less than 30 after 1 hour had a better prognosis than those with a

Table 6. Hypothetical Benefit from Elective Irradiation
by Renal Vein Involvement/ESR/Sex

	Number	I Pulmonary Mets (%)	II C4 + L2 Mets (%)	I + II (%)
Renal vein -				
ESR < 30	♂38	8	8	16 (40)[a]
	♀24	5	4	9
ESR ≥ 30	♂22	27	9	36 (50)[a]
	♀19	11	16	27
Renal vein +				
ESR < 30	♂12	67	8	75
	♀14	8	15	23
ESR ≥ 30	♂26	35	8	43
	♀12	50	25	75

[a] In case of low degree of differentiation.

higher sedimentation rate. Sex and sedimentation rate factors were
not interrelated.

The T categories appeared to have no bearing on prognosis. It
could be assumed that the accuracy of radiodiagnostic assessment is
not sufficient. This suggestion is substantiated by the fact that
there is no correlation between T categories and the more correctly
microscopically assessable P categories. On the other hand, P categories also have no significant bearing on prognosis. The demonstrated prognostic influence of P categories is caused by the fact
that with increasing P category the chance of renal vein involvement
increases: patients with renal vein involvement have a significantly
worse prognosis than those without renal vein involvement. Growths
of low degree of differentiation predict a poorer outlook than those
with a high or medium degree of differentiation. In each degree of
differentiation the sedimentation rate overrules prognosis.

Prognosis in case of renal cancer - apart from inoperable or
only partially removable growths - is mainly determined by the
existence of micrometastases at the time of operation. Apparently
renal vein involvement increases the risk of micrometastases (4,5,6),

and their existence is expressed by elevated sedimentation rate (5).
A low degree of differentiation is not related to renal vein involvement but very much so to sedimentation rate; hence it apparently
reflects the risk of micrometastases caused not only through renal
vein involvement but also by other metastatic pathways (6). The
better prognosis of women might be attributed to hormonal factors:
hypothetically, hormones could suppress or even eradicate micrometastases in some instances and thus improve prognosis in circumstances otherwise comparable to those of males. Indirectly this
hypothesis may be supported by the fact that once metastases are
present, women respond less well to hormone therapy than men (7,8).

    As prognosis at the time of operation is apparently already
determined by existing subclinical metastasis, it is understandable
that preoperative irradiation to the primary cannot contribute ap-
preciably to improvement of prognosis.

    Until now no form of chemotherapy has been found which can deal
effectively with clinically established metastases; hence a trial
using elective hormone therapy or chemotherapy in high risk patients
(males with renal vein involvement and ESR $\geq$ 30) might be considered.
On the other hand, as pulmonary metastases and metastases to the
vertebral bodies from cervical 4 to lumbar 2 are frequent (Table 6),
elective irradiation of these regions could be considered with a
benefit ranging from 9% in the low risk group to 75% in the high
risk group. Without great problems such an irradiation could be
given by supervoltage machines.

SUMMARY

    A total of 174 patients underwent simple nephrectomy in case of
clinically operable kidney cancer without demonstrable metastases.
Of these 85 received preoperative irradiation to the kidney and the
regional lymph nodes (3000 - 4000 rad in 3 - 4 weeks). Prognosis
was not influenced by preoperative irradiation. The preoperatively
assessable prognostic criteria were sex and sedimentation rate:
ESR $\geq$ 30 and being male worsened prognosis. The clinical T categories of the UICC were not related to prognosis. Of the microscopic
examination of the nephrectomy specimen, renal vein invasion and to
a lesser extent a low degree of differentiation appeared to worsen
prognosis. The prognostic influence of the P categories was caused
by a higher incidence of renal vein involvement in case of higher
P category. The most important prognostic factors - ESR, renal
vein involvement, and sex - were not interrelated. Elective chemotherapy, radiation therapy, and hormone therapy could be considered
in certain high risk groups.

ADDENDUM (W.C.J. Hop, M.Sc.)

    Based on the presented data pertaining to the relevant prognostic
factors, a score for each factor was calculated by statistical methods
(9).

    The preoperatively assessable significant factors were sex and
sedimentation rate. In case of female, no number is given; in case
of male, 0.56 is attributed to the patient. To this initial figure
the sedimentation rate score is added, obtained by multiplying 0.02

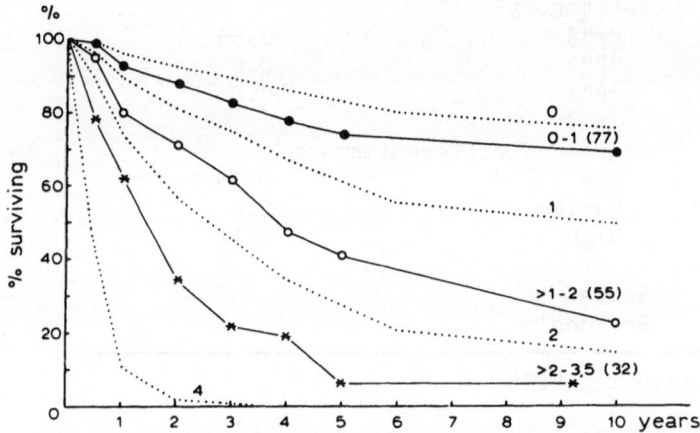

Fig. 9.   Survival by preoperative scores: M = 0.56; ESR = 0.02 x
          value. T4 = 0.7. (...) Expected survival by score;
          (—) actuarial uncorrected survival by score.

with the sedimentation rate after 1 hour; and in case of T4, 0.7 is
added. The sum of these two (or three) values is the final score to
be used as an indicator of prognosis of patients. Grouping patients
with a similar score resulted in survival curves as given in Figure 9.

    After nephrectomy more relevant data are available and a more
accurate prediction of prognosis becomes possible. The various
scores are added and the sum of the scores can be used as a post-
operative prognosticator. The postoperative scores are listed in
Table 7. Survival curves according to score are given in Figures
10 and 11.

Table 7.   Postoperative Scores for Prognosis

Sex	
Male	0.87
Female	0.0
ESR	0.02 x Value
Renal vein	
+	0.79
-	0.0
P-Category[a]	
"P"3	0.53
"P"2	0.0
"P"1	0.06
Degree of differentiation	
Low	0.39
Medium	0.0
High	0.14
Score	
Prognosis	

[a]Excluding "P"4

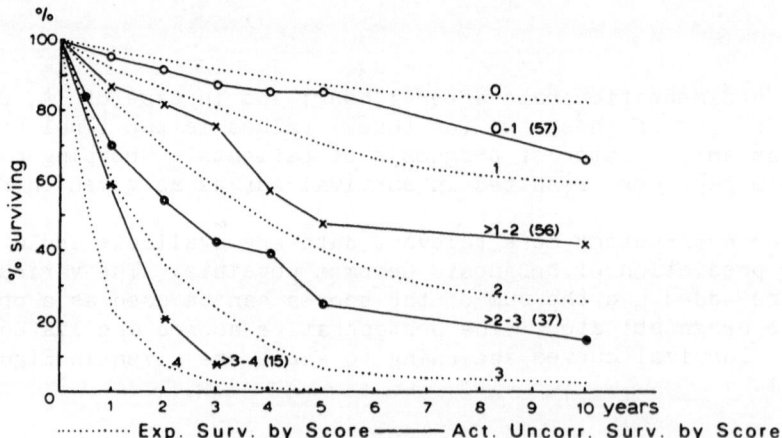

Fig. 10.   Survival by postoperative scores (excluding "P"4):
          M = 0.78; ESR = 0.02 x value; V = 0.9.

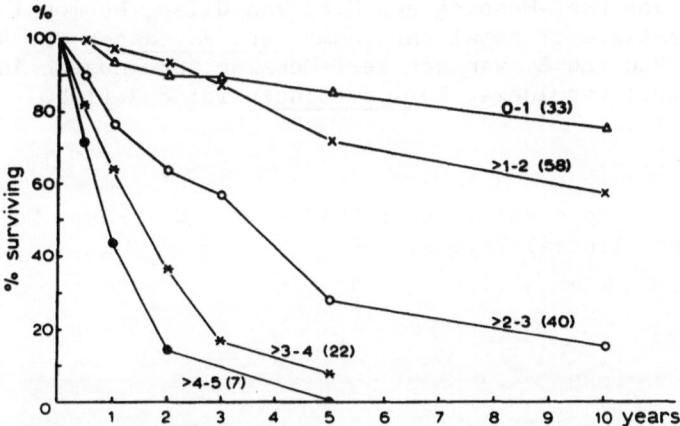

Fig. 11. Actuarial uncorrected survival by postoperative scores (excluding "P"4).

ACKNOWLEDGMENTS

The authors are grateful to all the Rotterdam urologists who contributed to the trial, to Miss P. de Haan who performed the secretarial work, to Mr. W. Hop (M.Sc.) and his department for statistical analysis, and to Mr. L. Ries and his department for drawing the graphs.

REFERENCES

1. B. van der Werf-Messing, Carcinoma of the kidney, Cancer 32: 1056 (1973).
2. Union Internationale Contre le Cancer (UICC), TNM Classification of Malignant Tumours (2nd ed.), Geneva (1974), p. 75.
3. J. Berkson and R.P. Gage, Calculation of survival rates for cancer, Proc. Mayo Clinic 25: 270 (1950).
4. O. Arner, C. Blanck, and T. von Schreeb, Renal adenocarcinoma. Morphology, grading and malignancy, prognosis; a study of 197 cases, Acta Chir. Scand. Suppl. 346: 25 (1965).
5. L.E. Böttiger, Prognosis in renal carcinoma, Cancer 26: 780 (1970).
6. E. Riches, Clinical features, in: "Tumours of the Kidney and Ureter, Vol. 5," E. Riches, ed., E. & S. Livingstone Ltd., Edinburgh and London (1964), p. 137.
7. H.J.G. Bloom, Hormone treatment of renal tumours: Experimental and clinical observations, in: "Tumours of the Kidney and Ureter, Vol. 5," E. Riches, ed., E. & S. Livingstone Ltd., Edinburgh and London (1964), p. 311.

8.   B. van der Werf-Messing and H.A. van Gilse, Hormonal treatment
      of metastases of renal carcinoma, Br. J. Cancer 25: 423 (1971).
9.   W.C.J. Hop and B. van der Werf-Messing, Prognostic indexes for
      renal cell carcinoma, Eur. J. Cancer 16: 833 (1980).

(Published by kind permission of Professor L.W. Brady, Editor-in-chief, Cancer Clinical Trials.)

RENAL CELL CARCINOMA: CLINICAL ASPECTS AND NATURAL HISTORY

J.P. Blandy, H.R. England and R.T.D. Oliver

The London Hospital and Institute of Urology
London
U.K.

We teach our medical students that the presenting features of
an adenocarcinoma of the kidney are haematuria, pain and a mass that
has been noticed either by the patient or the doctor.   We make the
diagnosis by discovering a mass in the urogram that is solid in the
ultrasound scan, typically vascular in the angiogram, or character-
istically dense in the CAT scan.   Pathologists tell us that one can
tell a cancer of the kidney from a benign adenoma not by the histological features of either of them, but by their size - tumours
smaller than 3 cm. in diameter being deemed benign, larger ones
malignant.   Treatment is nephrectomy: it is true that many of us
have added other adjuvant agents from time to time, but it is equally
true that none of them are (so far) of proven value.   This is the
conventional wisdom.   We thought it would be of value to examine
these well established truths in the light of the clinical experience of one centre over the last 15 years.

METHODS AND MATERIAL

A retrospective study was made of the records of 114 patients
admitted to the London Hospital with an index diagnosis of adenocarcinoma of the kidney from 1964 through 1979.   The list is probably incomplete, as we have had certain domestic difficulties in our
records department: nevertheless the results may still be of
interest.

It will not come as a surprise to find that there were nearly
twice as many males as there were females, or that cancer occurred
as often on one side as on the other (Table 1).   It is equally
unsurprising to see that cancer of the kidney was mainly a disease
of older people (Fig. 1).   We were surprised however to find that

611

Table 1. Present Series

	Right	Left	Total
Females	21	20	41
Males	38	33	71
Total	59	53	112*

(* Site of origin unclear at autopsy in 2 patients)

Table 2. Symptoms at Presentation to Hospital

Pain	11	9%
Haematuria	35	31%
Lump	7	6%
Combinations of pain, haematuria and lump	21	19%

Weight loss	2)		
Proptosis	1)		
Lung metastases	3)	14	12%
Bone metastases	6)		
Other metastases	2)		

Hypertension	3	3%
Insufficient information	23	20%

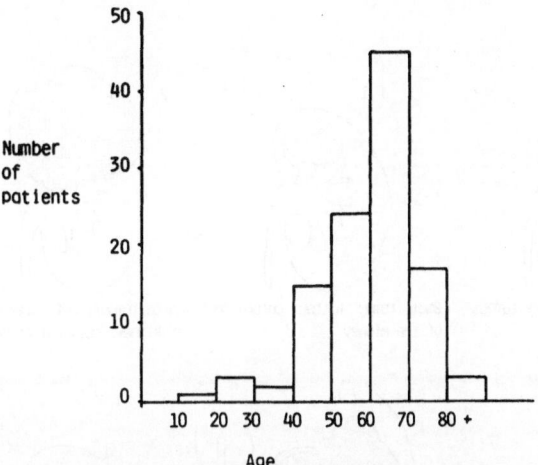

Fig. 1.   Age distribution of 114 cases of renal cell cancer.
           (Adenocarcinoma; The London Hospital, 1964-69).

so many presented with clinical features of late or metastatic
disease (Table 2).

Throughout this period, treatment was along conventional lines.
Nephrectomy was performed whenever possible, even when there were
distant metastases.   Early in the series, when it was still accepted
practice, our patients were given post-operative irradiation.   Later,
for a time, they received preoperative radiation as part of a clinical trial.   Today they get no radiation unless there has been an
obviously incomplete removal of the tumour though radiotherapy is
used when appropriate in the treatment of metastases.   Throughout
most of this period our patients (when they have developed metastases) have been given medroxyprogesterone acetate, mostly because
it is not known to do harm, rather than from any conviction that it
would do any good.

We have tried to stage the tumours in accordance with the TNM
system (1) but in doing so have probably erred on the side of understaging - since there were virtually no tumours in this series truly
in pT1 where the renal contour was not deformed (Fig. 2) and most
of our patients should perhaps really be placed in pT2 (Table 3).
Prognosis was clearly related to the stage of the disease (Table 4,
Fig. 3).   Unfortunately only a small proportion of our patients
were diagnosed when their tumours were in the early stage pT1 or pT2.
As shown in an earlier study from this department (2) the outlook is
good for tumours that are still confined to the kidney.

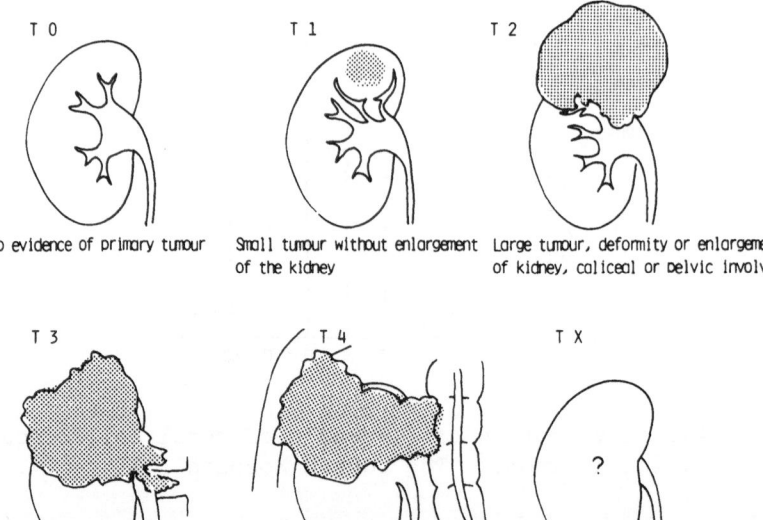

Fig. 2. T-staging of carcinoma of the kidney based on findings at
operation.   Diagram based on UICC TNM Classification of
Malignant Tumours, 3rd Edition, 1978.

Table 3. pT Staging in 144 Cases of Adenocarcinoma of Kidney.

	pTX	pT1	pT2	pT3	pT4	Total	
Males	7	5	11	27	24	73	
M1	5	0	4	7	7	23	32%
Females	8	8	6	11	8	41	
M1	4	0	1	2	2	9	22%
Total	15	13	17	38	31	114	
M1	9	0	5	9	9	32	28%

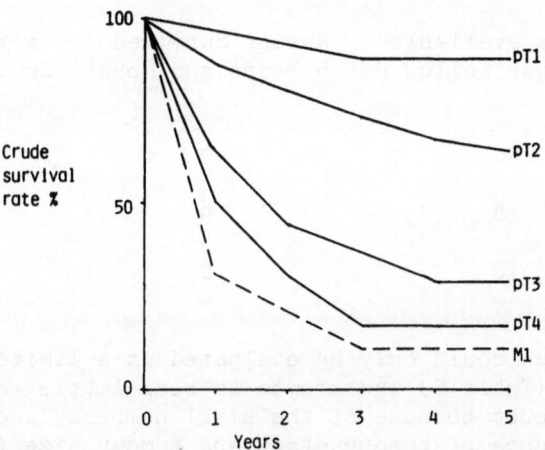

Fig. 3. Crude survival rate % according to pT stage of renal
         cell carcinomas.   (Adenocarcinoma;   The London Hospital,
         1964-69).

Table 4.   pT Staging and Survival

pT stage	Available for 5 Year Follow Up	Survived 5 yrs.	5 year Crude Survival Rate %
pT1	9	8	89%
pT2	14	9	64%
pT3	32	9	28%
pT4	31	5	16%
pTX	15	1	7%
M1	31	3	10%

Table 5.   Tumour Grade and Prognosis

Grade	Number available For 5 Year Follow Up	Number Survived 5 Years and More	5 Year Crude Survival Rate %
G1	30	9	30%
G2	18	9	50%
G3	16	6	38%

Tumour grade could only be evaluated in a limited number of these patients (Table 5) and seemed to bear little relationship to prognosis, no doubt because of the small numbers, and the more important influence of tumour stage and tumour size (Table 6). Indeed, perhaps the most striking finding in this study has been the consistently enormous size of these tumours (Fig. 4).   As a general rule, when they were relatively small, their outlook was good, but the very large ones did badly.

Table 6.   Tumour Stage and Grade, Where Data Available

	Grade	pTX	pT1	pT2	pT3	pT4	Total	M1	
	G1	0	1	3	13	9	26	7	
Females	G2	0	2	5	4	6	17	3	
	G3	0	1	0	5	2	8	3	
	G1	1	4	2	3	2	12	1	
Males	G2	0	1	1	2	0	4	0	
	G3	2	0	2	1	3	8	2	
All	G1	1	5	5	16	11	38	8	22%
	G2	0	3	6	6	6	21	3	13%
Cases	G3	2	1	2	6	5	16	5	38%
Total		3	9	13	28	22	75	16	23%

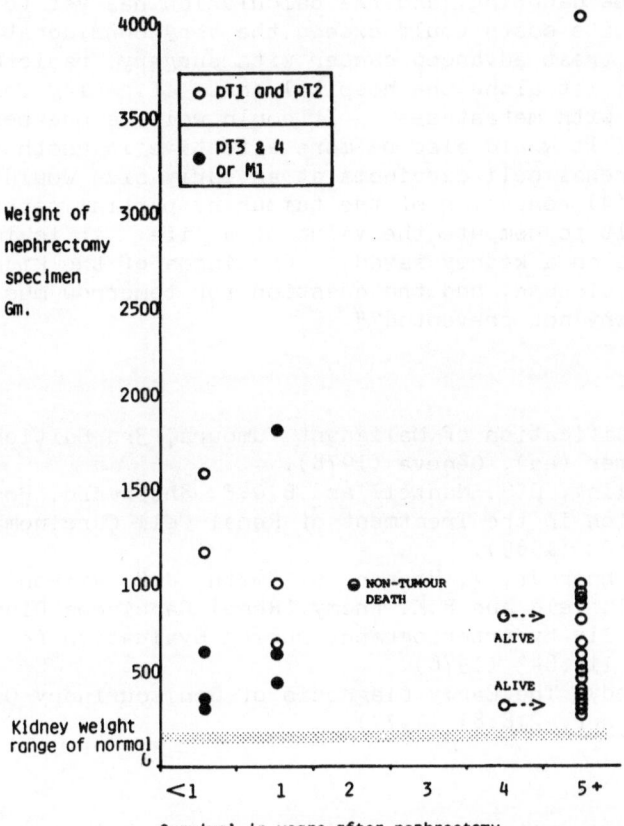

Fig. 4. Survival and weight of tumour specimen at nephrectomy.
The shaded band indicates the normal range of renal
weight.   (Adenocarcinoma;   The London Hospital, 1964-69).

DISCUSSION

    There are no grounds for complacency in the contemporary detec-
tion of carcinoma of the kidney: we are only finding these cases
when they are too late, and yet we already have the capacity to pick
them up when they are so small (under 3 cm. diameter) as to fall
within the pathologists category of benign adenoma, or at least into
a critical limit less than which metastases virtually never occur.
If detected at this level by chance radiography (3) the prognosis is
excellent.

    The expense and the difficulty of arranging annual radiological
or ultrasound screening of the population at risk for cancer of the

kidney would be daunting, and the calculation has yet to be made
as to whether its costs would exceed the very considerable costs of
attempting to treat advanced cancer with surgery, radiotherapy and
chemotherapy; let alone the hospital costs of caring for the
patient dying with metastases.   It could well be cheaper, let alone
more humane.   It would also be more effective in another way, for
detection of renal cell carcinoma at an early size would permit
conservative (4) resection of the tumour by partial nephrectomy.
It is difficult to compute the value of a life: it is impossible
to put a price on a kidney saved.   Carcinoma of the kidney is now
a preventable disease, and the question for tomorrow must be, "If
preventable, why not prevented?".

REFERENCES

1.   TNM Classification of Malignant Tumours, 3rd Edition,
      M.H. Harmer (ed), Geneva (1978).
2.   W.B. Peeling, B.S. Mantell and B.G.F. Shepheard, Post-Operative
      Irradiation in the Treatment of Renal Cell Carcinoma, Brit. J.
      Urol. 41:23 (1969).
3.   F.K. Kirchner Jr, V. Braren, C. Smith, J.P. Wilson, J.H. Foster,
      J.W. Hollifield and R.K. Rhamy, Renal Carcinoma Discovered
      Incidentally by Arteriography During Evaluation for Hypertension
      J. Urol. 115:643 (1976).
4.   J.P. Blandy, The Early Diagnosis of Genitourinary Carcinoma,
      Practitioner, 218:81 (1977).

CARCINOMA OF THE KIDNEY: BIOLOGICAL MARKERS

M.R.G. Robinson, D. Daponte and C. Chandrasekaran

The General Infirmary
Pontefract
U.K.

During the development and progression of malignant disease, certain biological products (markers) are produced by, or in response to, the tumour.   They may be specific for a particular tumour, or non-specific, and have a potential value in diagnosis, screening, staging, prognosis, the choice of treatment, monitoring disease progression, and evaluation of the response to treatment.   Improved biochemical and immunological techniques have made possible their identification, characterisation and availability for clinical use (1).

Ideal criteria for the reliability of tumour markers have been defined by Javadpour (2).   These are specificity for malignant disease, detectability in body fluids and tissue extracts, short biological half-life and correlation with the presence of tumour.

The ideal tumour marker does not exist.   Urologists are familiar with their clinical application in the management of carcinoma of the prostate (acid phosphatase) and testicular tumours (alpha-feto-protein and human chorionic gonadotrophin).   Measurable biological tumour markers include:-

     Foetal antigens
     Tumour associated antigens
     Hormone related substances
     Enzymes:-
               Specific isoenzymes
               Foetal isoenzymes
               Placental isoenzymes
     Acute phase reactant proteins
     Polyamines

Tumour markers of carcinoma of the kidney have not been extensively investigated. This is probably because, as yet, no population group at particular risk of developing this disease has been identified and there is not yet available effective adjuvant or secondary therapy for relapsed cases. The progression of this malignancy is, however, unpredictable and a good marker has potential clinical value in forecasting prognosis and in detecting relapse.

During the last decade occasional reports have appeared in the medical literature identifying possible kidney tumour markers. The ideal marker should be specific for renal adenocarcinoma and because this neoplasm may be associated with systemic metabolic and endocrinological syndromes due to the excessive production of substances normally elaborated in the kidney, as well as the ectopic production of hormones such as chorionic gonadotrophin and parathormone, Surfin et al (3) investigated plasma hormones as tumour markers in renal cancer. They reported that Renin was elevated in 21 of 57 patients (37%) who had poorly differentiated, advanced clinical stage, poor prognosis renal cancer. Erythropoetin was elevated in 36 (63%) but its assay did not correlate with histological grade or clinical stage. Chorionic gonadotrophins (Total and B subunits) were not elevated in any of the patients. Renin and Erythropoetin may be of value as specific tumour markers, although Erythropoetin is sometimes elevated in other tumours, e.g. neoplasms of the brain, liver and uterus (4). Surfin and his colleagues could not identify the renal tumour as the source of these markers (3). It is possible that elevated levels are due to stimulation of the contralateral kidney or a decreased rate of degradation.

Another approach to identify a specific tumour marker is to measure antibodies to tumour associated antigens. DeKernion, Ramming and Gupta (5) measured such antibodies in patients with renal cancer and found them elevated in 94%. They were, unfortunately, also elevated in 20% of controls and 20-70% of patients with other tumours. Therefore, their sensitivity for kidney cancer is high (6% false negative) but specificity is low (20-70% false positives) and they have no value as specific markers. Their prognostic potential, however, needs further evaluation. In patients with metastatic disease their titre remains high in long survivors but falls with disease progression in poor prognosis patients.

Non-specific biological markers which have been investigated include carcinoembryonic antigen, polyamines, prostaglandins and acute phase reactant proteins. In 1974, Chu et al (6) reported that plasma carcinoembryonic antigen levels were slightly elevated in one of three patients with non-metastatic disease and significantly elevated in seven of eight patients with metastases. They were also elevated in four of 12 patients with local recurrence of renal carcinoma. Levels tended to fall following nephrectomy and during chemotherapy with CCNU.

Sanford et al (7) studied the urinary polyamines (putrescine, spermine and spermidine) in renal parenchymal carcinoma.   In situations of rapid growth, these organic cations, which are related to ribonucleic acid synthesis, accumulate rapidly.

In the urine their concentration was increased in 9/11 patients with renal tumours.   They are also concentrated in other urinary tract malignancies but not in benign urological disease.   Therefore, as markers, their diagnostic value is limited but they may have a role in monitoring disease progression and response to treatment.

Prostaglandins can be identified in renal cell cultures, extracts of primary and secondary renal tumours, and in renal blood collected from the veins of kidneys with adenocarcinoma (8).   Serum prostaglandin E is inactivated by passage through the lungs but has been reported to be elevated in two patients with pulmonary metastases and hypercalcaemia.   It may, therefore, be a possible marker of renal lung metastases.   Prostaglandin A was found to be elevated in a patient whose essential hypertension was suppressed when he developed a renal carcinoma (9).   This prostaglandin was a potent antihypertensive agent (10).   Further studies of prostaglandins as markers of renal cancer are indicated.

Acute phase reactant proteins are a group of proteins whose plasma concentrations are altered in response to such stimuli as tissue injury, acute and chronic inflammation, and neoplasia (11). One of these, haptoglobin, was studied by Vickers (12) in 36 patients with abnormal renal masses.   None of ten patients with renal cysts had elevated levels.   High levels were found in 14 of 16 patients with localised renal carcinoma and in all six cancer patients with visceral metastases.   In two thirds of the cancer patients, a rise after treatment was diagnostic of recurrence.

The Yorkshire Urological Group (13) have studied the acute phase reactant proteins C-reactive (C-RP), α_1 chymotrypsin (ACTH) and α_1 glycoprotein (AGP) in renal adenocarcinoma.   A progressive rise of these variants indicates progressive metastatic disease.   Elevated but stable levels are found in patients with stable non-progressive metastatic disease.   In the same group of patients the enzyme phosphohexose isomerase, which reflects glycolytic activity was measured in the plasma.   This was elevated in 62% of advanced metastatic tumours and only in 17% of patients with localised disease.

CONCLUSIONS

This paper has reviewed some of the potential tumour markers for renal adenocarcinoma.   The ideal marker has not yet been determined and the application of markers in clinical practice needs further investigation and evaluation.   Potentially, however, biological markers, both tumour specific and non-specific, have an important role to play in the future management of renal cancer.

REFERENCES

1.   B. Wahren, Tumour Markers in Urology: Aids in Cancer Diagnosis
     and Management, Urol. Res. 7:56 (1979).
2.   N. Javadpour, Tumour Markers in Urologic Cancer, Urology, 16:127,
     (1980).
3.   G. Surfin, E.A. Mirona, R.H. Moore, T.M. Chu and G.P. Murphy,
     Hormones and Renal Cancer, J. Urol. 117:433 (1977).
4.   L.F. Altaffer and O.W. Chenault, Paraneoplastic Endocrinopathies
     Associated with Renal Tumours, J. Urol. 122:573 (1979).
5.   J.B. DeKernion, K.P. Ramming and R.K. Gupta, The Detection and
     Clinical Significance of Antibodies to Tumour-Associated
     Antigens in Patients with Renal Cell Carcinoma, J. Urol. 122:300
     (1979).
6.   T.M. Chu, S.K. Shukla, A.O. Mittleman and G.P. Murphy, Plasma
     Carcinoembryonic Antigen in Renal Cell Carcinoma Patients, J.
     Urol. 111:742 (1974).
7.   E.M. Sanford, J.R. Drago, T.J. Rohner, G.F. Kessler, L. Sheehan
     and A. Lipton, Preliminary Evaluation of Urinary Polyamines in
     the Diagnosis of Genitourinary Tract Malignancy, J. Urol. 113:218
     (1975).
8.   K.B. Cummings and R.P. Robertson, Prostaglandin: Increased
     Production by Renal Cell Carcinoma, J. Urol. 118:720 (1977).
9.   R.M. Zusman, J.J. Snider, A. Cline, B.V. Caldwell and L.
     Speroff, Antihypertensive Function of a Renal Cell Carcinoma.
     Evidence for a Prostaglandin A Secreting Tumour, New Eng. J.
     Med. 29:843 (1974).
10. J. Lee, H. Konnegiesser, J. O'Toole and E. Westura, Hypertension
     and Renomedullary Prostaglandins: A Human Study of Antihyper-
     tensive Effects of PGA, Ann. N.Y. Acad. Sci. 180:218 (1971).
11. E.H. Cooper and A. Milford Ward, Acute Phase Reactant Proteins
     as Aids to Monitoring Disease, Invest. Cell. Path. 2:293 (1979).
12. M. Vickers, Serum Haptoglobins: A Pre-Operative Detector of
     Metastatic Renal Carcinoma, J. Urol. 112:310 (1974).
13. B. Richards, M.R.G. Robinson, N.B. Pidcock and E.H. Cooper,
     Serum Protein Profiles in Carcinoma of the Kidney, Eur. Urol.
     (in press).

REGRESSION OF HYPERNEPHROMAS

W. E. Goodwin

University of California
Los Angeles
U.S.A.

Clear cell carcinomas of the kidney (hypernephromas) do regress within the kidney under certain circumstances. The Swedish pathologists, Bartley and Hultquist (1), have clearly shown this and illustrated it when they reviewed the literature and reported their own cases in 1950.

It is also clear that in some cases, although very few, distant metastases of renal cell carcinomas have been known to regress or disappear (2, 3). This has recently been summed up very clearly by Freed (4) who described 51 acceptable cases.

One of the clearly most acceptable cases with a reported autopsy showing regression was described by Jenkins (5) as a regression at eight years and then death at 13 years with an autopsy illustrating the regressed pulmonary lesions (6). Garfield and Kennedy (7) described a 16 year regression and reversal of liver disease. Braren et al (8) described reversal and regression of a skin lesion which they could clearly see and which they had biopsied.

Johnson et al (9) studied their cases and concluded that nephrectomy in the presence of metastases was justified only in cases with regression of bony metastases (2).

Usow and Silbar (10) reported regression of a pulmonary metastasis after nephrectomy and chemotherapy with 5FU, 600 mg. per week, Methotrexate, 25 mg. intravenously per week, Chlorambucil, 2 mg. three times a day and Provera, 10 mg. three times per day. Despite this encouraging report, there is no clear evidence that any chemotherapy is truly effective in renal cell carcinoma.

The growth of renal tumors and their metastases must be extremely variable and there are some reports of appearance of metastases at very long intervals after the original nephrectomy. Bradham et al (11) described a renal cell carcinoma metastasis 25 years after nephrectomy. They stated that the longest survival between recognition of a renal cell carcinoma and eventual death from metastasis is 37 years in a patient in whom the neoplasm was considered inoperable and left in place.

There has continued to be a great deal of speculation as to the possibility of some immunologic mechanism. There can be no doubt that there are well authenticated cases of regression, if not cure. The real unanswered question is "why and how", and what factors could be brought into play to make this phenomenon occur more frequently.

REFERENCES

1.   O. Bartley and G.T. Hultquist, Spontaneous Regression of Hypernephromas, Acta Path. Microbiol. Scand. 27:448 (1950).
2.   W.E. Goodwin, M.M. Mims, J.J. Kaufman, A.T.K. Cockett and D.C. Martin, Under What Circumstances Does "Regression" of Hypernephroma Occur?, in "Renal Neoplasia", J.S. King (ed), Little, Brown & Co., Boston (1967) p.13.
3.   W.E. Goodwin, Regression of Hypernephromas, JAMA 204:22 (1968).
4.   S.Z. Freed, J.P. Halperin and M. Gordon, Idiopathic Regression of Metastases from Renal Cell Carcinoma, J. Urol. 118:538 (1977).
5.   G.D. Jenkins, Regression of Pulmonary Metastasis Following Nephrectomy for Hypernephroma: Eight Year Follow Up, J. Urol. 82:37 (1959).
6.   G.D. Jenkins, Final Report: Regression of Pulmonary Metastasis Following Nephrectomy for Hypernephroma: Thirteen Year Follow Up, J. Urol. 94:99 (1965).
7.   D.H. Garfield and B.J. Kennedy, Regression of Metastatic Renal Cell Carcinoma Following Nephrectomy, Cancer 39:190 (1972).
8.   V. Braren, J.N. Taylor and W. Pace, Regression of Metastatic Renal Carcinoma Following Nephrectomy, Urology 3:777 (1974).
9.   D.E. Johnson, K.E. Kaesler and M.L. Samuels, Is Nephrectomy Justified in Patients with Metastatic Renal Carcinoma? J. Urol. 114:27 (1975).
10.   B.H. Usow and J.D. Silbar, Regression of Pulmonary Metastasis from Adenocarcinoma of the Kidney, Urologists Letter Club, Vol. XX, No. 38 (1972).
11.   R.R. Bradham, C.C. Wannamaker and H.R. Pratt-Thomas, Renal Cell Carcinoma Metastases 25 Years After Nephrectomy, JAMA 223:921 (1973).
12.   J. Holland, Natural History and Staging of Renal Cell Carcinoma, Ca-A Cancer Journal for Clinicians 25:121 (1975).

SPONTANEOUS REGRESSION OF METASTATIC RENAL CELL CARCINOMA AND ITS SIGNIFICANCE IN ASSESSING RESPONSE OF SUCH PATIENTS TO CHEMOTHERAPY

R.T.D. Oliver, R. Stuart-Harris, P.F.M. Wrigley

Institue of Urology and
St. Bartholomew's Hospital
London
England

INTRODUCTION

Spontaneous complete regression of tumour metastases received recognition as a genuine phenomenon following the carefully documented study of literature reports by Everson and Cole (1). Renal cell carcinoma was the tumour most frequently reported to undergo spontaneous complete regression, although in that series for only four of 26 patients was there histological documentation that the lung shadows contained malignant cells. In the recent review by Fairlamb (2) at least 15/67 lived five years although half subsequently died of recurrence of their disease up to 15 years later.

Apart from a series reported by Werf-Messing and Van Gilse (3), who observed partial regression of lung metastases in 8 of 33 (24%) of patients when frequent chest X-rays were performed and the control series of Tykka et al (4), who observed partial regression of pulmonary metastases in one of 12 patients there are few carefully followed series of renal cell carcinoma in which it is possible to establish a reliable estimate of the frequency with which spontaneous regression occurs, although in reviews of the literature Bloom (5) reported three out of 606 patients and Fairlamb (2), two out of 173 patients undergoing such regression.

Equally, there is no series in which biopsy of probable pulmonary metastases has been performed systematically in patients with renal adenocarcinoma to establish the frequency of positive histology. Nonetheless, given the fact that there are histologically proven lung and extra-pulmonary metastases where spontaneous regression has occurred, it is sensible to take account of this possibility in assessing the response of this disease to any form of therapy.

It is the purpose of this paper to review our recent experience of chemotherapy, endocrine therapy and immunotherapy in the light of this fact.

CLINICAL MATERIAL AND TREATMENT

Twenty-four patients have been treated. All had bidimensional measurable lung or lymph node metastases; a few had in addition bone metastases. Although the majority had several examinations confirming that the metastases were growing, some patients, usually due to the presence of extensive metastases, were treated at first diagnosis.

Patients were treated between September 1977 and February 1981 and all have had a minimum of six months' follow-up. Because of the low frequency of referral, no single protocol has been followed and patients receiving chemotherapy were treated according to whatever therapy was currently under investigation in the department or suggested from literature studies current at the time the patient presented. Patients on Provera received 100 mg three times a day for a minimum of six weeks. Patients on BCG received 2 Heaf gun punctures through 40 μl of standard Glaxo BCG every two weeks for three months then monthly for one year or until there was evidence of tumour progression.

Assessment of response was by a greater than 50% reduction of the product of the two maximum diameters of all metastases for longer than one month. Patients with stable disease showed no measurable change in size of any metastases and no symptoms suggestive of new metastases for $\geqslant$ 6 months.

RESULTS

The response to treatment is shown in Table 1.

The single patient who 'responded' to BCG had a solitary metastasis 1 cm in diameter in the left lung present at the time of diagnosis. His primary tumour was removed one week after renal infarction using gelfoam. The metastasis took six weeks to regress completely but within three months of starting treatment the patient developed bone metastases and subsequently developed metastases in the opposite lung. Following radiotherapy to a lytic lesion in the right humerus, further metastases developed in the lung including one at the site of the original lesion which had regressed. He is currently still alive 11 months after diagnosis with progressively growing metastases.

As mentioned in the introduction, the chemotherapy used in this study was not standard. Table 2 presents results according to the type of drugs used and whether given as primary treatment or following disease progression after Provera or BCG. The majority of these patients received single agent therapy, although one patient receiving Vinblastine received CCNU in addition (Table 2).

There were no responses and none of the patients had stable disease for six or more months as was seen for three patients receiving Provera.

Table 1

	N	Response	Stable Disease ≥6 months
Provera	14	0	3
Chemotherapy*	7	0	0
BCG	3	1	0

* for details see Table 2

Table 2

	Previously untreated		Treated after progression on Provera and/or BCG	
	N	Response	N	Response
Cyclophosphamide (0.75 - 1G weekly)	2	0	1	0
Vinca Alkaloid	3*	0	8*	0
Chlorambucil	2	0	1	0

* Vinblastine n =,8, Vindesine n = 2, Vincristine n = 1
  $(6mg/m^2/2-3$ wkly) $(3-4mg/m^2/wkly)$ (2mg/wkly)

DISCUSSION

Recent reviews of endocrine treatment in patients with metastatic renal cell carcinoma have reported a regression rate of 7% in 643 cases while for chemotherapy the average for all cases reviewed (n = 486) was 10%, although for the best drug (Vinblastine) it averaged 25% (6,7). In contrast, for all series of patients receiving immunotherapy, either by BCG or by chemically altered tumour extract (n = 139), 27% have responded (8), and in the small series of 16 patients with lung metastases in the study reported by Tykka et al (4), 8 responded, 6 with total disappearance of all evidence of disease after treatment with a vaccine of autologous tumour cells polymerised with ethyl-chloroformate combined with tuberculin or candida albicans antigen depending on the state of pre-existing immunity in the patients.

Although the data presented in this paper are not adequate as a definitive study, they are worth reporting as they emphasise the need for accurate information about spontaneous regression and the incidence of prolonged stabilisation of disease - points which have not been adequately emphasised in the majority of previously reported studies of chemotherapy, endocrine therapy or immunotherapy in patients with renal cell carcinoma.

Prolonged stabilisation of disease is well recognised in patients with metastatic renal cell carcinoma even without active treatment. This observation, taken together with the less frequent but well documented occurrence of spontaneous regression, means that assesment of any treatment on the basis of regression rate or duration of response is invalid unless there are concurrent untreated controls who have assessment of their metastases as frequently as the treated patients. It is pertinent in this context to note that there was no evidence of stable disease amongst the patients receiving chemotherapy as primary or secondary treatment. In fact, one of the main reasons for the small number of patients treated by any of the drugs investigated was the extremely rapid progression of metastases which occurred in all patients once chemotherapy was initiated, almost as though the drugs were acting as fertilisers for tumour growth.

In the literature reviewed by Everson and Cole (1) only four of 26 cases of spontaneous regression had histological documentation of lesions which subsequently regressed. Although we did not obtain histological confirmation in the only patient who showed definite but short-lived regression, it is reasonable to accept this as a temporary tumour response since, when further metastases developed, the original lesion reappeared. Nevertheless, it would improve confidence on reports of tumour response if there was histological confirmation, as non-malignant conditions can produce changes similar to those produced by metastases. The increasing accuracy of fine needle aspiration biopsy should make this a realistic possibility in future studies.

SUMMARY

Retrospective analysis of the results of treating 24 patients with metastatic renal cell carcinoma emphasised the difficulty of using measurements of tumour response to assess the results of treatment and suggests that only by using large scale randomised control studies will bias due to chance inclusion of an occasional case of spontaneous regression be excluded. Equally, only by using randomised controlled trial will it be possible to exclude the possibility that treatment accelerates tumour growth.

REFERENCES

1. T.C. Everson and W.H. Cole, "Spontaneous Regression of Cancer," W.B. Saunders Co., Philadelphia (1966), p. 11.
2. D.J. Fairlamb, Spontaneous Regression of Metastases of Renal Cancer, Cancer, 47: 2102 (1981).
3. B. Van der Werf-Messing and H.A. Van Gilse, Hormonal Treatment of Metastases of Renal Carcinoma, Br. J. Cancer: 3: 423 (1971).
4. H. Tykka, K.J. Oravisto, T. Lehtonen, S. Sarna, and T. Tallberg, Active Specific Immunotherapy of Advanced Renal Cell Carcinoma, Eur. Urol. 4: 250 (1978).
5. H.J.C. Bloom, Renal Cancer, in: "Endocrine Therapy in Malignant Disease," B.A. Stoll, ed., W.B. Saunders Co., London (1972), p. 339.
6. G.P. Bodey, Current Status of Chemotherapy in Metastatic Renal Carcinoma, in: "Cancer of the Genitourinary Tract," D.E. Johnson and M.L. Samuels, eds., Raven Press, New York (1979), p. 67.
7. W.J. Hrushesky and G.P. Murphy, Current status of the therapy of advanced renal carcinoma, J. Surg. Oncol. 9: 277 (1977).
8. S.A. Brosman, Immunotherapy for Renal Carcinoma, in: "Cancer of the Prostate and Kidney," P.H. Smith and M. Pavone-Macaluso, eds., Plenum Press, London and New York (1982).

RENAL CELL CARCINOMA, SURGICAL TREATMENT

OF THE PRIMARY LESION

W. E. Goodwin

University of California
Los Angeles
U.S.A.

Our management of the surgical approach to renal cell carcinoma
is essentially the same as that outlined by Kaufman and Mims (1) in
"Current Problems in Surgery, 1966". The most common approach was,
with the patient in the flank position, to make an extraperitoneal,
extrapleural, subdiaphragmatic approach through a flank incision
below the twelfth rib. Although this is satisfactory, it does not
really give good enough exposure for radical surgery, which is
indicated in renal cell carcinoma which so frequently has extension
or regional lymph node involvement. Modifications include removal
of the twelfth rib or an incision between the eleventh and twelfth
rib.

We believe that thoracoabdominal nephrectomy first described by
Mortenson (2) is the approach of choice. The patient is placed in
the flank position with the flank extended, and an incision is made
between the tenth or eleventh interspace. After the pleura is
opened, the diaphragm is divided far enough laterally so there is no
injury to the phrenic nerve. The peritoneum is opened and the abdomen
is inspected and palpated to determine the presence or absence of
metastases.

Following this, the colon is reflected anteriorly toward the midline and the retroperitoneal space is entered. The kidney is pushed
forward and the renal hilus is dissected free. The renal artery
which lies posterior to the renal vein is identified and ligated.
When the renal vein is occluded before the renal artery, there can be
excessive bleeding. The renal vein is then exposed and should be
palpated to determine the presence of a tumor thrombus before ligating
it.

The renal artery is doubly ligated with 2 - 0 silk, and then the vein is doubly ligated and both structures are transected.

As Robson has pointed out, the best results are obtained in a truly radical nephrectomy when the entire kidney with Gerota's fascia intact is removed together with the regional lymph nodes. (3) When the tumor is excessively large, it is sometimes necessary to remove the kidney before dissecting the lymphatics which should be removed from the diaphragm down the the lower abdominal aorta. If there is involvement of the superior pole of the kidney, it is sometimes necessary to remove the adrenal with the "en-bloc" specimen. After the renal cell carcinoma is removed and the lymph node dissection is completed, the colon falls back into the empty space and the diaphragm is closed with interrupted sutures. The chest is closed in a conventional fashion, and I usually use a chest tube during the immediate post-operative period. The lungs should be inflated by positive pressure from the anaesthetist when the final closing sutures are placed.

The important thing is to remove all of the tumor after primary ligation of the renal artery and to do a dissection of the hilar lymph nodes and, if there is evidence of extension into the lumbar muscles or even into the diaphragm, to remove the areas of extension.

REFERENCES

1. J.J. Kaufman and M.M. Mims, Tumors of the Kidney, in: "Current Problems in Surgery," Yearbook Medical Publishers, Inc., Chicago. (1966).
2. H. Mortensen, Transthoracic nephrectomy, J.Urol. 60:855 (1948).
3. C.J. Robson, Radical nephrectomy for renal cell carcinoma, J.Urol. 89:37 (1963).

Editorial Note (M.P.)

Dr Goodwin expresses his personal preference for the large thoraco-abdominal approach. Undoubtedly this route gives an excellent exposure and in my view is the approach of choice in the case of large cancers of the upper poles of the kidneys. Many surgeons are however inclined to believe that this is perhaps too extensive a procedure, which does not appear to be necessary in renal cancer of category T1 and T2, especially if it is located in the lower pole.

An extended lumbar approach still advocated by some authors, is probably adequate only for relatively small cancers. Many surgeons are nowadays in favour of an anterior transperitoneal route in most cases, with primary ligation of the renal artery at its origin from the aorta, followed by ligation of the renal vein, before mobilizing

the kidney en bloc with perirenal fat. Ligation of the renal vein
prior to the artery is acceptable if preoperative embolisation has
been performed. Some authors feel, however, that an attempt at
primary ligation of the artery should be performed even after
successful embolisation.

KIDNEY CANCER - SURGERY OF METASTASES

J.P. Blandy, H.R. England and R.T.D. Oliver

The London Hospital Medical College
London
U.K.

The management of the solitary metastasis from renal cell cancer
is not in dispute: it is agreed that where the anatomical site of
the metastasis lends itself to surgical excision, the metastasis ought
to be resected, and it is equally clear that when surgical removal is
not feasible, then radiotherapy may give immediate relief of pain and
sometimes prolonged freedom from recurrence. The only thing that
perhaps deserves a comment, a propos solitary metastases, is their
astonishing vascularity - a fact which is little mentioned in text-
books and which seems to be one of those things which we all have to
learn by experience. Nobody who has had to face the unbelievable
torrent of haemorrhage that may follow biopsy of a metastasis from a
Grawitz tumour will ever undertake such a minor procedure lightly, or
without plenty of blood in reserve to meet such a dramatic crisis.
The main topic for debate is the management of the patient who presents with multiple metastases: is it justifiable to attempt to take
out the kidney? (1,2). The literature is unhelpful on the topic.
Surgeons who have a patient whose metastases have disappeared after
removal of the primary in the kidney tend to report such an unexpected
miracle. Those of us who are less successful do not report our
failures. There are two separate but cognate questions: (a) how
often does removal of the primary cancer seem to prolong life or make
metastases go away? and (b) how great a price does the patient pay
in terms of pain and mortality for this small chance of benefit? It
is to these two questions that we have addressed ourselves in this
study.

CASE MATERIAL

In the 114 patients recently reviewed in our department 98 underwent nephrectomy, and in 12 others, an exploratory operation was

Table 1.   The London Hospital.   Adenocarcinoma of Kidney   1964-79.

		Nephrectomy	Laparotomy	Palliation only
Males	73	63	8	2
Females	41	35	4	2
Total	114	98	12	4

started in the hope that nephrectomy could be completed (Table 1).
Overall, the operative mortality for nephrectomy in our hospital has
been 2% when performed for carcinoma: one of these died four weeks
after operation from his cerebral and other metastases and the other
presented with a huge carcinoma in a horseshoe kidney which was
impossible to remove completely, and whose attempted removal impaired
the blood-supply to the remaining half-kidney.   In neither instance
was there an error of surgical technique, though with hindsight, there
was certainly an error of surgical judgment.

RESULTS

In this series 34 patients had metastases at presentation (Table
2); of these we set out to perform a nephrectomy in 27.   It was
impossible in five, and we contented ourselves with a biopsy - often
not a minor procedure - so that nephrectomy was achieved in 22 patients who presented with widespread metastases.   As we have seen,
one of these died of his cerebral and other metastases à month after
operation.   This gives 4% operative mortality for this "faint hope"
operation.   Most of the patients continued to go downhill and died
of their metastases.   But three survived for more than five years
(11%) (Table 3).   The first of these had shadows in the lung, never
proven by biopsy, that remained unaltered for eight years until she
died at the age of 83 from bronchopneumonia unproven by post-mortem
examination.   The second presented with a painful lump in the chest
wall which was found to be a metastasis from a silent primary in the
kidney, and lived for another five years after nephrectomy only to
develop other and widespread metastases which swiftly killed him.
The third patient survived for five years, but was intensively treated
- though with radiotherapy and provera - now regarded as probably
useless - only to die in the end of his disease.

The difficulty is to know whether these anecdotes mean anything.
It is well known that patients can live a long time after their metastases have cropped up.   We have three such patients (Table 4) who
have respectively survived 12, five and four years from the emergence
of their metastases, at varying intervals from nephrectomy of one to
two years.

Table 2. The London Hospital. Adenocarcinoma of Kidney 1964-79.

Is it justified to attempt nephrectomy when there are distant metastases at the time the patient comes to Hospital? Nephrectomy for M1.

Patients presenting with advanced mets, terminal, or unfit to consider nephrectomy	7	
Nephrectomy achieved	22	(1 op. death, male 46 yrs. pT4.G1.M1 cerebral mets.)
Nephrectomy not possible biopsy only.	5	(Op. deaths nil)
Total operated on with intention of nephrectomy	27	(Op. mortality 1 [4%])
5 year survivals	3	(5 yr. crude survival rate 11%)

DISCUSSION

At a moment in surgical history when we have nothing else to offer the patient with widespread metastases from renal cell carcinoma an 11% chance of doing good - even if doing good only means prolonged life for five years - may seem worth while. Clearly it is not good enough. Equally clearly, there may be other reasons for trying to

Table 3. The London Hospital. Adenocarcinoma of Kidney 1964-79.

Unexpected prolonged survival of patients presenting with metastases (M1).

DP. f. 75 pT2. G2. M1.	Nephrectomy. 2 lung mets (not biopsied) remained unchanged for 8 years. Death from 'bronchopneumonia'. No P.M.
AM. m. 63 pT4. GX. M1.	Nephrectomy. Presented with lump in rib - excised, showed metastasis. Lived 5 years, then 2nd metastasis in femur. RT. Died 2 months later with widespread mets.
MP. m. 68 pT3. G3. M1.	Presented with supraclavicular nodes, biopsied then IVU revealed tumour. Nephrectomy, R.T. local lymph nodes N4. Provera, Prednisolone. Lived for 5 years, died with widespread mets.

Table 4.   The London Hospital.   Adenocarcinoma of Kidney   1964-79.

Prolonged survival after late appearance of metastases.

W. deS-L m. 55   1967 pT3.G3.MO Left nephrectomy. 760 g.
                       post-op R.T.
                  1969 Met. in right upper lobe of lung.
                       lobectomy.
                  1974 Mets. in left supraclavicular nodes
                       biopsy and R.T.
                  1981 Alive and well.

M.D. f. 53   1966 pTX.G2.MO Left nephrectomy.
                       post-op R.T.
                  1968 Chest mets. Provera.
                  1972 Path. fracture left humerus. Mets
                       left femur. R.T.
                  1973 Died. Widespread mets. (7 years)

G.O. f. 64   1977 pT3.GX.MO. Left nephrectomy.
                  1978 Chest mets. No treatment.
                  1981 Chest clear. Alive and well (4 years).

take the kidney out - pain, haematuria, clot colic and so on.   But
the price of this small chance is a 4% operative mortality, added to
the inevitable pain and suffering of a big transabdominal operation.
After our review of our experience we remain optimistic, and unrep-
entant, but at the same time we are deeply aware that there must be
something better just around the corner.

SUMMARY

Twenty-seven patients were explored with the object of removing
the kidney for carcinoma that had already given rise to widespread
metastases.   One patient died (4%): three survived for five years
(11%).

REFERENCES.

1.   J. DeKernion and D. Berry, The Diagnosis and Treatment of Renal
     Cell Carcinoma, Cancer, 45:1947 (1980).
2.   D.J. Fairlamb, Spontaneous Regression of Metastases from Renal
     Cancer, Cancer, 47:2102 (1981).

ADENOCARCINOMA OCCURRING IN A SOLITARY KIDNEY

S.A. Brosman

University of California
Los Angeles
U.S.A.

Although many instances of adenocarcinoma occurring in the solitary kidney have been reported in the English literature, it has only been in recent years that the natural history and therapeutic options for this condition have been evaluated. To compare survival, prognosis and therapy, patients can be divided into three categories. The first group consists of those in whom one kidney was originally removed for a benign disease or those born with a solitary kidney. The second group includes patients in whom one kidney was removed at a previous time because of cancer (asynchronous renal carcinoma). The third group includes patients who have bilateral renal carcinoma at the time of diagnosis (synchronous renal carcinoma).

One of the first comprehensive reports on this subject was by Wickham [1]. He reviewed the literature and evaluated data on 51 patients with cancer in a solitary kidney who had been diagnosed from 1942 - 1974 [1]. There were 25 patients whose original nephrectomy was performed for benign disease. Seventeen (68%) were alive (mean time of 30 months), six (24%) had died of renal cancer (mean time of 8 months), and there was no follow-up on two patients. There were 27 patients whose contralateral kidney was removed because of renal cancer. Ten (37%) were alive (mean time of 26 months), 15 (55%) had died (mean time of 8 months), and there was no follow-up on two patients. Nineteen of the patients in this group had been diagnosed since 1968 but only seven patients in the entire group had surgical excision of their neoplasm in an effort to provide a cure.

This poor survival in patients with asynchronous renal cancer stands in contrast to the results reported by Novick et al [2] who reviewed the experience from the Cleveland Clinic. The records of the 353 patients with renal carcinoma were evaluated and 21 patients

with carcinoma in a solitary kidney were found who had received
surgical therapy. There were ten patients whose other kidney was
removed because of benign disease and five were alive five years
after surgery with evidence of recurrence. Four of seven patients
with asynchronous carcinoma had no tumor recurrence. It is important
to note that the original nephrectomies in this group were performed
11 - 19 years earlier.

Schiff, Bagley and Lytton (3) reviewed the literature subsequent
to 1968, and included seven patients of their own. These 62 selected
patients had undergone surgical treatment that resulted in complete
tumor removal. There were 48 patients (77%) who were alive without
evidence of recurrence at an average follow-up period of 45.7 months.
They found no differences in survival whether the contralateral kidney
was involved with carcinoma or was removed for benign disease.

Jacobs and associates (4) reviewed the literature and the results
of 61 patients with synchronous carcinoma who were treated with surgical excision. Hereditary types of carcinoma were found in 12
patients; six had Von Hippel-Lindau syndrome, five had familial renal
adenocarcinoma and one patient had tuberous sclerosis. Ten patients
had such extensive disease that bilateral nephrectomy was required.
Six patients were placed on dialysis and four died of cancer while
one had metastatic disease at the time of the report. Only two of
four patients who had renal transplantation remained alive.

There were 51 patients who were candidates for total resection
of their tumors with preservation of renal tissue. Only 11 patients
died of their disease (79% survival). Ex-vivo surgery was utilized
in 16 patients and 13 remained alive (82% survival). Of 34 patients
with in situ surgery 26 remained alive at five years (75% survival).

Smith et al (5) reported on 33 patients treated at UCLA. Complete surgical excision was possible in 29 patients. There were 12
operable patients whose contralateral kidney was removed for benign
disease. Ten remained alive without recurrence at five years. One
death resulted from surgical complications and the others from recurrent cancer.

There were 12 patients with asynchronous cancer and eight with
synchronous cancer. Three of these 20 patients had such extensive
disease thay they were not candidates for surgical therapy. An
additional three patients died from causes unrelated to their cancer.
Eleven patients remained alive after five years following surgery,
but two have evidence of metastases. There was no difference in
survival between those with asynchronous or synchronous cancer.

Compiling the list of patients included in this report and other
isolated case reports permits a calculation of crude survival data
from a total of 182 patients (Table 1). There is an overall five

Table 1. Carcinoma in the solitary kidney; cumulative
          5 year survival

Type of Carcinoma	No. of Patients	5-Year Survival	
		No. of Pts.	%
Solitary kidney*	60	45	75
Asynchronous	34	23	67
Synchronous	88	58	66
	182	126	69

*contralateral kidney congenitally absent or
 removed for benign disease.

year survival of 69%. This includes 45/60 (75%) patients with contralateral benign disease, 23/34 (67%) of patients with synchronous
disease and 58/88 (66%) patients with synchronous carcinoma.

Patients with synchronous carcinoma occurring within five years
of the contralateral nephrectomy for carcinoma have the poorest prognosis (47% five year survival). Early recurrence is generally associated with multiple sites of metastases. Late recurrence tends to
be associated with a solitary metastasis and a good prognosis.

Both synchronous and asynchronous renal carcinoma represent
metastatic disease. Therefore, it is not surprising that survival
in these patients is not quite as good as those whose other kidney
was removed for benign disease, although the differences are not
statistically significant. All groups of patients without evidence
of widespread metastatic disease deserve an attempt to eradicate
their disease with surgery. Stage for stage, the disease seems to
be no more virulent in a patient with cancer in a solitary kidney
than in patients with two kidneys. The extent of the disease is far
more important than the reason the other kidney was removed. Unfortunately, there is not any clear data which relates stage to survival
but the presumption is that patients with low stage disease have
longer survival than those with high stage disease. The good survival
in these patients may be explained by the early detection of a solitary metastasis. Lung and osseous metastases are generally silent
until they reach a large size. Renal metastases tend to produce
hematuria early in the course of their development.

Current diagnostic techniques allow an accurate assessment of
the extent of the tumor within the kidney and permit the surgeon

to carefully plan the operative procedure. We have found that upper
pole tumors and extremely large tumors are easiest to approach through
a thoracoabdominal incision. Transabdominal and extrapleural retroperitoneal approaches through the tenth and eleventh rib beds are
also satisfactory.

Most carcinomas recurring in the solitary kidney can be managed
by in-vivo surgery. Even though there has been a great deal of
interest in 'bench surgery' in recent years, this type of surgical
procedure is not usually necessary. However, the capability of performing ex-vivo surgery should be available before contemplating the
removal of a large tumor or one that is located in the midportion of
the kidney. The major disadvantages of ex-vivo surgery are the com-
plexity of the technique, the need for vascular and possible ureteral
anastomosis, increased operating time and the potential of ischemic
damage to the kidney and increased patient morbidity.

Survival does not seem to be influenced by in-vivo surgery.
Jacobs et al (4) found that there were only three cancer deaths among
16 patients treated with ex-vivo surgery (survival 82%), compared to
eight deaths in 34 patients treated with in-vivo surgery (survival
76%).

The surgical principles which should be followed in the in-vivo
excision of these tumors are those generally applied to all types of
cancer surgery. The wound and surgical areas should be protected
from possible tumor spill by appropriate drapes. All of Gerota's
fascia can be removed but should not be stripped away from the tumor.
The adrenal gland may need to be removed with the upper pole tumors
since it is often a part of the tumor mass. When the adrenal is not
removed, it should be carefully inspected for possible metastases.
The renal artery and its major branches do not need to be stripped of
surrounding tissues. This may induce serious vasospasm and compro-
mise the residual normal tissue. The artery to the segment of the
kidney containing the carcinoma may be identifiable and if so, can
be ligated prior to occluding the renal artery; a Mannitol-induced
diuresis is beneficial for the preservation of renal function. In
some instances renal perfusion with cell-preserving agents such as
those used in renal transplantation may be necessary. Generally,
with the use of local hypothermia from iced saline slush, the renal
artery can be occluded for an hour without serious long-term renal
impairment. A Swan-Ganz catheter placed in the renal artery pre-
operatively can be used for vascular control as well as renal perfusion. Intraoperative angiograms may be necessary particularly
with ex-vivo surgery. Delicate reconstructive surgery is sometimes
necessary and is facilitated by the presence of appropriate instruments, magnifying loupes, or even an operating microscope. The use
of Avitene on the cut surface of the kidney has been a benefit in
providing hemostasis.

A staging regional lymphadenectomy is usually advocated to help determine prognosis. Removal of the ipsilateral nodal tissue adjacent to the kidney is sufficient. Following completion of the tumor removal and kidney reconstruction, the operative area should be thoroughly irrigated with distilled water.

CONCLUSION

Patients with carcinoma in a solitary kidney are potential candidates for curative surgery. Their prognosis depends on the stage of their disease and correlates with the cause of the contralateral nephrectomy. Those whose other kidney was removed for carcinoma do not have as good a prognosis as those whose kidney was removed for a benign disease. Patients with asynchronous tumors whose recurrences developed within five years of the original nephrectomy do not have as good a prognosis as those whose recurrence appeared later or those with synchronous disease in whom there are no other metastases.

Most operations can be done in-vivo. The operative team should be experienced in the various technical aspects, including ex-vivo surgery. Current diagnostic and operative techniques have improved the prognosis for patients with carcinoma in a solitary kidney.

REFERENCES

1. J.E.A. Wickham, Conservative Renal Surgery for Adenocarcinoma. The Place of Bench Surgery. Brit. J. Urol. 47: 25 (1975).
2. A.C. Novick, B.H. Steward, R.A. Straffon, and L.H. Banowsky, Partial Nephrectomy in the Treatment of Renal Adenocarcinoma, J. Urol. 118: 932 (1977).
3. M.S. Schiff, D.H. Bagley, and B. Lytton, Treatment of Solitary and Benign Renal Carcinoma, J. Urol. 121: 581 (1979).
4. S.C. Jacobs, S.I. Berg, and R.K. Lawson, Synchronous Bilateral Renal Cell Carcinoma: Total Surgical Excision. Cancer 46: 2341 (1980).
5. R.B. Smith, J.B. DeKernion, D.G. Skinner, and J.J. Kaufman, Management of Bilateral Renal Cell Carcinoma and Renal Cell Carcinoma in the Solitary Kidney (in press) (1981).

LYMPHADENECTOMY IN RENAL CANCER

G. Carmignani, E. Belgrano, P. Puppo,
C. Giberti and A. Cichero

Urological University Clinic
Genoa
Italy

ABSTRACT

On the basis of the experience of the Urological University
Clinic of Genoa (104 cases of renal cancer operated on in the last
10 years) the problems related to the rationale, the technique and
the indications for retroperitoneal lymphadenectomy in renal
cancer are reviewed and discussed.

It is concluded that, although lymphadenectomy adds little
morbidity and constitutes a fundamental part of radical nephrectomy
performed through an anterior transperitoneal approach, no actual
benefit can yet be demonstrated.

The generally accepted management of renal cancer is radical
nephrectomy, which includes perifascial nephrectomy through an
anterior transperitoneal approach, adrenalectomy and retroperitoneal lymphadenectomy (1). However it is possible to question
the benefits of lymphadenectomy, the technique and the extension
of nodal dissection and the indications for nodal extirpation in
high stage tumors. In this paper we shall discuss our experience
at the Urological University Clinic of Genoa, based on 104
consecutive cases of renal cancer operated on during the last
10 years and we will attempt to define the role of lymphadenectomy
in the treatment of renal cell carcinoma.

The rationale of lymphadenectomy

The indications for lymphadenectomy in every neoplastic
disease are:

- to allow accurate staging, which is indispensable to the planning of the postoperative treatment and to the evaluation of long-term results, and
- to improve the radicality of surgery and therefore to improve the survival rate.

However, immunological studies in renal cancer patients have drawn attention to the fact that routine lymphadenectomy, by abolishing the regional lymph node barrier, could impair the immunological defences of the host against the tumor. As yet there are no convincing arguments which support this opinion and we are not able to shed further light on this matter.

Our figures which show a 77% overall five year survival in patients without distant metastases at the time of surgery, submitted to extended nephrectomy with lymphadenectomy reveal no evidence of any unfavourable influences of lymph node excision. Moreover, the fact that 34.6% of patients without distant metastases, but with nodal involvement, in whom nodal metastases were extirpated, survived five years suggests that retroperitoneal lymphadenectomy might have a beneficial effect.

Incidence of regional nodal involvement

It is well known that renal cancer metastasizes by both blood-borne and lymphatic routes. The generally reported incidence of positive regional nodes during radical nephrectomy is about 20% (2-5). In our patients we found 32.6% to have positive nodes. If we consider these data in relation to the stage (Table 1) we can see that positive nodes are present in 6% of low stage tumors, but in a higher percentage of high stage tumors. At present we have no data either about the number of involved nodes or about the magnitude of the tumoral infiltration, which varied from microscopic foci to massive invasion.

Table 1: Incidence of regional lymph node involvement
          in renal cancer patients submitted to
          radical surgery.

	P2	P3	M+	V+M+
N+/Total	2/33	13/28	13/21	6/9
	(6%)	(46.4%)	(61.9%)	(66.6%)

The extent of lymphadenectomy

The extent to which nodes should be removed is also controversial (1,6,7). The accepted steps of the involvement of regional
nodes in renal cancer are - renal, hilar, ipsilateral para-aortic
or paracaval and later the mediastinal nodes. However the pattern of
the nodal involvement is unpredictable and although the iliac nodes
are not involved unless by retrograde embolism, contralateral and
supraclavicular metastases are not rare.

We assume that the very extensive lymphadenectomy advocated by
Robson et al (6) and by Angervall et al (2) does not add greatly
to survival and probably implies major morbidity for the patient.
Our practice is to carry out a more limited lymphadenectomy, which
extends from the diaphragm to the aortic or caval bifurcation and
includes the ipsilateral lumbar nodes, the retro-aortic or retro-
caval nodes and the interaortico-caval nodes (Fig. 1 a,b,c).

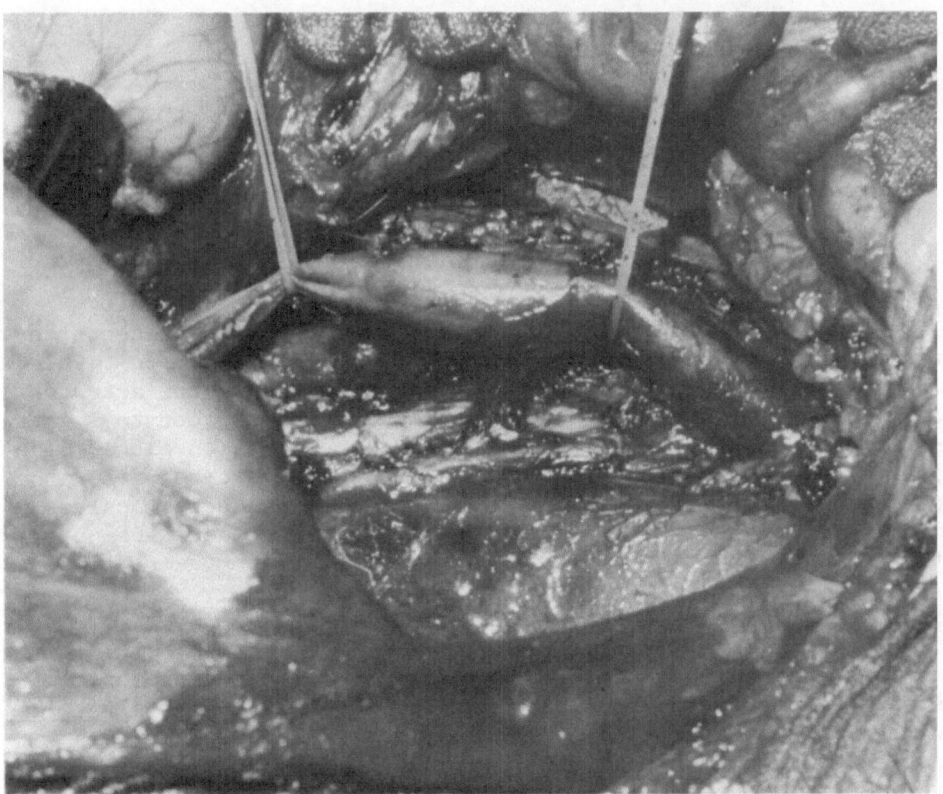

Fig. 1. Latero-caval lymphadenectomy

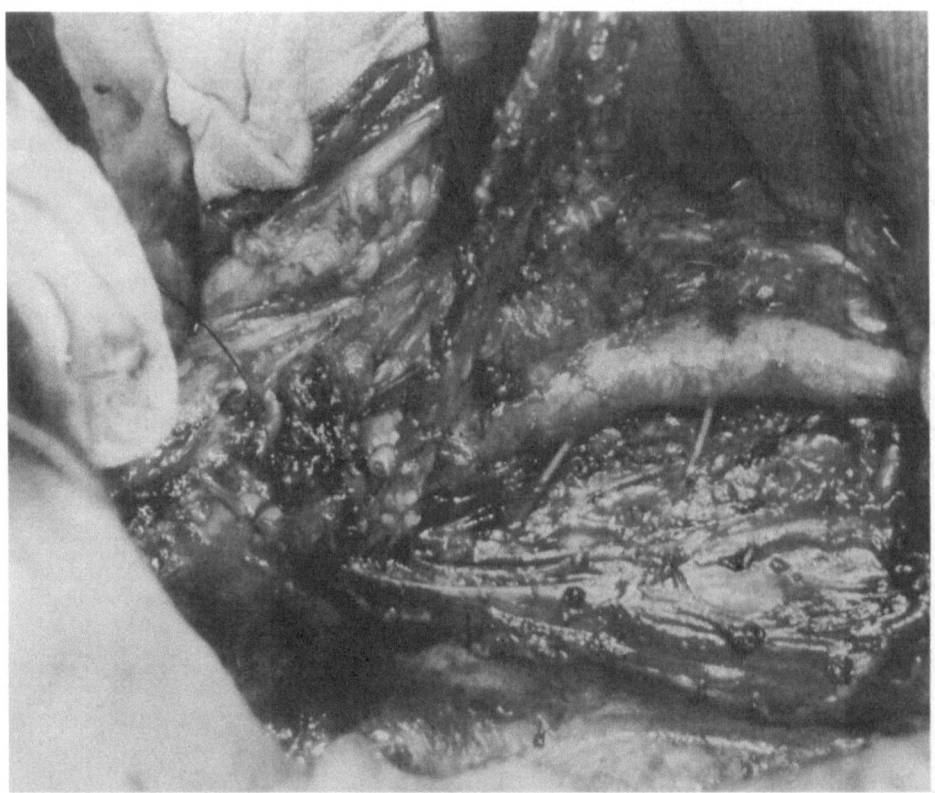

Fig. 1b.   Latero-aortic lymphadenectomy

In our series we did not note any significant morbidity
related to lymphadenectomy, which, on the contrary, represents an
integral part of the intervention.   Indeed the inter-aorto-caval
lymphadenectomy is indispensable to correctly expose the anterior
face of the aorta and vena cava, so allowing the surgeon to ligate
first the renal artery at its origin from the aorta on either side
(1).   Lateral and retroaortic or caval nodes are excised after the
nephrectomy. We do not perform an iliac node dissection, unless
lumbar nodes are clearly involved.   Contralateral nodes are not
extirpated.

Lymphadenectomy in patients with distant metastases

Aggressive management of renal carcinoma in the presence of
distant metastases has been advocated by several authors (1,5,8).
However, in the majority of reports no mention is made of the
practice of lymphadenectomy in these cases.   In our patients nodal
involvement in the presence of distant metastases was found in
52.4% of the cases.

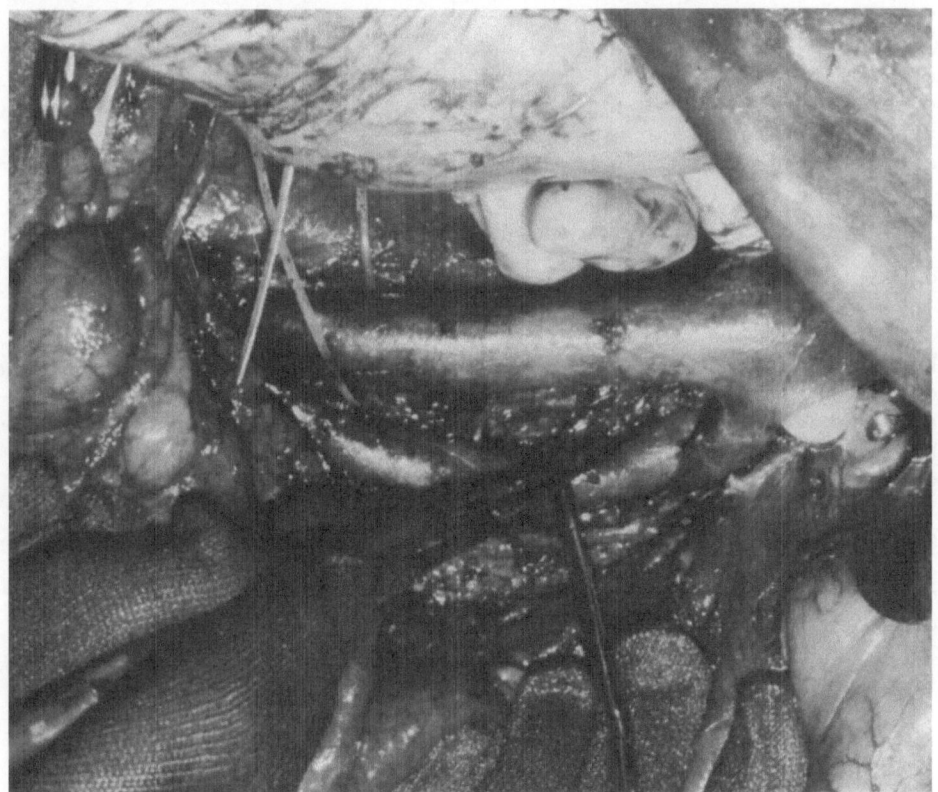

Fig. 1c.   Interaortico-caval-lymphadenectomy

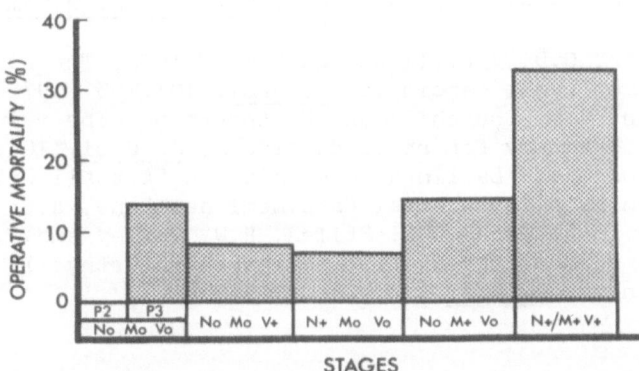

Fig. 2.   Renal cancer - operative mortality rate according to the stage of the tumor

We are of the opinion that lymphadenectomy should be performed
in these cases as part of the concept of reductive surgery, surgical
toilette and prevention of local renal fossa recurrences. When we
face a solitary metastasis, lymphadenectomy becomes of greater
importance in the effort to achieve a radical excision. In the
presence of multiple metastases, its goal is to give better
possibilities to chemotherapeutic treatment. On the other hand, it
is true that operative mortality is increased in patients with
distant metastases from 9.6 to 14% (Fig. 2).

Conclusions

We continue to advocate and to practice lymphadenectomy,
although no actual benefit from it can be demonstrated. On the other
hand, we have never observed any significant morbidity which could
be attributed to it and in skilled hands it adds little time to the
operation. However, there are as yet no reports in the literature
which satisfactorily define the problems related to its practice.
Additional information regarding the metastatic patterns of renal
cancer and tumoral lymphatic drainage and the effective contribution
of lymphadenectomy to the survival of renal cancer patients are
needed and we hope that a prospective clinical trial to provide
information on the role of lymphadenectomy will soon be started.

REFERENCES

1. L. Giuliani, Le vie di accesso, in "Attuali Orientamenti nella
    Diagnosi e Terapia dei Carcinomi del Rene," Atti SIU (1976).
2. L. Angervall, L. Wahlquist, Follow-up and prognosis of renal
    carcinoma in a series operated by perifascial nephrectomy
    combined with adrenalectomy and retroperitoneal lymphadenectomy,
    Eur. Urol. 4:13 (1978).
3. J.B. deKernion, Lymphadenectomy for renal cell carcinoma:
    therapeutic implications, Urol. Clin. N. Am. 7:697 (1980).
4. P.C. Peters, and G.L. Brown, The role of lymphadenectomy in the
    management of renal cell carcinoma, Urol. Clin. N. Am.
    7:705 (1980).
5. D.G. Skinner, C.D. Vermillion and R.B. Colvin, The surgical
    management of renal carcinoma, J. Urol. 107:705 (1972).
6. C.J. Robson, B.M. Churchill and W. Andersson, The results of
    radical nephrectomy for renal carcinoma, J. Urol. 101:297 (1969).
7. S. Rocca Rossetti, La linfadenectomia, in "Attuali Orientamenti
    nella Diagnosi e Terapia dei Carcinomi del Rene, Atti SUI (1976).
8. R.O. Klugo, M.Detmers, R.E. Stiles, R.W. Talley and J.C. Cerny,
    Aggressive versus conservative management of stage IV renal
    cell carcinoma, J. Urol. 118:244 (1977).

TECHNIQUES OF EMBOLIZATION IN RENAL CANCER

G. Carmignani, E. Belgrano, P. Puppo, S. Quattrini,
and A. Cichero

Urological University Clinic
Genoa
Italy

ABSTRACT

Embolization has now been widely accepted as a step in the management of large kidney tumours. Herein the technical problems of embolization are described and discussed.

As yet Cyanoacrylates are the best substances available for kidney embolization. A coaxial catheterisation system is not always necessary. Isobutyl-2-cyanoacrylate (IBC), which is the most used acrylic resin, can be made radiopaque by mixing it with Lipiodol Ultrafluid.

Radical nephrectomy should be carried out within 24 hours of embolization. The complications of embolization of kidney tumors are, in our experience, very few.

INTRODUCTION

Transcatheter embolization of renal tumours is a procedure that has gained more and more worldwide acceptance among urologists and its indications are now well defined (1,2). What is still debated is the technique of embolization, and especially the choice of embolic material to be used. A variety of different embolic materials have been utilized including finely fragmented pieces of autologous muscle (3), particles of gelatin foam (1,4), microspheres (5), special devices such as the Gianturco coil (6), complex apparatus such as an electromagnet in ferromagnetic silicone vascular occlusion (7) and finally the tissue adhesives (2,8,9).

Table 1.   TNM Categorization of 62 Renal Tumours
           treated by Preoperative Embolization
           at the Urological University Clinic of
           Genoa from 1975-1980.

$$T_1 \cdots 0 \qquad V_0 \cdots 39$$

$$T_2 \cdots 8 \qquad V_1 \cdots 16$$

$$T_3 \cdots 41 \qquad V_2 \cdots 7$$

$$T_4 \cdots 13$$

We have investigated, developed and perfected this last technique (2,8,9) and we report herein on the technical aspects of 62
cases of renal tumour embolization by cyanoacrylates performed at
the Urological University Clinic of Genoa during the last five years
(1975-1980).   (Table 1)

USE OF TISSUE ADHESIVES

Tissue adhesives are acrylic acid derivatives which, liquid in
a monomer form, rapidly polymerize, instantly solidifying as soon as
they come in contact with blood or other biological or electrolytic
fluids. Owing to their fluid nature they can be injected even
through very small catheters and the embolus can be brought downstream in the arterial tree to the capillary bed, so producing a
complete and distal embolization by forming a non-resorbable "cast"
of the arterial tree. This offers undoubted advantages over other
embolic materials such as gelatin foam, which is quickly reabsorbed,
Gianturco's device, which only produces a proximal embolization and
is difficult to place correctly in certain cases as for example when
there is early bifurcation of the renal artery. In selected
instances the use of a balloon catheter can prove very useful, but
generally it is not necessary. The recourse to a complicated
system of a detachable balloon to be used as an embolus (10) is still
in the experimental phase and, in this type of embolization, does not
seem to offer particular advantages.

Pitfalls in the use of Tissue Adhesives

The only disadvantage of the acrylic emboli is that they are
not easy to handle and do not allow any mistake, so that a very
experienced operator is needed. Previous practice in laboratory
animals is highly advisable.

The Choice of the Catheter: Coaxial or Conventional System?

Initially we thought that a coaxial catheterisation system was necessary (9) for fear that the catheter's tip might remain trapped within the sticky thrombus and owing to the need to control the effect of embolization by a subsequent injection of contrast medium through the outer loading catheter, since the inner one was occluded by the polymerization of the acrylic fluid and the cyanoacrylates are radiolucent substances.

The former danger proved to be groundless, whilst the latter problem could have been overcome by a trick that made the substance radiopaque.

How is one to make IBC radiopaque? In order to make IBC radio-opaque, so facilitating the control of the embolization procedure, Dotter and Rösch proposed the use of tantalum powder (11). However this substance is not easily available and is difficult to sterilise and we have proposed and adopted the addition to the IBC of an equal quantity of Lipiodol Ultrafluid^R(2), which, being a non-ionic substance, does not cause IBC polymerization.

Technique of Embolization

It is extremely important to flush the catheter carefully with five per cent dextrose in water prior to embolization (2) in order to prevent polymerization within its lumen. After careful and prolonged flushing of the catheter, a 2.5 ml plastic syringe containing the embolic mixture - 1 ml of IBC plus 1 ml of Lipiodol - is connected through a two way plastic stopcock and the embolus is slowly and completely injected under fluoroscopic control.

Owing to the radiopacity of the embolus, the entire procedure can be very easily controlled. The IBC Lipiodol mixture is quickly transported by the blood flow downstream to the finest arterial branches, so producing a very distal embolization.

In order to eject completely the embolic material out of the catheter a further small amount of five per cent dextrose in water is injected, until the circulation appears completely stopped.

The catheter is then withdrawn, while the radiopaque cast persists unmodified and clearly evident within the renal artery (Figs. 1a,b,c). Operation is usually carried out 24 hours after embolization.

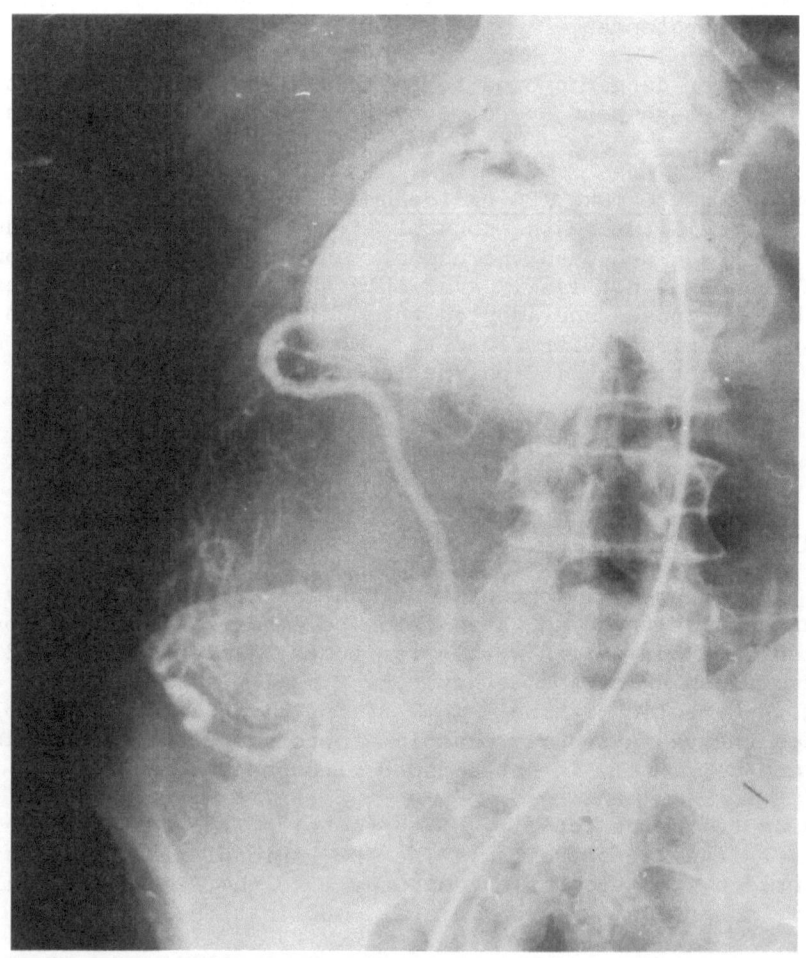

Fig. 1a.   Angiography and embolization of a very large right
           renal tumour.

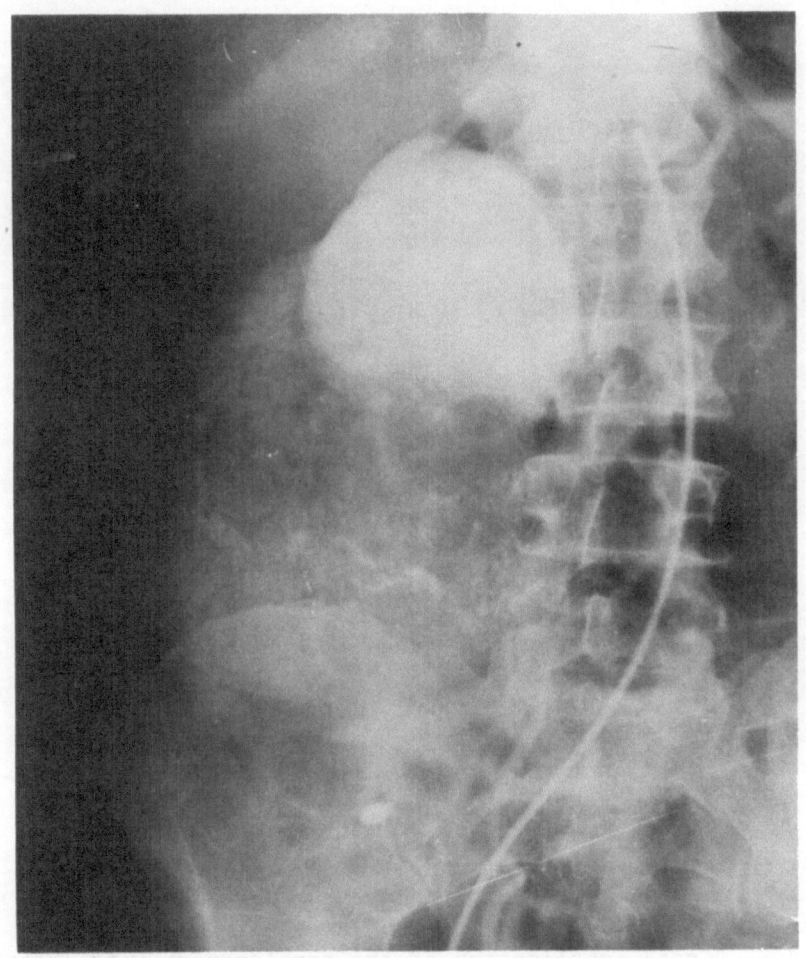

Fig. 1b.   Parenchymal phase.

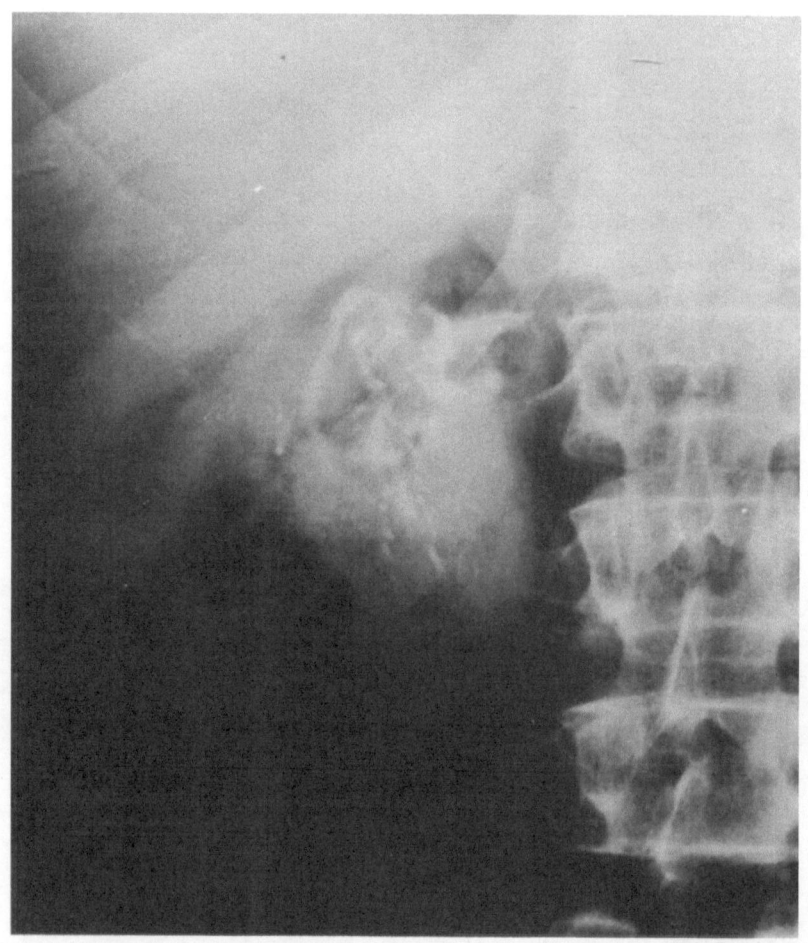

Fig. 1c. "Cast" embolization of the renal artery with Isobutyl-
          2-Cyanoacrylate.

COMPLICATIONS

The only complication we have seen is a certain degree of lumbar pain, which generally subsides following the administration of analgesics. Mild hyper-pyrexia was observed in 30 per cent of cases.

The search for new materials which give complete and lasting embolization is fully justified, because the "ideal" embolic material has not yet been found. In our opinion, and experience, IBC represents the best currently available embolic material for renal tumour embolization.

REFERENCES

1. L. Giuliani, G. Carmignani, E. Belgrano, and P. Puppo, Therapeutic embolization of renal cell carcinoma, Eur. Urol. 3:197 (1977).
2. L. Giuliani, G. Carmignani, E. Belgrano, and P. Puppo, Transcatheter embolization in urological tumors: the use of Isobutyl-2-Cyanoacrylate, J. Urol. 121:630 (1979).
3. L.E. Almgård, I. Fernstrom, M. Haverling, and A.J. Ljungquist, Occlusion of renal circulation facilitating later nephrectomy for carcinoma of the kidney, Scand. J. Urol. Nephrol. 77:521 (1971).
4. A. Hlava, L. Steinhart, and P. Navratil, Intraluminal obliteration of the renal arteries in kidney tumors, Radiology 121:323 (1976).
5. K. Barth, E. Bischoff, and G. Wenzel, Dauerhafte Ausschaltung der Nierendruchblutung durch Embolisation mit Mikrospheren, Vorläufige Mitteilung, Urologe A 14:250 (1975).
6. H.M. Goldstein, S. Wallace, J.H. Anderson, R.L. Bree, and C. Gianturco, Transcatheter occlusion of abdominal tumors, Radiology 120:539 (1976).
7. R.D. Turner, R.W. Rand, J.R. Bentson, and J.A. Mosso, Ferromagnetic silicone necrosis of hypernephromas by selective vascular occlusion to the tumor: a new technique, J. Urol. 113: 455 (1975).
8. G. Carmignani, E. Belgrano, P. Puppo, and L. Guiliani, Cyanoacrylates in transcatheter renal embolization, Acta Radiol. Diagn. 19:49 (1978).
9. L. Giuliani, G. Carmignani, E. Belgran, and P. Puppo, Embolization of renal cell carcinomas with Isobutyl-2-Cyanoacrylate, Urology 10:197 (1977).
10. R.L. White, S.L. Kaufman, K.H. Barth, V. DeCaprio, and J.D. Strandbert, Embolotherapy with detachable silicone balloons, Radiology 131:619 (1979).
11. C.T. Dotter, L.M. Goldman, and J. Rösch, Instant selective arterial occlusion with Isobutyl-2-cyanoacrylate, Radiology 114:227 (1975).
12. R. Küss, R. Bories, J.J. Merland, and M. LeGuillou, L'emboli-

13. G. Carmignani, P. Puppo, E. Belgrano, and P. Cornaglia, T and B lymphocyte levels in renal cancer patients: influence of preoperative transcatheter embolization and radical nephrectomy, <u>J. Urol</u>. 118:941 (1977).

HOW OFTEN IS EMBOLIZATION OF RENAL CANCER USEFUL NOWADAYS?

S. Khoury, F. Richard, and R. Kuss

Hôpital de la Pitié
Paris
France

Renal tumor embolization has many advantages which are summarized in Table 1. Embolization alone does not affect paraneoplastic manifestations (1) and any immunological advantages are
still hypothetical. Embolization destroys normal kidney tissue but
induces little or no histological change in the tumor itself.

Unfortunately embolization also has disadvantages:-

1. It is an additional procedure, especially since arteriography
is no longer necessary for the diagnosis of kidney tumors.

2. One should embolize all arteries going to the kidney and since
there may be several and also, because embolization to be effective
must be as distal as possible to the main artery, it is sometimes
a lengthy procedure.

3. Embolization lengthens the period of hospitalisation and adds
to the costs.

4. It also has complications including pain, fever and ectopic
embolization. Pain always occured in our cases, obliging us to
keep patients under sedatives and to program operation 24 to 48
hours after embolization. This might disturb the organization of
busy operating room schedules and we are now doing renal embolization under epidural anaesthesia, leaving the epidural catheter in
place to maintain anaesthesia until the time of operation. Fever
is also a common manifestation after embolization.

Ectopic embolization (in areas other than the diseased kidney)
is sometimes a very serious complication. Even in the best hands

659

this complication still happens. In our experience it has occured
in 3% of cases.

In arteriosclerotic patients (as most of them are) the manipulations may provoke endoarterial lesions. Embolization needs an
experienced vascular radiologist if a prohibitive level of complications is to be avoided.

The only aim of embolization is to enable the surgeon more
easily to remove the diseased kidney. In these circumstances any
disadvantage detracts from the value of the technique. The benefit
of embolization is marginal in T1 and T2 tumors, which account for
approximately 40% of all our patients. We have therefore always
limited our indications to cases where local difficulties at surgery
are to be expected and until 1977 we selected for embolization
patients who had one or more of the criteria listed in Table 2,
which encompassed nearly 30% of all patients. Embolization was
very often combined with the diagnostic arteriography.

With time, our enthusiasm for embolization has decreased. We
now rely on CT scan for the final diagnosis cf kidney tumors in 95%
of cases and very rarely carry out arteriography for diagnostic
reasons. We now believe that the usefulness of embolization is
limited to certain patients with T3 and T4 tumors.

Our criteria of selection have thus changed in the last two
years and, apart from very large tumors, a major lymph node involvement at CT scan or massive thrombosis of vena cava or renal vein,
our indications are based on the combination of more than one of the
conditions stated in Table 2. Our most common indication is the
association of a large tumor with lymph node involvement or renal
vein thrombosis.

Given this more selective attitude our indications for embolization dwindled down to 12% in our last 100 radical nephrectomies,
as compared with 26 in a previous series of 100 cases.

This personal opinion might change with different local factors
and is dependent upon the skill of the radiologist, the possibility of
 a rapid appointment for embolization, and whether one still depends
on arteriography for diagnosis. However even in the most optimal
conditions we do not believe that embolization is of any great value
in more than 20% of all cases.

Embolization is sometimes indicated as a palliative measure
when surgery is not practicable, e.g. in cases of intractable
haematuria for unresectable tumors. In some such cases control of
haematuria was satisfactory in five. In cases where patients had
metastases no regression of these lesions was noticed.

Table 1. Advantages of Renal Tumor Embolization

1. Reduction of the size of the tumor.

2. Permits ligation of renal vein prior to ligation
   of artery.

3. Reduction of distension of capsular veins.

4. Decrease in operative blood loss.

5. Improves surgical dissection planes.

Table 2. Indications for Embolization

1. Large tumors.

2. Massive renal vein thrombosis and vena cava
   extension.

3. Enlarged nodes on CT scan.

4. Palliative procedure in non resectable tumors
   with intractable haematuria.

Embolization also has experimental indications. We are now
working on the elaboration of microcapsules of antimitotic agents
having a slow release effect, and we are doing animal experiments,
trying to embolize the kidney and other organs with these microcapsules. The major drawback in kidney tumors is that we do not
have a potent antimitotic agent at the moment and that the use of
non potent agents intra-arterially is not likely, in our opinion, to
change the outcome and the potency of the drug.

In some cases kidney tumors have been embolized by radioactive
material. This obviously can only be a palliative procedure and we
do not believe that any palliative effect can justify the potentially
dangerous use of isotopes as a treatment modality. In addition, some
researchers in California are embolizing kidney tumors with a ferrite
compound and will use an external magnetic field to heat the kidney.
They call this technique electro magnetic surgery and will report
their results at the coming meeting on kidney tumors in Paris next
November.

REFERENCES

1.   G.D. Chisholm, The effect of embolisation/nephrectomy for renal
      carcinoma on the paraneoplastic syndromes, in: "Cancer of the
      Prostate and Kidney," P.H. Smith and M. Pavone-Macaluso, eds.,
      Plenum Press, London and New York (1982).

THE EFFECT OF EMBOLISATION/NEPHRECTOMY FOR

RENAL CARCINOMA ON THE PARANEOPLASTIC SYNDROMES

G.D. Chisholm, J.R. Hindmarsh, and T.B. Hargreave

Western General Hospital
Edinburgh
Scotland

INTRODUCTION

The presentation of renal carcinoma may be considered under four
headings:-

1. A triad of loin pain, mass or haematuria. The components
of this triad more commonly present separately; thus haematuria is
the presenting feature in 62%, loin pain in 50% and a renal mass in
34% (1). It is unusual for all three features to occur together, and
most series report the triad occurring in approximately only 10-15%
of cases.

2. Metastatic disease. There is almost no organ in the body
where a metastasis from renal carcinoma has not been found and in
many of these it is the presenting feature of the tumour. A secondary tumour in a bone is the most common site but the diagnosis is not
usually made until the biopsy is examined.

3. Autopsy findings. It is well recognised that a renal
carcinoma may be an incidental finding at autopsy. This incidence is
low, <1% of all autopsies (2). However, in a recent study by
Hellsten (3) a detailed study of kidneys in an area with a very high
autopsy rate showed a much higher incidence than previously reported.

4. Paraneoplastic syndromes. A very wide range of clinical
and laboratory abnormalities have been described in association with
renal tumours (4). The diversity of these abnormalities has led
them to be described either as systemic effects or as tumour markers.
A classification of these paraneoplastic syndrome is as follows:

1. Non-specific (toxic) syndromes

    - Haematological syndromes (e.g. anaemia)
    - Biochemical syndromes (e.g. abnormal liver function tests)
    - Metabolic syndromes (e.g. fever)
    - Immunological syndromes (e.g. neuromyopathy)

2. Specific endocrine (humoral) syndromes

    - Hypersecretion of a substance usually associated with the
      kidney (e.g. renin, erythropoietin)
    - Hypersecretion of substances not normally associated with
      the kidney (e.g. parathormone, gonadotrophins)

3. Miscellaneous syndromes

    - including mucin secretion and salt losing nephritis

The clinical importance of recognising these abnormalities is
that they are often the early signs or symptoms of a renal carcinoma.
It is well recognised that many of these apparently non-specific
abnormalities can lead to extensive medical investigation before the
link with a renal tumour is established. What is less well recognised is that the presence of these abnormalities does not
necessarily mean that there is metastatic renal carcinoma. For
example, the abnormalities of liver function, first described by
Stauffer in 1961 (5), are almost always not due to metastases because
they disappear following removal of the tumours. Using α2 globulin
as an example, the abnormal level of this substance usually returns
to normal after nephrectomy but can again rise with the development
of a metastasis. On the other hand, if the α2 globulin level does
not return to normal after nephrectomy this is good evidence of
metastatic disease.

Thus some of the paraneoplastic syndromes can be useful not only
for diagnostic purposes but also for monitoring the course of the
disease.

The possibility that embolisation and/or nephrectomy may have
specific immunological effects has been raised but not well substantiated (6,7,8). Assessment of anti renal carcinoma antibodies by
microcomplement fixation assays has suggested that a high percenage
of these patients mount an adequate antitumour response which falls
only when the malignancy becomes overwhelming; persistently elevated
titres are associated with the longest survival (9).

We have studied the effect of embolisation and/or nephrectomy on
the paraneoplastic syndromes and extended the study to examine the
effects especially on the immunoglobulins.

PATIENTS AND METHODS

Between 1978-80 20 patients (14 male, 6 female) presented with renal carcinoma. Half of these patients had metastatic disease at presentation. The presenting symptoms and signs were: Haematuria (6), haematuria + loin pain (5), haematuria, pain and mass (1), mass (2), tiredness (2), dysuria (1), polycythaemia (1), hypertension (1), bone pain (1).

All these patients were assessed by urography, chest x-ray, ultrasound, Technetium bone scan and renal arteriography. Laboratory measurements consisted of haemoglobin, white cell count, ESR, blood urea, lactic dehydrogenase, bilirubin, alkaline phosphatase, calcium, phosphate, total protein, globulins, and immunoglobulins.

The management policy for these patients consisted of renal arterial embolisation at the time of renal arteriography with nephrectomy, (3-5 days later), at which time the kidney was removed with its envelope but no formal node dissection was made. The decision to undertake nephrectomy in those patients with metastases at initial presentation depended upon the general state of the patient; this was an arbitrary decision and was influenced by the age of the patient and the activity level, thus two of the patients were treated by embolisation alone.

RESULTS

The initial assessment showed the following abnormalities:

Haematological

    ESR   75%
    Anaemia   50%

Liver function

    Lactic dehydrogenase   35%
    Alkaline phosphatase   20%

Bone

    Calcium ↑ 20%

Proteins

    Albumen ↓   55%
    Globulins   α2↑   55%
                 β ↑   60%
                 γ ↑   20%
    Immunoglobulins IgM   40%

There was no difference in the number of abnormal measurements in patients with metastases and without metastases.

The initial data and the follow up of six patients who underwent embolisation and nephrectomy are detailed in Table 1; none received progestogen. In all six patients at least one of the "marker" measurements was abnormal. At three months, nearly all of these abnormalities had returned to normal. Two patients had a raised ESR, three had mildly raised globulin fractions and two had raised IgM levels. Three patients had a raised gamma globulin at three months (but not pre operatively).

At six months, the two patient with persistently raised IgM showed further abnormalities (Table 1). One patient developed a raised serum calcium, then paraesthesia of the right hand followed by a lytic lesion of the first rib. Another patient developed a raised alkaline phosphatase and ESR at six months: one year later she had developed liver metastases.

In the two patients treated by embolisation alone, the one with bony metastases developed a marker elevation of gamma globulin, IgG and Ig M three months after embolisation but these had returned to normal by six months. This patient remains alive after 15 months but developed a positive bone scan one year after embolisation. The other patient with soft tissue metastases showed no response to embolisation and was started on chemotherapy.

DISCUSSION

The role of the paraneoplastic syndromes in renal carcinoma has not yet been clarified. Despite the range of abnormalities, most of them are non specific and can occur in association with other malignancies and other chronic diseases. The specific humoral abnormalities are uncommon and their exact incidence is uncertain since it requires renal arterial, venous and tumour tissue concentrations to be certain of an abnormal production by the tumour of a hormone. It is possible that these abnormalities are more common than reported, but few centres are able to pursue these studies in the detail required to answer this question.

A raised sedimentation rate remains the most common abnormality (10,11) but this is often found in other malignancies and may be associated with other medical conditions. The abnormalities of liver function described by Stauffer (4) are common in renal tumours, but they can also occur in the non-malignant condition of tumefactive xanthogranulomatous pyelonephritis. A raised $\alpha 2$ globulin spike has been described as a characteristic association with renal carcinoma (12) and this is probably the most useful 'marker' for renal tumours; changes in the $\alpha 2$ globulin correlate well with the course of this tumour.

Table 1. Abnormal serum tumour markers pre and post embolisation and nephrectomy

Initial Abnormality*	At 3 months		Recent Abnormality	Outcome	
	Normal	Still Abnormal		Metastases	No metastases
1. E.S.R	E.S.R	IgM	Ca^{++} γglobulin	Bone 8/12 Died 15/12	
2. IgM		IgM		Liver 18/12	
3. Haemoglobin E.S.R. Albumin↓ α2 & β globulin	Haemoglobin Albumin α2 globulin	E.S.R. β globulin	6/12 alkaline phosphatase E.S.R.		9/12
4. E.S.R. L.H. Calcium↓ β globulin IgM	L.H. Calcium	E.S.R. β globulin IgM	γglobulin IgA		12/12
5. Anaemia Calcium↓ Albumin↓ Bilirubin	Calcium Bilirubin	Albumin↓	γglobulin IgA		8/12
6. Anaemia E.S.R. Calcium α1 α2 βγ globulins IgA	Anaemia E.S.R. Calcium α1 α2 β γglobulins IgA		L.H.		6/12

* "Markers" represent increased concentration of the relevant substance except when specified (↓)

An extra renal triad that occurs commonly with renal tumours comprises fever, anaemia and hyperhaptoglobinemia (13). However many patients do not have all components of this triad so that its usefulness is limited.

In the present study we have looked for changes that might correlate with the treatment by embolisation/nephrectomy. There was no special pattern seen in these data as a group but the numbers are few and the follow up limited. However, each patient acts as his own control so that serial monitoring identifies marker changes. This study needs to be extended before a conclusion can be reached. In addition further studies of the paraneoplastic syndrome need to be undertaken so that a more complete picture of their role in renal carcinoma can be determined. A reliable tumour marker, or a pattern of markers is a great advantage in the diagnosis and treatment of an increasing number of tumours; the aim must be to define those paraneoplastic syndromes which can be of use in the management of renal carcinoma.

REFERENCES

1. E.N. Riches, I.H. Griffiths, and A.C. Thackray, New growth of kidney and ureter, Brit. J. Urol. 23:297 (1951).
2. H.M. Cameron and E. McGoogan, A prospective study of 1152 hospital autopsies: II Analysis of inaccuracies in clinical diagnoses and their significance, J. Pathol. 133:285 (1981).
3. S. Hellsten, T. Berge, and L. Wehlin, Unrecognized renal cell carcinoma, in:"Cancer of the Prostate and Kidney," P.H. Smith and M. Pavone-Macaluso, eds., Plenum Publishing Co., London and New York (1982).
4. G.D. Chisholm, Nephrogenic ridge tumors and their syndromes, Ann. N.Y. Acad. Sci. 230:403 (1974).
5. M.H. Stauffer, Nephrogenic hepatosplenomegaly, Gastroenterology 40:694 (1961).
6. J.B. DeKernion, Y. Katsuoka, and K.P. Ramming, Immunology of renal adenocarcinoma, in:"Renal Adenocarcinoma, UICC Technical Report Series," G. Sufrin and S.A. Beckley, eds., UICC, Geneva, (1980), Vol. 49, p.96.
7. D.J. Johnson, Percutaneous transfemoral renal artery occlusion in the management of advanced renal carcinoma, Henry Ford Hosp. Med. J. 27:92 (1979).
8. D.A. Swanson, S. Wallace, and D.E. Johnson, The role of embolization and nephrectomy in the treatment of metastatic renal carcinoma, Urol. Clin. North Am. 7:719 (1980).
9. J.B. DeKernion, K.P. Ramming, and R.K. Gupta, The detection and clinical significance of antibodies to tumor-associated antigens in patients with renal cell carcinoma, J. Urol. 122:300 (1979).
10. G.D. Chisholm, Clinical and biochemical markers in renal

carcinoma, in:"Renal Adenocarcinom, UICC Technical Report Series,"
G. Sufrin and S.A. Beckley, eds., UICC, Geneva, (1980), Vol. 49,
p.182.

11. B. Van der Werf Messing, R.O. Van der Heul, and R. Ch. Ledeboer,
Prognostic factors in renal cancer, in:"Cancer of the Prostate
and Kidney," P.H. Smith and M. Pavone-Macaluso, eds., Plenum
Publishing Co., London and New York (1982).

12. P. McPhedran, S.C. Finch, Y.R. Nemerson, and M.G. Barnes,
Alpha-2 globulin "spike" in renal carcinoma, Ann. Intern. Med.
76:439 (1972).

13. H.S. Bowman and E.J. Martinez, Fever, anemia and hyperhaptoglobinemia: an extrarenal triad of hypernephroma, Ann. Intern.
Med. 68:613 (1968).

RADIOTHERAPY OF RENAL CANCER: PRINCIPLES AND INDICATIONS

M. A. Bagshaw

University School of Medicine
Stanford
U.S.A.

INTRODUCTION

This paper will deal with the question of the usefulness of
radiotherapy in renal adenocarcinoma (hypernephroma), and will not
be concerned with renal sarcoma or with Wilms' tumor. There is a
lack of definitive knowledge about the role of radiation therapy in
the treatment of renal cell carcinoma (1-4). There are several
reasons for this:

(1) This uncommon tumor accounts for only 2% of all malignant
tumors in man.
(2) Definitive studies have been few, and the design of many
which have been done was compromised by the low incidence of the
disease.
(3) Pretreatment staging procedures have not been perfected,
further hampering the design of careful research studies, and
making comparison of results from different studies difficult.
(4) The liver, the gastrointestinal tract, and the spinal
cord, because of their radiosensitivity and their close anatomical
relationship to the kidney, present barriers to aggressive pre- or
postoperative radiotherapy.
(5) Renal adenocarcinomas are considered to be relatively
radioresistant.
(6) Diagnosis is established late in the disease, partially
due to the inaccessible anatomical location of the kidney, and
partially due to the lack of cardinal symptoms, such as pain,
swelling, or other obvious manifestations.

Earlier reports of the use of radiotherapy (whether pre- or
postoperative) are conflicting (5-9). The small number of

TABLE I

Comparison: Preoperative Irradiation + Surgery vs. Surgery alone in the Treatment of Renal Cell Carcinoma Without Metastases at Time of Treatment.

Major Study Location: Title	Author	Date of last report	No. Pts. randomized (evaluable)	Radiation dose	Differences in 5 year survival
U.S.: The Genito-urinary Group	Cox, C.*	1981	150	4500	No differences.
Holland: Rotterdam. Carcinoma of Kidney Trial, 1965	Van der Werf-Messing, B.	1973	141	3000	No differences (but decrease in renal fossa recurrence & in distant mets in P3 patients).
Finland: Helsinki University Central Hospital Clinical Trial, 1968.	Juusela, H.	1977	88	3300	No differences.

* Personal communication

patients and lack of consistent staging, or of controls, make these earlier reports difficult to evaluate.

PREOPERATIVE RADIATION AS A SURGICAL ADJUVANT

In the 'sixties and early 'seventies several more stringent clinical trials were carried out. Three studies, all of which were designed to compare radical surgery plus preoperative radiation versus radical surgery alone, have been completed in the last decade (see Table I) (10-13). All three were done on patients with no evidence of local or distant metastases at the time of treatment. Comparable numbers of patients were studied, and radiation doses ranged from 3000 to 4500 rads.

These recent studies were well designed in that three important criteria were met. The patients were studied prospectively, they were properly randomized into the two treatment groups, and they were not lost to follow-up.

Results of Prospective Studies: Overall, actuarial survival at five years was not affected by preoperative radiotherapy in any of the studies. The usual pattern of decreasing survival with increasing P category was observed (Table II). The P1 survival rate at 5 years was generally very high, around 90%, followed closely by the P2 group, who, at 5 years, were at the 75% level. In the P3 group, a much poorer result, about 25% survival, was typical. These five year survival figures agree with most studies of this tumor after surgery alone.

TABLE II

Definition of stages of renal cell carcinoma
by P-categories of the U.I.C.C. 1978*

P CATEGORY	DEFINITION
P_1	Tumor confined within the kidney
P_2	Extension of tumor beyond the kidney
P_3	Tumor involves vascular or lymphatic structures

* U.I.C.C.   1978 TMN Classification of Malignant Tumours, Geneva.

The early postoperative course of the disease was however affected by radiotherapy, according to van der Werf-Messing (13). In the P3 group of that study, residual tumor occurred frequently in the surgery alone group and there was clearly improved survival during the first 18 months postoperatively in the irradiated patients who had metastatic disease discovered postoperatively. Of 33 patients with such metastatic disease, 100% of those irradiated versus 62% of those who had surgery only were alive at 12 months post treatment. At 18 months post-treatment the figures were 78% survival for the combined treatment versus 28% for those with surgery alone. The explanation for this was thought to be that the follow-up procedures in the radiotherapy unit were better at identifying metastases earlier than in the surgical clinic, where those treated by surgery alone were followed.

POSTOPERATIVE RADIATION

The literature on the use of postoperative irradiation illustrates that it has been less well studied. Tumors which are found to extend beyond the kidney (Stage II or P2), or which extended to the regional lymph nodes (Stage III or P3), can be presumed to have residual microscopic disease after surgical removal of the diseased kidney. There are numerous reports of the use of radiation in such cases (9,14-17), but most of these are hampered by the lack of controls. Overall, it appears that radiation is best used postoperatively to treat residual disease in the renal fossa or for selected attack on solitary metastases.

CONCLUSIONS

Overall, the data on the outcome of radiation therapy in renal cell carcinoma are too few to warrant strong recommendations. Surgical treatment is still recommended as the primary treatment (1,2).

Radiation may be indicated (a) for residual disease after surgical resection and (b) for selected solitary metastases found postoperatively.

REFERENCES

1. J.B. deKernion and D. Berry, The diagnosis and treatment of renal cell carcinoma, in Proceedings of the American Cancer Society's National Conference on Urologic Cancer, Los Angeles, April 4-6 1979, Cancer 45:1785 (1980).
2. W.B. Waters and J.P. Richie, Aggressive surgical approach to renal cell carcinoma: Review of 130 cases, J. Urol. 122:306 (1978).

3. D.G. Skinner and J.B. deKernion, Clinical manifestations and treatment of renal parenchymal tumors, in: "Genitourinary Cancer," D.G. Skinner and J.B. deKernion, eds., W.B. Saunders, Philadelphia (1978).

4. D.G. Skinner, R.B. Colvin, C.B. Vermillion, R.C. Pfister and W.F. Leadbetter, Diagnosis and management of renal cell carcinoma, Cancer 28:1165 (1971).

5. R.H. Flocks and M.C. Kadesky, Malignant neoplasms of the kidney, J. Urol. 79:196 (1958).

6. B. Windemeyer and E. Riches, Radiotherapy and combined treatment in adults, in: "Tumors of the Kidney and Ureter," E.W. Riches, ed., E. & S. Livingston, Edinburgh (1964).

7. V. Paces, V. Doleckova and J. Zamecnik, Preoperative irradiation of renal carcinoma in adults (controlled clinical trial), Int. Urol. Nephrol. 10:77 (1978).

8. R.K. Royce and A.R. Tormey, Jr., Malignant tumors of the renal parenchyma in adults, J. Urol. 74:23 (1955).

9. E. Riches, The place of radiotherapy in the management of parenchymal carcinoma of the kidney, J. Urol. 95:313 (1966).

10. C.E. Cox, Personal communication, May 1981.

11. C.E. Cox, S.S. Lacy, W.G. Montgomery and W.H. Boyce, Renal carcinoma: 28 year review with emphasis on rationale and feasibility of preoperative radiotherapy, J. Urol. 104:51 (1970).

12. H. Juusela, K. Malmio, O. Alfthan and K.J. Oravisto, Preoperative irradiation in the treatment of renal adenocarcinoma, Scand. J. Urol. Nephrol. 11:277 (1977).

13. B. van der Werf-Messing, Carcinoma of the kidney, Cancer 32:1056 (1973).

14. R.C. Chan, Renal cell carcinoma, in: "Textbook of Radiotherapy," Third Edition, G.H. Fletcher, ed., Lea and Febiger, Philadelphia (1980).

15. J.C. Paradelo, Renal cell carcinoma, in: "Genitourinary Cancer Surgery," E.D. Crawford and J.A. Borden, eds., Lea and Febiger, Philadelphia (in press).

16. D.G. Bratherton and B. Chir, The place of radiotherapy in the treatment of hypernephroma, Brit. J. Radiol. 37:141 (1964).

17. S. Rafla, Renal cell carcinoma: Natural history and results of treatment, Cancer 25:26 (1970).

COMBINED CHEMOTHERAPY AND IRRADIATION OF PULMONARY METASTASES IN PATIENTS WITH RENAL ADENOCARCINOMA

F. Edsmyr, L. Andersson, and I. Näslund

Karolinska Sjukhuset
Stockholm
Sweden

INTRODUCTION

In the records of patients treated for renal adenocarcinoma and followed at the Radiumhemmet in Stockholm since 1940, no cases of spontaneous regression of metastases have been observed, either in the lungs or elsewhere. All patients with metastases died of their malignancies. During one period in the 1960s, hormone therapy, mainly provera in high doses, was given to patients with metastases from their primary kidney tumor. A short term objective regression was observed in 1.7% of patients.

In 1975 a chemotherapy pilot study was started in Stockholm in which patients in whom progressive pulmonary metastases appeared following primary nephrectomy for renal adenocarcinoma were treated with vincristine, bleomycin and irradiation.

All patients had bilateral, multiple metastases in the lungs which had been shown to be progressing on two chest X-rays taken prior to therapy. In some patients fine needle aspiration biopsy had been carried out to verify the diagnosis.

METHOD

Combined therapy with vincristine, bleomycin and irradiation was given twice weekly. Vincristine 0.5 mg IV was administered, followed six hours later by bleomycin 15 mg i.m.

Irradiation was delivered by a conventional 200 kV X-ray unit with a central dose in both lungs of 1000 rad (10 Gy) given in one month five days weekly; when the patient received the chemotherapy irradiation was given one hour after the bleomycin.

Chest X-rays have been performed every one to two months after the completion of therapy.

RESULTS

Of twenty patients treated, partial remission of the metastases has been observed in twelve and a stabilization of the lesions in seven. In one patient there was no effect observed. The mean duration of partial remission and stabilization was 5 months (1 - 24 months).

The subjective response in terms of pain relief and improved well-being was good and the side effects of the combined therapy were negligible.

CONCLUSION

Short term objective remission of pulmonary metastases have been seen following combined treatment with vincristine, bleomycin and irradiation in 12 of 20 patients treated. Subjective improvement also occurred.

On the basis of this investigation a randomized study has started, to compare the above-mentioned combined schedule with inferferon given in daily doses of 8 million international units.

Editorial Comment (P.H.S.)

A 60% partial response rate following chemotherapy and radiotherapy of pulmonary metastases in an institute in which spontaneous regression of metastases has not been observed for forty years is truly remarkable and deserves to be repeated, preferably with further evidence of the details of the subjective responses seen.

PREOPERATIVE IRRADIATION AND NEPHRECTOMY IN POORLY DIFFERENTIATED CARCINOMA OF THE KIDNEY (A PRELIMINARY STUDY)

L. Andersson, F. Edsmyr, S. Franzén

Karolinska sjukhuset
Stockholm
Sweden

INTRODUCTION

In the late 1960's we started to investigate whether post-nephrectomy survival in renal carcinoma is improved by preoperative irradiation. It was intended to study especially those patients with poorly differentiated cancer. However, a few cases of moderately or even well differentiated cancer were included in the investigation.

METHODS AND MATERIAL

Malignancy Grading

Fine needle aspiration of the tumor was performed after the diagnosis had been established by urography and nephroangiography. The puncture was done under television - monitored fluoroscopy and with the patient in the prone position. The kidney was located by intravenous urography.

Irradiation

The irradiation was given by a 6 MeV linear accelerator with a three-field technique to give an average irradiation dose to the kidney tumour of 3,500 rad, in about 35 days. Extrafascial nephrectomy was carried out 3 - 4 weeks after cessation of irradiation. No extensive lymphadenectomy was done.

Clinical Material

This investigation comprises 34 patients with carcinoma of the kidney operated on in the period 1968 - 1971. The cytologic smears

were reviewed by one cytologist (S.F.). In 24 cases the cancer was
initially evaluated as poorly differentiated, in 9 as moderately well
and in one case as well differentiated.

RESULTS

In 11 cases judged as poorly differentiated carcinoma before
irradiation, only moderately well or well differentiated carcinoma
was found in the operative specimen. In one case diagnosed as moderately well differentiated cancer before irradiation only well differentiated tumour was found in the operative specimen. In another case
of moderately well differentiated cancer in the biopsy, poorly differentiated tumour was found in the specimen. In the remaining cases
there was either the same malignancy grade in the biopsy and operative
specimen, or incomplete data were available (9 cases).

There was no operative mortality in this series. The postoperative survival of the 24 patients with poorly differentiated carcinoma
is presented in Figure 1. The postoperative survival of 103 patients
with poorly differentiated carcinoma, subjected to nephrectomy in the
same hospital without previous irradiation and previously reported by
Arner, Blanck and von Schreeb (1) is demonstrated for comparison. In
the latter series, operative deaths are excluded from the calculations.

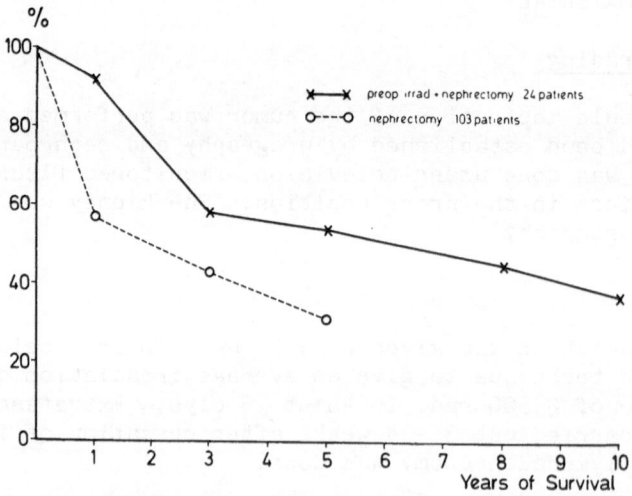

Fig. 1. Postnephrectomy survival in patients with poorly differ-
         entiated renal cell carcinoma after preoperative irrad-
         iation, compared with survival in patients treated by
         surgery alone.

Average five year survival in the patients given preoperative irradiation was 54%, in the other group 31%.

    The group of moderately well differentiated carcinoma was too
small, only 9 cases, to allow any definite conclusions. With this
reservation in mind, it may be mentioned that survival in this small
group was approximately the same as survival rate in a series of 55
non-irradiated cases of moderately well differentiated carcinoma
reported by Arner, Blanck and von Schreeb (1). Five year survival
in the patients given irradiation was 67%; in the other group 63%.

    With the technique used here there was no damage to the contra-
lateral kidney but some patients with right-sided tumours had a
slight to moderate, but temporary, disturbance of liver function
following irradiation.

DISCUSSION

    It is noteworthy that in 12 cases the kidney tumour had a lower
malignancy grade at nephrectomy a month after irradiation than on
the preirradiation biopsy. Whilst allowance must be made for
certain personal variations in the evaluation of cytologic and histo-
pathologic patterns, a previous investigation (2) has shown, however,
that with the technique used in this study there is good conformity
between the percutaneous aspiration biopsy and the histopathologic
findings of the nephrectomy specimen. It would therefore appear that
in certain cases the preoperative irradiation may eradicate cell
populations of high malignancy grade.

    From this small series it would also appear that in cases of
poorly differentiated renal carcinoma, preoperative irradiation may
improve postoperative survival. Investigation of a larger patient
series is in progress.

SUMMARY

    Thirty-four patients with carcinoma of the kidney were treated
by preoperative irradiation (3,500 rad) followed by nephrectomy 3 -
4 weeks later. In some cases the malignancy grade of the operative
specimen was lower than on puncture biopsy of the tumour before
irradiation, indicating possible eradication of highly malignant
cell populations. The postoperative survival in cases of poorly
differentiated tumour cases was higher than in a previous series of
patients operated on without preoperative irradiation. In a small
number of patients with moderately well differentiated carcinoma
there was no difference between patients given preoperative irradiation and those treated by surgery alone.

REFERENCES

1. O. Arner, C. Blanck, and T. von Schreeb, Renal adenocarcinoma.
    Morphology - Grading of malignancy - Prognosis. A study of 197
    cases., Acta Chir. Scand. 346 (1965).

2. T. von Schreeb, S. Franzén, and A. Ljungquist, Renal adeno-
    carcinoma. Evaluation of malignancy on a cytologic basis: A
    comparative cytologic and histologic study., Scand. J. Urol.
    Nephrol. 1: 265 (1967).

Editorial Note (M.P.)

        This paper by Professor Andersson and his associates is closely
related to another work by the same group, published in this book
under the title of "Aspiration biopsy and cytology of renal cancer".

        These stimulating articles raise some questions. The indication
for a fine needle aspiration-biopsy of renal cancer lies in the fact
that the finding of a high grade tumor should favour the decision of
performing preoperative irradiation prior to nephrectomy. The
validity of this approach will become clear if some doubts can be
solved. In the first place, the accuracy of a grading solely based
on cytology from fine needle aspirates does not yet appear to be
established with certainty. As the authors point out from their own
personal data, which stem from the work of very experienced cytologists, the correlation between cytological and histological grading
is far from being satisfactory. Agreement was obtained only in 36
of 47 cases, i.e. there was disagreement in 23.4% of all cases. The
disparity was sometimes of one, but occasionally even of two grades.
Cytology tended to produce an "overgrading", as shown by the fact
that only four cases were classified as "high grade" by histology,
whereas eight cases were assigned to the high grade category by
cytology. As the grading was determined by the highest malignancy
grade found in both the histological specimen and in the cytology
smear, it is obvious that a larger number of cells can be visualised
by histology, so that even small foci of more atypical cells can be
identified. This seems to amplify the risk for "overgrading" by
cytological technique in this particular tumour. This conclusion
is supported by the fact that the percentage of high grade tumors
in the present series based on cytology (70.6%) is much higher than
that reported in other reports (see Tannenbaum and Tannenbaum in
this volume: only 18% of G3 renal adenocarcinomas). If these considerations are correct, then the finding of a lower malignancy
grade at histology of the nephrectomy specimen as compared to the
higher grade on cytology of the pre-nephrectomy aspirate can hardly
be considered as a criterion for response and the suggestion that
the preoperative irradiation may eradicate populations of high
malignancy grade remains hypothetical. On the other hand the fact
that survival was better in this series of patients treated with

preoperative irradiation followed by nephrectomy than in a previous
series of patients operated upon without irradiation, is not a definitive argument in favour of preoperative irradiation, but suffers
from the weakness inherent in all comparisons based on historical
controls. Therefore, neither the need for needle aspiration biopsy
nor for preoperative irradiation is based, in my opinion, on un-
shakable evidence. However the idea is very attractive and further
studies are certainly warranted. Their results will be awaited with
the greatest interest.

It should be emphasized that no untoward effects were produced
by percutaneous puncture of renal tumors, contrary to a widespread
fear. This is certainly a very important observation.

IMMUNOTHERAPY FOR RENAL CARCINOMA

S.A. Brosman

University of California
Los Angeles
U.S.A.

Adenocarcinoma of the kidney may be uniquely suited for attempts at immunotherapy. The natural history of this neoplasm is unusual because these patients may have long periods of time between excision of the primary tumor and development of metastases. We have observed patients in whom the primary tumor existed for 15 to 20 years before treatment was initiated. Following removal of the primary tumor, metastases rapidly appeared. Temporary regression of metastases and long term stabilization of tumors has been described. These findings suggest the presence of immune response which is able to control the development of the tumor.

Considerable evidence has been amassed to suggest the presence of cellular and immune response in patients with renal cell carcinoma (1). These observations, along with the usual clinical behavior of the tumor which suggest an important role of host immunity, prompted a variety of immunotherapy trials.

The first efforts at passive immunotherapy of renal carcinoma were in the form of serotherapy. Horn et al (2) infused plasma from a patient previously cured of renal carcinoma into a family member with diffuse metastases. The patient remained clinically free of tumor for 20 months, after which he died of cerebral metastases. Another patient with extensive pulmonary metastases received plasma infusion from a family member who previously had undergone curative nephrectomy for a renal carcinoma. One pulmonary metastasis completely resolved and two others remained stable. The serum of the treated patients showed significant levels of serum blocking activity prior to immunotherapy, but were demonstrated to have unblocking activity during periods of regression or stabilization of tumor. The serum donors also appeared to have specific unblocking

activity (3).   These preliminary attempts at serotherapy have not
been expanded into formal clinical trials.   Adoptive immunotherapy
in the form of transfer factor and immune RNA have been used more
extensively than any other form of immunotherapy for renal carcinoma.
Montie et al reported early results in a few patients with metastatic
renal carcinoma treated with transfer factor (4).   Although they
reported some objective responses, which included stabilization of
measurable lesions, the number of patients was too small to make a
true assessment of the value of this agent.

In a subsequent report from the same institution, transfer
factor was combined with other modalities (5).   These were not randomized trials but three different regimens were employed at different times.   Nine patients received transfer factor alone, of which
one had a complete response.   There were no partial responders.   A
second group received transfer factor plus Tice strain BCG by scarification.   Two of the eight patients treated had partial regression
of measurable metastases.   A third group received transfer factor
plus CCNU plus Megace.   Of the 14 so treated, one had a complete
response and four had partial responses.   Toxicity was apparently
acceptable.   Before attributing the regressions to the therapy, it
will be important to perform randomized clinical trials.   Furthermore, the duration of response and survival of treated patients must
be compared either to untreated controls or to historically matched
controls from the same institution.   Nonetheless, the incidence of
complete response (two out of 31) and partial responses (six out of
31) is higher than would be expected from that due to inherent natural
history characteristics.   It is also interesting to note that in
this study and in those by Schapira et al (6) and Tykka et al (7)
most patients who responded to therapy were those with pulmonary
metastases.

DeKernion described experiments using immune RNA in the treatment of renal cell carcinoma.   Initially, lysis of human renal carcinoma tumor cells by allogeneic peripheral blood lymphocytes which
were stimulated with immune RNA were reported (8).   Subsequently,
20 patients with metastatic renal cell carcinoma and nine patients
with minimum residual disease who had a high risk for recurrence
following nephrectomy   received weekly intradermal injections of
4 mg. of immune RNA.   The RNA was extracted from lymphoid organs
of sheep which had been immunized with human cell carcinoma.   Toxicity of therapy was minimal and consisted of erythema and a flu-like
syndrome in six patients.   Total doses of over 700 mg. and single
doses of 64 mg. did not produce severe toxicity.   Complete tumor
response was not observed in any patients with metastases.   Seven
patients had a partial response which was defined as less than 50%
regression of stability of measurable, previously growing tumors
for over three months (9).

The most commonly used agents have been non-specific immuno-

stimulants, especially BCG.   We have treated 12 patients with far-
advanced renal cell carcinoma and compared survival to 10 patients
who did not receive immunotherapy (10).   Although survival of the
treated patients was somewhat increased, the difference was not significant.   Eidinger and Morales treated eight patients with metastatic
renal carcinoma with BCG (11).   They reported objective improvement
in five of eight patients, although the criteria for improvement
included stabilization of growth of metastatic foci in one patient.
Also, all of these responses were transient in this non-randomized
study and the mean duration of follow-up was brief.

Lange treated patients with metastatic renal carcinoma by multiple intradermal BCG injections after removing the bulk of the
tumor (12).   Tumor stabilization or regression occurred temporarily
in only 15% of patients, and they concluded that survival was not
increased by this method of surgery plus immunotherapy.   Minton et al
reported clinical responses in four of nine patients with metastatic
renal carcinoma to the lungs treated with intradermal BCG (13).
Antibody-dependent cell cytotoxicity was correlated with clinical
control of the tumor.   Sera from the responders induced lysis of old
tuberculin-treated red blood cells by normal human peripheral lymphocytes, whereas sera from non-responders did not.

Tykka et al treated 31 patients with metastatic renal cell carcinoma with active specific immunotherapy after palliative nephrect-
tomy (7).   A soluble fraction of autologous tumor prepared by hypo-
tonic cell lysis was polymerised into small particles by addition of
ethylchlorformiate.   The polymerised tumor was injected intradermally
with PPD tuberculin or candida antigen as adjuvants.   Survival of
treated patients was improved over that of controls, although only
20% of treated patients were alive at five years.   The major effect
was noted in patients with pulmonary metastases, which disappeared
in six of 16 treated patients.

Although these results appear to be encouraging, it is unclear
whether patients were prospectively randomized or selected for reasons
such as unavailability of tumor or other criteria.   Some patients
had only microscopic tumor, others had solitary lesions which were
excised, and some had no measurable disease.   Although control and
treatment groups were similar with respect to stage of disease, it
is not stated whether they were matched with respect to site and
number of metastases and the use of polymerised tumor.   Anti-tumor
antibodies could not be detected in the sera of treated patients and
no difference in migration inhibition assay was noted between treated
patients and controls.   It is therefore not possible to conclude from
these data that this form of immunotherapy is effective.   However,
results are sufficiently better than those expected for patients with
this stage of renal carcinoma to warrant a prospective randomized
trial.

Several reports of active immunotherapy with allogeneic lymphocytes (14) and microsomal renal carcinoma cell fractions (15) were
reported to show possible efficacy in renal carcinoma, but have not
been expanded into clinical trials from which definite conclusions
could be derived.

DeKernion from UCLA has begun a study in cooperation with
investigators from Roswell Park and the University of Rochester.
The Method of immunotherapy proposed in this study is based on the
combination of a tumor cell vaccine with a non-specific adjuvant.
One of the classic immunologic techniques for priming the immune
system is to inject intradermally, the foreign antigen bathed in an
adjuvant such as Freund's adjuvant.   This is particularly useful
when the antigen itself is poorly immunogenic.   The adjuvant concept
was applied to animal neoplasia beginning in the early 1970's.   When
poorly immunogenic animal tumors are prepared as a cell suspension
in medium containing an adjuvant and injected intradermally, a
systemic, long-lasting antitumor effect can consistently be produced.
Bartlett and Zbar demonstrated that BCG could be effectively used as
an adjuvant in their model of guinea pig hepatoma (16).   Scott
demonstrated that C. parvum could be used as the adjuvant in a mouse
mastocytoma system (17).   When tumor cells and a bacterial adjuvant
are injected, two distinct categories of an immune response occur:
a local inflammatory response and a systemic tumor-rejecting specific
immunity which is cell-mediated.

C. parvum was selected as the adjuvant for this trial because
of the possibility of decreased toxicity in human trials.   Based
upon animal studies, variables have been observed which determine
success or failure of specific immunotherapy with bacterial adjuvants.
These are: a) proper ratio of C. parvum to tumor cells: b) serial
immunizations rather than a single dose: c) adequate quantities of
tumor cells in the immunizing doses: d) an effective method of cryo-
preserving tumor tissues.   Others have demonstrated that this immunizing procedure is highly specific for the individual tumor and
required autologous (syngeneic) rather than allogeneic tumor
cells (18).

The phase II study in metastatic renal carcinoma included 16
patients (19).   Objective regression of metastases occurred in five
patients and a sixth had symptomatic improvement and no progression
of tumor for greater than 27 months.   Six patients survived 20
months or greater which is better than one would expect in that group
of patients.

The major shortcoming of this modality is the necessity of
obtaining autologous tumor cells.   In view of the current practice
of palliative nephrectomy in patients with metastases, removal of
the primary tumor is a reasonable approach.   In addition to the
expectation for palliation and perhaps temporary cessation of growth

of metastases, further justification is cited for the prospect of
offering the patient an immunotherapeutic modality.

Allogeneic cells do not seem to be appropriate in such a study.
Animal data suggests significant antigenic disparities among various
tumors of similar cell types, in spite of the reported evidence of
the presence of shared tumor associated antigens.   In addition,
the potential for toxicity, including hepatitis, is increased with
the use of allogeneic cells.

Brown and co-workers have recently reported their experience
using a tumor vaccine consisting of a single cell suspension of tumor
cells prepared by mechanical disaggregation and complexed with di-
methyldiotadecyl ammonium bromide (DDA) (20).   DDA is a potent
macrophage activator and depending on the techniques of administration gives some selectivity in promoting delayed hypersensitivity
or humoral responses.

Twenty-seven patients with metastatic carcinoma were treated
with radical nephrectomy followed by specific immunotherapy.   They
received monthly injections of a vaccine which was placed intradermally near regional lymph nodes.   A vaccine dose of 25 mg. of autologous or allogeneic tumor protein complexed with two micromoles of
DDA was used.

The longest follow-up was 131 weeks with a median follow-up of
41 weeks.   Seven patients have died of their disease.   Three patients have developed complete remission but the duration of this
remission is not reported.   Utilizing life table analysis, Brown
et al reported a one year survival of 69% with a predicted median
survival of 131 weeks.   This group of patients was compared to two
groups of historical controls.   Thirty-six patients who received
nephrectomy alone had a one year survival of 48% and a median
survival of 36 weeks.   The second group received no surgery and
only palliative therapy.   Their one year survival was 32% with a
median survival of 18 weeks.

Neidhart et al report their results in 24 patients with metastatic renal carcinoma who were treated with a tumor vaccine similar
to that described by Tykka et al (21).   Aggregated soluble tumor
antigens were admixed with tuberculin or phytohemagglutinin.
Initially the patients own tumor was used to prepare the antigen
but later allogeneic cells were used.   In contrast to Tykka's study,
scarification with BCG was added to ensure maximum reactivity to
tuberculin.

Two patients demonstrated a complete response to therapy and
were tumor free after four and 56 weeks.   Two patients had a partial
response at 12 and 32 weeks and 11 patients had stable disease at

14-111 weeks.   These responses are similar but not quite as good as those of Tykka.

All of these various immunotherapy studies in patients with metastatic disease indicate that there are patients who may have a beneficial response to selective immunotherapy.   The results are as good as, and in some cases better than, current chemotherapy.

REFERENCES

1.   J.B. DeKernion, Y. Katsuoka and K.P. Ramming, Immunology of Human Renal Adenocarcinoma, UICC Technical Report Series 49:96, (1980).
2.   L. Horn and H.L. Horn, An Immunological Approach to the Therapy of Cancer, Lancet 2:466 (1971).
3.   I. Hellstrom, K.E. Hellstrom and H.O. Sjogren, Serum Factors in Tumor-Free Patients Cancelling the Blocking of Cell-Mediated Tumor Immunity, Int. J. Cancer 8:185 (1971).
4.   J.E. Montie, R.M. Bukowski, S.D. Deodhar, J.S. Hewlett, B.H. Stewart and R.A. Straffon, Immunotherapy of Disseminated Renal Cell Carcinoma with Transfer Factor, J. Urol. 117:553 (1977).
5.   R.M. Bukowski, C. Groppe, R. Relmer, J. Weick and J.S. Hewlett, Immunotherapy (IT) of Metastatic Renal Cell Carcinoma, Proc. Amer. Assoc. Cancer Res. of Amer. Soc. of Clin. Oncol. 20:402 (1979).
6.   D.V. Schapira, C.S. McCune and E.C. Henshaw, Treatment of Advanced Renal Cell Carcinoma with Specific Immunotherapy Consisting of Autologous Tumor Cells and C. Parvum, Proc. Amer. Assoc. Cancer Res. of Amer. Soc. of Clin. Oncol. 20:348 (1979).
7.   H. Tykka, K.J. Oravisto, T. Lehtonen, S. Sharna and T. Tallberg, Active Specific Immunotherapy of Advanced Renal Cell Carcinoma, Eur. Urol. 4:250 (1978).
8.   P.A. Brower, J.B. DeKernion and K.P. Ramming, Immune Cytolysis of Human Renal Cell Carcinoma Mediated by Xenogeneic Immune Ribonucleic Acid, J. Urol. 115:243 (1976).
9.   K.P. Ramming and J.B. DeKernion, Immune RNA Therapy for Renal Cell Carcinoma: Survival and Immunologic Monitoring, Ann. Surg. 186:459 (1979).
10.   S. Brosman, Non-Specific Immunotherapy in GU Cancer, Proc. Chic. Symp. Plubl., Franklin Inst. Press., Chic.   (1977) p. 97.
11.   A. Morales and D. Eidinger, Bacille Calmette-Guerin in the Treatment of Adenocarcinoma of the Kidney, J. Urol., 115:377 (1976).
12.   P.H. Lange, Lymphocyte-Mediated Cytotoxicity in Patients with Renal and Transitional Cell Carcinoma Receiving BCG, Natl. Cancer Inst. Monogr. 49:343 (1978).
13.   J.P. Minton, K. Pennline, J.F. Nowrocki et al, Immunotherapy of Human Kidney Cancer, Proc. Am. Soc. Clin. Oncol. 17:301 (1976)

14. L.J. Humphrey, D.R. Murray and O.R. Boehm, Effect of Tumor Vaccines in Immunizing Patients with Lung Cancer, <u>Surg. Gynecol. Obstet.</u> 132:437 (1971).

15. R.C. Nairn, J. Phillip, T. Ghose et al, Production of a Precipitin Against Renal Cancer, <u>B.M.J.</u> 1:1702 (1963).

16. G.L. Bartlett and B. Zbar, Tumor-Specific Vaccine Containing Mycobacterium Bovis and Tumor Cells: Safety and Efficacy, <u>J. Natl. Cancer Inst.</u> 48:170 (1972).

17. M.T. Scott, Potentiation of the Tumor-Specific Immune Response by Corynebacterium Parvum, <u>J. Natl. Cancer Inst.</u> 55:65 (1975).

18. R.L. Tuttle and R.J. North, Mechanisms of Antitumor Action of Corynebacterium Parvum: The Generation of Cell-Mediated Tumor Specific Immunity, <u>J. Reticulothelial Soc.</u> 20:197 (1976).

19. C.S. McCune, D.V. Schapira and E.C. Henshaw, Specific Immunotherapy of Advanced Renal Carcinoma, <u>Cancer</u> 47:1984 (1981).

20. G.L. Brown, P.C. Peters, M.D. Prager and S. Baechtel, Specific Immunotherapy of Metastatic Human Renal Cell Carcinoma, Presented at Amer. Urol. Assoc. Annual Meeting, Boston, Mass, (1981).

21. J.A. Neidhart, S.G. Murphy, L.A. Henrick and H.A. Wise, Active Specific Immunotherapy of Stage IV Renal Carcinoma with Aggregated Tumor Antigen Adjuvant, <u>Cancer</u> 46:1128 (1980).

CHEMOTHERAPY OF ADVANCED RENAL CELL CARCINOMA: RESULTS OF TREATMENT

WITH METHYL-GLYOXAL BIS-GUANYLHYDRAZONE (methyl-GAG): AN EORTC STUDY

J.A. Child*, G. Stoter,S.D. Fosså, A.V. Bono, M. de Pauw
and EORTC Urological Group

*The General Infirmary at Leeds
 England
 U.K.

INTRODUCTION

The range of drugs which have been thoroughly tested in advanced
renal cancer is still limited.   Few oncologists have been able to
accumulate sufficient experience of the treatment of adequate numbers
of patients.   Results of single agent therapy have recently been
reviewed by Bodey (1) and de Kernion (2).   It is uncertain whether
any agent yet tested can be regarded as effective but there is some
evidence to suggest that vinblastine may be, Hrushesky and Murphy (3)
reporting a 25% objective response rate - including three complete
remissions of up to four years duration - in a series of 135 patients.
Other reports on the activity of vinblastine have been less encouraging (2).   In recent studies, methodichlorophen has been shown to be
inactive (4) as has 4-epi-adriamycin (5).   A variety of chemotherapeutic combinations have been investigated with disappointing results.
A combination of adriamycin, vincristine and medroxyprogesterone
acetate with BCG was reported as giving a 33% overall response (6)
and vinblastine plus CCNU a 24% response (7).   There is no evidence
that any combination studied is superior to vinblastine when used as
a single agent.   It is clear that there is a continuing urgent need
to evaluate untested, especially new, chemotherapeutic agents in
renal cell carcinoma.   It may then be possible to study the most
promising agents in combined schedules.   Further investigation of
the vinca alkaloids, in particular, the newer analogue vindesine,
seems indicated.   Study of combinations with other agents found to
have significant activity would then be a logical next step.

Methyl-GAG was first synthesised in 1958 and was used in the

treatment of the leukaemias in the early 1960's (8,9).   Toxicity
with daily administration was considerable but recently, weekly
administration schedules have been shown to cause much less toxicity
and to produce responses in a variety of solid tumours, including
kidney cancer (10-14).   The drug has an anti-proliferative effect
on cancer cells which probably reflects two principal properties (15,
16):   selective binding to mitochondria with resulting structural and
functional damage;   and inhibition of polyamine synthesis, notably
the inhibition and depletion of spermidine.

It was against this background that the EORTC Urological Group
formulated a protocol for a phase II study of the anti-tumour effect
of methyl-GAG in patients with renal cell carcinoma with measurable
metastases not amenable to surgery.   A secondary objective was to
assess the morbidity of the treatment.

MATERIAL AND METHODS

It was required that the patients should be under 75 years of
age with a Karnofsky index > 60%.   Concurrent, but not previous,
treatment excluded, as did the existence of brain metastases and
evidence of significant bone marrow depression or renal failure.
Measurable metastases of histologically or cytologically proven
renal cell carcinoma were necessary.

Methyl-GAG (supplied to the EORTC for the study by Riom
Laboratories, France) was administered weekly in a dose of 500 mg/m^2
by intravenous infusion over 30 minutes.   Dose modifications were
not allowed but delay of up to 3 weeks was permissable in the event
of bone marrow depression (wbc < 3000/mm^3) or renal dysfunction (serum
creatinine > 1.5 mg/100 ml.).

Physical examination, whole blood count, biochemistry profile
and roentgenographic examinations were done before the start of
therapy and at regular intervals during treatment.   Full description
and measurement of indicator lesions were recorded.   Investigations
necessary for the assessment of indicator lesions were repeated as
appropriate but were required in all cases after seven treatment
cycles.

WHO criteria (17) were applied with complete remission necessitating disappearance of all lesions and partial remission a 50% or
more decrease in the product of the two largest perpendicular
diameters of all measurable lesions.   Complete and partial remissions
had to be maintained for no less than four weeks with no new lesions
appearing.   Stable disease and progression were the other two
recognised categories.   Arbitrarily patients were considered
evaluable for response if they had received a minimum of four treatment cycles with methyl-GAG.

RESULTS

Forty-five patients were entered into the study. Only three of these were completely non-evaluable because of lack of data or protocol violation. Thirty patients had received four or more treatment cycles, and were evaluable for response. Twelve patients were only partially evaluable, i.e. for assessment of toxicity.

Of the 30 fully evaluable patients, three achieved partial remission, 11 showed no significant change and in 16 the disease progressed. No complete remissions were observed (Table 1). The duration of the partial remissions in no case exceeded eight weeks.

The nature and severity of the toxicity encountered in 42 patients are presented in Table 2. The commonest side effects were anorexia, nausea and vomiting (43%), moderate or severe in 19% of all patients. Neuropathy, myopathy and myalgia also proved troublesome in some patients and was encountered in 21% overall (moderate or severe in 14% of all patients). Mucositis was moderate or severe in 7%. Six patients had to be taken off treatment because of polyneuropathy (two), mucositis (one), arthralgia (one), nausea, vomiting and diarrhoea (one) and vasculitis (one). Evidence of bone marrow depression was unusual and leucopenia necessitated delay in treatment in only three patients.

DISCUSSION

The results of this EORTC study add to information which is accumulating as to the effects of methyl-GAG in advanced renal cancer. The data from SWOG furnished by Knight et al (10-12) indicated significant responses to methyl-GAG in a weekly dose of 500 mg/m^2 with 100 mg/m^2 dose escalation per treatment cycle, occuring both within four and after four treatment cycles. One complete and two partial remissions were seen in 23 patients. Todd et al (13), who also gave 500 mg/m^2 weekly but with 50 mg/m^2 escalation, reported one complete and three partial remissions among 18 patients. All these remissions occurred within four weeks. However, in a more recent study, Zeffren et al (18) observed no remissions in 30 patients, in whom toxicity was apparently severe - including muscle weakness, lethargy, myalgia, mucositis and skin rashes. In the study reported here, where a fixed

Table 1. Results of Methyl-GAG in Metastatic Renal Cell Cancer

Patients Evaluable/ Patients Entered	Partial Remission	Stable Disease	Progression
30/45	3	11	16

Table 2.   Toxicity of Methyl-GAG 500 mg/m^2/wk.
           (42 patients)

	Number of patients		
Side Effects	Mild	Moderate	Severe
Anorexia, nausea, vomiting	10	5	3
Neuropathy, myopathy, myalgia	3	4	2
Mucositis	3	2	1
Skin reactions	2	2	1
Leucopenia	2	2	0
Diarrhoea	2	1	1

dose was adopted, three partial remissions have been recorded among the 30 patients receiving at least four treatment cycles.   The toxicity observed was moderate to severe in some patients, necessitating cessation of treatment in six patients.   Knight et al (11) and Todd et al (13) encountered rather more side effects presumably because of their dose escalation schedule.

Currently, there is good evidence that methyl-GAG has limited activity of short-term duration in renal cell cancer.   However, the degree of toxicity encountered with the use of this drug may well preclude further study.

REFERENCES

1.   G.P. Bodey, Current Status of Chemotherapy in Metastatic Renal Carcinoma, in "Cancer of the Genitourinary Tract," D.E. Johnson and M.L. Samuels (eds), Raven Press, New York. (1979) p.67.
2.   J.B. de Kernion, Renal Cell Carcinoma, in "Cancer Treatment," C.H. Haskell (ed), Saunders, Philadelphia. (1980) p.392.
3.   W.J. Hrushesky and G.P. Murphy, Current Status of the Therapy of Advanced Renal Carcinoma, J. Surg. Oncol. 9:277 (1977).
4.   J.R. Hindmarsh, R.R. Hall and A.E. Kulatilake, Renal Cell Carcinoma: A Preliminary Clinical Trial of Methodichlorophen, Clin. Oncol. 5:11 (1979).
5.   S.D. Fossa, B. Wik, E. Bae and H.H. Lien, 4'-Epi-Adriamycin in Metastatic Renal Cancer, in "Cancer of the Prostate and Kidney," P.H. Smith and M. Pavone-Macaluso (eds), Plenum, London and New York. (1982).

6. D.R. Ishmael, L.J. Burop and R.H. Bottomley, Combined Therapy of Advanced Hypernephroma with Medroxyprogesterone, BCG, Adriamycin and Vincristine (Abstract C-403), <u>Proc. Am. Assoc. Cancer Res. Am. Soc. Clin. Oncol</u>. 19:407 (1978)

7. T.E. Davis and F.B. Manado, Combination Chemotherapy of Advanced Renal Cancer with CCNU and Vinblastine (Abstract C-39), <u>Proc. Am. Assoc. Cancer Res. Am. Soc. Clin. Oncol</u>. 19:316 (1978).

8. R.H. Levin, E. Henderson, M. Karon and E.J. Freireich, Treatment of Acute Leukaemia with Methylglyoxal Bis Guanylhydrazone (methyl-GAG), <u>Clin. Pharmacol. Ther</u>. 6:31 (1964).

9. P.P. Carbone, E.J. Freireich, E. Frei III, D.P. Rall, M. Karon and C.O. Brindley, The Effectiveness of Methylglyoxal Bis Guanylhydrazone in Human Malignant Disease, <u>Acta Unio Internat. Contra Cancrum</u>, 20:340 (1964).

10. W.A. Knight III, R.B. Livingston, C. Fabian and J. Costanzi, Methylglyoxal Bis-Guanylhydrazone (methyl-GAG, MGBG) in Advanced Human Malignancy, <u>Proc. Am. Assoc. Cancer Res</u>. 20:319 (1979).

11. W.A. Knight III, R.B. Livingston, C. Fabian and J. Costanzi, Phase I-II Trial of Methyl-GAG: A Southwest Oncology Group Pilot Study, <u>Cancer Treat. Rep</u>. 63:1933 (1979).

12. W.A. Knight III, R.B. Livingston, C. Fabian and J. Costanzi, Methyl-Glyoxal Bis-Guanylhydrazone (methyl-GAG, MGBG) in Advanced Renal Carcinoma, <u>Proc. Am. Assoc. Cancer Res</u>. 21:367 (1980).

13. J. Killin, D. Hoth, F. Smith, P. Schein and P. Woolley, Methyl-Glyoxal Bis-Guanylhydrazone (NSC 32946)(methyl-GAG) Phase II Experience and Clinical Pharmacology, <u>Proc. Am. Assoc. Cancer Res</u>. 21:368 (1980).

14. R.F. Todd, M.D. Garnick and G.P. Canellos, Chemotherapy of Advanced Renal Adenocarcinoma with Methyl-Glyoxal Bis-Guanylhydrazone (methyl-GAG), <u>Proc. Am. Assoc. Cancer Res</u>. 21:340 (1980).

15. C.W. Porter, D. Mikles-Robertson, D. Kramer and C. Dave, Correlation of Ultrastructural and Functional Damage to Mitochondria of Ascites L1210 Cells Treated <u>In Vivo</u> with Methylglyoxal Bis (Guanylhydrazone) or Ethidium Bromide, <u>Cancer Res</u>. 39:2414 (1979).

16. V.T. Oliverio, R.H. Adamson, E.S. Henderson and J.D. Davidson, The Distribution, Excretion and Metabolism of Methylglyoxal Bis (Guanylhydrazone C^{14}), <u>J. Pharmacol. & Exper. Therap</u>. 141:149, (1963).

17. WHO Handbook for Reporting Results of Cancer Treatment, Definitions of Objective Response, <u>WHO Offset Publication</u>, 48:23 (1979).

18. J. Zeffren, A. Yagoda, R.C. Watson, R.B. Natale, M.S. Blumenreich and J. Howard, Phase II Trial of Methyl-Glyoxal Bis-Guanylhydrazone in Advanced Renal Cancer, <u>Cancer. Treat. Rep</u>. 65:525 (1981).

4'-EPI-ADRIAMYCIN IN METASTATIC RENAL CANCER

S.D. Fosså,[1] B. Wik,[2] E. Bae,[1] H.H. Lien[1]

1. The Norwegian Radium Hospital
    Oslo, Norway

2. Ulleval Hospital
    Oslo, Norway

INTRODUCTION

4'-epi-Adriamycin (4'-epi-ADR) is a stereoisomer of Adriamycin Preliminary observations have indicated cytostatic activity of 4'-epi-ADR in metastatic renal cancer (1). A phase II study was therefore performed in order to define the efficacy of 4'-epi-ADR in this malignancy.

MATERIAL AND METHODS

During a nine month period 21 consecutive patients with histologically proven metastatic renal cancer were treated with 4'-epi-ADR (75 mg/m^2 intravenously as a push injection, together with a 500 ml normal saline infusion, repeated every third week). All patients had at least one bidimensionally measurable tumour manifestation for monitoring the response to 4'-epi-ADR treatment. Details concerning the patients are given in Table 1.

After at least two treatment courses efficacy has been evaluated using the WHO criteria for response (2). If progression occurred, 4'-epi-ADR was discontinued after the second course. In case of stable disease after two treatment courses the patients received an additional (third) injection of 4'-epi- ADR. If no tumour regression was observed in these patients after three courses, 4'-epi-ADR was discontinued in most of the patients.

The toxicity of 4'-epi-ADR treatment was evaluated using the WHO recommendations (2). Hemoglobin, leukocytes, thrombocytes,

Table 1. Details of 21 Patients with Metastatic Renal
          Cancer Treated with 4'-epi-Adriamycin

Total No. of Patients   21

Age (years)   Mean: 60.1
                                         Range: 40-70

Karnofsky Index   Mean: 84.5
                                         Range: 60-100

Interval between initial diagnosis   Mean: 15.7
and demonstration of metastases (months) Range: 0-76

Interval between initial diagnosis   Mean: 23.0
and start of 4'-epi-ADR treatment (months) Range: 1-92

No. of nephrectomized patients   18

No. of patients with previous cytostatic
treatment   8
                          CCNU-Vinblastine   4
                          Methyl-GAG*   3
                          Ifosfamide   1

Localization of indicator
lesions: Lung   12
                          Retroperitoneal and/or
                          mediastinal lymph nodes**   5

                          External lymph nodes   2
                          Kidney (primary tumour)   2
                          Cutis/subcutis   1
                          Os pelvis***   1

Progression of indicator lesions
prior to start of 4'-epi-ADR: <2 months   8
                              <6 months   1
                              >6 months   2
                              Unchanged within 6 months 7
                              Not evaluable   3

*   Methyl-Glyoxal Bis-Guanylhydrazone
**   Measurable by CT Scan
***   Surrounded by a soft tissue tumour, measurable
      by CT scan.

hematological liver function tests and serum creatinine were analyzed prior to each treatment course. In order to define the myocardial toxicity of 4'-epi-ADR an electrocardiogram was performed before each 4'-epi-ADR injection. Furthermore, the systolic time interval (STI) was determined prior to each treatment course and at treatment discontinuation. The grade of gastrointestinal toxicity and the degree of hair loss were also estimated regularly during the treatment period.

RESULTS

One patient died after the first treatment course due to progressive disease (early death). For the remaining twenty patients the response rates are given in Table 2. No tumour remissions were obtained. Four patients received 4 - 6 courses without reduction of the indicator lesions. "No change" was observed in two of eight patients with indicator lesions which were progressing during the two months preceding treatment with 4'-epi-ADR.

Toxicity was generally mild to moderate (Table 3). In particular, no major myocardial toxicity was observed. STI remained unchanged during 4'-epi-ADR treatment in all patients. Two patients however complained of increased angina pectoris after two and three courses of 4'-epi-ADR respectively. One of these patients died of myocardial infarction three days after the third treatment course. The lowest values of leukocytes were observed in patients who had received cytostatic treatment prior to 4'-epi-ADR therapy. Anemia was most frequent and most severe in patients with widespread metastatic disease, and was not clearly related to the accumulated total dose of 4'-epi-ADR. The degree of hair loss increased with increasing total accumulated doses of 4'-epi-ADR.

DISCUSSION

This study did not confirm previous preliminary results showing anticancer activity of 4'-epi-ADR in renal cancer (1). Objective response was not observed in any of the twenty evaluable patients.

Even in untreated patients with metastatic renal cancer periods of progressive disease may alternate with intervals of stable disease lasting for several months. Therefore "no change" of even previously progressive metastatic renal cancer observed during treatment with an anticancer drug does not necessarily indicate activity of the cytostatic drug. In renal cancer the efficacy of a cytostatic drug can only be demonstrated by the frequency of clearly defined objective remissions (partial response, complete response) obtained in measurable indicator lesions.

Used at the above dose schedule the overall acute and subacute toxicity of 4'-epi-ADR seems less than the side effects of Adriamycin

Table 2.   Response to 4'-epi-Adriamycin in Patients with
           Metastatic Renal Cancer

Evaluation	C.R.	P.R.	N.C.	Progression	No. of Observed Patients
After 2 courses	0	0	13	7	20[x]
After 3 courses	0	0	11	1	12

[x]One additional patient died after the first course
due to progressive disease (early death).

C.R. = Complete Response
P.R. = Partial Response
N.C. = No Change

Table 3.   Acute and Subacute Toxicity in 59 Courses of
           4'-epi-Adriamycin (75 mg/m^2) i.v. q 3 weeks

	Grade 0	Grade 1	Grade 2	Grade 3
Anemia	29	12	16	2
Leukopenia	45	7	4	3
Thrombopenia	59	-	-	-
Nausea Vomiting	-	41	18	-
Alopecia	-	23	26	10
Cardiac Arhythmia	59	-	-	-
Cardiac Dysfunction	59	-	-	-

in comparable doses. It is unlikely that the ischaemic heart disease observed in two of our patients (angina pectoris, myocardial infarction) was due to treatment with 4'epi-ADR. In general, anthracyclines do not cause this type of cardio-toxicity. These drugs lead to a primary damage of the myocardium with the clinical symptoms of congestive heart failure (3).

However, we cannot define the long-term toxicity of 4'-epi-ADR as most of our patients did not receive more than two to four courses. As with Adriamycin, cardio-myopathy may represent a problem when higher accumulated doses of 4'-epi-ADR are used (4). Furthermore, STI determinations probably do not represent the optimal method of determining anthracycline-induced myocardial toxicity, biopsies from the myocardium (4) or assessment of the radionuclide ejection fraction (3) being modern techniques to evaluate anthracycline-induced cardiomyopathy.

CONCLUSIONS

4'-epi-ADR does not seem to have a cytostatic effect in metastatic renal cancer. Due to the relative mildness of toxicity, 4'-epi-ADR seems to be especially useful for the cytostatic treatment of out patients. 4'-epi-ADR should therefore be evaluated more extensively in other malignant diseases.

REFERENCES

1. V. Bonafante, G. Bonadonna, F. Villani, G. Di Fronzo, A. Martini, and A.M. Casazza, Preliminary Phase I Study of 4'-Epi-Adriamycin, Cancer Treat. Rep. 63: 915 (1979).
2. A.B. Miller, B. Hoogstraten, M. Staquet, and A. Winkler, Reporting Results of Cancer Treatment, Cancer 47: 207 (1981).
3. J.L. Ritchie, J.W. Singer, D. Thorning, S.G. Sorensen, and G.W. Hamilton, Anthracycline Cardiotoxicity, Cancer 46: 1109 (1980).
4. M.R. Bristow, J.W. Mason, M.E. Billingham, and J.R. Daniels, Doxorubicin cardiomyopathy, evaluation by phoncardiography, endomyocardial biopsy, and cardiac catheterization, Ann. Intern. Med. 88: 168 (1978).

IS RENAL CANCER A HORMONE-DEPENDENT TUMOUR AND HOW DOES IT

RESPOND TO HORMONAL TREATMENT?   ROUND TABLE REPORT

J. Altwein

Bundeswehrkrankenhaus Ulm
Ulm
West Germany

Despite the lack of clinical data to support the concept of renal cell carcinoma (RCC) as a "hormone dependent tumour" - the title of a paper from Concolino in Cancer Research in 1978 (1) - hormone therapy is still being used in many institutions.

There are three simple reasons -

1.   In metastatic RCC there are few, if any, therapeutic alternatives.

2.   Hormone treatment is easy to administer and produces few adverse side effects.

3.   It often produces a remarkable improvement in the well-being of the patient.

The recent availability of synthetic ligands for receptor measurements is another reason for the renewed interest in the endocrine relationships of this rather relentless tumour.

THE NORMAL KIDNEY AS ENDOCRINE TARGET ORGAN

There is some evidence that the normal kidney is a target for hormones of the pituitary, adrenal, parathyroid and gonad.   It contains receptors and enzymes capable of degrading testosterone.   However, the progesterone and estrogen receptor concentrations in the normal is low, as is the capability to degrade testosterone (2).

HORMONE RELEASE OF THE NORMAL KIDNEY AND RCC

The kidney is an active endocrine organ secreting erythropoietin, parathormone-like compounds and PGE2.   The secretion by RCC of a variety of hormones has been demonstrated.   Of interest in this context is the ectopic secretion of HCG, Prolactin and ACTH in 5% of the afflicted patients.

Dunzendorfer et al (3) measured the circulating peptide hormones in 25 patients with RCC.   None of the patients had a paraneoplastic syndrome.   47% had increased prolactin (PRL) values which dropped to normal in M0 disease after nephrectomy.   TSH which is controlled like PRL by a releasing hormone was high in 29% without correlation to PRL.

ETIOLOGY OF RCC: HORMONES?

There is circumferential evidence that hormones have some influence, since RCC has not been observed at times of endocrine hyperactivity, e.g. pregnancy, and is less common in younger women (see below).

$$M : F = 3 : 1 \text{ in pts } < 40 \text{ yrs, but}$$

$$M : F = 2 : 1 \text{ in pts } > 40 \text{ yrs.}$$

Van der Werf-Messing reported a M : F ratio 1.2 : 1 in 174 M0-RCC (4), but the women had a significantly better prognosis than the men.   There are three case reports suggestive of an estrogen induced RCC in men being treated for prostatic cancer: one by Bellet et al (5) and two by Nissenkorn et al (6), but no obvious cause-and-effect relationship could be demonstrated.

Finally, if vital isolated RCC cells were exposed to estradiol 5/10 were stimulated, but the other five were inhibited as determined by H^3-thymidine-incorporation.   The same applied to progesterone (7).   Thus, there is no strong evidence that hormones are involved.

RECEPTOR CONTENT OF RCC AND ITS SIGNIFICANCE
IN PREDICTING HORMONE RESPONSIVENESS

Some RCC contain low concentrations of high affinity binding sites to estrogen and progesterone.   Estrogen treatment does not induce receptors in humans, as opposed to the finding of Li et al in hamsters (8).   Androgen and glucocorticoid receptors binding to gestagen have recently also been demonstrated.

Pizzocaro (I.N.T. Milan) reported that 12/31 RCC had estrogen receptors.   Of five RCC patients with metastases, two had stable

disease whilst on medroxyprogesterone acetate.   In a randomised
trial they collected 62 Mo-RCC, of whom 10% had estrogen and androgen
receptors.   Of the 46 evaluable Mo patients, four relapsed, of whom
three had been treated with MPA.   All MO - locally extensive disease - relapses occurred in receptor-negative cases.   Twelve Ml-RCC
were treated with MPA: four patients had stabilization, but no
objective response was seen.   There was no correlation between
receptor content and stabilization.   Concolino (Rome) found estrogen
and progesterone receptors in 17 of 55 RCC without clear relation to
hormone treatment response.

    Macchia (New York) developed a system in which testosterone is
bound to albumin and labelled by fluoresceine.   Subsequent Immunofluorescence is regarded as an indicator of binding.   Cyproterone
acetate reduces the visible fluorescence probably by competitive
inhibition.   Thirty-six RCC were studied: nine showed no binding,
four low binding for estrogen, one moderate and eight high binding
(= more than 50% cells fluorescent).   Determining specifity and
intensity appeared to be problematic.   Furthermore the binding sites
cannot as yet be defined.

HORMONAL TREATMENT OF RCC

    It was emphasized that stabilization does not constitute a
response.   Furthermore, spontaneous regression, though infrequent
(0.4% of 1340 RCC from the literature) could be present.

RESULTS

    Hrushesky and Murphy (9) observed that, between 1967 and 1971,
228 patients were treated with Progesterone with 17% remissions, but
of 415 patients treated between 1971 and 1976 only 2% had a remission.
The difference is due to a different definition of remission rates.
In a recent prospective trial of progesterone plus androgens versus
no treatment, De Kernion treated 110 patients without a single remission.   The South West Oncology Group Study of Tamoxifen showed 4%
remissions but 28% subjective improvement (1).   Finally, there is
a report of the Eastern Cooperative Oncology Group, where 41 RCC have
been randomized to MPA or Nafoxidine, producing 5% and 15% partial
remissions, respectively (11).

IMMUNOTHERAPY AND HORMONES

    Ishmal et al (12) treated 31 patients with Vincristine, Adria-
mycin, BCG + Provera and claimed a 33% response.   At the Cleveland
Clinic a regimen of Megestrol acetate + CCNU + Transfer Factor + BCG
was used in 33 patients (13).   Six (19%) had a partial remission of
short duration.

CHEMOTHERAPY AND HORMONES

In the literature are reports of 11% responses with MeCCNU + MPA in 38 patients and of 8% responses with VLB + MPA in 38 patients (14).

CONCLUSIONS

There is some evidence that a weak hormone dependence may exist in RCC, but at the present time hormonal treatment does not induce remission in M1-RCC.   However, MPA is well tolerated and leads to a remarkable subjective improvement.

REFERENCES

1.   G. Concolino, A. Marrachi, C. Conti, R. Tenaglia, F. Di Silverio and U. Bracci, Human Renal Cell Carcinoma as a Hormone-Dependent Tumor, Cancer Res. 38:4340 (1978).
2.   M. Marberger Jr., J.E. Altwein and F. Orestano, The Influence of the Progestagen Gestonorone Caproate on Testosterone Turnover in Renal Cell Carcinoma, Invest. Urol. 13:302 (1976).
3.   U. Dunzendorfer, D. Drahovsky, H. Schmidt-Gayk and H.P. Zahradnik, Klinische Bedeutung der Peptilhormone LH, FSH, TSH, Prolaktin, HCG, Parathormon, Calcitonin, Prostaglandin F_2 beim Nierenkarzinom, Z. Urol. Nephrol. 74:13 (1981).
4.   B. van der Werf-Messing, Prognostic Factors in Renal Cancer, in "Cancer of the Prostate and Kidney", P.H. Smith and M. Pavone-Macaluso (eds), Plenum Publishing Company Ltd., London and New York (1982).
5.   R.E. Bellett and A.P. Squitieri, Estrogen-Induced Hypernephroma, J. Urol. 112:60 (1974).
6.   I. Nissenkorn, C. Servadio and I. Avidor, Oestrogen-Induced Renal Cell Carcinoma, Brit. J. Urol. 51:6 (1979).
7.   H. Bojar, K. Marz and W. Staib, The Endocrine Background of Renal Cell Carcinoma I, Urol. Int. 34:302 (1979).
8.   J.J. Li, S.A. Li and J.L. Cuthbertson, Nuclear Retention of All Steroid Hormone Receptor Classes in the Hamster Renal Carcinoma, Cancer Res. 39:2647 (1979).
9.   W.J. Hrushesky and G.P. Murphy, Current Status of the Therapy of Advanced Renal Carcinoma, J. Surg. Oncol. 9:277 (1977).
10.   J.B. DeKernion and D. Berry, The Diagnosis and Treatment of Renal Cell Carcinoma, Cancer 45:1947 (1980).
11.   S.S. Legha, N. Slavik and S.K. Carter, Nafoxidine - An Anti-estrogen for the Treatment of Breast Cancer, Cancer 38:1535 (1976).
12.   D.R. Ishmael, L.J. Burpo and R.H. Bottomley, Combined Therapy of Advanced Hypernephroma with Medroxyprogesterone, BCG, Adriamycin and Vincristine, Proc. Am. Assoc. Cancer Res. Am Soc. Clin. Oncol. 19:407 (1978).

13. S. Brosman, Immunotherapy for Renal Carcinoma, <u>in</u> "Cancer of
     the Prostate and Kidney", P.H. Smith and M. Pavone-Macaluso (eds)
     Plenum Publishing Company Ltd., London and New York (1982).
14. G.P. Bodey, Current Status of Chemotherapy in Metastatic Renal
     Carcinoma, <u>in</u> "Cancer of the Genitourinary Tract, D.E. Johnson
     M.L. Samuels (eds), Raven Press, New York (1979) p. 67.

STRATEGY OF THERAPY IN RENAL CARCINOMA - ROUND TABLE REPORT

J. P. Blandy[1] and F. Edsmyr[2]

1. The London Hospital
   London, U.K.

2. Karolinska Hospital
   Stockholm, Sweden

Schmidt began with a comprehensive review of the state of the art, drawing attention to some of the more notable gaps in our contemporary approach to renal cell cancer. This was followed by a lively discussion, which fell into three parts:

1. The need for earlier diagnosis

There was universal agreement that the diagnosis was too often being made too late, and that we should aim to detect these tumours when small and non-invasive, and before they had metastasized, ie., pT1/pT2, M0, but nobody had any new notion how this was to be achieved. Clearly to screen the entire population at risk by ultrasound, CAT or urography would be logistically impossible. Smith reminded us again of the fallacies of conventional diagnosis, illustrating this by one example where a huge tumour remained unchanged for many years, and another in whom an enormous mass appeared within a few months. In the face of this unpredictable rate of growth, conventional clinical signs and symptoms were of even less value. Nor were the para-neoplastic syndromes of any greater value: certainly internists needed to be reminded of their existence, but it was seldom that they denoted early disease. Those alterations of the plasma albumen/globulin ratio including elevation of the $\alpha 2$ globulin fraction that resulted in a raised ESR, were not features of early disease. Van der Werf-Messing found that elevation of the ESR signified a poor prognosis and appeared to denote occult micro-metastases. We still have no easy means of detecting these tumours at an early stage, and none that could be used on a large scale.

2.   Management of the local lesion in the kidney

    (a)   A no-nephrectomy group? We discussed the interesting
suggestion of Denis that there was a place for refraining from
nephrectomy in patients over the age of 75 who had no symptoms.
Considerable anxiety was expressed about the risk of untoward late
morbidity. Perhaps this might form the subject of a well designed
clinical trial.

    (b)   Embolisation The initial burst of enthusiasm for pre-
operative embolisation had obviously been tempered by experience;
now only a minority of urologists continued to employ angiography,
let alone embolisation, for every case. It clearly had value in
limiting blood loss when the tumour was very large or where there
was evidence of caval invasion, in which case a cavogram should
be added.

    (c)   Lymph node dissection There was even more discussion as
to the place of lymph node dissection. Its enthusiastic advocacy
by Carmignani received little support. Pavone questioned whether
the inevitable morbidity of this procedure in the hands of the
average surgeon could ever be justified when lymphadenectomy could
never be more than a staging manoeuvre. To this Goodwin retorted
that some patients might benefit by removal of a single lymph node
metastasis: perhaps a more limited node resection could give
equally useful staging information without heroic dissection behind
the great vessels. The suggestion was made that the advantages now
being claimed for node dissection needed to be tested for the only
hard data that were available (1) came from a retrospective study
of a very selected series in which node dissection appeared to confer
an advantage (3 year actuarial survival 73% versus 64%). This is
certainly a question that will not go away and if we do not set
about answering it in the near future, it will continue to hang
around and worry us for years to come.

    (d)   Radiotherapy - not a dead issue? There was general
agreement that there was no place either for pre-operative or
post-operative radiotherapy, but Andersson caused us to discuss
whether in the anaplastic group (detected cytologically by fine-
needle aspiration) pre-operative radiotherapy might deserve a
second look. When tumour was known to be left behind after
nephrectomy, radiotherapy was probably justified, particularly when
modern techniques were used, and the residual mass was carefully
monitored by CAT scanning. At the other end of the scale it was
again suggested that we should reconsider the role of partial
nephrectomy for pT1 tumours.

3.   Management of metastases (M1)

    (a) Hormone therapy In the absence of any acceptable

evidence to support the use of androgens or progestational agents in patients with metastases, de Vere White pointed out that this futile practice was hindering the active search for more effective treatment, and perpetuated the myth of the 20% response to hormone therapy. Clinical trials should put an end to this practice. No alternative hormone therapy appeared to be on the horizon, and anyway the evidence that kidney cancer is hormone-sensitive appears to be limited to one species.

(b) <u>Chemotherapy</u> Stoter's grave recapulation of the scrupulous EORTC and other trials of single-agent chemotherapy showed that no agent so far tested was effective. Nevertheless the method of the clinical trial, discouraging as it sometimes seems, is the only means whereby these desirable agents can ever be detected.

(c) <u>Interferon</u> In the face of the news media excitement about Interferon Edsmyr warned us against unjustified euphoria and observed that much more work was needed.

(d) <u>Immunotherapy</u> Equal caution was necessary in interpreting the results of immunotherapy. The claims for pre-nephrectomy embolization followed by BCG needed to be ratified in carefully supervised trials before it was adopted or abandoned. Brosman pointed out that the promising autologous tumour vaccine developed by Tykkä et al (2) was still very experimental. Premature enthusiasm, even for clinical trials, would risk premature disrepute. In our quest for immunological suppression of tumour growth we must never forget that immunology is two edged, and that its undesirable edge was tumour enhancement.

Before the session closed de Voogt entered an impassioned protest at the "negative" attitude, expressed by the many participants who had listened to such a long and dismal recitation of negative results. He urged a more "positive" view and reproached us for failing to give sufficient attention to cell kinetics from which he sensed, alas without any evidence, that something good would come.

<u>Summary</u>

It seemed that five "questions for today" could be identified:

1. The need for some method, whether a "marker" or a method of screening, which could pick up the early pT1 M0 cancer.
2. Whether or not it was legitimate to refrain from nephrectomy in the symptomless patient over 75 years of age.
3. To test in properly designed clinical trials the current claims that lymphadenectomy improved survival.
4. To continue the painstaking search, by means of well-regulated

clinical trials, for effective chemotherapeutic agents. The search
was likely to be long - but this was no good reason for giving up.
Rome, let alone Erice, was not built in a day.
5. Current claims for immunotherapy needed to be tested by
similarly well-controlled clinical trials.

REFERENCES

1. A. Sigel, S. Chlepas, P. Hermanek and A. Herrlinger,
    Stagnation in der Therapie der Nierentumoren - chancen einer
    Besserung, in: "Diagnostik und Therapie das Nierenkarzinomas.
    Klinische und Experimentelle Urologie (Band 2), E. Schmiedt
    und H. W. Bauer, eds., W. Zuckschwerdt, Munich (1981)
2. H. Tykkä, K.J. Oravisto, T. Lehtonen, S. Sarna and T. Tallberg,
    Active specific immunotherapy of advanced renal cell carcinoma,
    Eur. Urol. 4:250-258 (1978).

TREATMENT OF RENAL CANCER

J. D. Schmidt

University of California Medical Centre
San Diego
U.S.A.

The therapy of renal-cell carcinoma has evolved slowly. The earlier reports of increased benefit from radiotherapy, as adjuvant to nephrectomy, were tempered by the improved survival afforded to patients using a radical or extrafascial nephrectomy, (1-6). In this procedure the kidney, with its tumor, is removed along with the accompanying adrenal gland, perinephric fat and perinephric fascia of Gerota. An ipsilateral regional lymphadenectomy, removing tissue from the diaphragmatic crus to the bifurcation of the aorta or vena cava has been espoused by many. At this point, lymphadenectomy can be considered important for more accurate staging and therefore of prognostic value, but it is unlikely that many patients with tumor involvement in the regional lymph nodes (Stage III) are cured by this manoeuvre alone. Pre- or postoperative irradiation is not indicated.

Radical nephrectomy is best performed via a transperitoneal or thoracoabdominal route. Simple nephrectomy via a flank or retroperitoneal route is generally reserved for the older patient with a renal cancer who is not a good risk for the extrafascial procedure. Operative mortality for radical nephrectomy should be less than 5%.

The value of surgery in renal cancer has been emphasized in patients with multiple tumors, bilateral tumors or a tumor in a solitary kidney. Rather than total or bilateral nephrectomy requiring hemodialysis and possible transplantation, renal conserving operations have benefited many patients. Choices available to the urologist have included partial nephrectomy, wedge resection of renal parenchyma and local excision (Table 1).

An exciting adjuvant to radical nephrectomy is the use of

715

TABLE I

Surgery for Renal Cell Carcinoma

Local Excision

Partial Nephrectomy

Simple Nephrectomy

Radical Nephrectomy

Regional Lymphadenectomy

Resection of Metastases

angiographic embolization and infarction preoperatively (7). We
currently employ this technique in large and medium-sized
hypernephromas, usually the day prior to or on the morning of
the planned surgery. The shrinkage of the kidney and tumor has
been impressive (Figures 1-2). The surgery is facilitated as
1)   the mass is smaller, 2)   the renal artery or arteries are

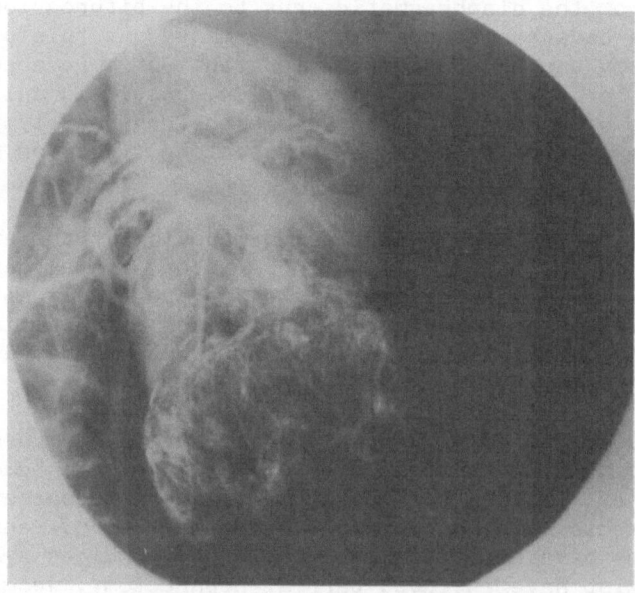

Fig. 1.   Magnification aortogram demonstrating typical
hypervascular left lower pole mass.

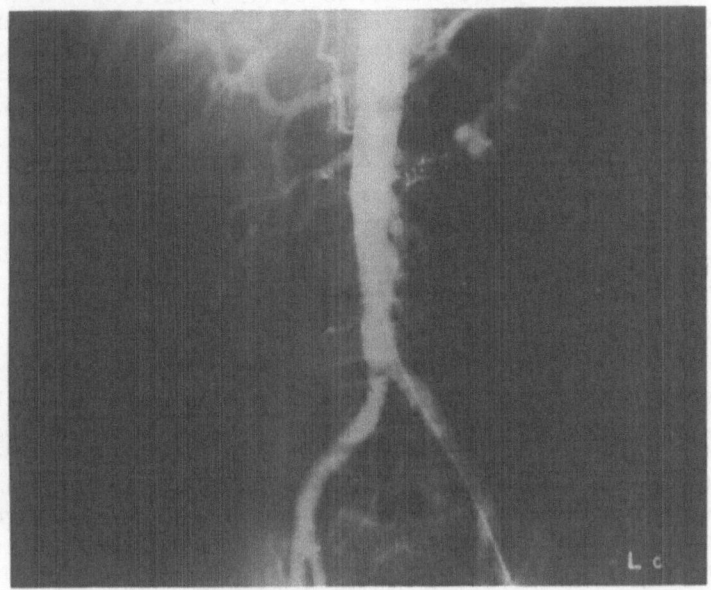

Fig. 2. Aortogram of same patient as in Fig. 1. following
        embolization using Gianturco coil.

already occluded allowing the early ligation and division of the
renal vein, and   3) the dissection seems to be improved by the
reactive edema created.

     In patients who have not undergone operation immediately
there has been a variable degree of ipsilateral flank pain, fever
and ileus related to the infarction. Materials used for the angioinfarction include the Gianturco coil, particles of Gelfoam and
Ivalon sponges. We have also utilized angioinfarction in place of
surgery in a few instances: in patients refusing surgery or in
those with advanced disease having complications such as severe
renal hemorrhage.

HORMONAL AND CHEMOTHERAPY

     Progestational agents have been associated with a small but
significant response rate in advanced (Stage IV) renal cancer
(8-9). We recommend the use of medroxyprogesterone acetate
(Depo-Provera), 400 mg intramuscularly twice weekly or 800 mg IM
once weekly for twelve consecutive weeks. Although the use of
androgen therapy, for example testosterone proprionate, 25-50 mg
two- to three-times weekly, has also been reported to be occasionally effective, this author has not seen such responses.
Progestational agents are relatively nontoxic and thus well
accepted by the patient.

Over the last ten years numerous studies have been reported
regarding chemotherapy of advanced renal cancer. To date there is
no clear-cut evidence that any single drug or combination of agents
is effective. Yet responses have been documented for vinblastin
sulfate (Velban), 5-10 mg intravenously weekly for twelve weeks and
for methyl-CCNU or CCNU 130-200 mg/m^2 orally every six weeks. Of
significance are the disappointing results using cis-platinum (DDP),
a drug shown to be of value in both prostatic and bladder cancer.
It is postulated that the tendency for hypernephroma to be slow-
growing explains its relative radioresistance and resistance to
chemotherapy.

IMMUNOTHERAPY

Scattered reports continue to be published regarding the
effective use of adjuvant immunotherapy, generally in advanced renal
cancer. These agents include immune-RNA and Bacillus Calmette-
Guerin (BCG) (10). Although of interest, for the most part these
studies have not been randomized or controlled. The employment of
angioinfarction seven to ten days prior to radical nephrectomy may
be considered a form of immunotherapy when the infarction of both
normal and neoplastic tissue may incite an immunological response.
Such a study is currently underway in the United States. Although
the theory is inviting, there has been no evidence that spontaneously induced tumor infarction as evidenced by fever has been associated with regression of metastases or improved survival.

REFERENCES

1. R. H. Flocks and M. C. Kadesky, Malignant neoplasms of the kidney:
An analysis of 353 patients followed five years or more, J. Urol.
79:196 (1958).
2. E. W. Riches, The place of radiotherapy in the management of
parenchymal carcinoma of the kidney, J. Urol. 95:313 (1966).
3. C. J. Robson, Radical nephrectomy for renal cell carcinoma,
J. Urol. 89:37 (1968).
4. C. J. Robson, B. M. Churchill, and W. Anderson, The results of
radical nephrectomy for renal cell carcinoma, Trans. Am. Assoc.
Genitourin. Surg. 60:122 (1968).
5. D. G. Skinner, R. B. Colvin, C. D. Vermillion, R. C. Pfister,
and W. F. Leadbetter, Diagnosis and management of renal cell
carcinoma: a clinical and pathologic study of 309 cases, Cancer
28:1165 (1971).
6. R. G. Middleton, and A. J. Presto III, Radical thoracoabdominal nephrectomy for renal cell carcinoma, J. Urol. 110:
36 (1973).
7. H. M. Goldstein, H. Medellin, M. T. Beydorn, and S. Wallace,
Transcatheter embolization of renal cell carcinoma, Am. J.
Roentgenol. 123:557 (1975).
8. H. J. G. Bloom, Adjuvant therapy for adenocarcinoma of the

kidney: Present position and prospects, <u>Br. J. Urol</u>. 45:237 (1973).

9. R. Talley, Chemotherapy of adenocarcinoma of the kidney, <u>Cancer</u> 32:1062 (1973).

10. K. P. Ramming and J. B. deKernion, Immune RNA therapy for renal carcinoma: Survival and immunologic monitoring, <u>Ann. Surg</u>. 186: 459 (1977).

RENAL CANCER - CLINICAL STUDIES IN THE U.S.A.

J.D. Schmidt

University of California Medical Center
San Diego
California, U.S.A.

SURVIVAL FACTORS

The five year survival for untreated renal cell cancer is approximately 2%. This increases to 30 - 47% following simple nephrectomy whereas the overall five year survival following radical (perifascial) nephrectomy is 57 - 80%. Ten year survivals for renal cell cancer overall are 17 - 27% for simple nephrectomy and 40 - 66% following radical nephrectomy (1-5).

Employing the staging system as seen in Table 1, the five year survival rates for radical nephrectomy stage by stage are: Stage I 59 - 80%, Stage II 51 - 64%, Stage III 34 - 48% and for Stage IV 5% (5,6). The ten year survival rates for radical nephrectomy are for Stage I 39 - 70%, Stage II 17 - 66%, Stage III 20 - 38% and for Stage IV 2%. The addition of regional lymphadenectomy may increase these figures by another 6 - 9%.

Survival has also been related to histologic cell type. Pure clear cell carcinoma accounts for 25% of all cases of hypernephroma; five year survival for pure clear cell tumor is approximately 58%. Granular and mixed cell types account for 15 and 46%, respectively, of all renal cancers; the five year survival for the granular cell or mixed type is 46%. Finally, spindle cell tumors account for 14% of all renal cell cancers and are associated with a five year survival rate of only 23%. The lesser survival of spindle cell, granular cell and mixed cell types relates more to these tumors being of higher grade compared to the lower grade propensity of pure clear cell lesions.

Table 1.   Comparison of Robson and TNM
Staging for Renal Cell Carcinoma

Robson	TNM Clinical	Pathological	Extent of Tumor
I	T1	pT1	Tumor within capsule (small)
	T2	pT2	Tumor within capsule (large)
II	T3	pT3	Tumor contained within perinephric fascia
III	T3	pV1	Tumor in renal vein
	N1-N3	pN1-N3	Tumor in regional nodes
	-	pV2	Tumor in vena cava
IV	T4	pT4	Tumor in adjacent organs
	M1	pM1	Distant metastases
	N4	pN4	Tumor in nodes beyond regional group

The current concepts for renal adenoma and oncocytoma are that the tubular adenoma should be considered a small malignancy whereas the oncocytoma, in spite of its often attaining a large size, is a benign tumor. The "spoke wheel" pattern on angiography earlier thought to be pathognomonic for renal oncocytoma is no longer felt to be specific for this lesion.

Studies of inferior vena caval involvement reveal this to occur in 5 - 10% of all patients with hypernephroma, but this incidence increases to 25% in the group of patients with renal vein involvement. Of interest, the five and ten year survival statistics for patients with vena caval involvement and no other involvement are similar to Robson Stages I and II: 55% at five years and 43% at ten years.

CLINICAL PRESENTATIONS

About one third of patients present with some conbination of flank pain, hematuria, and abdominal mass. Yet this "classic triad" is seen in only 10% of all patients with hypernephroma. Another one third present with symptoms from metastatic disease. The remaining one third have symptoms of a constitutional nature, e.g. fever or

weight loss. A varicocele, mostly left-sided, has been noted in only
1% of cases.

Spontaneous regression of the primary tumor is rare. Spontaneous regression of metastatic lesions has been reported in over
50 cases; 88% have involved pulmonary metastases and three fourths
of cases have been in men, about equal to the usual sex distribution
of hypernephroma. Few of the cases of spontaneous regression of
metastases have had histologic confirmation of their malignant nature.
Regression has generally been related to nephrectomy but has also
been reported without such surgery. To date there is little evidence
that a nephrectomy influences survival in the face of metastatic
disease; however, there may be a slight advantage in survival for
patients with osseous metastases.

It is of interest to compare the interval between nephrectomy
and the appearance of metastasis and subsequent survival. If metastases occur within six months post-nephrectomy, survival has been
only 8% at two years. On the other hand, if metastases occur 24
months or longer after operation, the two year survival measured
from that point is increased to 32% (5).

SPECIFIC CLINICAL TRIALS

In the late 1960's the Renal Cell Carcinoma Cooperative Study
Group began a trial comparing radical nephrectomy alone to the combination of 4500 rads of external beam irradiation in 4 - 6 weeks
followed by radical nephrectomy for clinically localized hypernephroma. Although early results seemed to favor the combined treatment,
later data showed no significant difference in survival (7). However,
external beam irradiation to the tumor may shrink the lesion, making
nephrectomy possible if not easier.

At the M.D. Anderson Hospital and Tumor Clinic, a study of angioinfarction related to nephrectomy and other treatments is currently
being pursued in patients with varying stages of renal cell cancer
(8). Immunologic studies so far have demonstrated an improvement in
the impaired baseline immunocompetence measured by delayed hypersensitivity following angio-infarction. However, concomitant
decreases in cellular immunity as measured by lymphocyte blasto-
genesis have been reported by the same team of investigators (9,10).
Humoral antibodies to the renal cell cancer have been identified in
59 - 94% of patients studied (11).

In the presence of metastatic disease, angioinfarction is
followed by medroxyprogesterone acetate (Depo-Provera) with or without an interval nephrectomy. The interval between angioinfarction
and nephrectomy has generally been two to ten days. Of 36 evaluable
patients with pulmonary metastases, responses have been seen in 21
(58%). Six responses have been complete; five have been partial

(50% or greater reduction in size of metastases). Nine patients
have either remained stable or demonstrated a less than 50% shrinkage
in the size of pulmonary metastases. Survival has been as long as
thirty months in patients with a complete response following angioinfarction, nephrectomy and progestational therapy. The early results
in 25 patients treated with embolization and hormones (no nephrectomy)
are less optimistic (9).

The use of immunotherapy in metastatic renal cell cancer has
been received with less enthusiasm recently. Using immune xenogenic
ribonucleic acid (RNA), no complete or partial regressions have been
reported (12). Stable disease has been noted in 35% of patients with
Stage IV tumors. In another study, transfer factor plus either
Bacillus Calmette-Guerin (BCG) or CCNU and megestrol acetate (Megace)
has been associated with a response rate of 26% with a ten month
median duration of response (13).

SUMMARY

The mainstay of therapy for renal cell carcinoma continues to
be surgery. The earlier reports of increased survival associated
with combinations of irradiation and simple nephrectomy have been
replaced by unassisted radical nephrectomy (perifascial nephro-
adrenalectomy) and/or regional lymphadenectomy. Current efforts
consist of evaluation of 1) angioinfarction techniques with either
nephrectomy or progestational agents as well as with the combination
of nephrectomy and hormones, 2) immunotherapy and 3) chemotherapy.

REFERENCES

1. C.J. Robson, Radical nephrectomy for renal cell carcinoma,
    J. Urol. 89: 37 (1968).
2. C.J. Robson, B.M. Churchill, and W. Anderson, The results of
    radical nephrectomy for renal cell carcinoma, J. Urol. 101:
    297 (1969).
3. D.G. Skinner, R.B. Colvin, C.D. Vermillion, R.C. Pfister, and
    W.F. Leadbetter, Diagnosis and management of renal cell carc-
    inoma: a clinical and pathologic study of 309 cases, Cancer 28:
    1165 (1971).
4. J.B. deKernion and D. Berry, The diagnosis and treatment of
    renal cell carcinoma, Cancer 45: 1947 (1980).
5. G. Sufrin and G.P. Murphy, Renal adenocarcinoma, Urol. Surv. 30:
    129 (1980).
6. M.H. Harmer, "TNM Classification of Malignant Tumors", 3rd ed.,
    International Union Against Cancer, Geneva (1978).
7. C.E. Cox, S.S. Lacy, W.G. Montgomery, and W.H. Boyce, Renal
    adenocarcinoma: 28-year review, with emphasis on rationale and
    feasibility of preoperative radiotherapy, J. Urol. 104: 53 (1970).

8. E.M. Hersh, S. Wallace, D.E. Johnson, and R.B. Bracken,
    Immunologic studies in human cancer, in: "Cancer of the Genito-
    urinary Tract," D.E. Johnson and M.L. Samuels, eds., Raven
    Press, New York (1979), p. 47.

9. S. Wallace, V. Chuang, B. Green, D.A. Swanson, R.B. Bracken,
    and D.E. Johnson, Diagnostic radiology in renal carcinoma, in:
    Cancer of the Genitourinary Tract," D.E. Johnson and
    M.L. Samuels, eds., Raven Press, New York (1979), p. 33.

10. D.A. Swanson, The current immunologic studies of renal carcinoma,
    Cancer Bull. 31: 36 (1979).

11. T.R. Hakala, A.E. Castro, A.Y. Elliott, and E.E. Fraley,
    Humoral cytotoxicity in human renal cell carcinoma, Invest.
    Urol. 11: 405 (1974).

12. K.P. Ramming and J.B. deKernion, Immune RNA therapy for renal
    cell carcinoma: Survival and immunologic monitoring, Ann. Surg.
    186: 459 (1977).

13. R.M. Bukowski, C. Jroppe, R. Reimer, J. Weich, and J.S. Hewlett,
    Immunotherapy (IT) of metastatic renal cell carcinoma, Proc.
    Amer. Soc. Clin. Oncol. 20: 402 (1979).

CONSERVATIVE MANAGEMENT OF RENAL TUMOURS

C. Selli and M. Carini

Department of Urology
University of Florence
Italy

INTRODUCTION

Although the conservative treatment of renal tumors is an option attracting increasing interest, it is still, in our experience, an uncommon event. During the last eight years we have carried out 250 nephrectomies for tumours in our institution and we have adopted a conservative approach in a further 11 cases (less than 5% of the cases).

This form of treatment was initially reserved for those patients in whom the preservation of functioning renal parenchyma seemed more relevant than radical surgical excision, ie, in patients with bilateral renal cell carcinoma and in cancer in a solitary kidney. The favourable results obtained have allowed us to extend the indications to include patients with contralateral renal damage. Conservative surgery may also be performed for small tumours discovered within renal cysts, or on the surface of kidneys operated upon for different reasons. The available surgical techniques consist of polar resection and tumour enucleation; both may be performed either in-situ or extracorporeally. Each technique finds its indications according to the size and location of the neoplasm.

The rationale for performing conservative surgery is related to the unusual way in which renal tumours grow, at least in the initial stages, since they are often surrounded by a pseudocapsule of fibrosis and compressed tissue.

PATIENTS AND METHODS

Indications for conservative surgery in our 11 patients were:

simultaneous bilateral tumours in two cases, tumours in solitary
kidney in three (one surgical, two functional), tumours with a
damaged contralateral kidney in three cases (one UPJ obstruction, two
stones), two small tumours associated with a cyst, and a pseudo-
encapsulated small tumour with normal contralateral kidney. Polar
resection was performed in six patients and tumour enucleation in
five. Pathology revealed nine renal cell carcinomas (three consisting of granular cells), one oncocytoma and one renal adenoma.

All patients are alive, with a follow-up ranging between two
months and eight years (mean: three years and six months). The
first eight cases were reviewed in September 1980 (mean follow-up
at that time: 44 months) and were without evidence of metastases.
No significant impairment of renal function was observed postoperatively.

DISCUSSION

When one has to face the difficult choice between radical
excision of a neoplasm and preservation of renal function, various
therapeutic solutions have been proposed. We believe that only
surgery can be considered as an effective treatment.

A radical procedure, rendering these patients anephric, commits
the patient to subsequent chronic dialysis and possible renal transplantation, which nowadays implies a 40 to 50% 5-year survival.
This is definitely better than has been observed in untreated renal
cancers, but worse than the results reported for conservative
surgery (1).

Polar resection, removing the tumour with an area of surrounding normal tissue, is apparently safer, but presents some drawbacks,
such as difficulties in haemostasis, possible infarction of the
underlying parenchyma and at times excessive sacrifice of functioning tissue. Enucleation could theoretically leave behind some
neoplastic cells, but presents the advantages of being a simple and
fast technique which seldom requires hypothermia and pedicle clamp-
ing and sacrifices a minimal amount of normal tissue. In our
opinion it is always worthwhile to try it first (2).

Extracorporeal surgery finds it main indication in the treatment of central bulky renal masses; this procedure allows efficient
haemostasis, meticulous reconstruction of the excretory system and
ample time for pathologic reports on the section surface. It is
often used by surgical teams familiar with transplant techniques.

In patients with bilateral renal tumours we favour a midline
transperitoneal approach, first removing the smaller tumour
conservatively, then performing a radical contralateral nephrectomy
during the same procedure.

The results of conservative surgical management of renal tumours seem promising. Palmer and Swanson (3) reported a 78% survival after an average follow-up of 45 months which compares favourably with a 65% 5-year survival rate for radical nephrectomy in cases of cancer confined to the kidney. Obviously a longer trial period is still required, particularly if we consider the unpredictable behaviour of renal tumours. An accurate pathological review is also necessary, since we cannot group renal cell carcinoma with other tumours which have a more benign prognosis.

REFERENCES

1. S. C. Jacobs, S. I. Berg and R. K. Lawson, Synchronous bilateral renal cell carcinoma: total surgical excision, Cancer 46:2341 (1980).
2. M. Carini, C. Selli, G. B. Muraro, A. Trippitelli, G. Masini, and D. Turini, Conservative surgery for renal cell carcinoma, Eur. Urol. 7:19 (1981).
3. J. M. Palmer and D. A. Swanson, Conservative surgery in solitary and bilateral renal carcinoma: indications and technical considerations, J. Urol. 120:113 (1978).

SPEAKERS

C.C. Abbou, Creteil, France.
A. Akdas, Ankara, Turkey.
J. Altwein, Ulm, West Germany.
L. Andersson, Stockholm, Sweden.
M.A. Bagshaw, Stanford, USA.
D. Beccati, Ravenna, Italy,
J.P. Blandy, London, UK.
J.H.M. Blom, Rotterdam,
  The Netherlands.
C. Bollack, Strasbourg, France.
C. Bouffioux, Liege, Belgium.
S.A. Brosman, Los Angeles, USA.
D.P. Byar, Bethesda, USA.
F. Calais da Silva, Lisbon,
  Portugal.
G. Carmignani, Genoa, Italy.
J.A. Child, Leeds, UK.
G.D. Chisholm, Edinburgh, UK.
F.M.J. Debruyne, Nijmegen,
  The Netherlands.
L. Denis, Antwerp, Belgium.
F. Edsmyr, Stockholm, Sweden.
S.D. Fossa, Oslo, Norway.
W.E. Goodwin, Los Angeles, USA.
S. Hellsten, Malmö, Sweden.
A.C. Jobsis, Amsterdam,
  The Netherlands.
S. Khoury, Paris, France.
M. Kralj, Ljubljana, Yugoslavia.

G. Lindgardh, Orebro, Sweden.
R.J. Macchia, New York, USA.
J. Naucler, Göteborg, Sweden.
R.T.D. Oliver, London, UK.
M. de Pauw, Brussels, Belgium.
M. Pavone-Macaluso, Palermo,
  Italy.
G. Pizzocaro, Milan, Italy.
H. Rauschmeier, Innsbruck,
  Austria.
B. Richards, York, UK.
M.R.G. Robinson, Pontefract, UK.
J.C. Romijn, Rotterdam,
  The Netherlands.
J.D. Schmidt, San Diego,
  California, USA.
F.H. Schröder, Rotterdam,
  The Netherlands.
C. Selli, Florence, Italy.
G. Stoter, Amsterdam,
  The Netherlands.
R. Sylvester, Brussels, Belgium.
M. Tannenbaum, New York, USA.
B. van der Werf-Messing,
  Rotterdam, The Netherlands.
R. de Vere White, New York, USA.
H.J. de Voogt, Amsterdam,
  The Netherlands.